Food Oxidants
and Antioxidants
Chemical, Biological, and Functional Properties

Chemical and Functional Properties of Food Components Series

SERIES EDITOR

Zdzisław E. Sikorski

Food Oxidants
and Antioxidants
Chemical, Biological, and Functional Properties

EDITED BY
Grzegorz Bartosz

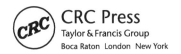

CRC Press
Taylor & Francis Group
Boca Raton London New York

CRC Press is an imprint of the
Taylor & Francis Group, an **informa** business

CRC Press
Taylor & Francis Group
6000 Broken Sound Parkway NW, Suite 300
Boca Raton, FL 33487-2742

First issued in paperback 2016

© 2014 by Taylor & Francis Group, LLC
CRC Press is an imprint of Taylor & Francis Group, an Informa business

No claim to original U.S. Government works

Version Date: 20130214

ISBN 13: 978-1-138-19969-9 (pbk)
ISBN 13: 978-1-4398-8241-2 (hbk)

Library of Congress Cataloging-in-Publication Data

Food oxidants and antioxidants : chemical, biological, and functional properties / edited by
  Grzegorz Bartosz.
    pages cm. -- (Chemical & functional properties of food components)
    Summary: "This volume discusses the effects of naturally occurring and process-generated
pro-oxidants and antioxidants on various aspects of food quality. It emphasizes the chemical
nature and functional properties of these compounds and their interactions with other food
components in storage and processing, specifically focusing on the sensory quality, nutritional
value, health promoting activity, and safety aspects of foods. It demonstrates the analysis of
pro-oxidants and antioxidants in foods, their mechanism and activity, their chemistry and
biochemistry, and the practical considerations of healthy food production and marketing"--
Provided by publisher.
    Includes bibliographical references and index.
    ISBN 978-1-4398-8241-2 (hardback)
    1. Food additives. 2. Oxidizing agents. 3. Antioxidants. I. Bartosz, G. (Grzegorz)

    TX553.A3F64 2013
    613.2'86--dc23   2012048741

Visit the Taylor & Francis Web site at
http://www.taylorandfrancis.com

and the CRC Press Web site at
http://www.crcpress.com

Contents

Preface

Food antioxidants are of primary importance for the preservation of food quality during processing and storage. They are also of considerable interest for consumers, who seek antioxidant-rich food items hoping for the prevention of diseases and postponement of aging. However, the status of food depends on the balance of prooxidants and antioxidants, the former being usually neglected when discussing food antioxidants. This book comprises, in one volume, a selection of topics covering both prooxidants and antioxidants occurring in food, which can be interesting, first of all, for food technologists and chemists and students in these fields.

After a general introduction to the problem (Chapter 1), Chapter 2 characterizes the main oxidants present in food, including both nonenzymatic oxidants (hemoproteins, redox active metals, and photosensitizers) and enzymes (lipoxygenases, myeloperoxidases, lactoperoxidases, and polyphenol oxidases). While the idea of antioxidant activity/capacity/potential has become popular, that of oxidation potential, equally useful, is much less known; it is presented in Chapter 3. Chapters 4 and 5 discuss the mechanisms of oxidation of main food components, lipids and proteins, respectively, including factors affecting this process, such as the presence of prooxidants and antioxidants, light, temperature, oxygen, and food composition. In many cases, exogenous oxidants are added to food during processing; this practice, as well as the effects of such physical agents as irradiation, freeze–thawing, and high hydrostatic pressure during food processing, is presented in Chapter 6. Chapter 7 discusses the effects of oxidation on the sensory characteristics of food components; these effects are usually unwanted, but there are also cases where they can be beneficial. Chapter 8 analyzes how the oxidation of main food components (lipids, proteins, and carbohydrates) and antioxidants affects the nutritive and health-promoting features of food components. Chapter 9 discusses natural antioxidants present in food, especially those that are less known, such as antioxidant amino acids, peptides, proteins, and polysaccharides and oligosaccharides. Chapter 10 presents antioxidants generated in food as a result of processing. The mechanisms of antioxidant activity and the main antioxidant enzymes are discussed in Chapter 11. The next two chapters deal with the measurement of the antioxidant activity of food components (Chapter 12) and their application to a specific material (apple products, Chapter 13). Many food components are classified as antioxidants but under certain conditions may have prooxidant activity; this question is described in Chapter 14. The bioavailability and antioxidant activity of two important groups of antioxidants, curcuminoids and carotenoids, are discussed in Chapter 15. Chapter 16 deals with case studies on selected natural food antioxidants, presenting novel extraction methods for optimal preservation of antioxidant activities, such as supercritical fluid extraction, pressurized liquid extraction, subcritical water extraction, and microwave- and ultrasound-assisted extraction, as well as their application to specific raw materials. Functional antioxidant foods and beverages are presented in Chapter 17.

The last chapter contains some general ideas concerning mainly the effects of food on the redox homeostasis of the organism.

The authors of the book are renowned scientists from Australia, Denmark, Germany, Italy, Lithuania, Poland, Slovakia, Spain, and the United States. I am deeply indebted for their contributions and cooperation. I hope that the book can provide basic information for students and newcomers to the field but also be of use to more experienced readers interested in the problems of food prooxidants and antioxidants.

Editor

Grzegorz Bartosz received his MS and PhD degrees from the University of Łódź and his DSc degree from the Jagiellonian University of Cracow (Poland). He spent his postdoctoral fellowship at Texas A&M University; was a research fellow at the University of Düsseldorf and Macquarie University in Sydney; and for short terms, visited various European universities and institutions. Presently, he is a professor at the Department of Molecular Biophysics of the Faculty of Biology and Protection of the Environment at the University of Łódź and at the Department of Biochemistry and Cell Biology of the Faculty of Biology and Agriculture of the University of Rzeszów (Poland). His research interest concentrates on reactive oxygen species and antioxidants. He is a corresponding member of the Polish Academy of Sciences and of the Polish Academy of Arts and Sciences and chairman of the Committee of Biochemistry and Biophysics of the Polish Academy of Sciences. He is on the editorial boards of *Acta Biochimica Polonica*, *Acta Physiologiae Plantarum*, *Free Radical Biology and Medicine*, and *Free Radical Research*. In 2011–2012 he was president of the Society for Free Radical Research–Europe. He is an author of more than 300 journal publications, 2 books, and 8 book chapters.

Contributors

Caroline P. Baron
Technical University of Denmark
(DTU)
National Food Institute
Kgs Lyngby, Denmark

Grzegorz Bartosz
Department of Biochemistry and Cell
Biology
University of Rzeszów
Rzeszów, Poland

and

Department of Molecular Biophysics
University of Łódź
Łódź, Poland

Izabela Sadowska-Bartosz
University of Rzeszów
Rzeszów, Poland

Louise Bennett
Animal, Food and Health Sciences
Commonwealth Scientific and
Industrial Research Organisation
Victoria, Australia

Susan Brewer
University of Illinois at
Urbana–Champaign
Urbana, Illinois

Alejandro Cifuentes
Institute of Food Science Research
Consejo Superior de Investigaciones
Cientificas and Universidad
Autónoma de Madrid
Madrid, Spain

María Dolores del Castillo
Institute of Food Science Research
Consejo Superior de Investigaciones
Cientificas and Universidad
Autónoma de Madrid
Madrid, Spain

Rosa M. Delgado
Instituto de la Grasa
Consejo Superior de Investigaciones
Científicas
Seville, Spain

Juana Fernández-López
Miguel Hernández University
Orihuela, Spain

Jan Frank
Institute of Biological Chemistry and
Nutrition
University of Hohenheim
Stuttgart, Germany

Anna Gliszczyńska-Świgło
Faculty of Commodity Science
Poznań University of Economics
Poznań, Poland

Tilman Grune
Institute of Nutrition
Friedrich-Schiller-University Jena
Jena, Germany

Miguel Herrero
Institute of Food Science Research
Consejo Superior de Investigaciones
Cientificas and Universidad
Autónoma de Madrid
Madrid, Spain

Francisco J. Hidalgo
Instituto de la Grasa
Consejo Superior de Investigaciones
    Científicas
Seville, Spain

Francisca Holgado
Instituto de Ciencia y Tecnología de
    Alimentos y Nutrición
Consejo Superior de Investigaciones
    Científicas
Madrid, Spain

Elena Ibáñez
Institute of Food Science Research
Consejo Superior de Investigaciones
    Cientificas and Universidad
    Autónoma de Madrid
Madrid, Spain

Klaudia Jomova
Constantine the Philosopher University
Nitra, Slovakia

Alexa Kocher
Institute of Biological Chemistry and
    Nutrition
University of Hohenheim
Stuttgart, Germany

Anna Kołakowska
Department of Biochemistry and
    Human Nutrition
Pomeranian Medical University
Szczecin, Poland

Michael Lawson
Slovak Technical University
Bratislava, Slovakia

Amy Logan
Animal, Food and Health Sciences
Commonwealth Scientific and
    Industrial Research Organisation
Victoria, Australia

Gloria Márquez-Ruiz
Instituto de Ciencia y Tecnología de
    Alimentos y Nutrición
Consejo Superior de Investigaciones
    Científicas
Madrid, Spain

Isabel Medina
Instituto de Investigaciones Marinas
Consejo Superior de Investigaciones
    Científicas
Vigo, Spain

José A. Mendiola
Institute of Food Science Research
Consejo Superior de Investigaciones
    Cientificas and Universidad
    Autónoma de Madrid
Madrid, Spain

Jan Oszmiański
Department of Fruit and Vegetable
    Processing
Wrocław University of Environmental
    and Life Sciences
Wrocław, Poland

Manuel Pazos
Instituto de Investigaciones Marinas
Consejo Superior de Investigaciones
    Científicas
Vigo, Spain

Jose A. Pérez-Álvarez
Miguel Hernández University
Orihuela, Spain

Christina Schiborr
Institute of Biological Chemistry and
    Nutrition
University of Hohenheim
Stuttgart, Germany

Takayuki Shibamoto
University of California, Davis
Davis, California

Netsanet Shiferaw-Terefe
Animal, Food and Health Sciences
Commonwealth Scientific and
    Industrial Research Organisation
Victoria, Australia

Tanoj Singh
Animal, Food and Health Sciences
Commonwealth Scientific and
    Industrial Research Organisation
Victoria, Australia

Marian Valko
Slovak Technical University
Bratislava, Slovakia

Joaquín Velasco
Instituto de la Grasa
Consejo Superior de Investigaciones
    Científicas
Seville, Spain

Petras Rimantas Venskutonis
Kaunas University of Technology
Kaunas, Lithuania

Manuel Viuda-Martos
Miguel Hernández University
Orihuela, Spain

Robyn Warner
Animal, Food and Health Sciences
Commonwealth Scientific and
    Industrial Research Organisation
Victoria, Australia

Iwona Wawer
Medical University of Warsaw
Warsaw, Poland

Daniela Weber
Institute of Nutrition
Friedrich-Schiller-University Jena
Jena, Germany

Rosario Zamora
Instituto de la Grasa
Consejo Superior de Investigaciones
    Científicas
Seville, Spain

Emanuela Zanardi
Dipartimento di Scienze degli Alimenti
Università degli Studi di Parma
Parma, Italy

Abbreviations

AAA:	α-aminoadipic acid
AAS:	α-aminoadipic semialdehyde
ABTS:	2,2′-azino-bis(3-ethylbenzothiazoline-6-sulfonic acid)
ACA:	aldehyde/carboxylic acid
ACE:	angiotensin converting enzyme
ADP:	adenosine diphosphate
AGEs:	advanced glycation end products
ALA:	alpha-lipoic acid
ALEs:	advanced lipid oxidation end products
AMP:	adenosine monophosphate
AOX:	antioxidant
APCI:	atmospheric pressure chemical ionization
ARA:	arachidonic acid
AsA:	ascorbic acid
ATP:	adenosine triphosphate
AUC:	area under curve
AVA:	avenanthramide
BHA:	butylated hydroxyanisole
BHT:	butylated hydroxytoluene
CAP:	captopril
Car:	carotenoid
cGMP:	cyclic guanosine monophosphate
CLA:	conjugated linoleic acid
CMLys:	carboxymethyllysine
CMP:	caseinomacropeptide
COPs:	cholesterol oxidation products
CPP:	casein phosphopeptides
CumOOH:	cumene hydroperoxide
CYP:	cytochrome P450
DAG:	diacylglycerol(s)
DHA:	docosahexaenoic acid
DHLA:	dihydrolipoic acid
DNPH:	dinitrophenylhydrazine
DOPA:	3,4-dihydroxyphenylalanine
DP:	degree of polymerization
DPPH:	1,1-diphenyl-2-picrylhydrazyl
DSF:	defatted soy flour
DTNB:	5,5′-dithiobis-(2-nitrobenzoic acid), Ellman's reagent
ECD:	electron-capture detector
EDTA:	ethylenediaminetetraacetic acid
EFB:	empty fruit bunches
EGC:	epigallocatechin
EGCG:	epigallocatechin gallate
EPA:	eicosapentaenoic acid
ESR:	electron spin resonance
FA:	fatty acid(s)

FI:	flow ice
FID:	flame ionization detection
FFA:	free fatty acid(s)
FOS:	fructo-oligosaccharide
FOX:	ferrous oxidation-xylenol orange
FRAP:	ferric reducing/antioxidant power
FPH:	fish protein hydrolysates
FTC:	ferric thiocyanate
GC:	gas chromatography
GGC:	γ-glutamylcysteine
GGS:	γ-glutamic semialdehyde
GPx:	glutathione peroxidase
GRAS:	generally recognized as safe
GSH:	glutathione
GST:	glutathione *S*-transferases
Hb:	hemoglobin
HCA:	hydroxycinnamic acid(s)
HDLc:	high-density lipoprotein-associated cholesterol
HHE:	4-hydroxy-2-hexenal
HHP:	high hydrostatic pressure
HMF:	hydroxymethylfurfural
HMW:	high molecular weight
HNE:	4-hydroxy-2-nonenal
H(p)ETE:	hydro(pero)xyeicosatetraenoic acid
HPL:	hydroperoxide lyase(s)
HPLC:	high-performance liquid chromatography
HPSEC:	high-performance size-exclusion chromatography
La:	lactalbumin
LA:	linoleic acid
LDH:	lactate dehydrogenase
LMW:	low molecular weight
LOX:	lipoxygenase(s)
LPO:	lactoperoxidase
MAE:	microwave-assisted extraction
MAG:	monoacylglycerol(s)
MALDI-TOF:	matrix-assisted laser desorption ionization-time of flight
MAP:	modified atmosphere packaging
Mb:	myoglobin
MCL:	methyl conjugated linoleate
MDA:	malondialdehyde
metHb:	methemoglobin
metMb:	metmyoglobin
ML:	methyl linoleate
MMP:	matrix metalloproteinase
MPO:	myeloperoxidase
MRP:	Maillard reaction product(s)
MS:	mass spectroscopy
MUFA:	monounsaturated fatty acids
MW:	molecular weight
NAC:	N-acetylcysteine
NQO1:	NAD(P)H-quinone oxidoreductase

OFI:	flow ice system including ozone
OMWW:	olive-mill wastewater
ONE:	4-oxo-2-nonenal
OP:	oxidation potential
ORAC:	oxygen radical absorbance capacity
OS:	oligosaccharide(s)
PAD:	pulsed amperometric detection
PAGE:	polyacrylamide gel electrophoresis
PDA:	photodiode array detection
PEF:	pulsed electric field
PHWE:	pressurized hot water extraction
PIR:	protein interaction report
PLE:	pressurized liquid extraction
POBN:	(4-pyridyl-1-oxide)-*N*-*tert*-butylnitrone
POD:	polyphenol peroxidase
PPF:	palm pressed fibers
PPO:	polyphenol oxidase(s)
PS:	polysaccharide(s)
PUFA:	polyunsaturated fatty acid(s)
PV:	peroxide value
RNS:	reactive nitrogen species
ROS:	reactive oxygen species
RTE:	ready to eat
SDG:	secoisolariciresinol diglucoside
SDS:	sodium dodecyl sulfate
SECO:	secoisolariciresinol
Sen:	sensitizer
SFE:	supercritical fluid extraction
SO:	sunflower oil
SPI:	soy protein isolate
SWE:	subcritical water extraction
TAC:	total antioxidant capacity
TAG:	triacylglycerol(s)
TAnC:	total anthocyanin content
TBA:	thiobarbituric acid
TBARS:	thiobarbituric acid reactive substances
TBHQ:	tertiary butyl hydroquinone
TE:	Trolox equivalent(s)
TEAC:	Trolox equivalent antioxidant capacity
TO:	Tonalin oil
TPC:	total phenolic content
TRAP:	total radical-trapping antioxidant parameter
TRX:	thioredoxin
UAE:	ultrasound-assisted extraction
UGT:	uridine-5′-diphospho glucuronosyltransferase
UV:	ultraviolet
WEPO:	water extraction and particle formation online
WOF:	warmed-over flavor
WPC:	whey protein concentrate
WSP:	water-soluble proteins

1 Oxidation of Food Components
An Introduction

Anna Kołakowska and Grzegorz Bartosz

CONTENTS

Remember that thou goest in the midst of snares,
and that thou walkest upon the battlements of the city

Sirach 9.13

1.1 INTRODUCTION

Oxidation in food has its source in the physiological mechanisms of the oxidation processes in plants and animals, which are raw materials for food products. In the chain of food production, under the influence of biological, environmental, and technological factors and the additives used, the status of the oxidation and antioxidant

1

changes. Oxidation in food systems is a detrimental process. It deteriorates the sensory quality and nutritive value of a product and poses health hazards by the presence of toxic oxidation products. Oxidation affects all food components, but its impact on food quality is not uniform.

Oxidation processes that occur naturally in the human body contribute to the development of most major diseases due to an insufficient defense system. The presence of toxic oxidation products in food and its reduced nutritional value and decreased antioxidant content, which are supplied in the diet, can significantly affect the health of the consumer. It can be expected that a diet rich in oxidized food components leads to a lowering of the antioxidant or oxidant status in an organism, increasing the risk of disease.

1.2 FREE RADICALS AND REACTIVE OXYGEN SPECIES

The sources of oxidative processes in living organisms are free radicals and other reactive oxygen species (ROS), which are formed in every living cell. A free radical is any atom or molecule that has at least one unpaired electron in its outermost shell. Any free radical containing oxygen is then referred to as a ROS, but a ROS can also include species that are not free radicals (such as hydrogen peroxide H_2O_2, singlet oxygen $^1O_2$, ozone O_3, hypochlorite ^-OCl, and peroxynitrite $ONOO^-$). The most commonly formed ROS are the superoxide anion radical $\left(O_2^{\cdot-}\right)$ and hydrogen peroxide, and the hydroxyl radical is the most reactive ROS. Nitric oxide ($NO^{\cdot}$) is also a free radical. A reaction $O_2^{\cdot-}$ anion with $NO^{\cdot}$ produces peroxynitrite $ONOO^-$, a strong oxidant (Figure 1.1). The main source superoxide is the one-electron leakage of the mitochondrial respiratory chain and, in plant cells, of the chloroplasts redox

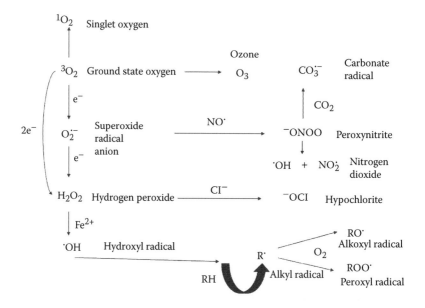

FIGURE 1.1   Main ROS occurring in biological systems

system. Free radicals can also be produced by many cells as a defensive mechanism (phagocytes) or for signaling purposes. Neutrophils produce free radicals to attack and destroy pathogens. NO$^\bullet$ plays mainly a signaling role in the body.

While ROS are predominantly implicated in causing cell damage, they also play a major physiological role in several aspects of intracellular signaling and regulation. ROS interfere with the expression of a number of genes and signal transduction pathways and, depending on the concentration, cause either a positive response (cell proliferation) or a negative cell response (growth arrest or cell death). ROS can thus play a very important physiological role as secondary messengers (Valko et al. 2006; Bartosz and Kołakowska 2011).

1.3 PEROXIDATION OF LIPIDS

1.3.1 INITIATION

All types of biological molecules are damaged by ROS, but lipid oxidation plays a special role in this process because the energy barrier to initiate lipid peroxidation is lower than those to initiate oxidation of proteins, carbohydrates, or nucleic acids. Nevertheless, there is interplay between oxidative reactions of various biomolecules. Free radicals of other molecules may initiate lipid oxidation while products of lipid oxidation modify proteins and nucleic acids and deplete antioxidants. Different mechanisms are able to induce lipid peroxidation: free-radical reactions, photooxidation, enzyme action, and oxidation catalyzed by trace metals.

1.3.2 AUTOXIDATION

Autoxidation is a radical-chain process involving three steps: initiation, propagation, and termination. In the initiation step, a hydrogen atom is removed from a molecule LH and a free-radical form of lipid alkyl radical L$^\bullet$ is formed. Heat, ultraviolet (UV), and visible light and metal catalysts can accelerate this step. It is usually initiated by hydroxyl, peroxyl, or hydroperoxyl radicals (but not superoxide or hydrogen peroxide) or hemoproteins activated to the ferryl state.

In the propagation step, an alkyl radical reacts with oxygen to form a peroxyl radical (LOO$^\bullet$):

$$L^\bullet + O_2 \rightarrow LOO^\bullet$$

which, in turn, can abstract a hydrogen atom from another lipid molecule:

$$LOO^\bullet + LH \rightarrow LOOH + L^\bullet$$

thus causing an autocatalytic chain reaction. The peroxyl radical combines with H to give a lipid hydroperoxide.

Alternatively, peroxyl radicals [especially those formed from polyunsaturated fatty acids (PUFAs), such as arachidonic acid (ARA) or eicosapentaenoic acid (EPA)] can be transformed in the organism into cyclic peroxides or even cyclic endoperoxides.

Reaction between two radicals terminates the reaction

$$LOO^{\bullet} + L^{\bullet} \rightarrow LOOL$$

$$L^{\bullet} + L^{\bullet} \rightarrow LL$$

1.3.3 Photooxidation

Oxygen can be excited to the singlet state ($^1O_2$) by light energy (photooxidation) promoted by pigments that act as sensitizers. As singlet oxygen ($^1O_2$) is highly electrophilic, it can react rapidly with unsaturated lipids but by a different mechanism than free-radical autoxidation. In the presence of sensitizers (chlorophyll, porphyrins, myoglobin, riboflavin, bilirubin, erythrosine, rose bengal, methylene blue, etc.), the double bond of a fatty acid (FA) residue interacts directly with singlet oxygen produced from O_2 by light or UV radiation. The photooxidation is a faster reaction than autoxidation; it was demonstrated that photooxidation can be 30,000 times faster than autoxidation in the case of oleic acid and can be 1000–1500 times faster in the case of polyenes.

Lipid hydroperoxides, the main intermediates of the peroxidation reactions, accumulate in the bilayer and induce changes in the structure and biophysical organization of membrane lipid components, especially oxidation of phospholipid FA residues, including the loss or rearrangement of double bonds. The main biophysical consequences of the lipid membrane include changes in membrane fluidity and permeability, alteration of membrane thermotropic phase properties, and membrane protein activities (Mosca et al. 2011).

1.3.4 Enzymatic Peroxidation

Lipoxygenases (LOXs) (EC 1.13.11.12), a family of non-heme iron-containing FA dioxygenases, are widely distributed in plants, animals, and microorganisms. LOX-catalyzed lipid oxidation differs from the free-radical reaction by the formation of hydroperoxides in a defined position of FA chains. LOXs use molecular oxygen to catalyze the stereospecific and regiospecific oxygenation of PUFAs with 1-*cis*,4-*cis*-pentadiene moieties. The newly formed FA peroxy free radical abstracts hydrogen from another unsaturated FA molecule to form a conjugated hydroperoxy diene. Hydroperoxy dienes are responsible for the off-flavor in frozen vegetables; for lipid oxidation in cereal products, rapeseed, pea, and avocado; and for "beany" and bitter flavors. If the oxidation reactions proceed to a low degree only, they may be considered as desirable. For example, the typical flavors of cucumbers and virgin olive oil are results of lipid oxidation products (Pokorny and Schmidt 2011). LOXs in fish are also responsible for the formation of a desirable fresh fish flavor, the seaweed flavor, from n-3 PUFA. Soybean LOX has been used to bleach flour to produce white bread crumbs and to improve the dough-forming properties and baking performance of wheat flour by oxidizing free lipids.

In both plants and animals, cyclooxygenase enzymes catalyze the addition of molecular oxygen to various polyunsaturated FAs, which are thus converted into biologically active endoperoxides, intermediates in the transformation of FAs to prostaglandins. Among the cytochrome-P450 catalyzed reactions, the FA epoxygenase activity produces epoxide derivatives. These monoepoxides can be metabolized into diepoxides, epoxy-alcohols, or oxygenated prostaglandins.

1.3.5 Peroxidation Catalyzed by Trace Metals and Heme Compounds

Transition metal ions, first, participate in the Fenton reaction believed to be the main source of the hydroxyl radical ($^{\bullet}$OH) in biological systems. Another contribution of transition metal ions to lipid peroxidation is a result of their role in the decomposition of lipid hydroperoxides. These primary products of peroxidation may slowly decompose spontaneously, especially at elevated temperatures, but transition metal ions accelerate their decomposition, resulting in formation of alkoxyl (RO$^{\bullet}$) and peroxyl (ROO$^{\bullet}$) radicals (Bartosz 2003):

$$ROOH + Fe^{2+} \rightarrow RO^{\bullet} + HO^- + Fe^{3+} \quad \text{(fast reaction)}$$

$$ROOH + Fe^{3+} \rightarrow ROO^{\bullet} + H^+ + Fe^{2+} \quad \text{(slow reaction)}$$

Metal ions found naturally in food components and gained from the environment or metal equipment can initiate lipid peroxidation in foods. Higher concentrations of hemoglobin and myoglobin iron in meat and in fish are associated with higher rates of lipid oxidation. In meat, lipid oxidation and myoglobin oxidation can occur concurrently. The oxidation of oxymyoglobin (OxyMb) to metmyoglobin (MetMb) generates reactive intermediates capable of enhancing further oxidation of OxyMb and/or unsaturated FAs. Specifically, a superoxide anion is formed and dismutates enzymatically or nonenzymatically, producing hydrogen peroxide. The latter can react with the MetMb concurrently generated in this oxidation sequence to form an activated MetMb complex capable of enhancing lipid oxidation. Heme or iron can be released from the myoglobin and hemoglobin during postmortem handling and storage, thereby also promoting lipid oxidation (Min et al. 2010; Faustman et al. 2010).

Compared to LOX, iron and hemoglobin cause slower lipid oxidation in the initial phase but result in a severe oxidized oil odor, and LOX is associated with a strong fishy odor (Fu et al. 2009).

1.3.6 Secondary Oxidation Products

Lipid hydroperoxides, the primary products of oxidation, are highly unstable and, under conditions of elevated temperature and illumination and in the presence of prooxidants, tend to decompose via β-scission reaction, giving rise to secondary products, such as aldehydes, ketones, lactones, alcohols, keto acids, hydroxy acids, epidioxides, and other volatile compounds. Some of these secondary products can be toxic to humans and are responsible for the undesirable rancid odor typical of oxidized oils (Decker 2010).

The most important of these products are short-unsaturated aldehydes because of the reactivity of the aldehyde group. They exhibit biological activity *in vivo* and interact easily with cell and food components, causing a loss of the nutritional value of food. For years, malonodialdehyde (MDA), the most abundant aldehyde, which results from lipid peroxidation in food, has been found to be the main culprit. Its concentration in meat and fish products could even reach 300 μM (Kanner 2007). Since the 1990s, trans-4-hydroxy-2-nonenal (HNE) has been viewed as the quintessential toxic lipid peroxidation product. In addition to the formation of HNE, the hydroperoxides of ARA and linoleic acid are precursors of the highly electrophilic γ-keto aldehyde trans-4-oxo-2-nonenal (4-ONE). Lipid oxidation of n-3 PUFA generates a closely related compound, 4-hydroxy-2-hexanal (HHE), whose concentration in several foods, such as fish products, could reach 120 μM (Long and Picklo 2010). Analysis of aldehyde products resulting from docosahexaenoic acid (DHA) oxidation identified at least 15 aldehydes, including HHE, glyoxal, malondialdehyde, 4-hydroxy-2,6-nonadienal, 2-pentenal, and others (Kanner 2007).

These aldehydes are capable of producing damage to the biological macromolecules even at a distance from the formation site (Traverso et al. 2010). They are durable and easily absorbed from food (Gracanin et al. 2010; Goicoechea et al. 2011).

Because of its ability to interact with DNA and proteins, such as MDA, HNE has often been considered as a potentially genotoxic agent able to cause mutations. Moreover, MDA toxicity also is directed toward cardiovascular system stability through the intermolecular crosslinking of collagen, which contributes to the stiffening of cardiovascular tissue.

There seems to be a dual influence of 4-HNE on the physiology of cells: Lower intracellular concentrations (around 0.1–5.0 μM) seem to be beneficial to cells, promoting proliferation, and higher concentrations (around 10–20 μM) have been shown to be toxic and involved in the pathology of several diseases.

1.3.7 Oxysterols

Oxidized derivatives of cholesterol and phytosterols can be generated in the human organism through different oxidation processes, some requiring enzymes. Furthermore, oxysterols are also present in food as a result of lipid oxidation reactions caused by heat treatments, contact with oxygen, exposure to sunlight, etc. Cholesterol oxides are present in our diet, particularly in foods high in cholesterol. Storage, cooking, and processing tend to increase the cholesterol oxidation products contain. Their concentration is particularly high (10–100 μM, i.e., 10–150 μg/g dry weight) in dried egg, milk powders, heated butter (ghee), precooked meat and poultry products, and heated tallow. Oxysterols can be absorbed from the diet at different rates, depending on their side chain length. In the organism, oxysterols can follow different routes: They may be secreted into the intestinal lumen, esterified, and distributed by lipoproteins to different tissues or degraded, mainly in the liver (Kanner 2007). Cholesterol oxidation products show cytotoxicity (especially the 7-oxygenated species) and apoptotic and proinflammatory effects, and they have also been linked with chronic diseases, including atherosclerotic and neurodegenerative processes. In the case of phytosterol oxidation products, more research on their toxic effects is needed. Nevertheless, current knowledge suggests they may also exert cytotoxic and proapoptotic effects although at higher concentrations than oxycholesterols (Otaegui-Arrazola et al. 2010; Wąsowicz and Rudzińska 2011).

1.4 PROTEIN OXIDATION

Reactive oxidants generated continuously in biological systems are expected to react mainly with proteins as a result of the high abundance of proteins (approximately 70% of the dry mass of cells) and rapid rates of their reactions with many oxidants. The occurrence of protein oxidation in biological systems has been known and studied for approximately 50 years as a result of the connection between the oxidative damage to proteins and the development of age-related diseases. The oxidation of food proteins is one of the most innovative research topics within the food science field having only been studied for approximately 20 years (Estévez 2011).

Protein oxidation occurs as a result of either direct attack by ROS or photooxidation or indirectly through peroxidation of lipids that further degrade and attack proteins.

Numerous ROS, such as the superoxide $(O_2^{\cdot-})$, the hydroperoxyl $(HO_2^{\cdot})$, and hydroxyl (HO$^{\cdot}$) radicals and other nonradical species, such as hydrogen peroxide (H_2O_2) and hydroperoxides (ROOH), are potential initiators of protein oxidation. As a direct consequence of the abstraction of a hydrogen atom from a susceptible target (PH), a carbon-centered protein radical (P$^{\cdot}$) is formed. The initial P$^{\cdot}$ is consecutively converted into a peroxyl radical (POO$^{\cdot}$) in the presence of oxygen and to an alkyl peroxide (POOH) by abstraction of a hydrogen atom from another susceptible molecule. Further reactions with ROS, such as the $HO_2^{\cdot}$ radical or with reduced forms of transition metals (M^{n+}), such as Fe^{2+} or Cu^+, lead to the formation of an alkoxyl radical (PO$^{\cdot}$) and its hydroxyl derivative (POH) (Estévez 2011):

$$PH + HO^{\cdot} \rightarrow P^{\cdot} + H_2O$$

$$P^{\cdot} + O_2 \rightarrow POO^{\cdot}$$

$$POO^{\cdot} + PH \rightarrow POOH + P^{\cdot}$$

$$POOH + HO_2^{\cdot} \rightarrow PO^{\cdot} + O_2 + H_2O$$

$$POOH + M^{n+} \rightarrow PO^{\cdot} + HO^- + M^{(n+1)+}$$

$$PO + HO_2^{\cdot} \rightarrow POH + O_2$$

$$PO^{\cdot} + H^+ + M^{n+} \rightarrow POH + M^{(n+1)+}$$

The common protein targets for ROS are the peptide backbone and the functional groups located in the side chains of amino acid residues. It has been shown that a single hydroxyl radical is capable of causing damage of up to 15 amino acids of a peptide chain. Certain amino acids, such as cysteine and methionine, would be first oxidized because of the high susceptibility of their sulfur centers. Tryptophan residues are also promptly oxidized. Susceptible to oxidation are also amino acids with a free amino, amide, and hydroxyl group (lysine, arginine, and tyrosine).

Lipid radicals abstract hydrogen mainly from the side chains of the protein molecule, in particular, from lysine, arginine, histidine, tryptophan, cysteine, and cystine residues, to form protein radicals (P·) that initiate formation of further radicals interacting with the protein, causing formation of protein radicals or protein–protein and protein–lipid adducts, or they react also with other food components (Sikorski 2007):

$$P + L^{\cdot} \rightarrow P^{\cdot} + L$$

$$P + LO^{\cdot} \rightarrow P^{\cdot} + LOH, LO^{\cdot}P$$

$$P + LOO^{\cdot} \rightarrow P^{\cdot} + LOOH, LOO^{\cdot}P$$

$$P + LOH \rightarrow LO^{\cdot} + P^{\cdot} + {\cdot}OH + H^{\cdot}$$

These processes generate various byproducts, among them oxidized amino acids, carbonyls, and fragmentation products. The formation of carbonyl compounds is principally a result of the oxidation of threonine, proline, arginine, and lysine residues. The total protein carbonyl content is estimated to be ≈1–2 nmol/mg protein in a variety of human and animal tissues, which represent modification of about 10% of the total cellular protein. The result of protein oxidation is the loss of the native structure and functionality of protein molecules (Estevez 2011; Gracanin et al. 2010).

1.5 CONSEQUENCES OF LIPID AND PROTEIN OXIDATION *IN VIVO*

Once free radicals are generated, they are often capable of giving rise to chain reactions, that is, reactions that create new radicals that, in turn, trigger new reactions. Despite the numerous lines of defense, protection against free radicals is never complete, and more or less severe random damage continually takes place within living organisms.

Considering that the sites responsible for the greatest production of oxygen radicals are localized on biological membranes, the components of the membrane themselves (phospholipids and proteins) are among the principal targets. The fundamental roles of free radicals have been suggested in aging and numerous pathological situations regarding several organs; among these, for instance, are inflammation; ischemia–reperfusion syndromes; atherosclerosis; degenerative cerebral syndromes, particularly Alzheimer's disease; cataracts; retinopathy; diabetic complications; and cancer (Traverso et al. 2010; Bartosz and Kołakowska 2011).

Proteins are structurally altered by oxidation under oxidative stress conditions; their oxidation leads to the generation of disulfide bridges, unfolding and increasing exposure of the polypeptide chain to the hydrophilic environment (Chaudhuri et al. 2002).

As a result of oxidation, carbonyls are introduced into proteins either by direct oxidation of amino acids or, indirectly, by covalent attachment of a carbonyl-containing moiety, such as HNE or MDA. The proteins, when oxidized at the level of sulfur-containing amino acids, can be repaired. Cells have limited mechanisms for protein repair and mechanisms for getting rid of damaged proteins (mainly proteasomes). Protein damage may include, for example, disulfide bridges; cysteine sulfenic acid; methionine sulfoxide; hydroxylation and carbonylation of Arg, Lys, Pro, Thr, Leu, etc.; nitrosylation of Cys; nitration of Tyr, Try, and His; lipid peroxidation adducts to His, Cys, and Lys; glycation/glycoxidation adducts to Lys and Arg; and protein aggregation (Friguet 2006). Accumulation of oxidized forms of protein is observed in aging and age-related diseases (Valko et al. 2006).

A consequence of the harmful protein oxidation processes is the formation of lipofuscin, which accumulates intracellularly with age (e.g., in the liver, kidney, heart muscle, adrenals, nerve cells, eyes, and brain). It is an aggregate containing highly oxidized and covalently cross-linked proteins (30%–58%), oxidized lipids (19%–51%), and low amounts of saccharides. These yellowish-brown pigment granules are products that result from the interaction of oxidatively modified proteins and lipids, in which a major cross-linking agent are carbonyls (aldehydes as MDA, HNE, HHE) of lipids and proteins. Carbohydrates form only a minor structural component (Höhn et al. 2011; Traverso et al. 2010). Oxidative stress is a major promoter for lipofuscin formation *in vitro* and *in vivo* (Breyer and Pischetsrieder 2009).

Similarly colored melanoidin-like polymers from oxidized lipids and proteins are formed in food. In these reactions, the main active amino acid is the lysine as it possesses a free amine group, and aldehydes are the most active groups in oxidized lipids. Another sensitive amino acid is tryptophan because of the indole group (Pokorny et al. 2011).

1.6 FACTORS AFFECTING LIPID AND PROTEIN OXIDATION IN FOOD

Susceptibility of lipids and/or protein oxidation in food depends on the composition of the foods: content and composition of lipids and proteins, the presence of prooxidants and antioxidants, oxygen levels, light, temperature, and a number of biological and technological factors.

FA composition. The hydrogen atom bound to the carbon atom separating the C=C bond is the easiest to detach; therefore, PUFAs containing such residues are most prone to peroxidation. If we assume the rate of this reaction for stearic acid as 1, it would be 100 for oleic acid, 250 for linoleic acid, and 2500 for linolenic acid. FAs may be autoxidized either in free form or, mostly, as components of glycerolipids or glycolipids. PUFAs were shown to be more stable to oxidation when located at the *sn*-2 position of triacylglycerol compared to *sn*-1.

Fortification of food with LC n-3 PUFAs can make it more prone to protein oxidation. For example, dairy products enriched with n-3 PUFAs can lead to severe changes, including oxidation of the side chain groups, backbone fragmentation, aggregation, and loss of nutritional value and functional properties of the proteins (Cucu et al. 2011).

Temperature. The increase in temperature during storage and food processing accelerates the oxidation process and changes its course. Primary lipid oxidation products decompose more easily and interact more quickly with other components of food. Heating above 100°C is critical for the oxidation of cholesterol. The frying temperature above 170°C causes oxidation of not only the frying oil but also of lipids in the fried food, especially in foods rich in PUFAs.

Water activity. Rate of oxidation decreases as the water activity (a_w) is lowered. The rate of many lipid oxidation reactions increases under very low a_w (<0.2). Rancidity becomes a major problem in dehydrated foods and in frozen foods rich in PUFAs, such as fish.

Light. Light is a source of energy that can lead to the formation of radical initiators. UV irradiation is particularly harmful. The influence of light on lipid oxidation depends on the wavelength, the depth of penetration into the product, sensitizer content, and the content of carotenoids, which are a barrier to the photooxidation. Reduced-fat dairy products often seem more sensitive to oxidation compared to dairy foodstuffs with a higher lipid content, demonstrating the important role of proteins and lipid–protein interaction in this chemical decay (Mestdagh et al. 2011). In the processing of fish intended for long frozen storage, where the process-initiated lipid oxidation cannot be effectively inhibited, certain technological operations are performed in rooms with artificial lighting. The appropriate choice of food packaging, forming a barrier against oxygen and light, is important.

Technological process. Susceptibility to oxidation of raw materials (plant and animals) is affected by many biological factors (species, variety, race, sex, age, etc.) and many others. For example, environmental pollutants may induce oxidative stress (Braconi et al. 2011; Grosicka-Maciąg 2011). In technological processes, increased susceptibility to oxidation through mechanical processing (milling, mixing) and salt addition may occur (Sakai et al. 2004). This problem may be especially important in technologies such as irradiation, drying, and microwaves that produce ROS (Zanardi et al. 2009). Microwaves can break disulfide bonds, thus inducing subunit disaggregation, which can cause protein unfolding and formation of smaller aggregates in the solution (Guan et al. 2011). Lipid oxidation in microwave-cooked food is difficult to detect because of the participation of lipid oxidation products in interactions with proteins (Kołakowska 2011). As a result of microwave heating of fish's lipids–albumin system, almost half of the lipids were not available for extraction (covalently bound to a protein). In a system containing partly oxidized lipids, as much as 76% of the lipids after microwave heating have been covalently bound to a protein; DHA was bound.

1.7   WHAT IS OXIDIZED FIRST: LIPIDS OR PROTEINS?

Until recently, protein oxidation in food was primarily interpreted as a secondary result of lipid oxidation. In the presence of linoleate, bovine serum albumin was not oxidized by the direct action of HO• radicals but was undergoing a secondary oxidation by nondienic lipid hydroperoxides and/or lipid radical intermediates, arising from the HO•-induced linoleate oxidation. However, linoleate was secondarily oxidized by oxidized species of albumin (Collin et al. 2010). However, the •OH radical would react faster and preferentially with certain proteins, such as albumin ($k = 8 \times 10^{10}$ dm^3 mol^{-1} s^{-1}) or collagen ($k = 4 \times 10^{11}$ dm^3 mol^{-1} s^{-1}), than with unsaturated lipids, such as linoleic acid ($k = 9 \times 10^9$ dm^3 mol^{-1} s^{-1}) (Davies 2005). According to Soyer and Hultin (2000), reactions of ROS with lipids and proteins in fish tissue proceed simultaneously. Lipid and protein oxidation appeared to occur simultaneously in chicken meat during frozen storage (Soyer et al. 2010) and in minces from horse mackerel during processing and storage, but it was not possible to determine at which level these two reactions were coupled (Eymard et al. 2009). During storage of frozen fatty fish, lipid oxidation symptoms occur significantly ahead of changes in proteins; therefore, the last were assumed to be a result of lipid oxidation. But in lean fish, where the ratio of protein to lipid is about 20:1, protein denaturation changes were observed already in the initial period of frozen storage while rancidity was noticeable after a period of several times longer. With the increase of lipid oxidation in herring, the antioxidant activity of tissue decreases. Therefore, even in fatty fish rich in PUFAs, the primary target of ROS appears to be protein (Kołakowska 2011; Aranowska 2011).

The free radical transfer from oxidizing lipids to protein and amino acids has been observed in dry (lyophilized) products. These interactions may initiate the reactions leading to protein degradation (Schaich 2008). On the other hand, free radicals may transfer from proteins to lipids and initiate lipid oxidation. Furthermore, free radicals may transfer from proteins to other biomolecules, such as other proteins and peptides. Hence, the free radical interactions in food systems may be important in determining the stability and shelf life of dry foods, in particular, in irradiated freeze-dried products. The interactions between the particles of different powdered ingredients in soup powder increased the rate of reactions, leading to a higher rate of radical reactions than in powdered ingredients stored separately (Raitio et al. 2011).

1.8 CARBOHYDRATE OXIDATION

Classical nonenzymatic browning (Maillard reactions) is traditionally attributed to reactions of reducing sugars with amine-containing compounds, and it is uncertain whether these free-radical reactions are accompanied by the oxidative processes of saccharides. Free radicals do not play a significant role in the browning reactions of amine groups of ethanolamine and PUFA and in a saccharide–lecithin system (Nguyen et al. 2002). The presence of radicals and the oxidation of saccharides have been shown in an oxidative model system copper–carbohydrate (Cerchiaro et al. 2005) and in the iron-containing xanthine oxidase and hypoxanthine (Fe-XO/HX)–saccharide system. Saccharide molecules, such as glucose, fructose, and sucrose, are essential for generating radicals ($R^•$) as no $R^•$ were detected in the absence of saccharides (Luo et al. 2001).

$$\text{Saccharide chain (R)} - \text{H} + \text{OH}^• \rightarrow \text{saccharide derivatives} + R^• + H_2O$$

Free radicals formed during irradiation of lactose (Lyutova and Yudin 2006) and during the industrial oxidation of starch (Łabanowska et al. 2011). Various stable and short-living radical species were formed upon thermal treatment (at 180°C–230°C) of pressurized starches (Błaszczak et al. 2008, 2010). A stable radical was detected in dark beers and in sweet wort produced with dark malt. The radical is formed during the roasting of malt (Jehle et al. 2011). When roasting coffee, free radical-mediated reactions could be important processes during both the heating and cooling phases of a roasting cycle (Goodman et al. 2011). Interactions at the free-radical level were observed between dry ingredients in cauliflower soup powder, prepared by dry mixing of ingredients and rapeseed oil (Raitio et al. 2011). Spices are subjected to irradiation. In irradiated black pepper, cellulose, starch, phenoxyl, and peroxyl radicals were observed (Yamaoki et al. 2011). Therefore, the Maillard reaction and lipid oxidation follow parallel mechanisms. ROS are capable of activating glucose and other α-hydroxy aldehydes (or α-hydroxy ketones), rendering them more reactive and favoring the attack of biological macromolecules; ultimately, ROS are capable of accelerating the Maillard reaction. Equally, the reducing sugars, Amadori products, and other intermediaries of a Maillard reaction can, in the presence of metallic transition ions, lead to autoxidation generating oxygen free radicals (Adams et al. 2011; Traverso et al. 2010).

In comparison with the lipid and protein oxidation, oxidation of saccharides has no significant effect on ROS in mitochondria (Sanz et al. 2006). In the food, formation of saccharide radicals requires drastic conditions (irradiation, high temperature, the presence of strong metal catalysts).

Carbohydrates in foods act as antioxidants. Some of the Maillard reaction products (glycated proteins) and complexes of oxidized lipids with proteins, such as moderate properties, also have such properties (Pokorny et al. 2011). It has been reported that polysaccharides from different resources extracted from plants and seaweed have strong antioxidant properties (free-radical scavenging, transition-metal binding) and can be explored as novel potential antioxidants (Zhang et al. 2011; Waraho et al. 2011). Polysaccharides extracted from marine algae, chitosan, and its derivatives are effective antioxidants (Feng et al. 2008; Redouan et al. 2011). Scavenging ability on hydroxyl radicals was found to be in the order of chitosan > hyaluronan > starch (Yang et al. 2010).

1.9 CONSEQUENCES OF FOOD COMPONENT OXIDATION

While ROS play multiple, both beneficial and deleterious, roles in living organisms, their reactions in food are almost always harmful, leading to loss of sensory quality, nutritional value, and health risks. This also changes the usefulness of raw materials for processing. It is difficult to find a food component that would not be capable of affecting the oxidation process.

In food, $^1O_2$ reacts with vitamins and other compounds, causing a loss of nutritive value. Riboflavin is a photosensitizer but also reacts with $^1O_2$. Milk exposed to sunlight for 30 min may lose up to 30% of its riboflavin; an 80% loss has been reported in milk stored under light. Light of wavelength 450 nm (maximum absorption of riboflavin) is the most destructive to this compound. Ascorbic acid is also reactive with singlet oxygen ($k = 3.1 \times 10^8$ M^{-1} s^{-1}); as a result, vitamin C is also easily destroyed by light. Losses of 80%–100% of ascorbic acid have been reported upon 60 min of exposure of milk to sunlight (Min and Boff 2002). Vitamin D reacts effectively with $^1O_2$ (reaction rate $k = 2.2 \times 10^7$ M^{-1} s^{-1}), which leads to its photodestruction. Lipid-soluble vitamins are particularly susceptible to oxidation resulting from physical factors (temperature, sunlight, UV light, and oxygen or air), chemical factors (radicals, peroxides, metal ions, e.g., Cu^{2+}, Fe^{3+}), and enzymes, mainly oxidases, for example, LOX, and the process is further accelerated by the presence of oxidized fats. These factors, acting jointly, could cause even greater vitamin losses in foodstuffs during technological processes and, afterward, during storage. Processes in which radicals are generated, such as irradiation and microwave heating, significantly affect vitamin losses, depending on the applied dose and the environmental conditions (Nogala-Kałucka 2011).

Oxidation of pigments (carotenoids, anthocyanins, myoglobin) in foods manifested by discoloration, or bleaching, lowers the attractiveness of the product. This takes place during the storage of raw materials and heat treatment, especially in the presence of oxygen, light, and copper or iron ions. Carotenoids in fruits, vegetables, some invertebrates, and fish (meat and skin), in the presence of PUFAs, undergo oxidation. Despite the nutritional and biological functions of carotenoids, several of the oxidation products of these pigments are deleterious (Benevides et al. 2011). It can also lead to a change in the composition of carotenoids. The dominant carotenoid in trout is astaxanthin with canthaxanthin representing approximately 20% of total carotenoids in freshly cooked trout. Trout cooked after 2 weeks of storage showed an increase in lipid oxidation, and canthaxanthin content increased up to 50% of total carotenoids (Kołakowska and Łomaszewska 2006).

It is generally accepted that, apart from microbial spoilage, lipid oxidation is the primary process by which muscle food spoilage occurs. The oxidative deterioration of lipids leads to the development of rancidity; off-odor, off-flavor compounds; polymerization; and other reactions causing the reduction of shelf life, nutritional quality, and safety. Lipid oxidation leads to loss of essential FAs. However, apart from bulk oils and fat, even in fish products, when rancidity is sensorily detectable, the LC n-3 PUFA losses are relatively small (Kołakowska 2011).

The western diet contains large quantities of oxidized lipids because a high proportion of the diet is consumed in a fried, heated, processed, or stored form. It is important to what extent lipid oxidation products contained in a diet may contribute to the *in vivo* destructive activity of ROS. The gastrointestinal tract is constantly exposed to dietary oxidized food compounds; after digestion, a part of them are absorbed into the lymph or directly into the bloodstream. Hydroperoxides are generally thought to be decomposed in the stomach from where they are not transported any further. On the other hand, the human gastric fluid may be an excellent medium for enhancing the oxidation of lipids and other dietary constituents. It is possible that, at low doses, FA hydroperoxides are converted to the corresponding hydroxy FA in the mucosal membrane before they are transported to the blood. Gastric mucosa, under stress conditions, exhibits intensification of lipid peroxidation (an increase of MDA and 4-HNE) (Kwiecień et al. 2010).

The secondary products of lipid autoxidation contain cytotoxic and genotoxic compounds; after digestion, a part of them is absorbed into the lymph or directly into the bloodstream and may cause an increase in oxidative stress and deleterious changes in lipoprotein and platelet metabolism. The aldehydes occur in free form or conjugates with amino acids being bioaccessible in the gastrointestinal tract and so are able to reach the systemic circulation. Besides, it was evidenced that during digestion of Maillard products, esterification and oxidation reactions take place (Goicoechea 2011). The absorbable aldehydes form adducts with protein from the diet that are less toxic than free aldehydes. Oxidized cholesterol in the diet was found to be a source of oxidized lipoproteins in the human serum. Some of the dietary advanced lipid oxidation end products, which are absorbed from the gut to the circulatory system, seem to act as injurious chemicals that activate an inflammatory response, which affects not only the circulatory system but also the liver, kidney, lungs, and the gut itself. However, Ottestad et al. (2011) reported that 9 g/day daily intake of highly oxidized cod liver oil (capsules) for 7 weeks does not significantly change the level of circulating oxidation products or affect oxidative stress markers. This can probably be attributed to the specific composition of this oil and the role of LC n-3 PUFAs (Kołakowska et al. 2002).

Protein oxidation's effect on the loss of nutritional value of food by the loss of essential amino acids decreased proteolytic susceptibility and impaired digestibility (Soyer et al. 2010; Estévez 2011). Loss of digestibility was correlated with oxidative parameters of proteins resulting from hydrophobicity change, aggregation, and carbonylation. The analysis of the *in vitro* digestibility of semidry sausages showed no correlation between pepsin activity and protein oxidation; however, a highly significant correlation was observed with trypsin and α-chymotrypsin activity (Sun et al. 2011). The destruction of labile amino acids, such as cysteine and methionine, and their cross-linking of covalent bonds significantly reduces the biological value of protein (Sikorski 2007).

However, the most significant oxidation effect on the loss of nutritional value is a result of the interaction of oxidized components in food (Table 1.1). This applies in particular lipid–protein interactions (Hęś and Korczak 2007; Pokorny et al. 2011; Sikorski 2007). Most covalent bonds formed in the interaction are not hydrolyzed by proteases under the conditions of digestion in human subjects. The 6-amine group of bound lysine is particularly sensitive to interaction with carbonylic oxidation products, such as aldehydes or ketols, and the resulting imine bonds substantially reduce the lysine availability. Other amino acids, such as tyrosine, tryptophan, and methionine, are also partially converted into unavailable products (Pokorny et al. 2011). The interaction preferentially involves most unsaturated FAs. During microwave cooking of fish lipids (oxidized)-albumin, as much as 95% of DHA was covalently bonded. While in systems with fresh and added DHA, respectively, 81% and 75% DHA was bound covalently (Bienkiewicz 2001).

Oxidized lipids also interact with saccharides but generally form weak, reversible complexes. Polyunsaturated FAs, EPA, and DHA, in particular, proved to be most susceptible to binding amylose and amylopectin (Bienkiewicz and Kołakowska 2003, 2004). Up to 90% of the DHA from fish lipids are complexed with amylopectin as a result of homogenization. Compared to fresh fish lipids, those lipids, which were oxidized to a higher extent, were shown to be more amenable to complexing with amylopectin, but they were also more readily released from these complexes (Bienkiewicz and Kołakowska 2003). Thermal treatments, such as heating, microwave cooking, or freezing, exert a significant, differential effect on the fish lipid–starch interaction. This effect depends on the FA profile and degree of oxidation of lipids on the type of starch used.

Saccharide–protein interactions, although of great importance to food quality and shelf life, are not a direct result of oxidation.

TABLE 1.1

Effect of Lipid, Protein, and Carbohydrate Oxidation and the Interaction between Them on the Quality of Food

	Lipid L	Protein P	Interactions (L–P)	Carbohydrate S	Interactions (P–S)
		Undesirable Effects			
Sensory Attributes					
Development of					
Off-odor	LLL	P	(LL–P)	S	(P–S)
Off-flavor	LLL	P	(LL–P)		(P–S)
Discoloration	LLL		(L–P)		(P–SS)
Undesirable texture	L	PPP	(L–PP)		(P–S)
Nutritional Value					
Losses in					
PUFA	L		(L–P)		
Vitamins	LL				
Carotenoids	LL				
Phytosterols	LL				
Other antioxidants	LL	PPP	(L–P)		
Digestibility	L	PPP	(L–PP)		(P–S)
Enzymatic activity		PPP	(L–PP)		(P–S)
Damage of					
Proteins		PPP	(L–PP)		(P–S)
Blocking of essential amino acids		PP	(LL–PP)		(P–S)
Oxidation of amino acids		PPP			
S–S bonding		PPP			
Toxicity					
Generation of					
Radicals	LLL	PP	(L–P)	S	
Peroxides	LLL				
Aldehydes	LLL	PP			
Epoxides	LL				
Oxycholesterols	LL				
Trans FAs	LL				
Maillard-type product			(L–P)	SS	(P–SS)
Technological Suitability					
Decrease in					
Stability of the emulsion	LL	PP	(L–P)		
Protein solubility		PPP	(L–PP)		(P–S)
Protein gel		PPP	(L–PP)		(P–S)

(continued)

TABLE 1.1 (Continued)
Effect of Lipid, Protein, and Carbohydrate Oxidation and the Interaction between Them on the Quality of Food

	Lipid L	Protein P	Interactions (L–P)	Carbohydrate S	Interactions (P–S)
Desirable Effects					
Typical flavors of some vegetables, seafood	LL				
CLA	LL				
Antioxidants			(L–P)		(P–S)
Aroma compounds				SS	(P–S)
Blanching of flour	LL				
Improvement of breadmaking	L	P	(L–P)		(P–S) (L–P–S)
Bactericidal effects of ROS	L	P			

Note: Effects of L, P, S – weak; LL, PP, SS – medium; LLL, PPP, SSS – strong.

Oxidation affects all food components and their interactions. Determination of lipid oxidation and/or protein oxidation products does not sufficiently reflect the status of food oxidation. Similarly, instead of determining the antioxidant activity of individual antioxidants, antioxidant capacity assays are often used, and an overall estimate of the degree of oxidation is provided by the total content (in w.w.) of oxidation products in food (the oxidation index). There is always a very significant negative correlation between the total oxidation index and total antioxidant activity (Kołakowska and Bartosz 2011; Kołakowska 2011). *Antioxidative–oxidative status* (the ratio of total antioxidant activity to total oxidation index) allows us to control development of the oxidation process, taking into account changes in antioxidant activity (synergism, antagonism) during storage and processing of food (Aranowska 2011).

1.10   CONCLUDING REMARKS

Because of the natural presence of ROS in animal and plant raw material and the action of a catalytic factor, despite the presence of antioxidants, spontaneous oxidation reactions likely take place in each food. There are even reports on the harmless benefits of a small degree of food oxidation; however, in general, food oxidative processes are detrimental. The intensity and rate of these reactions are affected by the food composition and the processes to which food is subjected *from the farm to the plate*. Oxidation affects all food components, but their impact on food quality is not uniform. Among the main components, lipid and protein oxidation are the most important destructors of the quality of food. Carbohydrate oxidation does not play a significant role in determining the quality of food under conventional conditions, while the antioxidant properties of saccharides do. Oxidative processes apply to all food components, and the interaction between them affects the course of oxidation. There has also been a radical transfer between the food ingredients. Therefore, *remember that thou goest in the midst of snares, and that thou walkest upon the battlements of the city* (Sirach 9.13).

REFERENCES

Adams, A., Kitryte, V., Venskutonis, R. and De Kimpe, N. 2011. Model studies on the pattern of volatiles generated in mixtures of amino acids, lipid-oxidation derived aldehydes, and glucose. *J Agric Food Chem* 59: 1449–1456.

Aranowska, A. 2011. Effects of fish lipids oxidation on antioxidant activity fish-carrot system. Ph.D. thesis, West Pomeranian University of Technology, Szczecin (in Polish).

Bartosz, G. 2003. *The Other Face of Oxygen*. Polish Scientific Publishers, Warsaw [in Polish].

Bartosz, G. and Kołakowska, A. 2011. Lipid oxidation in food systems. In *Chemical, Biological, and Functional Aspects of Food Lipids,* Z.E. Sikorski, A. Kołakowska (eds), CRC Press, Boca Raton, FL, 163–184.

Benevides, C.M., Veloso, M.C., Pereira, P.A. and Andrade, J.B. 2011. A chemical study of β-carotene oxidation by ozone in an organic model system and the identification of the resulting products. *Food Chem* 126: 927–934.

Bienkiewicz, G. 2001. Influence of fish lipids–protein and fish lipids–starch interaction on extractability of lipids and content of n-3 polyunsaturated fatty acids, Ph.D. thesis, University of Agriculture Szczecin [In Polish].

Bienkiewicz, G. and Kołakowska, A. 2003. Effects of lipid oxidation on fish lipids–amylopectin interactions. *Eur J Lipid Sci Technol* 105: 410–418.

Bienkiewicz, G. and Kołakowska, A. 2004. Effects of thermal treatment on fish lipids–amylose interaction. *Eur J Lipid Sci Technol* 106: 376–381.

Błaszczak, W., Bidzińska, E., Dyrek, K., Fornal, J. and Wenda, E. 2008. Effect of high hydrostatic pressure on the formation of radicals in maize starches with different amylose content. *Carbohydr Polym* 74: 914–921.

Błaszczak, W., Bidzińska, E., Dyrek, K., Fornal, J. and Wenda, E. 2010. EPR study of the influence of high hydrostatic pressure on the formation of radicals in phosphorylated potato starch. *Carbohydr Polym* 82: 1256–1263.

Braconi, D., Bernardini, G. and Santucci, A. 2011. Linking protein oxidation to environmental pollutants: Redox proteomic approaches. *J Proteom* 74: 2324–2337.

Breyer, V., and Pischetsrieder, M. 2009. Influence of oxidative stress on the formation of advanced glycation end-products. *Congress on Free Radical Biology and Medicine,* Society for Free Radical Biology and Medicine (SFRBM) 16th Annual Meeting, 18–22 November 2009, San Francisco. Abstracts S118, 307.

Cerchiaro, G., Micke, G.A., Tavares, M.F.M. and Ferreira, A.-M. 2004. Kinetic studies of carbohydrate oxidation catalyzed by novel isatin–Schiff base copper(II) complexes. *J Mol Catalysis A: Chem* 221: 29–39.

Chaudhuri, A., Waal, E., Mele, J. and Richardson, A. 2002. Oxidative stress, protein oxidation and unfolding: A novel disulfide detection assay. In *Oxidation of Macromolecules, DNA, Lipid, Proteins, Carbohydrate*, 97th Annual Meeting of the Oxygen Society, November 20–24, 2002, Abstracts, S385, 249.

Collin, F., Hindo, J., Thérond, P., Couturier, M., Cosson, C., Jore, D. and Gardès-Albert, M. 2010. Experimental evidence of the reciprocal oxidation of bovine serum albumin and linoleate in aqueous solution, initiated by HO˙ free radicals. *Biochimie* 92: 1130–1137.

Cucu, T., Devreese, B., Mestdagh, F., Kerkaert, B. and De Meulenaer, B. 2011. Protein–lipid interactions during the incubation of whey proteins with autoxidizing lipids. *Int Dairy J* 21: 427–433.

Davies, M.J. 2005. The oxidative environment and protein damage. *Biochim Biophys Acta* 1703: 93–109.

Decker, E.A., Alamed, J. and Castro, I.A. 2010. Interaction between polar components and the degree of unsaturation of fatty acids on the oxidative stability of emulsions. *J Am Oil Chem Soc* 87: 771–780.

Estévez, M. 2011. Protein carbonyls in meat systems: A review. *Meat Sci* 89: 259–279.

Eymard, S., Baron, C.P. and Jacobsen, C. 2009. Oxidation of lipid and protein in horse mackerel (*Trachurus trachurus*) mince and washed minces during processing and storage. *Food Chem* 114: 57–65.

Faustman, C., Sun, Q., Mancini, R. and Suman, S.P. 2010. Myoglobin and lipid oxidation interactions: Mechanistic bases and control. *Meat Sci* 86: 86–94.

Feng, T., Du, Y., Li, J., Hu, Y. and Kennedy, J.F. 2008. Enhancement of antioxidant activity of chitosan by irradiation. *Carbohydr Polym* 73: 126–132.

Friguet, B. 2006. Oxidized protein degradation and repair in ageing and oxidative stress. *FEBS Lett* 580: 2910–2916.

Fu, X., Xu, S. and Wang, Z. 2009. Kinetics of lipid oxidation and off-odor formation in silver carp mince: The effect of lipoxygenase and hemoglobin. *Food Res Int* 42: 85–90.

Goicoechea, E., Brandon, E.F.A., Blokland, M.H. and Guillén, M.D. 2011. Fate in digestion *in vitro* of several food components, including some toxic compounds coming from omega-3 and omega-6 lipids. *Food Chem Toxicol* 49: 115–124.

Goodman, B.A., Pascual, E.C. and Yeretzian, C. 2011. Real time monitoring of free radical processes during the roasting of coffee beans using electron paramagnetic resonance spectroscopy. *Food Chem* 125: 248–254.

Gracanin, M., Lam, M.A., Morgan, P.E., Rodgers, K.J., Hawkins, C.L. and Davies, M.J. 2010. Amino acid, peptide, and protein hydroperoxides and their decomposition products modify the activity of the 26S proteasome. *Free Radic Biol Med* 15: 389–399.

Grosicka-Maciąg, E. 2011. Biological consequences of oxidative stress induced by pesticides. *Post Hig Med Dośw* 65: 357–366.

Guan, J.-J., Zhang, T.-B., Hui, M., Yin, H.-Ch., Qiu, A.-Y. and Liu X.-Y. 2011. Mechanism of microwave-accelerated soy protein isolate–saccharide graft reactions. *Food Res Int* 44: 2647–2654.

Hęś, M. and Korczak, J. 2007. Wpływ produktów utleniania lipidów na wartość odżywczą białka. *Nauka Przyr Technol* 1: 1–14.

Höhn, A., Jung, T., Grimm, S., Catalgol, B., Weber, D. and Grune, T. 2011. Lipofuscin inhibits the proteasome by binding to surface motifs. *Free Radic Biol Med* 50: 585–591.

Jehle, D., Lund, M.N., Ogendal, L.H. and Andersen, M.L. 2011. Characterisation of a stable radical from dark roasted malt in wort and beer. *Food Chem* 125: 380–387.

Kanner, J. 2007. Dietary advanced lipid oxidation end products are risk factors to human health. *Mol Nutr Food Res* 51: 1094–1101. Special Issue: Are Dietary AGEs/ALEs a Health Risk?

Kołakowska, A. 2011. Fish lipids. In *Chemical, Biological, and Functional Aspects of Food Lipids,* Z.E. Sikorski, A. Kołakowska (eds). CRC Press, Boca Raton, FL, 273–312.

Kołakowska, A. and Bartosz, G. 2011. Antioxidants. In *Chemical, Biological, and Functional Aspects of Food Lipids*, Z.E. Sikorski, A. Kołakowska (eds). CRC Press, Boca Raton, FL, 185–210.

Kołakowska, A. and Łomaszewska, S. 2006. The effect of cooking method on carotenoids in trout. In *Effect of Freshness on Loss of Nutritional Value of Proteins and Lipids During Thermal Processing of Trout.* Rep. Project 3PO6T 060 25. West Pomeranian University of Technology, Szczecin, pp. 116–119 [In Polish].

Kołakowska, A., Stypko, K., Bienkiewicz, G., Domiszewski, Z., Perkowska, A. and Witczak, A. 2002. Canned cod liver as a source of n-3 polyunsaturated fatty acids, with a reference to contamination. *Nahrung/Food* 46: 40–45.

Kwiecień, S., Pawlik, M.W., Brzozowski, T., Pawlik, W.W. and Konturek, S.J. 2010. Reactive oxygen metabolite action in experimental, stress model of gastric mucosa damage. *Gastroenterol Pol* 17: 2342–2343.

Łabanowska, M., Bidzińska, E., Pietrzyk, S., Juszczak, L., Fortuna, T. and Błoniarczyk, K. 2011. Influence of copper catalyst on the mechanism of carbohydrate radicals generation in oxidized potato starch. *Carbohydr Polym* 85: 775–785.

Long, E.K. and Picklo, M.J., Sr. 2010. Trans-4-hydroxy-2-hexenal, a product of n-3 fatty acid peroxidation: Make some room HNE. *Free Radic Biol Med* 49: 1–8.

Luo, G., Qi, D., Zheng, Y., Mu, Y., Yan, G., Yang, T. and Shen, J.-C. 2001. ESR studies on reaction of saccharide with the free radicals generated from the xanthine oxidase/hypoxanthine system containing iron. *FEBS Lett* 492: 29–32.

Lyutova, Z.B. and Yudin, I.V. 2006. Reaction pathways of the formation of molecular products upon dissolution of gamma-irradiated lactose crystals. *High Energy Chem* 40: 206–211.

Mestdagh, F., Kerkaert, B., Cucu, T. and De Meulenaer, B. 2011. Interaction between whey proteins and lipids during light-induced oxidation. *Food Chem* 126: 1190–1197.

Min, D.B. and Boff, J.M. 2002. Chemistry and reaction of singlet oxygen in foods. *Comp Rev Food Sci Food Safety* 1: 58–72.

Min, B., Nam, K.C. and Ahn, D.U. 2010. Catalytic mechanisms of metmyoglobin on the oxidation of lipids in phospholipid liposome model system. *Food Chem* 123: 231–236.

Mosca, M., Ceglie, A. and Ambrosone, L. 2011. Effect of membrane composition on lipid oxidation in liposomes. *Chem Phys Lipids* 164: 158–165.

Nguyen, H.T.T., Parkanyiova, L., Miyahara, M., Uematsu, T., Sakurai, H. and Pokorny, J. 2002. Interactions between phospholipids in non-enzymic browning reactions. *Int Congress Series* 1245: 443–444.

Nogala-Kałucka, M. 2011. Lipophilic vitamins. In *Chemical, Biological, and Functional Aspects of Food Lipids*, Z.E. Sikorski, A. Kołakowska (eds). CRC Press, Boca Raton, FL, 135–162.

Otaegui-Arrazola, A., Menendez-Carreno, M., Ansorena, D. and Astiasaran, I. 2010. Oxysterols: A world to explore. *Food Chem Toxicol* 48: 3289–3303.

Ottestad, I., Vogt, G., Myhrstad, M., Retterstřl, K., Nilsson, A., Haugen, J.-E., Ravn-Haren, G., Brřnner, K.W., Andersen, L.F., Holven, K. and Ulven, S. 2011. Health effects of oxidized cod liver oil in healthy subjects: A randomized controlled trial. *Atheroscler Suppls* 12: 13–184.

Pokorny, J. and Schmidt, S. 2011. Plant lipids and oils. In *Chemical, Biological, and Functional Aspects of Food Lipids,* Z.E. Sikorski, A. Kołakowska (eds). CRC Press, Boca Raton, FL, 249–272.

Pokorny, J., Kołakowska, A. and Bienkiewicz, G. 2011. Lipid-protein and lipid-saccharide interactions. In *Chemical, Biological, and Functional Aspects of Food Lipids,* Z.E. Sikorski, A. Kołakowska (eds). CRC Press, Boca Raton, FL, 455–472.

Raitio, R., Orlien, V. and Skibsted, L.H. 2011. Free radical interactions between raw materials in dry soup powder. *Food Chem* 129: 951–956.

Redouan, E., Petit, E., Pillon, M., Courtois, B., Courtois, J. and Delattre, C. 2011. Evaluation of antioxidant capacity of ulvan-like polymer obtained by regioselective oxidation of gellan exopolysaccharide. *Food Chem* 127: 976–983.

Sakai, T., Munasinghe, D.M.S., Kashimura, M., Sugamoto, K. and Kawahara, S. 2004. Effect of NaCl on lipid peroxidation-derived aldehyde, 4-hydroxy-2-nonenal formation in minced pork and beef. *Meat Sci* 66: 789–792.

Sanz, A., Gomez, J., Caro, P. and Baria, G. 2006. Carbohydrate restriction does not change mitochondrial free radical generation and oxidative DNA damage. *J Bioenerg Biomembr* 38: 327–333.

Schaich, K.M. 2008. *Lipid Oxidation Pathways.* Volume 2. AOCS Press, Champaign, IL: 183–274.

Sikorski, Z.E. 2007. Proteins-structure and properties. In *Food Chemistry* V.2, Z.E. Sikorski (ed). WNT, (Scientific and Technical Publisher) Warszawa, pp. 167–201 [in Polish].

Sirach 9.13 The Bible, Old Testament, wisdom of Sirach.

Soyer, A. and Hultin, H.O. 2000. Kinetics of oxidation of the lipids and proteins of cod sarcoplasmic reticulum. *J Agr Food Chem* 48: 2127–2134.

Soyer, A., Ozalp, B., Dalmıs, U. and Bilgin, V. 2010. Effects of freezing temperature and duration of frozen storage on lipid and protein oxidation in chicken meat. *Food Chem* 120: 1025–1030.

Sun, W., Cui, C., Zhao, M., Zhao, Q. and Yang, B. 2011. Effects of composition and oxidation of proteins on their solubility, aggregation and proteolytic susceptibility during processing of Cantonese sausage. *Food Chem* 124: 336–341.

Traverso, N., Balbis, E., Sukkar, S.G., Furfaro, A., Sacchi-Nemours, A.M., Ferrari, C., Patriarca, S. and Cottalasso, D. 2010. Oxidative stress in the animal model: The possible protective role of milk serum protein. *Mediterr J Nutr Metab* 3: 173–178.

Valko, M., Rhodes, C.J., Moncol, J., Izakovic, M. and Mazur, M. 2006. Free radicals, metals and oxidants in oxidative stress-induced cancer. Mini-review. *Chem Biol Int* 160: 1–40.

Waraho, T.D., McClements, J. and Decker, E.A. 2011. Mechanisms of lipid oxidation in food dispersions. *Trends Food Sci Technol* 22: 3–13.

Wąsowicz, E. and Rudzińska, M. 2011. Cholesterol and phytosterols. In *Chemical, Biological, and Functional Aspects of Food Lipids,* Z.E. Sikorski, A. Kołakowska (eds). CRC Press, Boca Raton, FL, 113–134.

Yamaoki, R., Kimura, S. and Ohta, M. 2011. Electron spin resonance characterization of radical components in irradiated black pepper skin and core. *Radiat Phys Chem* 80: 1282–1288.

Yang, S., Guo, Z., Miao, F., Xue, Q. and Qin, S. 2010. The hydroxyl radical scavenging activity of chitosan, hyaluronan, starch and their *O*-carboxymethylated derivatives. *Carbohydr Polym* 82: 1043–1045.

Zanardi, E., Battaglia, A., Ghidini, S., Conter, M., Badiani, A., Ianieri, A. 2009. Lipid oxidation of irradiated pork products, *LWT - Food Sci Technol* 42: 1301–1307.

Zhang, Z., Wang, X., Zhang, J. and Zhao, M. 2011. Potential antioxidant activities *in vitro* of polysaccharides extracted from ginger (*Zingiber officinale*). *Carbohydr Polym* 86: 448–452.

2 Oxidants Occurring in Food Systems

Manuel Pazos and Isabel Medina

CONTENTS

2.1 INTRODUCTION

Important food components such as unsaturated lipids, proteins, and vitamins are very prone to undergoing oxidative deterioration during processing and storage. Although several of these food constituents suffer important autoxidative reactions under certain conditions, in most foods, the rate and extent of oxidation are highly conditioned by the concentration and activity of oxidizing agents, which can be natural components of foods, food additives, and even substances generated during processing or storage. Food oxidation regularly causes a decrease in consumer acceptance, but in some cases, oxidative reactions of specific food components lead to an improvement in the product quality. An example is the enzymatic oxidation of polyunsaturated fatty acids (PUFAs) by lipoxygenases (LOXs) that is responsible for the fresh aromas in fish and vegetables or the oxidation developed during the ripening of several appreciated salted fish products that are related with the characteristic organoleptic properties of these foods (Andersen, Andersen and Baron 2007). On the contrary, the activity of oxidants, such as redox active metals and hemoproteins, on PUFA generates rancid off-flavors and diminishes nutritive value during processing and storage. This oxidative deterioration of PUFA dramatically restricts shelf life and consumer acceptance in a large variety of foodstuffs, such as meat, fish, milk products, and new functional products enriched in PUFA n-3. Therefore, the identification of the

TABLE 2.1
Principal Oxidants Occurring in Foods

Chemical Oxidants	Enzymatic Oxidants
Redox active metal (Fe, Cu)	LOX
Hemoproteins (hemoglobin, myoglobin)	MPO and LPOs
Singlet-oxygen sensitizers (riboflavin, porphyrins, and chlorophylls)	Catalase
Phenolics and reductants	PPOs

Note: LOX, lipooxygenases; MPO, myeloperoxidases; PPOs, polyphenol oxidase.

principal oxidants occurring in foods is essential to understanding the oxidative reactions suffered by food components and their implication on food quality.

Catalysts of oxidation in foods include both enzymatic and nonenzymatic compounds (Table 2.1). Most of these compounds exert vital functions for life in redox-balanced living organisms; however, foodstuffs exhaust their endogenous antioxidant defense systems during processing and storage, and in these conditions of impaired redox balance, the above substances are extremely reactive, promoting oxidation of lipids, proteins, and vitamins. The main aspects of their occurrence—pathways of oxidative action, influence of technological processing and storage on concentration and activity, and redox interactions with other food constituents—will be addressed in the following sections.

2.2   NONENZYMATIC OXIDANTS

2.2.1   REDOX-ACTIVE METALS

The transition metals iron and copper are endowed with a labile d-electron system able to catalyze oxidative modifications in foods. The most common redox state for iron, the ferric ion, exhibits a reduced solubility at pH values near neutrality. For this reason, iron ions exist in food systems chelated to other compounds to form soluble low-molecular-weight (LMW) complexes. Inorganic phosphates, nucleotides [Adenosine triphosphate (ATP); Adenosine diphosphate (ADP); Adenosine monophosphate (AMP)], peptides (carnosine), amino acids (glycine, histidine), and carboxylic acids (citric acid, oxalic acid, pyruvic acid) are potential iron-chelating agents in foods (St. Angelo 1992). Metal chelation may alter the catalytic activity of oxidation by changing metal accessibility and/or its redox potential (Table 2.1). In general, chelators that coordinate Fe(II) via oxygen ligands promote the oxidation of Fe(II), whereas the oxidation of ligated Fe(II) is retarded by chelators with nitrogen ligands (Welch, Davis, and Aust 2002). The capacity of iron complexed to nucleotides, citrate, or pyrophosphate to stimulate oxidation has been reported (Rush, Maskos, and Koppenol 1990; Rush and Koppenol 1990; Soyer and Hultin 2000; Pazos et al. 2006). Carnosine, an endogenous β-alanyl-histidine dipeptide in meat, has been suggested as an important inhibitor for iron-mediated oxidation via metal chelation, although the antioxidant mechanism of carnosine seems also to be a result of free radical scavenging (Chan et al. 1994; Decker and Faraji 1990).

LMW-iron concentrations vary depending on the food system, processing conditions, and even on the species and type of muscle tissue. Levels of LMW iron are initially low, being only 2.4%–3.9% of total muscle iron in beef, lamb, pork, and chicken (Hazell 1982). The analysis of light and dark muscles from mackerel indicated that about 7%–10% of the iron and 7%–38% of the copper are associated with fractions with molecular weights lower than 10 kDa (Decker and Hultin 1990). In general, the total content of LMW Fe is notably higher in dark muscle than in light muscle. The dark muscle from mackerel has approximately fivefold more LMW Fe than the light muscle (Decker and Hultin 1990). The distribution of redox-active metals in foods is modified during storage and processing as a result of the release from metal-containing proteins. The delivery of iron from the heme pocket of hemoglobin (Hb) and myoglobin (Mb) is a principal source of LMW Fe in processed and/or stored muscle-based foods. There is evidence of the increment in the levels of LMW Fe during the chilled storage of chicken, turkey, and fish muscle (Decker and Hultin 1990; Kanner, Hazan, and Doll 1988). The reduction of the levels of heme iron and the parallel increase in the non-heme iron content are noticeable in the fish muscle from tilapia and sea bass stored under refrigeration (Thiansilakul, Benjakul, and Richards 2010). Previous freeze–thawing processes enhance the accumulation of free iron and copper in refrigerated fish muscle (Decker and Hultin 1990). Cooking and other thermal treatments are able to increase the concentration of non-heme iron in beef, lamb, and chicken (Purchas et al. 2003; Min et al. 2008). Heating decreased heme iron, and the severity of the losses can be controlled by using milder processing conditions that do not weaken the anchorage of the heme group to the protein (Lombardi-Boccia, Martinez-Dominguez, and Aguzzi 2002).

Food fortification to prevent iron-deficiency anemia in at-risk populations can be an additional source of LMW Fe (Theuer 2008). To avoid unacceptable taste, color, and stability derived from the fortification, iron is stabilized by applying principles of colloid chemistry (encapsulation), chelation, antioxidant compounds, and electrochemical chemistry (redox modulation) (Mehansho 2006).

The progress of lipid oxidation may also change the proportion of LMW Fe. The interaction of Hb with lipid hydroperoxides, primary lipid oxidation products, or trans-2-pentenal, an aldehyde product of the decomposition of lipid hydroperoxides, triggers the liberation of hemin (an oxidized form of the heme group) from the hemoprotein (Maestre, Pazos, and Medina 2009). The capacity of lipid hydroperoxides and trans-2-pentenal to promote the loss of the heme group from Hb may be ascribed to their ability to accelerate the oxidation of hemoproteins to met- forms (Maestre, Pazos, and Medina 2009). Methemoglobin (MetHb) is endowed with a higher propensity to release the heme group than the reduced oxyHb species (Hargrove, Wilkinson, and Olson 1996; Maestre, Pazos, and Medina 2009). The electrophilic character of unsaturated aldehydes favors the establishment of covalent bonds with the amine groups of amino acids through a nucleophile/electrophile mechanism. The analysis of Mb adducts with 4-hydroxy-2-nonenal (HNE), an unsaturated aldehyde generated by lipid peroxidation, indicates that HNE establishes covalent bonds with the proximal (HIS 93) and distal (HIS 64) histidine associated with the heme group (Alderton et al. 2003). This hemoglobin–aldehyde interaction destabilizes the linkage heme–protein favoring the loss of hemin. The free heme group out of the protein globin core is notably made unstable by reaction with free radicals, resulting in the oxidative cleavage of the porphyrin ring and the liberation of ferric ion (Pazos, Andersen, and Skibsted 2008). Figure 2.1 illustrates the fast degradation of free hemin in the presence a cumene hydroperoxide, a source of free radicals by interaction by hemin.

In addition to the concentration, the redox state of metals is crucial for the oxidative stability of foods. The most common redox state for iron, the oxidized ferric [Fe(III)] ion, is significantly less prooxidant than the reduced ferrous [Fe(II)] state. However, several enzymatic and nonenzymatic food components or additives may convert the ferric iron to the more oxidizing ferrous form: enzymatic iron-reductase systems, ascorbic acid, glutathione, and phenolic compounds (Pierre and Fontecave 1999; Soyer and Hultin 2000; Petrat et al. 2003; Gülçin 2006). The reduction of the ferric to the ferrous state is the driving force for the catalysis of oxidation by iron, being thermodynamically possible for reductants whose one-electron reduction potential is lower than that of ferric iron. The redox potential of the Fe(III)/Fe(II) transition depends strongly on the chelating agent and pH. Iron coverts a wide physiological range of redox potentials, from approximately −0.5 to 0.6 V, depending on the ligand complexed to the metal (Table 2.2). Moreover, the reducing potential of the Fe(III)/Fe(II) pair is extremely pH-dependent. Acidic pH values favor the reduction of ferric because the transition to ferrous occurs at the standard redox potential of +0.77 V, whereas at pH 7.0, the transition redox potential is between +0.1 and +0.2 V. Accordingly, the reduction rate of ferric to ferrous iron by reducing agents increases noticeably as the pH decreases, and the prooxidative effect of phenolic

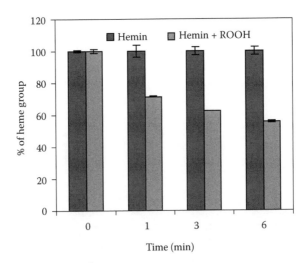

FIGURE 2.1 Effect of hydroperoxides, primary lipid oxidation products, on stability of free hemin: Hemin (40 μM) was incubated in presence or absence of 2000 μM cumene hydroperoxide (CumOOH), which was used as a model for lipid hydroperoxide. Hemin stability was monitored as absorbance at 390 nm, wavelength at which hemin is endowed of maximum absorption.

TABLE 2.2

Standard One-Electron Reduction Potential of Interest to Predict the Course of the Fe(III)/Fe(II) Transition by Interacting with Common Reducing Food Components

	Reduction Potential $(E°'; V)$[a]	Reference
Fe(III)-citrate/Fe(II)-citrate	0.6	Pierre, Fontecave, and Crichton 2002
Fe(III)$_{(aq)}$/Fe(II)$_{(aq)}$	0.1–0.2	Buettner 1993
Fe(III)-EDTA/Fe(II)-EDTA	0.12	Buettner 1993
Fe(III)-ADP/ Fe(II)-ADP	0.1	Buettner 1993
Fe(III)-transferrine/Fe(II)-transferrine	−0.4	Pierre, Fontecave, and Crichton 2002
Semiubiquinone·/ubiquinol	0.2	Buettner 1993
Ascorbate·/Ascorbate	0.28	Buettner 1993
EGCG·/EGCG	0.43	Jovanovic et al. 1995
α-Tocopheryl·/α-tocopherol	0.48	Buettner 1993
Caffeyl·/caffeic acid	0.54	Laranjinha et al. 1995
Catechin·/Catechin	0.57	Jovanovic et al. 1995

[a] Reduction potentials at pH 7.0 (vs. NHE).

antioxidants in the presence of iron is especially relevant in mayonnaises and other food systems marked by acid pH (pH < 5) (Hsieh and Hsieh 1997). Caffeic acid has demonstrated prooxidant activity in oil-in-water emulsion at pH 3.0 and pH 6.0, whereas the phenolics with higher reduction potential than caffeic acid and, therefore, with lower reducing power, as naringenin, rutin, and coumaric acid, exhibit a prooxidative capacity only at pH 3.0 (Sorensen et al. 2008). Ascorbic acid is also known for its high efficiency for Fe(III) reduction at both neutral and acidic pH values. At acid pH (pH 2.6), 2 mol of Fe(III) are reduced by 1 mol of ascorbic acid (Hsieh and Hsieh 1997). The reduction rate of Fe(III) by ascorbic acid decreases as the pH value increases (Hsieh and Hsieh 1997), but still at pH near neutrality (pH 7.4), ascorbic acid has a strong capacity to reduce Fe(III)–ATP complexes to the Fe(II) state (Petrat et al. 2003). The supplementation of ethylenediaminetetraacetic acid (EDTA), a chelating agent generally used as a food additive, prevents Fe(III) from being reduced by ascorbic acid at pH 2.6–6.0 (Hsieh and Hsieh 1997). In turkey muscle, ascorbic acid is recognized to be the main reductant that affects the iron redox cycle because the destruction of ascorbic acid totally inhibits lipid oxidation (Kanner 1994). Table 2.3 collects some of the food systems or food model systems in which the ascorbic acid combined with traces of iron causes oxidation of important food components, for example, lipids, proteins, α-tocopherol, or ubiquinol.

Iron-reducing enzymatic systems are also a relevant font of the reactive ferrous ions in meat-based foods not subjected to thermal treatments. Cellular membranes of

TABLE 2.3
Oxidative Targets of LMW Fe and LMW Cu in Food Systems

Food System or Food Model System	Oxidizing System	Oxidative Target	Reference
Pork mitochondrial system	Fe(III)/ascorbic	Lipid, α-tocopherol, and ubiquinol	Tang et al. 2005
Pork myofibrillar proteins	Fe(III)-ascorbate	Protein	Xiong et al. 2010
Pork myofibrillar proteins	Fe(III) and Cu(II) combined with H_2O_2	Protein	Estévez and Heinonen 2010
Fish muscle membranes	Fe(III)/ADP/ascorbate Fe(III)-ADP/NADH	Lipid and protein	Soyer and Hultin 2000
Fish muscle membranes	Fe(III)-ADP/ascorbate Fe(III)-ADP/NADH	Lipid	Pazos et al. 2006
Fish myofibrillar and sarcoplasmic proteins	Fe(II)/ascorbate	Protein	Pazos et al. 2011
Whey-based and casein-based infant formulas	Fe(II)	Lipid	Satue-Gracia et al. 2000
Emulsion containing linoleic acid	Fe(II)	Lipid	Sugiarto et al. 2010
Water–oil mixtures	Cu(II)	Lipid	Alexa et al. 2011
Oil-in-water emulsions	Fe(II), Fe(II)-EDTA, Fe-lactoglobulin (beta), Fe(II)-caseinate	Lipid	Guzun-Cojocaru et al. 2011

muscle foods contain NAD(P)H-dependent enzymatic systems with the capacity to transfer one electron to convert ferric to ferrous iron, such as ferredoxin, thioredoxin, and cytochrome P450 (Petrat et al. 2003). It is also relevant that these enzymatic reducing systems of membranes generate the oxidizing ferrous iron in an environment fundamentally consisting of highly unsaturated lipids, an essential oxidative substrate in foods. In the presence of iron, the iron-reducing systems of fish sarcoplasmic reticulum and microsomes, small particles consisting of fragments of ribosomes and endoplasmic reticulum obtained by sedimentation at ultracentrifugation, exert an important activity promoting oxidation of both lipids and proteins (Table 2.3). Comparing the oxidative efficiency with nonenzymatic iron-reducing systems, the iron-reducing system from fish sarcoplasmic reticulum has shown a lower ability than the ascorbate–iron system to promote the oxidation of lipids and proteins (Soyer and Hultin 2000). A similar tendency has been observed by studying the iron-reducing enzymes contained in fish microsomes, causing the ascorbate–iron system a faster lipid oxidation system compared to those enzymatic complexes (Figure 2.2).

The oxidative behavior of ferrous ions is in part attributable to their peroxidase activity to decompose hydroperoxides generating reactive peroxyl (ROO•), alkoxyl (RO•), and alkyl (R•) free radicals. Ferrous iron is 14 times more active than ferric iron in producing free radicals by decomposition of lipid hydroperoxides, but free iron ions are significantly less effective than heme proteins (O'Brien 1969).

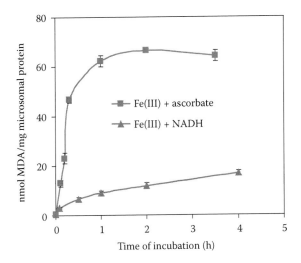

FIGURE 2.2 Activity of enzymatic iron [NADH-Fe(III)] and nonenzymatic iron [ascorbate-Fe(III)] in promoting lipid oxidation in fish microsomes. Fish microsomes were suspended in 0.12 M potassium chloride and 5 mM histidine (pH 6.8) to final concentration of 0.7 mg/mL. The membranes oxidized by enzymatic iron contained 20 μM Fe(III), 100 μM ADP, and 100 μM NADH, and NADH was substituted by 100 μM ascorbate in membranes oxidized by nonenzymatic iron. Lipid oxidation was monitored by the formation of aldehydes, secondary lipid oxidation products, by means of the thiobarbituric acid (TBA) reaction with aldehydes, using malondialdehyde (MDA) as standard.

Ferrous ions also have the capacity to generate the extremely powerful oxidizing hydroxyl radical (HO·) through the reaction with hydrogen peroxide via a Fenton-type mechanism:

$$Fe(II) + H_2O_2 \rightarrow Fe(III) + HO^{\bullet} + {}^-OH$$

The elevated oxidizing power of the hydroxyl radical is a consequence of its extremely high standard reduction potential ($E^{\circ\prime}HO^{\bullet}/H_2O = 2.31$ V) that makes it competent to steal one electron (or hydrogen atom) from compounds whose reduction potentials are lower, which are mostly lipids, proteins, and vitamins (Buettner 1993). The lower reduction potentials of allylic ($E^{\circ\prime}$ allylic$^{\bullet}$/allylic $-$ H $= 0.96$ V) and *bis*-allylic ($E^{\circ\prime}bis$-allylic$^{\bullet}$/*bis*-allylic $-$ H $= 0.6$ V) imply the capacity of a hydroxyl radical to initiate the oxidation of monounsaturated fatty acids (MUFAs) and PUFAs. Even though a hydroxyl radical is a very powerful oxidizing species with the ability to oxidize whichever of the 20 essential amino acids, it shows some selectivity in its reaction. The highest reaction rate of a hydroxyl radical is achieved by cysteine (3.4×10^{10} dm^3 mol^{-1} s^{-1}) and the aromatic amino acids tryptophan, histidine, and tyrosine (1.3×10^{10} dm^3 mol^{-1} s^{-1}), but it also provokes the fast oxidation of arginine, methionine, and phenylalanine [$(3.5–8.3) \times 10^9$ dm^3 mol^{-1} s^{-1}] (Davies and Dean 1997).

2.2.2 HEMOPROTEINS

The hemoproteins, hemoglobin (Hb) and myoglobin (Mb), have a decisive contribution to the oxidative degradation of muscle foods as a result of their elevated content in muscle tissues and their behavior as oxidizing agents. Table 2.4 reports some of the food systems or food model systems in which hemoproteins promote oxidation of important food components. Hb is a tetramer composed of four globin chains containing one heme group inside each polypeptide chain. Mb consists of a globin chain along with a porphyrin heme group (Shikama 1998). *In vivo* and during the early postmortem stages, hemoproteins are typically present in the ferrous state either with molecular bound oxygen (oxygenated state) or without bound oxygen (deoxygenated state). Hemoproteins undergo oxidation to a ferric state, also called the met-form, in muscle subjected to processing and long-term storage. The oxidized forms methemoglobin (metHb) and metmyoglobin (metMb) are unable to bind molecular oxygen, which gives a less compact structure of these proteins compared to that of their reduced ferrous forms.

The relative level of hemoproteins depends on the type of muscle and species. Pork and beef generally contain more Mb than Hb (Trout and Gutzke 1996), and Hb is the hemoprotein more abundant in chicken and some fish species (Kranen et al. 1999; Richards and Hultin 2002). Hb is the principal hemoprotein in mackerel light muscle (6 μmol Hb/kg muscle) and whole trout muscle (11 μmol Hb/kg). However, Mb is predominant in mackerel dark muscle, representing 65% of hemoproteins on a molar basis, although the tetrameric Hb supplies more heme units than monomeric Mb (*10*). Tuna also contains a higher proportion of Mb compared to Hb (Brown 1962; Sannier et al. 1996). Reddish-flesh fish as pelagic species have

TABLE 2.4
Oxidative Targets of Hb/Mb in Food Systems

Food System or Food Model System	Oxidizing System	Oxidative Target	Reference
Pork myofibrillar proteins	MetMb/H_2O_2	Protein	Xiong et al. 2010
Pork muscle membranes	Bovine oxyMb and metMb	Lipid	Bou et al. 2008; Bou et al. 2010
Pork myofibrillar proteins	Equine Mb/H_2O_2	Protein	Estévez and Heinonen 2010
Pork mitochondrial system	Equine oxyMb	Lipid, α-tocopherol, and ubiquinol	Tang et al. 2005
Isolated porcine myosin	Horse heart metMb/H_2O_2	Myosin	Frederiksen et al. 2008
Washed fish muscle	Fish Hb	Lipid	Richards and Hultin 2002
Washed fish muscle	Fish Hb	Lipid, protein and α-tocopherol	Larsson and Undeland 2010

more elevated Hb concentrations (3–12 µmol Hb/kg) than lean fish species, such as Atlantic cod (0.03–0.23 µmol Hb/kg) (Richards and Hultin 2002; Larsson, Almgren, and Undeland 2007; Maestre, Pazos, and Medina 2011). There is a direct dependence between Hb concentration and the ability to promote oxidation within the typical Hb concentrations found in muscle foods (Richards and Hultin 2002; Pazos, Medina, and Hultin 2005). Therefore, higher amounts of Hb cause a more rapid and extensive propagation of lipid oxidation. This observation can partially explain the poor oxidative stability of pelagic fish muscle during processing and storage and its underutilization to human food purposes compared to lean fish species. Experiments performed in a model system composed of washed muscle free of hemoproteins reveal the strong aptitude of the concentrations typically found in pelagic fish (3–12 µmol Hb/kg muscle) to activate lipid oxidation (Richards and Hultin 2002). The results also draw attention to the oxidizing activity of Hb concentrations as low as 0.06 µmol/kg of muscle.

On the other hand, the concentration is not the unique parameter relevant for understanding the oxidative action of hemoproteins. Hemoproteins have differential oxidizing power depending on the species considered but also on extrinsic factors, such as pH and thermal processing. The capacity of Hb from terrestrial animals, such as beef and chicken, in activating lipid oxidation is lower compared to that of fish species (Richards, Modra, and Li 2002; Richards and Dettman 2003; Aranda et al. 2009). Important differences are even found in the oxidizing ability of Hbs from different fish species. Pollock Hb is more effective than horse mackerel Hb in activating lipid oxidation, and both are less active than sea bass Hb (Maestre, Pazos, and Medina 2009). Other studies show the higher catalytic activity promoting lipid oxidation for pollock Hb followed, in decreasing order, by mackerel > menhaden > flounder (Undeland, Kristinsson, and Hultin 2004). Hb from mackerel and herring oxidizes fish muscle more rapidly as compared to trout Hb, whereas the latter is more oxidant than tilapia Hb, a warm-water fish species (Richards and Hultin 2003; Richards et al. 2007). The diversity of the prooxidative capacity of hemoproteins from different species has been related to two intrinsic factors of hemoproteins: (1) the redox instability to be converted to the ferric met- form and (2) the susceptibility to produce hemin. Hemin is the term used to describe the porphyrin ring coordinated to one ferric atom, and heme indicates the porphyrin ring with iron in the ferrous state. The ferric methemoglobin (metHb) and metmyoglobin (metMb) are formed spontaneously through the autoxidation of the corresponding reduced species, but their generation is accelerated in the presence of lipid oxidation products, such as hydroperoxides and aldehydes (Maestre, Pazos, and Medina 2009). Several lines of evidence indicate a straight correlation between the oxidizing activity of Hb and its vulnerability to be converted to metHb either spontaneously or when forced by the interaction with lipid oxidation products. Hbs with the most pronounced oxidizing activities are those that rapidly form metHb (Undeland, Kristinsson, and Hultin 2004; Pazos, Andersen, and Skibsted 2009). This observation is consistent with the stronger facility of metHb to promote oxidation in comparison to the reduced Hb form (Grunwald and Richards 2006). An extensive liberation of hemin has also been detected for those Hbs possessing greater prooxidative activity, in agreement with the poor hemin affinity observed for metHb species (Maestre, Pazos, and Medina 2009).

The two inherent properties of hemoproteins related to their oxidizing power, metMb generation and hemin liberation, are involved in the efficiency of the two principal prooxidative pathways ascribed to hemoproteins: (1) the formation of oxidizing ferrylHb radicals and (2) the generation of free radicals via scission of lipid hydroperoxides, including both heterolytic and hemolytic cleavage of the peroxide bond and a peroxidase-type mechanism. The interaction of metHb with hydrogen peroxide or lipid hydroperoxide results principally in the formation of the hypervalent ferrylHb [HbFe(IV) = O] and perferrylHb [$^{\bullet}$HbFe(IV) = O], which can initiate lipid peroxidation via abstraction of a hydrogen atom from the *bis*-allylic position of PUFA (Reeder and Wilson 1998; Kanner 1994). Hypervalent ferryl species are also active in transferring oxidative damage to the relevant muscle protein myosin by inducing thiyl, tyrosyl, and other unidentified protein radical species (Lund et al. 2008). In regard to the peroxidase mechanism, there is no difference in the free radical-generating activity of metHb and reduced Hb species (Pazos, Andersen, and Skibsted 2008). Therefore, the propensity of hemoproteins to be converted to metHb enhances the oxidizing behavior of hemoproteins through the formation of the highly oxidizing ferrylHb. Free hemin displays a more rapid and extensive generation of free radicals than Hb under low hydroperoxide concentrations (hydroperoxide/heme molar ratios ≤ 1:4), conditions found at the initial stages of lipid oxidation. Figure 2.3 represents the rapid kinetics of free radicals caused by free hemin versus Hb in conditions of low hydroperoxide concentrations (hydroperoxide/heme molar ratios = 1:8).

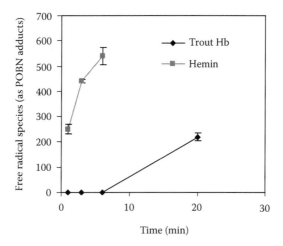

FIGURE 2.3 Capacity of free hemin (oxidized form of heme group) and Hb from rainbow trout (*Oncorhynchus mykiss*) to promote the formation of free radicals by interaction with low hydroperoxide levels (hydroperoxide/hemin molar ratio = 1:8). Free radicals were monitored as POBN-radical adducts, and cumene hydroperoxide (CumOOH) was used as a lipid hydroperoxide model. Heme-containing systems, CumOOH, and POBN were incubated at concentrations of 92 μM (heme basis), 11 μM, and 60 mM, respectively, in 50 mM phosphate buffer, pH 6.8.

By increasing the concentration of hydroperoxides or after successive exposures to hydroperoxides, hemin dramatically loses the efficiency to generate free radicals, and the radical generating activity of Hb is extraordinarily activated. The low free radical-generating efficiency of hemin in elevated free radical/hydroperoxide environments is ascribable to the hemin degradation and the subsequent liberation of the free ferric iron (Pazos, Andersen, and Skibsted 2008). Heme compounds are found to cleave hydroperoxides more rapidly than ferric or ferrous ions (O'Brien 1969). These data suggest a central role of free hemin during the initial stages of oxidation.

The oxidizing action of hemoproteins is often influenced by pH and thermal treatments. Several attempts have been made to identify the effect of heating on the oxidizing ability of hemoproteins. The capacity of several fish Hbs to generate hydroperoxide-derived free radicals has not been significantly affected by heating at 70°C for 10 and 45 min (Pazos, Andersen, and Skibsted 2009). Studies performed with bovine oxyHb and metHb show similar oxidizing activity for native Hb and that heated to 45°C, but the increment of heating temperature to 68°C and 90°C reduced the activity of Hb (Bou et al. 2010). The prooxidant activities of metHb heated at 68°C and 90°C were analogous, whereas the prooxidant activity of oxyHb heated at 68°C was higher than that heated at 90°C. The attenuation of the prooxidant activity of heat-denatured Hb is associated with a decrease in the solubility of heme iron and a reduced impact of free iron on the lipid oxidation. In the case of oxyMb, the native species is more efficient as a promoter of lipid oxidation than oxyMb heated at 45°C–95°C, being the heating temperatures of 90°C–95°C, which provoke lower oxidation (Bou et al. 2008). In contrast, bovine metMb incites a faster oxidation of lipids for Hb heated at 45°C–60°C than for the native form. Heating at temperatures immediately below the thermal denaturation of metMb induces structural changes in the heme protein, which increases its prooxidative activity (Kristensen and Andersen 1997). On the contrary, temperatures above the denaturation temperature of metMb decrease the prooxidant activity of the resulting species compared to native metMb.

It is important to bear in mind that Hb's oxygen binding affinity can decrease as conditions become acidic, a phenomenon known as the Bohr effect (Richards and Hultin 2000). Hbs from beef and chicken are fully oxygenated at pH 6.7 because of the low Bohr effect, and conversely, trout Hb is largely deoxygenated at the same pH value (Richards, Modra, and Li 2002). Hbs from fish species, such as rainbow trout and Atlantic cod, require pH values as high as 7.2–7.5 to be fully oxygenated (Richards, Modra, and Li 2002; Pazos, Medina, and Hultin 2005). In general, mammalian Hbs are endowed with a lower Bohr effect than those from fish species (Berenbrink 2006). The prevalence of the Bohr effect has been related to the proportion of anodic isoforms of Hb, whose oxygen affinity drops at acidic pH values, whereas cathodic Hb isoforms bind oxygen strongly independently of pH (Richards, Ostdal, and Andersen 2002). The Bohr effect enhances the oxidizing activity of Hb at the usual conditions of muscle-based food (pH value: 5–7) because the presence of deoxyHb accelerates metHb formation (Shikama 1998), and as indicated above, the ferric metHb is more oxidant than ferrous Hb species. Accordingly, the oxidizing activity of fish Hbs is pH-dependent, being more oxidant at acidic pH values (Pazos, Medina, and Hultin 2005; Richards and Hultin 2000). This pH dependence implies that the pH drop that naturally occurs during the rigor mortis of meat and fish may activate the oxidizing action of the Hbs with a strong Bohr effect. Therefore, the slaughtering methods that include a previous stunning procedure, which diminish the rate and extent of the postmortem pH reduction, should contribute to improving the oxidative stability of meat-based food by lessening the oxidative activity of Hb.

2.2.3 PHOTOSENSITIZERS

Riboflavin, porphyrins, and chlorophyll derivatives are photosensitizers naturally occurring in foods. Meat, fruit juice, and vegetable oils, together with dairy products, such as cheese, butter, and milk, are susceptible to photooxidation resulting from their natural content of photosensitizers.

Photosensitizers absorb light, becoming excited to one or more energy-rich state(s) (Figure 2.4). The excited sensitizer (Sen*) undergoes internal reactions that ultimately result in the oxidative alteration of a second molecule. The direct oxidative action of light, or photolytic autoxidation, is principally restricted to the production of free radicals primarily from the exposure of the primary substrate to UV radiation (Airado-Rodriguez et al. 2011). However, photosensitizers promote the photooxidation of diverse substrates when foods are exposed to visible light. Photooxidation by a photosensitizer can proceed through two major pathways, type I or type II reactions (Figure 2.4). Type I photosensitization proceeds through a free-radical mechanism in which the excited photosensitizer (Sen*) subtracts an electron or hydrogen atom from another component of the system. This reaction generates two radicals, a photosensitizer radical (Sen$^{\bullet-}$) and a substrate radical. If oxygen is present, both of these radicals can further react to produce oxygenated products. This type of reaction can lead to a loss of the sensitizer. An additional reaction is the direct transfer of the extra electron of the sensitizer radical (Sen$^{\bullet-}$) to molecular oxygen to produce an oxidant superoxide radical $\left(O_2^{\bullet-}\right)$, which can be converted via a dismutation process into another reactive oxygen species, hydrogen peroxide (H_2O_2). This reaction regenerates the sensitizer to the original ground state (Sen). In a type II reaction, the energy from the excited sensitizer is transferred to triplet oxygen, and

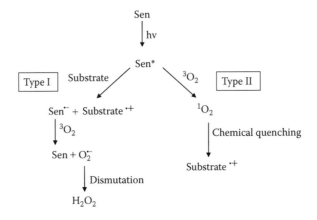

FIGURE 2.4   Type I and type II photosensitization process.

the very reactive singlet oxygen ($^1O_2$) is formed. Singlet oxygen reacts with electron-rich sites, such as unsaturated fatty acids, resulting in hydroperoxides and in the net reduction of oxygen (chemical quenching) (Huvaere et al. 2010). Singlet oxygen can also release its excess of energy (physical quenching). Compounds such as β-carotene and lycopene are able to remove the excitation energy of singlet oxygen without being damaged themselves. These reactions can occur at the same time in a competitive manner, the type II (singlet oxygen-mediated) mechanism being favored over the type I (radical) mechanism by lower substrate concentration and higher oxygen concentration (He, An, and Jiang 1998).

Lipids, proteins, DNA, or vitamins are chemical quenchers of singlet oxygen (Table 2.5). Ascorbate, α-tocopherol, and glutathione are among the vitamins or reductants oxidized by singlet oxygen. Guanosine is the DNA base most reactive with singlet oxygen. Unsaturated fatty acids and cholesterol are also targets of $^1O_2$-mediated oxidation because of the presence of electron-rich sites in their structure and the electrophilic nature of singlet oxygen. The triplet-excited riboflavin yields, directly or indirectly, radical species with the capacity to initiate oxidation of unsaturated fatty acid methyl esters, such as oleate, linoleate, and linolenate, but still the deactivation of the excited flavin by lipid derivatives is significantly slower than that observed by proteins (Huvaere et al. 2010; Huvaere and Skibsted 2009). The most susceptible places for proteins to quench singlet oxygen are cysteine, methionine, tryptophan, tyrosine, or histidine residues, which are holders of areas with high electron density, such as double bonds or sulfur moieties. Free amino acids have been reported to be superior to peptides in quenching singlet oxygen, and unfolded proteins have a higher quenching ability toward singlet oxygen than globular proteins (Dalsgaard et al. 2011).

Riboflavin has been traditionally considered as the active photosensitizer in dairy products. Riboflavin can initiate photooxidation of types I and II by exposure to UV radiation or visible light up to approximately 500 nm. Recent studies have shown the presence of five other photosensitizers in butter: protoporphyrin, hematoporphyrin, a chlorophyll a-like molecule, and two unidentified tetrapyrrols (Wold et al. 2006). Chlorophyll and porphyrin molecules absorb light in the UV and violet region with absorption peaks of approximately 410 nm (the Soret band). In addition, they absorb light pronouncedly in the red above 600 nm, and therefore, they may be responsible for the formation of off-flavors in dairy products exposed to light of wavelengths longer than 500 nm (Wold et al. 2006). Chlorophyllic compounds have also been recently suggested to contribute prominently to the major part of photooxidation in

TABLE 2.5
Principal Chemical Quenchers of Singlet Oxygen in Foods

Lipids	Proteins	Reductants	DNA
PUFA, cholesterol	Cysteine, histidine, methionine, tryptophan, tyrosine	ascorbate, glutathione, α-tocopherol	2′-deoxyguanosine

cow's milk (Airado-Rodriguez et al. 2011). In meats, heme porphyrins and riboflavin are the more relevant photosensitizers. Chlorophylls have importance in the photo-oxidation developed by vegetable oils.

2.2.4 POLYPHENOLS AND OTHER REDUCTANTS

As indicated above, the reducing ability of ascorbic acid to convert the less active ferric to the more oxidizing ferrous iron explains in part the oxidative effects observed by supplementing iron-rich foods with ascorbate. The dual antioxidant/prooxidant role of ascorbic acid is concentration-dependent. Ascorbic acid at higher doses acts as an antioxidant, but at lower concentrations, it enhances the catalytic effect of iron and copper (acting as a prooxidant) (Childs et al. 2001). Ascorbic acid can also induce oxidation because of its ability to induce lipid hydroperoxide decomposition to free radicals and aldehydes responsible for oxidative degradation of lipids, proteins, and vitamins (Lee, Oe, and Blair 2001).

Different phenolics are also able to generate oxidizing ferrous and cuprous ions, metal ions that yield the highly oxidizing hydroxyl radicals via a Fenton-type mechanism. Catechin, which is expected to have redox properties similar to epicatechin, gallic acid, and caffeic acid, has displayed prooxidant activity because of its ability to reduce ferric iron (Rodtjer, Skibsted, and Andersen 2006; Sorensen et al. 2008). Moreover, strongly reducing phenolic compounds, such as pyrogallol (three adjacent phenol groups) containing (–)-epigallocatechin gallate (EGCG) and (–)-epigallocatechin (EGC), are able to form the superoxide radical from molecular oxygen (Touriño et al. 2008). Recent studies have reported that EGCG and EGC cause protein carbonyl formation in proteins, and such prooxidant action has been related to their ability to be faster autoxidized to the quinone form (Ishii et al. 2010). The quinonic structure is reactive with the primary amine groups of proteins to render a protein–iminoquinone adduct, which undergoes hydrolysis to finally produce a protein carbonyl.

Therefore, the phenolic compounds that are commonly employed in antioxidant strategies to avoid deteriorative oxidations may also reduce the oxidative stability of foods. These antioxidant phenolic additives are endowed with one or more properties that result decisively to protect foods from oxidation, that is, radical-scavenging activity, metal-chelating action, regenerative ability on the endogenous antioxidant components, or deactivation of ferrylHb species (Iglesias et al. 2009). The promotion of oxidation by phenolics depends largely on the food system. Factors such as the type and concentration of prooxidants, antioxidants, oxidative substrates, pH, and T^a can modify the antioxidant effect of phenols and even render them prooxidants by favoring the pathways by which phenolics can activate oxidation: metal-reducing activity to ferrous or cuprous, hydroperoxide-derived free radicals through peroxidase activity, and generation of superoxide radicals via autoxidation.

2.3 ENZYMATIC OXIDANTS

Oxidative enzymes in food are of particular interest because they affect the flavor, color, and nutrient content of food. During food processing, their activity can be decreased but also enhanced, provoking off-flavor and off-odor in food because of its reaction with unsaturated fatty acids. They are widely described in plants, fungi, invertebrates, and mammals. These enzymes catalyze oxidation by a range of different reactions. As a general distribution, the two most common types of oxidative enzymes are catalases and peroxidases, which use hydrogen peroxide as the oxidizing substrate, and peroxidases, which use molecular oxygen, such as LOXs or cyclooxygenases (Table 2.1).

2.3.1 LIPOXYGENASES

LOXs consist of a structurally related family of non-heme iron-containing dioxygenases. Depending on its origin, LOX catalyzes the insertion of oxygen into PUFAs with a (Z,Z)-1,4-pentadiene structural unit to generate position-specific hydroperoxides. The reaction is stereospecific and regiospecific. The first LOXs were found in soybean seeds in the early 1970s. Nowadays, it is known that they are widely distributed in plants, fungi, invertebrates, and mammals (Brash 1999; Shibata and Axelrod 1995). Recently, LOXs have also been described in bacteria (Porta and Rocha-Sosa 2001). Although there are several forms of LOXs in plant and animal tissues, all of them are composed of a single polypeptide chain with a molecular mass of 75–81 kDa ($\approx$662–711 amino acids) in mammals and 94–103 kDa ($\approx$838–923 amino acids) in plants (Prigge et al. 1996). LOXs are characterized by preserved domains and sequence patterns, both aspects that determine different structures and the binding of the catalytic iron. The tridimensional configuration of the structural domain that regulates its catalytic action is formed by an α-helix with a single atom of non-heme iron near its center. The non-heme iron atom is coordinated with five amino acids, three histidines, one asparagine, and the carboxyl group of the carboxy-terminal isoleucine. The carboxy-terminal domain harbors the catalytic site of the enzyme (Minor et al. 1996).

The LOX enzymes are usually in the inactive ferrous (Fe^{2+}) form when isolated and must be oxidized to Fe(III) by the reaction product, fatty acid hydroperoxides or hydrogen peroxide, before activating as an oxidation catalyst (Andreou and Feussner 2009), and this form drives the reaction. LOX catalyzes the stereospecific hydrogen subtraction from a doubly allylic methylene group followed by a radical rearrangement and accompanied by a Z,E diene conjugation, depending on LOX specificity. The last step is dependent on the stereospecificity and implies the introduction of molecular oxygen and the reduction of the hydroperoxyl radical intermediate to the corresponding anion. The non-heme iron in the catalytic center of the LOX catalyzes the one-electron transitions.

The enzyme occurs in a variety of isoforms, which often vary in optimum pH as well as product and substrate specificity. Animal LOXs are classified according to their specificity of arachidonic acid (C-20) oxygenation, and plant LOXs are classified according to their positional specificity of linoleic acid (C-18). 9- and 13-LOXs (in plants) and 5-, 8-, 12-, and 15-LOXs (in mammals) have been widely described (Andreou and Feussner 2009). The general nomenclature is aimed at identifying the position of the dioxygenation, so the 12-LOX is that which oxidizes arachidonic acid at the C12 position, and 13-LOX is that which oxidizes linoleic acid at the C-13 position. The generated hydroperoxides may be subsequently cleaved to shorter chain length oxygenated products by LOXs themselves or by hydroperoxide lyases (HPLs). The cleavage products include volatile unsaturated aldehydes and alcohols and the corresponding unsaturated oxo fatty acids (Figure 2.5). Metabolites originating from these pathways are collectively named oxylipins. While higher plants use exclusively polyunsaturated C18 fatty acids for the production of oxylipins, animals and algae rely predominantly on the transformation of polyunsaturated C20 fatty acids, which are not ubiquitously found in the plant kingdom (Noordermeer, Veldink, and Vliegenthart 2001). Moreover, the formation of volatile short-chain aldehydes relies on the combined action of LOX and HPL species in higher plants, whereas animals and algae seem to be more flexible because they may use either the LOX/HPL system or specific LOX forms alone. The reaction is stereospecific with S-hydroperoxides being the predominant products of plant and mammalian LOXs, and R-epimers are formed predominantly by invertebrate LOXs. Most LOXs also exhibit high regiospecificity. Research on the sequence alignments has suggested that S-LOXs contain a conserved alanine residue at a critical position at the active site, but R-LOXs contain glycine (Gly) in this position. However, recent studies on the model vertebrate *Danio rerio* (zebra fish) by cloning have expressed a novel R-LOX isoform that carries Gly at this critical site, resulting in a predominant production of 12S-H(p)ETE [12S-hydro(pero)xyeicosatetraenoic acid] (Jansen et al. 2011). Research on the Ala-to-Gly exchange in human and animal LOXs resulted in different specificity for producing oxygenation products. In human LOXs, there was an increase of specific R-oxygenation products. However, in rabbits, orangutans, and mice, S-HETE (hydroxyeicosatetraenoic acid) isomers remained the major oxygenation products, whereas chiral R-HETEs contributed only 10%–30% to the total product mixture.

In plants, the most common LOX-resulting products from linoleic acid and linolenic acids lead to different bioactive mediators related to different functions, especially plant defense and development (Grechkin 1998). In mammals, the different

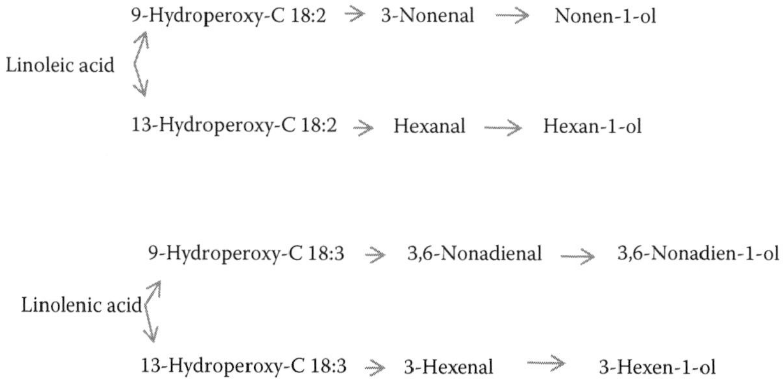

FIGURE 2.5 Representative oxidation products of linoleic (18:2 n-6) and linolenic (18:3 n-3) acids by action of 9-LOX and 13-LOX.

LOXs, mainly 5, 12, and 15, produce various eicosanoids (Funk 1996). They comprise a variety of bioregulators, including leukotrienes, hepoxilins, and HETEs, that are so numerous and have important biological activities involved in the survival and well-being of animals. All these molecules do not lead to the secondary scission products responsible for oxidized flavor, but they also have been shown to be implicated in a variety of human diseases, such as inflammation, fever, arthritis, and cancer. The production of small amounts of the hydroxylated derivatives is not, per se, a disruptive event. However, the enzymatic oxygenation of membrane lipids by the LOX may well provoke radical-mediated secondary reactions, which could lead to oxidative modification of membrane proteins. Such oxidative modifications to proteins are an important signal for their proteolytic breakdown (Wong et al. 1988). They are rapidly degraded by the proteases in reticulocytes. Also, the modification of membrane structures leads to structural changes that play a role in the maturation of various cell types, including erythrocytes, lens epithelial cells, and keratinocytes (Schewe and Kuhn 1991).

The position-specific hydroperoxides generated by LOXs can be further metabolized into various secondary oxidation products. Therefore, the LOX pathway is highly associated with both the development of fresh and off-flavors in many plant and animal food systems. Under postharvest conditions, the release of tissue LOXs from endogenous constraints could generate significant quantities of reactive lipid hydroperoxides, potential sources of free-radical species involved in lipid oxidation. As a result, the production of off-flavor and interaction products occurs and highly affects odor, color, and texture of food products.

LOX from soybean seed is the best characterized among plant LOXs. Soybean LOX provokes the rapid appearance of strong beany flavor in processed soybeans. Soybean LOX exists in eight different isoforms, and the primary lipid oxidation product by a LOX-catalyzed reaction in soy protein is 13-hydroperoxide of linoleic acid (Wu et al. 2009). This hydroperoxide formed has provoked alterations in soybean protein functionality, resulting in the generation of protein carbonyl derivatives, loss of protein sulfhydryl groups, and loss of native structure. Inactivation of LOXs eliminates the formation of the undesirable flavors and reactions in soybean preparations. This can be performed by heat treatments, but loss of protein solubility and other negative effects are also accompanied. Therefore, there is a strong interest in developing soybeans with reduced LOX activity suitable for human consumption, and significant genetic research has been made on this objective during the last several years. Different modified soybean lines lacking LOX isoforms have been developed, some of them having a high yield and a good and nutritional quality (Narvel, Fehr, and Welke 1998; Han, Ding, and Sun 2002).

Different LOX isoforms have already been observed in many vegetable products, such as potato, wheat germ, green beans, peas, tomato, etc. (Anese and Sovrano 2006). The LOX activity has been described as increasing during frozen storage and provoking color degradation in fruit products. Potato LOX has been identified as an unusual plant enzyme because it catalyzes the oxidation of the 20-carbon atom PUFA, arachidonic acid, to form 15-hydroperoxyeicosatetraenoic acid as the major product (Eskin, Grossman, and Pinsky 1977). LOXs have been reported to be involved in the ripening process of strawberry fruit, and thus, albino fruit have lower LOX activity because of poor color development in them (Sharma et al. 2006).

Early works by Winkler, Pilhofer, and German (1991) and Hsieh, German, and Kinsella (1988) described the presence of two distinct LOXs, 12 and 15, varying in specificity and stability on gills and skin tissues of marine and freshwater fish. Other PUFAs, such as EPA and DHA, highly abundant in fish species, are also subtracts for LOX activity. Teleost fish gills predominantly produce the 12-hydroxy derivative of arachidonic and eicosapentaenoic acids (Winkler, Pilhofer, and German 1991). A LOX enzyme was found in mackerel flesh, which oxidized linoleic and docosa-hexaenoic acids more efficiently than eicosapentaenoic or linolenic acids (Harris and Tall 1994). Recently, Margenat, Jachmanian, and Grompone (2005) have confirmed the presence of active LOXs in hake liver, but their activity was found to be 100,000 times lower than for soybeans.

LOXs are also found in a variety of cereal, such as rye, wheat, oat, barley, and corn. Unlike lipase and like most other enzymes, LOX activity is accelerated by adding water to cereal products (Barnes and Galliard 1991). Rice bran is particularly affected by LOX activity because LOX activity is localized in the bran fraction. The deterioration of rice bran by lipase and LOXs has been widely described to be affected by storage temperature and packaging conditions. The activity of some LOXs and lipases was negatively correlated during the deterioration of rice bran (Zhang et al. 2009).

2.3.2 MYELOPEROXIDASES AND LACTOPEROXIDASES

Myeloperoxidase (MPO) and lactoperoxidase (LPO) are mammalian peroxidase enzymes possessing similar structures and functions. They have a heme moiety attached through an imidazole nitrogen; their main function is to catalyze the H_2O_2-dependent oxidation of halides and pseudo halides to generate the corresponding hypohalous acid in the catalysis of oxidative reactions (Furtmuller et al. 2004). LPO is a monomeric protein with a single polypeptide chain of 78.5 kDa. It is found in many body secretions including milk, saliva, earwax, and lung surfactant (Pruitt and Reiter 1985). It catalyzes the oxidation of thiocyanate (SCN^-) and the production of hypothiocyanite ($OSCN^-$) by using hydrogen peroxide (H_2O_2). Bovine milk contains approximately 30 mg/L of the enzyme, and the concentration is fairly constant throughout the lactation. The LPO system is used as an antibacteriostatic agent for raw milk preservation and operates by the reactivation of the enzyme by the addition of thiocyanate and a source of peroxide (*Codex Alimentarius* 1991). It has also been used in reducing microflora in milk for cheese making. The effect has a limited duration, which is determined by temperature. It is fairly heat-resistant and is used as an indicator of overpasteurization of milk. Its applications as a control of post-culturing acidification of yogurt, a preservative of HTST pasteurized milk, and a stabilizer of caseinate stabilized emulsions at room temperature have been also described.

MPO, an abundant leukocyte enzyme, is a 150–165 kDa homodimer and uses chloride (Cl^-) as the preferred substrate to generate hypochlorous acid (HOCl) (Kiermeier and Petz 1967). It helps neutrophils and monocytes to destroy foreign substances because the hypochlorous acid generated is used for microbial killing by phagocytic cells. Its relevance in oxidative deterioration of foodstuffs is not significant.

Sulfhydryl oxidases have been also described in bovine milk (Podrez, Abu-Soud, and Hazen 2000). They catalyze disulfide bond formation at the expense of molecular oxygen and have been suggested to play significant roles in oxidative protein folding in mammals (Janolino and Swaisgood 1987). Quiescin-sulfhydryl oxidases have been also described in milk in addition to the iron-dependent oxidase (Jaje et al. 2007). It has been released from mammary epithelial cells during formation of the skim or cream phases of milk. Human milk sulfhydryl oxidase is rather stable at pH 2.5 and is resistant to degradation by pepsin, trypsin, and chymotrypsin.

2.3.3 POLYPHENOL OXIDASES

Polyphenol oxidases (PPOs) are a group of copper-containing metalloenzymes that were first discovered in mushrooms and have been found in most higher plants (Mathew and Parpia 1971). They are responsible for deleterious enzymatic browning in raw fruits, vegetables, and crustaceans, such as shrimp and lobster. However, browning by PPOs is now always an undesirable reaction. The desirable brown color of tea, cocoa, cider, and coffee is promoted by PPO during processing. PPOs are able to catalyze the oxidation of aromatic compounds by oxygen. There are two main types of PPO: tyrosinases and laccases (Hernández-Romero, Solano, and Sanchez-Amat 2005). Tyrosinases catalyze two kinds of reactions: *ortho*-hydroxylation of monophenols (cresolase activity) and the oxidation of the *ortho*-diphenols to *ortho*-quinones (catechol oxidase activity). Both reactions require the presence of molecular oxygen. Laccases are remarkably less specific than tyrosinases in regard to the substrate, being able to oxidize *ortho*-diphenols, such as catechol (for most laccases, but not all), but *p*-diphenols and methoxysubstituted phenols are the substrates preferred by laccases (Thurston 1994; Hernández-Romero, Solano, and Sanchez-Amat 2005). Laccases oxidize the phenolic structures to quinone groups. Therefore, the two enzymes may be distinguished based on the fact that laccases, unlike tyrosinases, do not have the capacity to hydroxylate monophenols to *ortho*-diphenols but are able to oxidize methoxy-activated phenols (McMahon et al. 2007). These enzymes are used as indicators for the adequacy of heat treatment of fruit-processed products.

The PPOs provide the formation of *ortho*-quinone structures that undergo rapid polymerization to yield black and brown pigments referred to as melanins. The formation of melanins in crustaceans is mainly a result of the oxidation of the amino acid L-tyrosine to yield L-3,4-dihydroxyphenylalanine (L-DOPA). In a second step, crustacean PPO oxidizes L-DOPA to the L-DOPA quinone. In pink shrimp (*Parapenaeus longirostris*), the PPO activity is higher in the carapace, followed by that present in the abdomen, exoskeleton, and cephalotorax (Zamorano et al. 2009). In the case of fruits and vegetables, a great variety of phenolics are involved in browning. Chlorogenic acid, catechins, caffeic acid, 3,4-dihydroxyphenylalanine (DOPA), *p*-coumaric acid, flavonol glycosides, and anthocyanins have been described as potential substrates for the enzymatic browning of fruits and vegetables.

Precooking at a sufficiently high temperature might be a means to prevent melanosis by full inactivation of PPO. When the shrimp were precooked at 80°C with a holding time of 30 s, the activity of PPO is significantly reduced (>95%) (Kusaimah et al. 2012). The resulting precooked shrimp possessed a lower melanosis score during 7 days of storage at 4°C. Other inactivation methods that can be applied to avoid enzymatic browning are based on the use of chemical additives with reducing (ascorbic acid, glutathione, cysteine) and chelating properties (phosphates, EDTA) or on the removal of essential components (most often oxygen) from the product (Almeida and Nogueira 1995). High-pressure treatment, a technique used in food processing to achieve microbial and enzyme inactivation, can also minimize the PPO activity (Liu et al. 2010). Inhibition of PPO gene expression can result in a reduction of discoloration (Anderson et al. 2006).

REFERENCES

Airado-Rodriguez, D., N. Intawiwat, J. Skaret, and J. P. Wold. 2011. Effect of naturally occurring tetrapyrroles on photooxidation in cow's milk. *J Agric Food Chem* 59: 3905–3914.

Alderton, A. L., C. Faustman, D. C. Liebler, and D. W. Hill. 2003. Induction of redox instability of bovine myoglobin by adduction with 4-hydroxy-2-nonenal. *Biochemistry-US* 42: 4398–4405.

Alexa, R. I., J. S. Mounsey, B. T. O'Kennedy, and J. C. Jacquier. 2011. Oxidative stability of water/oil mixtures as influenced by the addition of free Cu(2+) or Cu-alginate gel beads. *Food Chem* 129: 253–258.

Almeida, M. E. M., and J. N. Nogueira. 1995. The control of polyphenol oxidase activity in fruits and vegetables—A study of the interaction between the chemical-compounds used and heat-treatment. *Plant Foods Hum Nutr* 47: 245–256.

Andersen, E., M. L. Andersen, and C. P. Baron. 2007. Characterization of oxidative changes in salted herring (*Clupea harengus*) during ripening. *J Agric Food Chem* 55: 9545–9553.

Anderson, J. V., E. P. Fuerst, W. J. Hurkman, W. H. Vensel, and C. F. Morris. 2006. Biochemical and genetic characterization of wheat (*Triticum spp.*) kernel polyphenol oxidases. *J Cereal Sci* 44: 353–367.

Andreou, A., and I. Feussner. 2009. Lipoxygenases—Structure and reaction mechanism. *Phytochem* 70: 1504–1510.

Anese, M., and S. Sovrano. 2006. Kinetics of thermal inactivation of tomato lipoxygenase. *Food Chem* 95: 131–137.

Aranda, R., H. Cai, C. E. Worley, E. J. Levin, R. Li, J. S. Olson, G. N. Phillips, and M. P. Richards. 2009. Structural analysis of fish versus mammalian hemoglobins: Effect of the heme pocket environment on autooxidation and hemin loss. *Proteins Struct Funct Bioinform* 75: 217–230.

Barnes, P., and T. Galliard. 1991. Rancidity in cereal products. *Lipid Technol* 3: 23–28.

Berenbrink, M. 2006. Evolution of vertebrate haemoglobins: Histidine side chains, specific buffer value and Bohr effect. *Respir Physiol Neurobiol* 154: 165–184.

Bou, R., F. Guardiola, R. Codony, C. Faustman, R. J. Elias, and E. A. Decker. 2008. Effect of heating oxymyoglobin and metmyoglobin on the oxidation of muscle microsomes. *J Agric Food Chem* 56: 9612–9620.

Bou, R., N. Hanquet, R. Codony, F. Guardiola, and E. A. Decker. 2010. Effect of heating oxyhemoglobin and methemoglobin on microsomes oxidation. *Meat Sci* 85: 47–53.

Brash, A. R. 1999. Lipoxygenases: Occurrence, functions, catalysis, and acquisition of substrate. *J Biol Chem* 274: 23679–23682.

Brown, W. D. 1962. The concentration of myoglobin and hemoglobin in tuna flesh. *J Food Sci* 27: 26–28.

Buettner, G. R. 1993. The pecking order of free radicals and antioxidants: Lipid peroxidation, α-tocopherol and ascorbate. *Arch Biochem Biophys* 300: 535–543.

Chan, W. K. M., E. A. Decker, J. B. Lee, and D. A. Butterfield. 1994. EPR Spin-trapping studies of the hydroxyl radical scavenging activity of carnosine and related dipeptides. *J Agric Food Chem* 42: 1407–1410.

Childs, A., C. Jacobs, T. Kaminski, B. Halliwell, and C. Leeuwenburgh. 2001. Supplementation with vitamin C and N-acetyl-cysteine increases oxidative stress in humans after an acute muscle injury induced by eccentric exercise. *Free Radic Biol Med* 31: 745–753.

Codex Alimentarius. 1991. *Guidelines for the Preservation of Raw Milk by Use of the Lacto-peroxidase System* (CAC/GL 13-1991). Available at http://www.codexalimentarius.net/download/standards/29/CXG_013e.pdf.

Dalsgaard, T. K., J. H. Nielsen, B. E. Brown, N. Stadler, and M. J. Davies. 2011. Dityrosine, 3,4-Dihydroxyphenylalanine (DOPA), and radical formation from tyrosine residues on milk proteins with globular and flexible structures as a result of riboflavin-mediated photo-oxidation. *J Agric Food Chem* 59: 7939–7947.

Davies, M. J., and R. T. Dean. 1997. *Radical-Mediated Protein Oxidation. From Chemistry to Medicine*, Oxford: Oxford Science Publications.

Decker, E., and H. Faraji. 1990. Inhibition of lipid oxidation by carnosine. *J Am Oil Chem Soc* 67: 650–652.

Decker, E. A., and H. O. Hultin. 1990. Factors influencing catalysis of lipid oxidation by the soluble fraction of mackerel muscle. *J Food Sci* 55: 947–950.

Eskin, N. A. M., S. Grossman, and A. Pinsky. 1977. Biochemistry of lipoxygenase in relation to food quality. *CRC Crit Rev Food Sci Nutr* 9: 1–40.

Estévez, M., and M. Heinonen. 2010. Effect of phenolic compounds on the formation of alpha-aminoadipic and gamma-glutamic semialdehydes from myofibrillar proteins oxidized by copper, iron, and myoglobin. *J Agric Food Chem* 58: 4448–4455.

Frederiksen, A. M., M. N. Lund, M. L. Andersen, and L. H. Skibsted. 2008. Oxidation of porcine myosin by hypervalent myoglobin: The role of thiol groups. *J Agric Food Chem* 56: 3297–3304.

Funk, C. D. 1996. The molecular biology of mammalian lipoxygenases and the quest for eicosanoid functions using lipoxygenase-deficient mice. *Biochim Biophys Acta-Lipids Lipid Metab* 1304: 65–84.

Furtmuller, P. G., W. Jantschko, M. Zederbauer, C. Jakopitsch, J. Arnhold, and C. Obinger. 2004. Kinetics of interconversion of redox intermediates of lactoperoxidase, eosinophil peroxidase and myeloperoxidase. *Japan J Infect Dis* 57: S30–S31.

Grechkin, A. 1998. Recent developments in biochemistry of the plant lipoxygenase pathway. *Progr Lipid Res* 37: 317–352.

Grunwald, E. W., and M. P. Richards. 2006. Mechanisms of heme protein-mediated lipid oxidation using hemoglobin and myoglobin variants in raw and heated washed muscle. *J Agric Food Chem* 54: 8271–8280.

Gülçin, I. 2006. Antioxidant activity of caffeic acid (3,4-dihydroxycinnamic acid). *Toxicology* 217: 213–220.

Guzun-Cojocaru, T., C. Koev, M. Yordanov, T. Karbowiak, E. Cases, and P. Cayot. 2011. Oxidative stability of oil-in-water emulsions containing iron chelates: Transfer of iron from chelates to milk proteins at interface. *Food Chem* 125: 326–333.

Han, F.-X., A.-L. Ding, and J.-M. Sun. 2002. Development of new soybean variety with null trypsin inhibitor and lipoxygenase 2.3 genes-Zhonghuang 16 and its cultivation practices. *J Genet Genom* 29: 1105–1110.

Hargrove, M. S., A. J. Wilkinson, and J. S. Olson. 1996. Structural factors governing hemin dissociation from metmyoglobin. *Biochemistry-US* 35: 11300–11309.

Harris, P., and J. Tall. 1994. Substrate-specificity of mackerel flesh lipopolygenase. *J Food Sci* 59: 504–506.

Hazell, T. J. 1982. Iron and zinc compounds in the muscle meats of beef, lamb, pork and chicken. *J Sci Food Agric* 33: 1049–1056.

He, Y. Y., J. Y. An, and L. J. Jiang. 1998. EPR and spectrophotometric studies on free radicals (O-2(center dot-), Cysa-HB center dot-) and singlet oxygen (O-1(2)) generated by irradiation of cysteamine substituted hypocrellin B. *Int J Radiat Biol* 74: 647–654.

Hernández-Romero, D., F. Solano, and A. Sanchez-Amat. 2005. Polyphenol oxidase activity expression in *Ralstonia solanacearum*. *Appl Env Microbiol* 71: 6808–6815.

Hsieh, R. J., J. B. German, and J. E. Kinsella. 1988. Lipoxygenase in fish tissue—some properties of the 12-lipoxygenase from trout gill. *J Agric Food Chem* 36: 680–685.

Hsieh, Y. H. P., and Y. P. Hsieh. 1997. Valence state of iron in the presence of ascorbic acid and ethylenediaminetetraacetic acid. *J Agric Food Chem* 45: 1126–1129.

Huvaere, K., D. R. Cardoso, P. Homem-de-Mello, S. Westermann, and L. H. Skibsted. 2010. Light-induced oxidation of unsaturated lipids as sensitized by flavins. *J Phys Chem B* 114: 5583–5593.

Huvaere, K., and L. H. Skibsted. 2009. Light-induced oxidation of tryptophan and histidine: Reactivity of aromatic N-heterocycles toward triplet-excited flavins. *J Am Chem Soc* 131: 8049–8060.

Iglesias, J., M. Pazos, M. L. Andersen, L. H. Skibsted, and I. Medina. 2009. Caffeic acid as antioxidant in fish muscle: Mechanism of synergism with endogenous ascorbic acid and alpha-tocopherol. *J Agric Food Chem* 57: 675–681.

Ishii, T., T. Mori, T. Ichikawa, M. Kaku, K. Kusaka, Y. Uekusa, M. Akagawa, Y. Aihara, T. Furuta, T. Wakimoto, T. Kan, and T. Nakayama. 2010. Structural characteristics of green tea catechins for formation of protein carbonyl in human serum albumin. *Bioorgan Med Chem* 18: 4892–4896.

Jaje, J., H. N. Wolcott, O. Fadugba, D. Cripps, A. J. Yang, I. H. Mather, and C. Thorpe. 2007. A flavin-dependent sulfhydryl oxidase in bovine milk. *Biochemistry* 46: 13031–13040.

Janolino, V. G., and H. E. Swaisgood. 1987. Sulfhydryl oxidase-catalyzed formation of disulfide bonds in reduced ribonuclease. *Arch Biochem Biophys* 258: 265–271.

Jansen, C., K. Hofheinz, R. Vogel, J. Roffeis, M. Anton, P. Reddanna, H. Kuhn, and M. Walther. 2011. Stereocontrol of arachidonic acid oxygenation by vertebrate lipoxygenases newly cloned zebrafish lipoxygenase 1 does not follow the Ala-versus-Gly concept. *J Biol Chem* 286: 37804–37812.

Jovanovic, S. V., Y. Hara, S. Steenken, and M. G. Simic. 1995. Antioxidant potential of gallocatechins: A pulse radiolysis and laser photolysis study. *J Am Chem Soc* 117: 9881–9888.

Kanner, J. 1994. Oxidative processes in meat and meat products quality implications. *Meat Sci* 36: 169–189.

Kanner, J., B. Hazan, and L. Doll. 1988. Catalytic "free" iron ions in muscle foods. *J Agric Food Chem* 36: 412–415.

Kiermeier, F., and E. A. Petz. 1967. Sulfhydryl group-oxidizing enzyme in milk: III. Effect of heating temperature and heating time. *Z Lebensm Unters Forsch* 134: 149–156.

Kranen, R. W., T. H. Van Kuppevelt, H. A. Goedhart, C. H. Veerkamp, E. Lambooy, and J. H. Veerkamp. 1999. Hemoglobin and myoglobin content in muscles of broiler chickens. *Poultry Sci* 78: 467–476.

Kristensen, L., and H. J. Andersen. 1997. Effect of heat denaturation on the pro-oxidative activity of metmyoglobin in linoleic acid emulsions. *J Agric Food Chem* 45: 7–13.

Kusaimah, M., B. Soottawat, K. Kongkarn, and V. Wonnop. 2012. The effect of heating conditions on polyphenol oxidase, proteases and melanosis in pre-cooked Pacific white shrimp during refrigerated storage. *Food Chem* 131: 1370–1375.

Laranjinha, J., O. Vieira, V. Madeira, and L. Almeida. 1995. Two related phenolic antioxidants with opposite effects on vitamin E content in low density lipoproteins oxidized by ferrylmyoglobin: Consumption vs regeneration. *Arch Biochem Biophys* 323: 373–381.

Larsson, K., A. Almgren, and I. Undeland. 2007. Hemoglobin-mediated lipid oxidation and compositional characteristics of washed fish mince model systems made from cod (*Gadus morhua*), herring (*Clupea harengus*), and salmon (*Salmo salar*) muscle. *J Agric Food Chem* 55: 9027–9035.

Larsson, K. J., and I. K. Undeland. 2010. Effect of caffeic acid on haemoglobin-mediated lipid and protein oxidation in washed cod mince during ice and frozen storage. *J Sci Food Agric* 90: 2531–2540.

Lee, S. H., T. Oe, and I. A. Blair. 2001. Vitamin C-induced decomposition of lipid hydroperoxides to endogenous genotoxins. *Science* 292: 2083–2086.

Liu, X., Y. X. Gao, H. G. Xu, Q. F. Hao, G. M. Liu, and Q. Wang. 2010. Inactivation of peroxidase and polyphenol oxidase in red beet (*Beta vulgaris L.*) extract with continuous high pressure carbon dioxide. *Food Chem* 119: 108–113.

Lombardi-Boccia, G., B. Martinez-Dominguez, and A. Aguzzi. 2002. Total heme and non-heme iron in raw and cooked meats. *J Food Sci* 67: 1738–1741.

Lund, M. N., C. Luxford, L. H. Skibsted, and M. J. Davies. 2008. Oxidation of myosin by haem proteins generates myosin radicals and protein cross-links. *Biochem J* 410: 565–574.

Maestre, R., M. Pazos, and I. Medina. 2009. Involvement of methemoglobin (MetHb) formation and hemin loss in the pro-oxidant activity of fish hemoglobins. *J Agric Food Chem* 57: 7013–7021.

Maestre, R., M. Pazos, and I. Medina. 2011. Role of the raw composition of pelagic fish muscle on the development of lipid oxidation and rancidity during storage. *J Agric Food Chem* 59: 6284–6291.

Margenat, L., Y. Jachmanian, and M. A. Grompone. 2005. Determination of lipoxygenase activity in hake liver. *Grasas Aceites* 56: 205–208.

Mathew, A. G., and H. A. B. Parpia. 1971. Food browning as a polyphenol reaction. *Adv Food Res* 19: 75–145.

McMahon, A. M., E. M. Doyle, S. Brooks, and K. E. O'Connor. 2007. Biochemical characterisation of the coexisting tyrosinase and laccase in the soil bacterium *Pseudomonas putida* F6. *Enzyme Microb Technol* 40: 1435–1441.

Mehansho, H. 2006. Iron fortification technology development: New approaches. *J Nutr* 136: 1059–1063.

Min, B., K. C. Nam, J. Cordray, and D. U. Ahn. 2008. Endogenous factors affecting oxidative stability of beef loin, pork loin, and chicken breast and thigh meats. *J Food Sci* 73: C439–C446.

Minor, W., J. Steczko, B. Stec, Z. Otwinowski, J. T. Bolin, R. Walter, and B. Axelrod. 1996. Crystal structure of soybean lipoxygenase L-1 at 1.4 angstrom resolution. *Biochemistry* 35: 10687–10701.

Narvel, J. M., W. R. Fehr, and G. A. Welke. 1998. Agronomic and seed traits of soybean lines lacking seed lipoxygenases. *Crop Science* 38: 926–928.

Noordermeer, M. A., G. A. Veldink, and J. F. G. Vliegenthart. 2001. Fatty acid hydroperoxide lyase: A plant cytochrome P450 enzyme involved in wound healing and pest resistance. *Chembiochem* 2: 494–504.

O'Brien, P. J. 1969. Intracellular mechanisms for the decomposition of a lipid peroxide. I. Decomposition of a lipid peroxide by metal ions, heme compounds and nucleophiles. *Can J Biochem* 47: 485–492.

Pazos, M., M. L. Andersen, and L. H. Skibsted. 2008. Heme-mediated production of free radicals via preformed lipid hydroperoxide fragmentation. *J Agric Food Chem* 56: 11478–11484.

Pazos, M., M. L. Andersen, and L. H. Skibsted. 2009. Efficiency of hemoglobin from rainbow trout, cod, and herring in promotion of hydroperoxide-derived free radicals. *J Agric Food Chem* 57: 8661–8667.

Pazos, M., S. Lois, J. L. Torres, and I. Medina. 2006. Inhibition of hemoglobin- and iron-promoted oxidation in fish microsomes by natural phenolics. *J Agric Food Chem* 54: 4417–4423.

Pazos, M., I. Medina, and H. O. Hultin. 2005. Effect of pH on hemoglobin-catalized lipid oxidation in cod muscle membranes in vitro and in situ. *J Agric Food Chem* 53: 3605–3612.

Pazos, M., A. Pereira da Rocha, P. Roepstorff, and A. Rogowska-Wrzesinska. 2011. Fish proteins as targets of ferrous-catalyzed oxidation: Identification of protein carbonyls by fluorescent labeling on two-dimensional gels and MALDI-TOF/TOF mass spectrometry. *J Agric Food Chem* 59: 7962–7977.

Petrat, F., S. Paluch, E. Dogruöz, P. Dörfler, M. Kirsch, H.-G. Korth, R. Sustmann, and H. de Groot. 2003. Reduction of Fe(III) ions complexed to physiological ligands by lipoyl dehydrogenase and other flavoenzymes in vitro. *J Biol Chem* 278: 46403–46413.

Pierre, J. L., and M. Fontecave. 1999. Iron and activated oxygen species in biology: The basic chemistry. *Biometals* 12: 195–199.

Pierre, J., M. Fontecave, and R. Crichton. 2002. Chemistry for an essential biological process: The reduction of ferric iron. *Biometals* 15: 341–346.

Podrez, E. A., H. M. Abu-Soud, and S. L. Hazen. 2000. Myeloperoxidase-generated oxidants and atherosclerosis. *Free Radic Biol Med* 28: 1717–1725.

Porta, H., and M. Rocha-Sosa. 2001. Lipoxygenase in bacteria: A horizontal transfer event? *Microbiology-Sgm* 147: 3199–3200.

Prigge, S. T., J. C. Boyington, B. J. Gaffney, and L. M. Amzel. 1996. Structure conservation in lipoxygenases: Structural analysis of soybean lipoxygenase-1 and modeling of human lipoxygenases. *Proteins-Struct Funct Genet* 24: 275–291.

Pruitt, K. M., and B. Reiter. 1985. Biochemistry of peroxidase systems: Antimicrobial effects. In *The Lactoperoxidase System: Chemistry and Biological Significance*, edited by K. M. Pruitt and J. O. Tenovuo. New York: Marcel Dekker.

Purchas, R. W., D. C. Simcock, T. W. Knight, and B. H. P. Wilkinson. 2003. Variation in the form of iron in beef and lamb meat and losses of iron during cooking and storage. *Int J Food Sci Tech* 38: 827–837.

Reeder, B. J., and M. T. Wilson. 1998. Mechanism of reaction of myoglobin with the lipid hydroperoxide hydroperoxyoctadecadienoic acid. *Biochem J* 330: 1317–1323.

Richards, M. P., and M. A. Dettman. 2003. Comparative analysis of different hemoglobins: Autoxidation, reaction with peroxide, and lipid oxidation. *J Agric Food Chem* 51: 3886–3891.

Richards, M. P., and H. O. Hultin. 2000. Effect of pH on lipid oxidation using trout hemolysate as a catalyst: A possible role for deoxyhemoglobin. *J Agric Food Chem* 48: 3141–3147.

Richards, M. P., and H. O. Hultin. 2002. Contribution of blood and blood components to lipid oxidation in fish muscle. *J Agric Food Chem* 50: 555–564.

Richards, M. P., and H. O. Hultin. 2003. Effects of added hemolysate from mackerel, herring and rainbow trout on lipid oxidation of washed cod muscle. *Fisheries Sci* 69: 1298–1300.

Richards, M. P., A. M. Modra, and R. Li. 2002. Role of deoxyhemoglobin in lipid oxidation of washed cod muscle mediated by trout, poultry and beef hemoglobins. *Meat Sci* 62: 157–163.

Richards, M. P., N. M. Nelson, H. G. Kristinsson, S. S. J. Mony, H. T. Petty, and A. C. M. Oliveira. 2007. Effects of fish heme protein structure and lipid substrate composition on hemoglobin-mediated lipid oxidation. *J Agric Food Chem* 55: 3643–3654.

Richards, M. P., H. Ostdal, and H. J. Andersen. 2002. Deoxyhemoglobin-mediated lipid oxidation in washed fish muscle. *J Agric Food Chem* 50: 1278–1283.

Rodtjer, A., L. H. Skibsted, and M. L. Andersen. 2006. Antioxidative and prooxidative effects of extracts made from cherry liqueur pomace. *Food Chem* 99: 6–14.

Rush, J. D., and W. H. Koppenol. 1990. Reactions of Fe(II)-ATP and Fe(II)-citrate complexes with tert-butyl hydroperoxide and cumyl hydroperoxide. *FEBS Lett* 275: 114–116.

Rush, J. D., Z. Maskos, and W. H. Koppenol. 1990. Reactions of iron(II) nucleotide complexes with hydrogen peroxide. *FEBS Lett* 261: 121–123.

Sannier, F., C. LeCoeur, Q. Zhao, I. Garreau, and J. M. Piot. 1996. Separation of hemoglobin and myoglobin from yellowfin tuna red muscle by ultrafiltration: Effect of pH and ionic strength. *Biotechnol Bioeng* 52: 501–506.

Satue-Gracia, M. T., E. N. Frankel, N. Rangavajhyala, and J. B. German. 2000. Lactoferrin in infant formulas: Effect on oxidation. *J Agric Food Chem* 48: 4984–4990.

Schewe, T., and H. Kuhn. 1991. Do 15-lipoxygenases have a common biological role. *Trends Biochem Sci* 16: 369–373.

Sharma, R. R., H. Krishna, V. B. Patel, A. Dahuja, and R. Singh. 2006. Fruit calcium content and lipoxygenase activity in relation to albinism disorder in strawberry. *Sci Horticult* 107: 150–154.

Shibata, D., and B. Axelrod. 1995. Plant lipoxygenases. *J Lipid Mediat Cell Signal* 12: 213–228.

Shikama, K. 1998. The molecular mechanism of autoxidation for myoglobin and hemoglobin: A venerable puzzle. *Chem Rev* 98: 1357–1373.

Sorensen, A.-D. M., A.-M. Haahr, E. M. Becker, L. H. Skibsted, B. Bergenstahl, L. Nilsson, and C. Jacobsen. 2008. Interactions between iron, phenolic compounds, emulsifiers, and pH in omega-3-enriched oil-in-water emulsions. *J Agric Food Chem* 56: 1740–1750.

Soyer, A., and H. O. Hultin. 2000. Kinetics of oxidation of the lipids and proteins of cod sarcoplasmic reticulum. *J Agric Food Chem* 48: 2127–2134.

St. Angelo, A. J. (ed.) 1992. *Lipid Oxidation in Food.* ACS Symposioum 500. American Chemical Society. Washington, D.C.

Sugiarto, M., A. Q. Ye, M. W. Taylor, and H. Singh. 2010. Milk protein-iron complexes: Inhibition of lipid oxidation in an emulsion. *Dairy Sci Technol* 90: 87–98.

Tang, J. L., C. Faustman, T. A. Hoagland, R. A. Mancini, M. Seyfert, and M. C. Hunt. 2005. Interactions between mitochondrial lipid oxidation and oxymyoglobin oxidation and the effects of vitamin E. *J Agric Food Chem* 53: 6073–6079.

Theuer, R. C. 2008. Iron-fortified infant cereals. *Food Rev Int* 24: 277–310.

Thiansilakul, Y., S. Benjakul, and M. P. Richards. 2010. Changes in heme proteins and lipids associated with off-odour of seabass (*Lates calcarifer*) and red tilapia (*Oreochromis mossambicus * O. niloticus*) during iced storage. *Food Chem* 121: 1109–1119.

Thurston, C. F. 1994. The structure and function of fungal laccases. *Microbiology-Sgm* 140: 19–26.

Touriño, S., D. Lizarraga, A. Carreras, S. Lorenzo, V. Ugartondo, M. Mitjans, M. P. Vinardell, L. Julia, M. Cascante, and J. L. Torres. 2008. Highly galloylated tannin fractions from witch hazel (*Hamamelis virginiana*) bark: Electron transfer capacity, in vitro antioxidant activity, and effects on skin-related cells. *Chem Res Toxicol* 21: 696–704.

Trout, G. R., and D. A. Gutzke. 1996. A simple, rapid preparative method for isolating and purifying oxymyoglobin. *Meat Sci* 43: 1–13.

Undeland, I., H. G. Kristinsson, and H. O. Hultin. 2004. Hemoglobin-mediated oxidation of washed minced cod muscle phospholipids: Effect of pH and hemoglobin source. *J Agric Food Chem* 52: 4444–4451.

Welch, K. D., T. Z. Davis, and S. D. Aust. 2002. Iron autoxidation and free radical generation: Effects of buffers, ligands, and chelators. *Arch Biochem Biophys* 397: 360–369.

Winkler, M., G. Pilhofer, and J. B. German. 1991. Stereochemical specificity of the N-9 lipoxygenase of fish gill. *J Food Biochem* 15: 437–448.

Wold, J. P., R. Bro, A. Veberg, F. Lundby, A. N. Nilsen, and J. Moan. 2006. Active photosensitizers in butter detected by fluorescence spectroscopy and multivariate curve resolution. *J Agric Food Chem* 54: 10197–10204.

Wong, A., S. M. Hwang, M. N. Cook, G. K. Hogaboom, and S. T. Crooke. 1988. Interactions of 5-lipoxygenase with membranes—Studies on the association of soluble enzyme with membranes and alterations in enzyme-activity. *Biochemistry* 27: 6763–6769.

Wu, W., L. Hou, C. Zhang, X. Kong, and Y. Hua. 2009. Structural modification of soy protein by 13-hydroperoxyoctadecadienoic acid. *Eur Food Res Technol* 229: 771–778.

Xiong, Y. L., S. P. Blanchard, T. Ooizumi, and Y. Y. Ma. 2010. Hydroxyl radical and ferryl-generating systems promote gel network formation of myofibrillar protein. *J Food Sci* 75: C215–C221.

Zamorano, J. P., O. Martinez-Alvarez, P. Montero, and M. D. Gomez-Guillen. 2009. Characterisation and tissue distribution of polyphenol oxidase of deepwater pink shrimp (*Parapenaeus longirostris*). *Food Chem* 112: 104–111.

Zhang, Y., C. He, Y. Wu, J. Yang, H. Xuan, and X. Zhu. 2009. Effect of lipoxygenase activity and red seed coat on rice bran deterioration. *J Sci Food Agric* 89: 1904–1908.

3 Measuring the Oxidation Potential in Foods

Louise Bennett, Amy Logan,
Netsanet Shiferaw-Terefe, Tanoj Singh,
and Robyn Warner

CONTENTS

3.1 INTRODUCTION

Individual components of food, including lipids, pigments, proteins, DNA, carbo-hydrates, and vitamins (Kanner 1994), are susceptible to oxidation reactions that generate new chemical products. In some cases, such as oxidative cross-linking of proteins to manipulate viscosity and gelation in dairy products, this is desirable, but usually, oxidative processes are associated with anti-nutritional and adverse sensory outcomes. In meat, oxidative cross-linking of proteins causes toughness (Lund et al. 2011), reduced water-holding capacity in processed meat products, off-flavors and odors, and unwanted changes in color. The term "antioxidant" (AOX) is widely used in the context of food, being associated with the chemical stabilization of oxidative processes during storage, and AOX-rich foods are linked with a range of putative health benefits for the consumer. However, the concept of oxidation potential (OP) in foods is neither well defined nor in common use. The purpose of this chapter is to propose a definition of OP and propose a framework for measuring the OP of food components and whole foods. For the purposes of this work, OP will be defined as the extent or initial rate of oxidation of a suitable molecular marker present in a given food, which is sensitive to oxygen-mediated chemical change. This concept is distinct from that of oxidative stress in living organisms, which usually elicits an AOX biochemical response that may be supplemented by AOX-rich foods.

Oxidation of substrates present in foods involves the addition of oxygen or loss of hydrogen associated with conversion of primary hydroxyl groups (alcohols) to aldehyde to carboxylic acid functionality by either chemical or biochemically mediated oxidation. Susceptible residues are present on proteins, carbohydrates, and lipids. Radicals formed on oxygen or sulfur (in proteins) and oxygen excited-state species (singlet oxygen) generated by heat, light, or metal-catalyzed reactions target double bonds and generate reactive forms of these substrates (homoradicals). Subsequent cross-reactivity of intermediate species produces complex product matrices including auto-oxidative molecular products. In a mixed food system, lipids are most vulnerable to oxidation and initiate attack of nonlipid substrates. At a low temperature, the induction of lipid oxidation is variable and dependent on multiple variables, particularly those that catalyze electron transfer (Lundberg and Chipault 1947; Lea and Ward 1959); however, the rate of lipid oxidation increases significantly as a function of temperature (Lundberg and Chipault 1947). AOXs significantly delay or inhibit the oxidation of food molecules by scavenging species that initiate the formation of oxygen radical adducts (e.g., peroxides) by quenching singlet oxygen and by competing with homoradicals and thereby breaking autoxidative chain reactions. Oxygen scavenging by AOX species reduces localized oxygen concentration and protects the food substrate from oxidation. AOXs may also act by chelating metal ions and suppressing free radicals generated by single electron transfers, thereby suppressing oxidative chain reactions.

In this chapter, key oxidative pathways of major food components, including proteins, lipids, carbohydrates, and AOXs, will be described in addition to the oxygen-mediated cross-reactivity of these major molecular classes. Analytical methods used for detecting and quantifying products of food oxidation will be outlined before introducing the concept of measuring OP. This concept provides a framework for measuring the initial rate and trajectory of oxidation for a food ingredient or food system in its matrix. At completion of all oxidative processes, the trajectory maps the maximum extent of oxidation of a system and, by inference, the relative extent of need for oxidative stabilization. A practical use might be to measure the barrier to oxidation that the presence or addition of an AOX species is likely to confer. An experimental approach for quantitative evaluation of OP is also proposed.

3.2   PATHWAYS AND PRODUCTS OF FOOD PROTEIN OXIDATION

Oxygen-generated free radicals can attack either at the protein backbone or at the side chains of the most susceptible amino acids—His, Met, Cys, Trp, and Tyr residues—by pH- and reagent-dependent mechanisms. Reactivity between oxidized intermediates of amino acid side chains can generate a complex array of possible products (Davies 2005), which can lead to either cleavage of amide bonds or intermolecular covalent cross-linked derivatives (Lund et al. 2011). Protein oxidation is commonly manifested by formation of carbonyl groups at amino acid side chains, intermolecular (or intramolecular) cross-linking between cysteine or tyrosine residues, or hydrolytic cleavage (Figure 3.1). The protein-derived oxidation products associated with specific foods are summarized in Table 3.1. In a living organism, protein oxidation may be at least partly reversed by reducing agents or enzymatically controlled processes with consequent restoration of biological function (Manning, Patel, and Borchardt 1989), but reversal does not usually occur in food systems.

Meat systems provide particular opportunity for Fenton reaction (Fe)-mediated H-atom abstraction from protein-bound lysines and arginines to produce α-aminoadipic semialdehyde (AAS) and γ-glutamic semialdehyde (GGS, Figure 3.2). AAS can react with other amino acids or itself to yield a range of possible products (Estevez 2011). The oxidation of free thiols to form disulfides is also catalyzed by metal ions (e.g., Fe^{3+} and Cu^{2+}) in the presence of dissolved oxygen and hydroxide ions (Manning, Patel, and Borchardt 1989). Reactive oxygen species (ROS) produced under oxidative conditions will directly oxidize methionines and tryptophans (Kosen 1992).

Protein thiols are readily oxidized by oxygen into disulfide (or cystine) groups in a pH-sensitive reaction. Attack is mediated by the thiolate anion (RS^-) under neutral and alkaline conditions and by the sulfonium cation (RS^+) under acidic conditions. The product of reaction of either species with a disulfide group (RSSR') forms a mixed disulfide (Manning, Patel, and Borchardt 1989). The scrambling of disulfide linkages by the formation of intermolecular or intramolecular disulfide groups can produce structural isomers (Volkin and Klibanov 1987) and cause inactivation of proteins *in vitro* as shown for egg-white lysozyme (Ahern and Klibanov 1985) and ribonuclease (Zale and Klibanov 1986). Thiol-disulfide exchange may also occur in the absence of free thiols if the conformation favors the reaction, but catalytic quantities of free thiols, as produced by hydrolytic cleavage of disulfides or from β-elimination reactions, are usually required (Friedman 1973). Disulfide exchange is usually accelerated under conditions that promote denaturation (Mozhaev and Martinek 1982) and is suppressed by thiol-scavenging agents, which either chemically block the free thiol (e.g., *N*-ethylmaleimide, *p*-mercurobenzoate) or metal ion-mediated catalysis of air oxidation of the free thiol (Manning, Patel, and Borchardt 1989).

Protein oxidation is ideally exemplified by processes in meat for which oxidation is the key determinant of shelf life and quality for both fresh and processed meat products. In addition, the density of solids in meat provides opportunity for chain reactivity between lipid peroxyl radicals with the ability to attack nearby protein targets. Notwithstanding that lipid oxidation produces off-flavors and odors *per se*, the

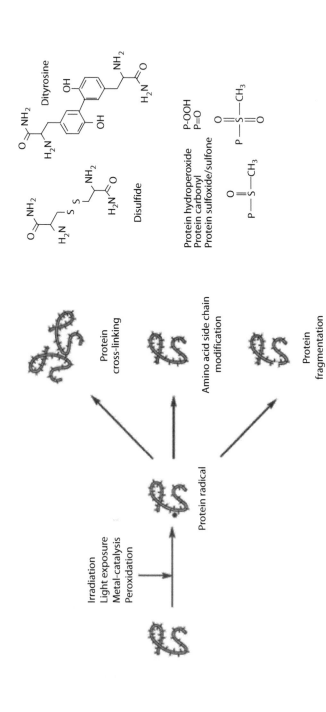

FIGURE 3.1   Modification of proteins by oxidation-driven processes. (From Lund, M. N. et al., *Mol Nutr Food Res* 55 (1): 83–95, 2011. With permission.)

TABLE 3.1

Summary of Oxidation Products Expected in Foods Based on Food Category and Chemical Class of Substrate Showing Possible Specific Substrates (or Reduced Forms) in Parentheses

Food Category	Protein-Derived	Lipid-Derived	Carbohydrate-Derived	Vitamin- and Other-Derived
Fruit and vegetables		Alcoholic, aldehydic, and carboxylic acid products formed from cleavage and hydrolysis of peroxide homodimers of fatty acids specific to particular types of fruit and vegetables	Aldonic, glycuronic, and aldaric acids (oligosaccharides); quinones (brown-colored products of polyphenolics); and derived polymers	Products of quinone reactions with proteins (primary and secondary amines, thiols), amino acids, ascorbic acid, sulfite dehydroascorbic acid (L–ascorbic acid)
Grains and pulses	Disulfide-cross-linked proteins (thiols in gluten)	Alcoholic, aldehydic, and carboxylic acid products formed from cleavage and hydrolysis of peroxide homodimers of the following fatty acids common to grains: oleic acid (18:1), linoleic acid (18:2), linolenic acid (18:3), ricinoleic acid (18:1, 9cis, 12OH), erucic acid (22:1)	Dimers of ferulate (ferulic acid) and oxidized forms of other phenolics and polyphenolics	
Meat	Disulfide-cross-linked proteins (thiols in myosin) Oxidized forms of taurine and carnosine; lysine, arginine side chains (carbonyls, AAS, GGS); calpain protease with cysteine-active site (inactivation of protease and failure to tenderize); tyrosine (protein cross-linkage); oxidized form of myoglobin (metmyoglobin)	Linoleic acid (hydroxynonenal) Malondialdehyde; lipid peroxides; peroxides and secondary oxidation products (aldehydes and ketones) of short, medium, and long chain PUFAs, e.g., 4-hydroxynonenal, 4-hydroxyhexenal, malondialdehyde, hexanal Lipid peroxide–protein adducts	Products of glycogen	Oxidized adducts form of vitamin E (alpha-tocopherol) and other AOX vitamins

(continued)

TABLE 3.1 (Continued)

Summary of Oxidation Products Expected in Foods Based on Food Category and Chemical Class of Substrate Showing Possible Specific Substrates (or Reduced Forms) in Parentheses

Food Category	Protein-Derived	Lipid-Derived	Carbohydrate-Derived	Vitamin- and Other-Derived
Dairy	Di-tyrosine; oxidized forms of cysteine, tryptophan (N-formylkynurenine and kynurenine) and methionine, dimethylsulfide, cystine-mediated cross-linked proteins, macroscopic evidence of protein aggregation, including viscosity and precipitation	Peroxides and secondary oxidation products (aldehydes and ketones) of short, medium, and long chain PUFAs, e.g., 4-hydroxynonenal, 4-hydroxyhexenal, malondialdehyde, hexanal	Lactobionic acid (lactose), galactic acid (lactose)	Oxidized forms of retinol, alpha tocopherol, riboflavin, beta carotene; dehydroascorbic acid (L-ascorbic acid)
Fish	Oxidized form of myoglobin methionines	Peroxides and secondary oxidation products (aldehydes and ketones) of long-chain PUFAs		
Eggs	Oxidized forms of yolk protein hydrolysate	Lipid peroxides of docosahexanoic, arachidonic, and linolenic acids; cholesterol oxidation products: 5 alpha-cholestane, 7-ketocholesterol, 7-β-hydroxycholesterol, 7-α-hydroxycholesterol, and others		Oxidized vitamin E, phosvitin-FeIII (phosvitin-FeII); oxidized forms of tocopherol, lutein, and other carotenoids
Bread	Cystine-cross-linked gluten proteins	Lipid peroxides and polymeric species		Dehydroascorbic acid (L-ascorbic acid), if used as a preservative

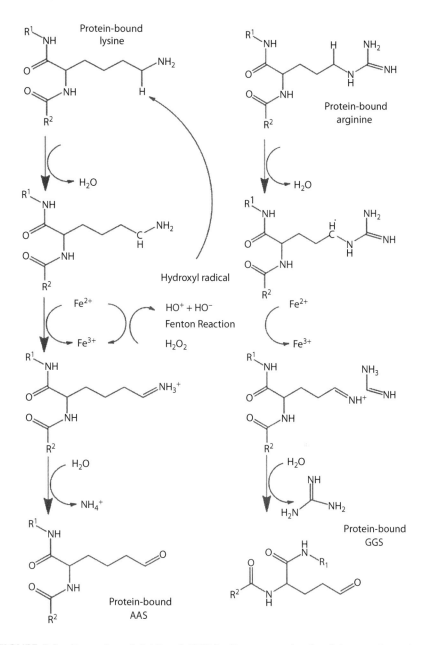

FIGURE 3.2 Formation of AAS and GGS by Fenton reaction involving non-heme iron. (From Lund, M. N. et al., *Mol Nutr Food Res* 55 (1): 83–95, 2011. With permission.)

catalysis of protein oxidation by lipids generates additional adverse effects on meat quality. For example, in meat, complexation of the oxidation product of linoleic acid, hydroxynonenal (HNE) with myoglobin-derived iron, promotes protein-localized browning and reduces shelf life (Faustman et al. 2010), and a similar process is also postulated to be mediated by free copper (Warner et al. 2010). Myofibrillar proteins in meat are also susceptible to carbonyl formation leading to denaturation and consequent loss of functionality and quality (Estevez 2011).

There are different consequences for oxidative degradation of different proteins in meat. For example, progressive oxidation of meat post-slaughter leads to irreversible inactivation of calpain, which is a key protease for regulating tenderization. However, oxidation of myosin leads to inhibition of the solubilization, gelation, and emulsification properties of meat used in comminuted products (Mitsumoto et al. 1993). Meats with elevated levels of polyunsaturated fatty acids (PUFAs) have an elevated tendency for oxidation and stimulation of protein oxidation (Faustman and Cassens 1990). Conversely, natural or fortified levels of vitamin E can provide effective suppression of oxidation processes in meat with the endogenous content of this species in the muscle resulting from the animal's diet being more efficacious than the introduction of vitamin E during meat processing (Mitsumoto et al. 1993). Finally, the storage conditions of slaughtered and processed meat, such as regulating atmospheric oxygen, temperature, light, and pH, represent important determinants to shelf life and quality primarily because of the regulation of oxidative processes (see also Chapter 5).

3.3   PATHWAYS AND PRODUCTS OF FOOD LIPID OXIDATION

With the exception of only a few foods, for example, sugar and honey, most foods contain lipids, primarily triacylglycerols, comprising three fatty acids joined at the carbonyl end to a backbone of glycerol. Each of the carbon atoms along the glyceride structure experiences a different stereospecific chemical environment (Richards et al. 2004) with differentiated susceptibility to oxidation (Wijesundera et al. 2008). The fatty acid profile determines the physical properties, oxidative stability, and nutritional value of a lipid and also provides a characteristic fingerprint. For example, most dietary oils contain proportional variations of the combination of fatty acids summarized in Table 3.2.

Oxygen attack at allylic positions of unsaturated fatty acids creates unsaturated lipid hydroperoxides. These products decompose via peroxyl and alkoxyl radicals to produce secondary oxidation products, including aldehydes, ketones, alcohols, acids, and lactones (Figure 3.3). Oxidative β-cleavage of lipids or fatty acids generates low mass volatile and higher mass nonvolatile products (Figure 3.4). These secondary oxidation products formed during auto-oxidation of unsaturated fatty acids are mostly responsible for the impaired taste, flavor, and texture in foods. Auto-oxidation occurs as a chain reaction via distinct induction, propagation, and termination phases. If no hydroperoxides (or other prooxidant species, such as metal ions, etc.) are present during the induction phase, the rate of oxygen uptake and formation of hydroperoxides is slow. In general, the ratio is 1 mol of oxygen for each mole of PUFA (Chan 1977; Porter 1980). The rate of auto-oxidation increases significantly once hydroperoxides

TABLE 3.2

Trivial and Systematic Names for Fatty Acids Commonly Found in Plant, Dairy, Marine, and Animal Sources

Trivial Name	Systematic Name (Acid)	Abbreviation
Butyric acid	Butanoic acid	4:0
Caproic acid	Hexanoic acid	6:0
Caprylic acid	Octanoic acid	8:0
Capric acid	Decanoic acid	10:0
Lauric acid	Dodecanoic acid	12:0
Myristic acid	Tetradecanoic	14:0
Palmitic acid	Hexadecanoic	16:0
Stearic acid	Octadecanoic acid	18:0
Arachidic acid	Eicosanoic acid	20:0
Oleic acid	*cis*-9-octadecenoic acid	18:1 Δ9 *cis*
Elaidic acid	*trans*-9-octadecenoic acid	18:1 Δ9 *trans*
Linoleic acid	*cis-cis*-9,12-octadecadienoic	18:2 Δ9,12 all *cis*
Conjugated-linoleic acid (CLA)	*cis-trans*-9,11-octadecatrienoic acid	18:2 Δ*cis*9, *trans*11
α-Linolenic acid (ALA)	*cis-cis-cis*-9,12,15-octadecatrienoic acid	18:3 Δ9,12,15 all *cis*
Arachidonic acid (AA)	*cis-cis-cis-cis*-5,8,11,14-eicosatetraenoic acid	20:4 Δ5,8,11,14 all *cis*
Eicosapentaenoic acid (EPA)	*cis-cis-cis*-5,8,11,14,17-eicosapentaenoic acid	20:5 Δ5,8,11,14,17 all *cis*
Erucic acid	*cis*-13-docosenoic acid	22:1 Δ 13 *cis*
Docosapentaenoic acid (DPA)	*cis-cis-cis*-7,10,13,16,19-docosapentaenoic acid	22:5 Δ7,10,13,16,19 all *cis*
Docosahexaenoic acid (DHA)	*cis-cis-cis*-4,7,10,13,16,19-docosahexaenoic acid	22:6 Δ4,7,10,13,16,19 all *cis*

are present. This is a result of the generation of reinitiating radicals produced as products of hydroperoxide decomposition (Labuza 1971). In addition, alkoxyl and peroxyl radicals generated during this process initiate further reaction chains with PUFAs resulting in highly reactive carbon-centered alkyl radicals. Under favorable conditions (low temperature, AOXs present, and absence of catalysts), hydroperoxides are relatively stable, but may otherwise catalyze auto-oxidation (Kamal-Eldin et al. 2002). At hydroperoxide concentrations beyond the critical level for a system, PUFA decomposition and oxidation rate increases rapidly. During propagation, the rate of formation is greater than the rate of decomposition, which is then reversed during the termination phase so that hydroperoxide decomposition is dominant.

The relative rate of oxidation increases as the number of double bonds within a fatty acid increases. In comparison to 18:1 (1 unit), Holman and Elmer (1947) reported the relative rates of oxidation for 18:2, 18:3, and 20:4 to be 40, 80, and 160, respectively. In addition to the number of double bonds, the supramolecular orientations of hydroperoxides may affect the degree of oxidation. For example, tuna oil was more stable to oxidation than soybean oil because the hydroperoxides of the tuna

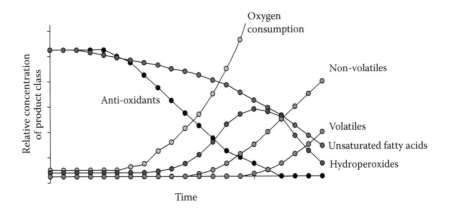

FIGURE 3.3 Kinetic curve of autoxidation of PUFAs over time. (Adapted from Labuza, T. P., *CRC Crit Rev Food Technol* 2 (3): 355–405, 1971.)

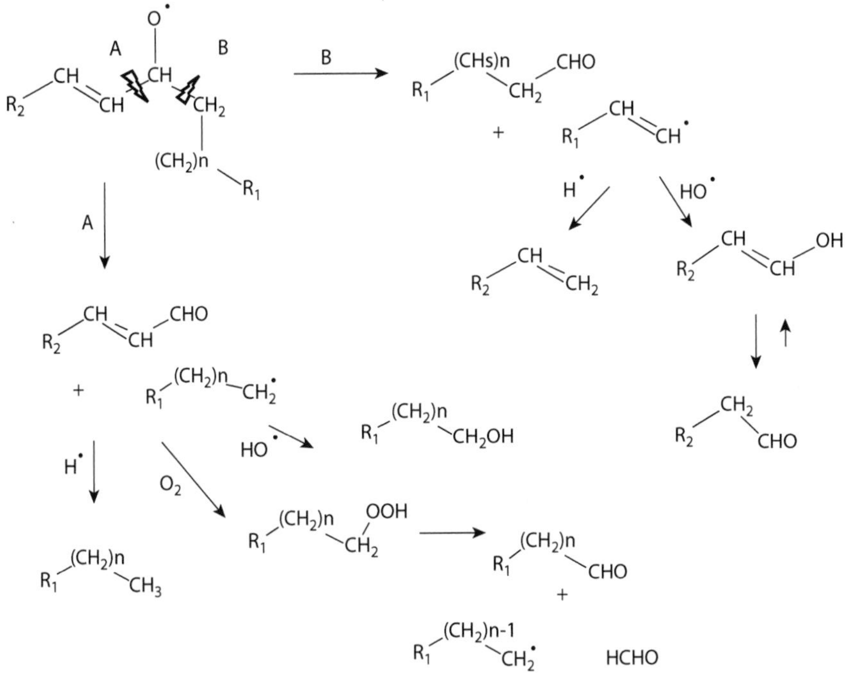

FIGURE 3.4 Alternative (A versus B) pathways of homolytic β-scission of monoperoxide fatty esters. Both pathways produce short-chain aldehydes and carbon-centered radicals that may either propagate or be quenched. (From Frankel, E. N., *Lipid Oxidation*, 2nd ed. Bridgewater, UK: The Oily Press, 2005. With permission.)

oil fatty acids were relatively "more bent," were more polar, and had an increased tendency to form micelles (Miyashita et al. 1995).

Temperature also regulates the rate of oxidation, increasing twofold for every 20°C rise from 40°C to 100°C (Lundberg and Chipault 1947). However, the variables that control the lipid oxidation at its initial stages may be poorly reproducible at low temperatures (Frankel 2005). This may include variations in the induction period (Lundberg and Chipault 1947; Lea and Ward 1959), which tend to become more stable as higher temperatures, up to 100°C, are approached (Kamal-Eldin et al. 2002). Lipid oxidation is frequently studied under accelerated conditions, such as in the Schaal oven, utilizing mild temperatures (40°C–60°C) (Wan 1995; Richards, Wijesundera, and Salisbury 2005). Other methods have been described for monitoring oxidation at elevated temperatures (≥100°C), such as the active oxygen method, Rancimat, oxidative stability index (OSI), and by the measurement of oxygen absorption rates. Apart from heating, lipid oxidation may also be accelerated by light exposure and metal-catalyzed oxidation. However, the array of products differs between low and high temperatures and other oxidative stimuli. In particular, light-induced photooxidation involves a different mechanism than auto-oxidation, driven by oxygen radicals.

Effects of accelerated stability tests at relatively low temperatures (40°C–60°C) were found to correlate well with storage at room temperature for predicting the shelf life of virgin olive oil (Gomez-Alonso, Salvador, and Fregapane 2004). However, increased temperature increased the rate of metal-catalyzed oxidation and promoted prooxidant activity by tocopherols naturally present in oils (Frankel 2005). Oxidation can be catalyzed by metal ions, in particular, copper and iron; however, the combination of metals and hydroperoxides is more reactive than metal alone (Frankel 1999). Conversely, some metal ions and trace levels of divalent sulfur, which can arise from glucosinolate decomposition, for example, in canola oil (Devinat, Biasini, and Naudet 1980), can behave as AOXs by stabilizing hydroperoxy radicals. The lipid-derived oxidation products associated with specific foods are summarized in Table 3.1 (see also Chapter 4).

3.4   OXIDATION PATHWAYS AND PRODUCTS OF FOOD CARBOHYDRATES

Carbohydrates represent a macronutrient whose purpose in food is to supply metabolizable energy to plants and animals (starch and glycogen, respectively) and non-metabolizable fiber (cellulose). Carbohydrates appear in the diet as either polysaccharides of 2 to 1000 monosaccharide units or as simple monosaccharide sugars per se. Monosaccharides, such as glucose and fructose, are found in fruits and honey, whereas galactose is released by the action of lactase on lactose. Disaccharides such as sucrose, maltose, cellobiose, and lactose are found in sugarcane, hydrolyzed starch, hydrolyzed cellulose, and milk, respectively. Polysaccharides such as starch are found in potatoes and corn, while cellulose is the key structural element of plant cell walls. Glycogen, a polysaccharide of glucose, is found in muscle tissue. In addition, oxidized forms of polysaccharides are widely used as food ingredients for texturizing, which are largely redox-stable in this form. The nature of oxidation processes and products relevant to food carbohydrates is discussed below. Strategically functionalized forms of monosaccharides are proposed to form the basis of new, "green" synthetic chemical processes for producing polymeric materials (Lichtenthaler and Peters 2004). The carbohydrate-derived oxidation products associated with specific foods are summarized in Table 3.1.

3.4.1 Carbohydrates in Plants

Living plants cycle energy in pathways that involve mobilization of carbohydrates and proteins and redox-coupled reactions. Vitamins E and C defend proteins and cell membranes against peroxidation, whereas plant wall celluloses are susceptible to oxidative hydrolysis in the presence of low levels of hydrogen peroxide as can be generated from NADH by cellular peroxidases (PODs) (Miller 1986). The suite of products includes oligosaccharides and low molecular mass reducing sugars with the rate of hydrolysis dependent on polysaccharide and pH (Miller 1986). Oxidation of sugars leads to a range of products with increasing unsaturation and consequent ability to behave as AOXs, which suppress ongoing oxidation (Russo et al. 2006). Soluble sugars are involved in metabolic reactions that regulate oxidative stress by either mediating production of ROS or stimulating synthesis of AOXs, such as carotenoids (Couee et al. 2006). The exposure of plants to biotic and abiotic stresses or normal ripening and senescence processes leads to progressive hydrolysis and oxidation of carbohydrates (Purvis 1997), the extent of which can be measured by the ratio of polysaccharides to simple (reducing) sugars and levels of polyphenol synthesis.

3.4.2 Carbohydrates in Milk

The major disaccharide in bovine milk, lactose, can be enzymatically oxidized to lactobionic acid using cellobiose dehydrogenase (Maischberger et al. 2008) or chemically oxidized by the use of metal catalysis (Chia, Latusek, and Holles 2008). However, thermal stressing of milk is more likely to generate oxygen-independent Maillard reaction products, such as hydroxyl-methyl furfural or furosine, or promote lactose crystallization (Thomsen et al. 2005).

3.4.3 Oxidation Chemistry of Sugars and Alcohols

The generic representation of sugars termed "aldoses" forms oxidation products of three classes (Figure 3.5). Aldonic acids are formed by either chemical, electrochemical, photochemical, or biochemical methods of oxidation. Lactobionic acid from lactose is an aldonic acid. Aqueous solutions of aldonic acids equilibrate between acid and either four-member or five-member ring lactones (De Lederkremer and Marino 2003), whereas under dehydrating conditions, intermolecular esterification is additionally possible.

Glucuronic acids are also susceptible to formation of lactones but usually occur as units of naturally occurring polysaccharides. Adducts of glucuronic acid of some drugs are formed in the liver to facilitate excretion. D-glucuronic acid is present in several

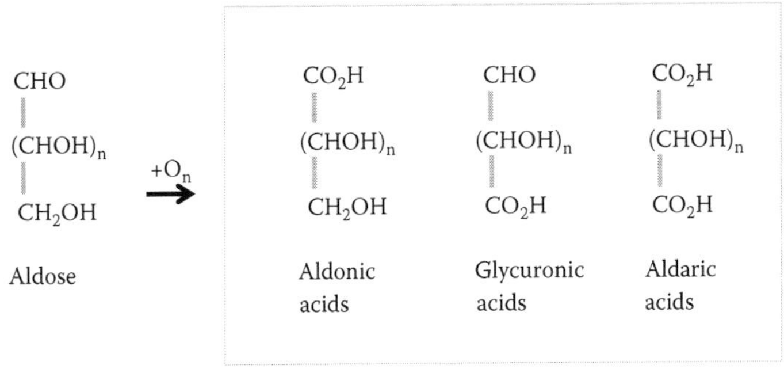

$$
\begin{array}{c}
\text{CHO} \\
| \\
\text{(CHOH)}_n \quad \xrightarrow{+O_n} \\
| \\
\text{CH}_2\text{OH} \\
\\
\text{Aldose}
\end{array}
\qquad
\begin{array}{c}
\text{CO}_2\text{H} \\
| \\
\text{(CHOH)}_n \\
| \\
\text{CH}_2\text{OH} \\
\\
\text{Aldonic} \\
\text{acids}
\end{array}
\qquad
\begin{array}{c}
\text{CHO} \\
| \\
\text{(CHOH)}_n \\
| \\
\text{CO}_2\text{H} \\
\\
\text{Glycuronic} \\
\text{acids}
\end{array}
\qquad
\begin{array}{c}
\text{CO}_2\text{H} \\
| \\
\text{(CHOH)}_n \\
| \\
\text{CO}_2\text{H} \\
\\
\text{Aldaric} \\
\text{acids}
\end{array}
$$

FIGURE 3.5 General structure of sugar acids that are oxidized forms of the corresponding aldose. Note that glycuronic acids are usually formed from a glycoside (i.e., glycone plus aglycone adduct). (Adapted from De Lederkremer, R. M., and C. Marino, *Adv Carbohydr Chem Biochem* 58: 199–306, 2003.)

important animal polysaccharides, such as heparin sulfate, chondroitin sulfates, and hyaluronic acid, and in the hemicelluloses of some plants. Glucuronic acids may also be present as a glycosidic linkage to plant flavonols and is a component of many bacterially expressed polysaccharides (De Lederkremer and Marino 2003). Aldaric acids require strong oxidizing conditions to form from their corresponding aldoses, such as treatment with hydrogen peroxide in the presence of iron salts (De Lederkremer and Marino 2003). Galactaric acid is the aldaric acid produced from lactose oxidation.

Primary hydroxyl groups are commonly present on neutral sugars (aldoses) and polysaccharides and represent an important target for oxidation into products with industrial significance. For example, aldehydes and hemi-acetals are useful precursors for further controlled polymerization, whereas polyuronic acids have thickening and gel-forming functionality when added to foods (Ponedel'kina, Khaibrakhmanova, and Odinokov 2010). These products would not normally undergo further oxidation in foods unless subjected to strongly oxidizing conditions.

3.5 OXIDATION PATHWAYS AND PRODUCTS OF ANTIOXIDANTS IN FOODS

AOXs delay or inhibit oxidation of food molecules by scavenging species that initiate peroxidation, by chelating metal ions so that they are unable to generate reactive species, by quenching singlet oxygen preventing formation of peroxides, by breaking auto-oxidative chain reactions, and by reducing localized oxygen concentration (Brewer 2011). These processes ultimately result in their sacrificial oxidation. Food AOXs are also highly susceptible to enzymatic and nonenzymatic oxidation during processing and storage of foods, which is one of the requirements of being a potent AOX (Shingai et al. 2011). The rate of oxidative degradation of AOX compounds depends on their chemical structure and physical form, oxygen concentration, presence of metals and enzymes, exposure to light, processing and storage temperatures, and the structure and composition of the food matrix. The major oxidation pathways of AOXs in foods, including phenolics, ascorbic acid, tocopherols, and carotenoids, are described below, and the AOX-derived oxidation products associated with specific foods are summarized in Table 3.1.

3.5.1 Phenolic Compounds

The main oxidation suppression mechanism of phenolic AOXs is free-radical scavenging (Shingai et al. 2011; Brewer 2011), although flavonoids can also chelate metal ions (Brewer 2011). As AOXs, phenolic compounds donate hydrogen to peroxy radicals resulting in phenolic radicals. The phenolic radicals react with each other to progressively form phenolic dimers or phenolic quinones with the regeneration of phenolic AOXs. The phenolic radicals may also further react with peroxy radicals to form phenolic peroxy species adducts, which undergo further degradation. Phenolic compounds are also oxidized by singlet oxygen (Choe and Min 2009).

Phenolic compounds are also susceptible to enzymatic oxidation during processing and storage. The main enzymes that are believed to be involved in the oxidation of phenolic compounds are polyphenol oxidase (PPO) and POD. PPO catalyzes two different reactions in the presence of molecular oxygen: the hydroxylation of monophenols to diphenols and the oxidation of diphenols to o-quinones. The o-quinones, which are yellow in color, are highly unstable and either react with high molecular weight polymers or form macromolecular complexes with amino acids and proteins. The nonenzymatic polymerization of these intermediate compounds and condensation of o-quinones give rise to heterogeneous black, brown, or red pigments commonly called melanins, which are the main cause of enzymatic browning of food products (Tomas-Barberan and Espin 2001). Anthocyanins, the glycosylated flavonoids, are not good substrates of PPO because of steric hindrance by the sugar moiety. However, the removal of the sugar moiety by the action of β-glucosidase results in the formation of anthocyanidins, which can be oxidized by PPO (Zhang et al. 2003). Anthocyanins also undergo co-oxidation in the presence of PPO and diphenols because the highly reactive PPO oxidation products, quinones, oxidize anthocyanins with the partial regeneration of the diphenolic cosubstrate (Patras et al. 2010). POD catalyzes the oxidation of phenolic compounds into quinones in the presence of hydrogen peroxide (Tomas-Barberan and Espin 2001). Nonenzymatic autoxidation of polyphenols into quinones and further degradation products also occurs during thermal processing and storage of food products (Cilliers and Singleton 1991; Talcott and Howard 1999; Patras et al. 2010).

3.5.2 Tocopherols

Tocopherols are fat-soluble AOXs, which are a family of derivatives of the monophenolic chromanol ring substituted by an aliphatic side chain (Figure 3.6), which permits penetration into biological membranes. Tocopherols donate hydrogen at the 6-hydroxy group on the chromanol ring to a peroxy radical resulting in a hydroperoxide and a tocopherol radical (Figure 3.6). The tocopherol radical can further react with a lipid peroxy radical to produce tocopherol quinone or react with another tocopherol radical to form a tocopherol dimer (Choe and Min 2009; Verleyen et al. 2001). The reaction of tocopherols with singlet oxygen produces tocopherol

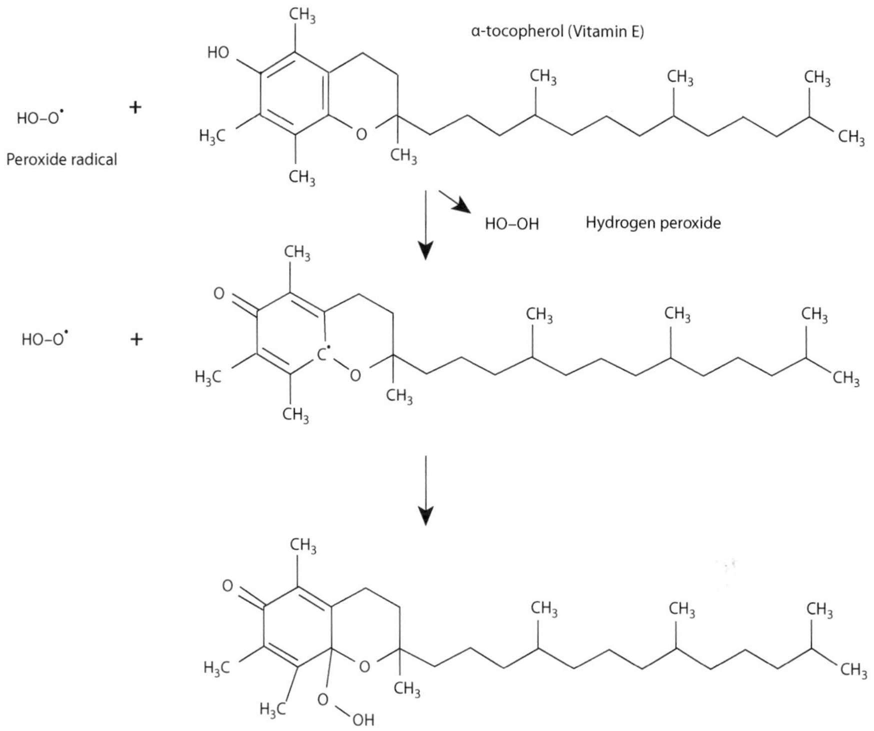

FIGURE 3.6 Structure of chromanol ring and mechanism of peroxide radical addition to α-tocopherols including vitamin E.

hydroperoxydienone, tocopherylquinone, and quinone epoxide (Choe and Min 2009). Tocopherols are relatively heat stable. Significant degradation of tocopherols occurs during processing mainly as a consequence of lipid oxidation (Hidalgo and Brandolini 2010; Tiwari and Cummins 2009). Co-oxidation of tocopherols occurs during the enzymatic peroxidation of unsaturated fatty acids by lipoxygenase (LOX), and the inactivation of the enzyme slows down the oxidative degradation of tocopherols (Hakansson and Jagerstad 1990).

3.5.3 ASCORBIC ACID

Ascorbic acid falls within the class of enolic lactones of glyculosonic acids. The most important member is vitamin C or *L*-ascorbic acid, which is water-soluble and widely present in citrus fruits. Ascorbic acid is reversibly oxidized to dehydroascorbic acid (Figure 3.7), and this redox couple mediates H-transfer at the 4-hydroxyl group (i.e., AOX) reactions with important consequences for plant and animal life. The hydroxyl groups on adjacent carbon atoms of ascorbic acid can also chelate metal ions and quench singlet oxygen (Brewer 2011). H-atom transfer from ascorbic acid to a food-based radical stabilizes the food component against oxidation. Further oxidation of

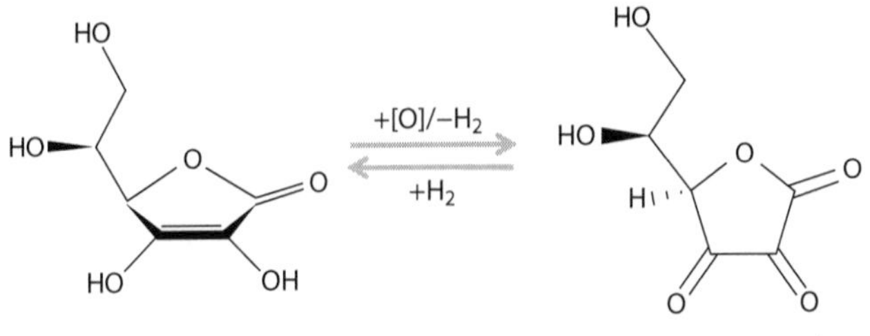

FIGURE 3.7 Structure of *L*-ascorbic acid (vitamin C) and its oxidation to dehydroascorbic acid.

dehydroascorbic acid leads to the irreversible formation of 2,3-diketogulonic acid, which further degrades into more than 50 types of degradation products containing less than five carbons (Deutsch et al. 1994). Ascorbic acid also reacts with singlet oxygen resulting in the formation of the unstable peroxide of ascorbic acid (Choe and Min 2009). Ascorbic acid in plants is highly susceptible to degradation during food processing and shelf storage (Phillips et al. 2010). Significant oxidation of ascorbic acid to dehydroascorbic acid also occurs during storage of vegetables (Podsedek 2007). Ascorbic acid oxidase is responsible for the enzymatic oxidation of ascorbic acid. Other enzymes, such as PPO and POD, are also believed to be involved in the oxidative degradation of ascorbic acid (Talcott et al. 2003).

3.5.4 CAROTENOIDS

Carotenoids are polyenoic terpenoids that have conjugated *trans* double bonds. By virtue of their conjugated double bonds, they are both free radical scavengers and quenchers of singlet oxygen (Choe and Min 2009). Carotenoids may donate hydrogen to lipid peroxy radicals producing a carotene radical. At low oxygen concentrations, the carotene radical may further react with a lipid peroxy radical to form nonradical carotene peroxides. Carotene radicals may also undergo oxygen addition and subsequent reaction with another carotene molecule producing carotene epoxides and carbonyl compounds of carotene (Choe and Min 2009) with 13, 11, 10, or 9 carbon atoms and retaining the terminal group of their carotenoid parent (Mendes-Pinto 2009). These carbonyl compounds are highly aromatic and include the family of ionones and damascones with oxygen at different positions (Mendes-Pinto 2009). Carotenoids are also involved in the chemical quenching of singlet oxygen. For instance, β-carotene reacts with singlet oxygen producing 5,8-endoperoxides of β-carotene (Choe and Min 2009). Carotenoids are, in general, relatively heat stable in their natural environment (Podsedek 2007). However, enzymatic oxidation of carotenoids takes place in plant-based products. Carotenoid cleaving deoxygenase catalyzes the enzymatic oxidation of carotenoids into aromatic carbonyl compounds (Mendes-Pinto 2009). Co-oxidation of carotenoids also occurs through the activities of LOX and PPO in the presence of free fatty acids and polyphenols, respectively (Aguedo et al. 2004; Dorantes-Alvarez and Chiralt 2000).

3.6 PATHWAYS AND PRODUCTS OF OXYGEN-MEDIATED CROSS-REACTIONS IN FOODS

In a mixed-food system, lipids are most vulnerable to oxidation and initiate attack of nonlipid substrates, either protein or carbohydrate. Cross-linking reactions can proceed rapidly in the absence of AOX termination, and the competition of radical attack between substrates reflects their relative abundance and physical proximity over the lifetime of the radical. Oxidative cross-reactivity of food systems will be discussed using meat and dairy products as examples.

Oxidation may be initiated by the formation of lipid peroxides. For example, in muscle meat, oxidation of linoleic acid produces HNE, which attacks myoglobin and propagates oxidation of the protein-bound iron (Faustman et al. 2010). Additionally, lipid oxidation results in a wide range of aldehyde products, which induce the oxidation of myoglobin to form metmyoglobin. Metmyoglobin formation is relatively accelerated by unsaturated versus saturated aldehydes of equivalent carbon chain length and for increasing aldehyde chain length (Faustman et al. 2010).

Bifunctional, usually α,β-unsaturated carbonyl compounds, such as HNE, 4-oxo-2-nonenal (ONE), and acrolein, generated from oxidation of PUFAs readily react with protein nucleophiles (Lee and Blair 2000). Analogous bifunctional aldehydes can produce intramolecular or intermolecular protein cross-links. Reorganization of initial adducts by tautomerization, oxidation, cyclization, dehydration, or condensation with a second aldehyde molecule (the same or different) can yield a range of possible stable advanced lipoxidation end products (ALEs) (Sayre et al. 2006).

Oxidation may also be driven by protein radicals, in particular, by divalent Fe complexed in the heme ring of myoglobin. The catalytic activity of oxidized myoglobin, metmyoglobin is promoted by hydrogen peroxide. The reaction between hydrogen peroxide and metmyoglobin results in the formation of two active hypervalent myoglobin species, perferryl-myoglobin and ferryl-myoglobin, which are responsible for lipid oxidation (Chaijan 2008) of oxymyoglobin; both superoxide anion and hydrogen peroxide are produced and further react with iron to produce hydroxyl radicals. The hydroxyl radical has the ability to penetrate into the hydrophobic lipid region and facilitate lipid oxidation (Chaijan 2008). Thus, in muscle meat, lipid oxidation and myoglobin oxidation can occur concurrently in a mutually catalytic manner (see also Chapter 2).

In milk systems, oxidative processes have been extensively studied following light induction in order to understand the deterioration of quality during storage (Borle, Sieber, and Bosset 2001; Dalsgaard et al. 2007). The oxidation of milk proteins has also been studied following induction by lactoperoxidase–hydrogen peroxide (Ostdal et al. 2000) and by Cu–hydrogen peroxide systems (Wiking and Nielsen 2004). Oxidative changes in milk proteins and amino acids result in the consumption of AOX vitamins and development of off-flavors (Cadwallader and Howard 1997), which is attributed to production of dimethylsulfide (van Aardt et al. 2005).

Unsaturated lipids in milk undergo auto-oxidation as well as light-induced oxidation, which can be suppressed by riboflavin and ascorbic acid (Cadwallader and Howard 1997) and which are also correlated with development of off-flavors (Hedegaard et al. 2006). However, apart from the interaction of AOXs with protein (Ostdal, Skibsted, and Andersen 1997) and possibly lipid-localized radicals in milk, cross-reactivity between protein and lipid oxidative radicals appears to be either less prevalent or less studied compared to meat. The initiation of a lipid attack by oxidized protein radicals in milk was proposed (Ostdal et al. 2000), although the evidence from studies in a model system of β-casein treated with either Cu–hydrogen peroxide or the lipid oxidation product malondialdehyde, in which hydrolysis of β-casein was promoted (Wiking and Nielsen 2004), inferred the opposite to occur, that is, that proteins could be substrates to lipid oxidation products. Although it is likely that oxidation of milk systems leads to cross-reactivity between proteins, lipids, AOXs, and other substrates, the actual reactivity is likely to reflect the relative abundance of respective components, which is highly variable in processed forms of dairy products.

3.7 ANALYSIS OF OXIDATION PRODUCTS OF FOOD COMPONENTS

3.7.1 ANALYSIS OF FOOD PROTEIN OXIDATION PRODUCTS

The oxidation chemistry of proteins in foods reflects the natural abundance of amino acids susceptible to oxidation (i.e., cysteine, tryptophan, methionine) and the potential for thiol-disulfide- and di-tyrosine-mediated bridging between proteins. Cross-linking of proteins resulting from advanced Maillard processes is not primarily driven by oxidation and will not be considered. Oxidized forms of free amino acids (e.g., taurine, carnosine) in meats and several amino acids in grains represent a distinct class of potential products. Metal-binding proteins, such as myoglobin in meat, are susceptible to accelerated oxidation resulting from the electron exchange between oxygen and ferrous ions that enhances redox lability and the rate of oxygen-driven reactivity. A range of other chemical processes, particularly Maillard chemistry involving attachment of sugars to proteins, can lead to cross-linking and may need to be analyzed in order to distinguish the specific contribution of non-Maillard oxidative processes to protein cross-linking.

A very wide range of experimental methods are known for probing changes in protein structure resulting from oxidation or other processes. These include detection of changes in accessibility of hydrophobic domains or "hydrophobicity" using fluorescent ligands or denaturation status, including characterizing native and non-native folding intermediates. Such methods may be useful provided that the effect is linked with an oxidative process. A summary of the methods used for analysis of oxidation products of proteins in foods is given in Table 3.3.

Analysis of oxidized forms of proteins can be achieved by either direct chemical analysis of products or the progress of oxidation monitored indirectly by detecting an effect on a physical, structural, sensory, or other property. Cross-linking between high mass protein molecules can be readily detected with size-based analytical techniques,

TABLE 3.3

Summary of Analytical Methods for Detecting Oxidation Products of Major Chemical Classes Present in Foods

Chemical Class	Target Analyte for Characterizing OP in Class	Analytical Methods	Indirect or Surrogate Methods
Proteins, peptides, and amino acids	Disulfide-cross-linked proteins and peptides; oxidized forms of taurine, carnosine, and tryptophan; dityrosine cross-linked proteins and peptides	PAGE, capillary gel electrophoresis, HPLC, LC-MS with PIR technology, fluorescence spectroscopy	Oxygen consumption, rheology, light scatter, solubility, molecular size
Lipids	Secondary oxidation products of short-, medium-, and long-chain fatty acids, malondialdehyde	HPLC (reverse and normal phase), HPLC-MS, GC-MS, GC-electronic nose	Oxygen consumption, sensory detection of rancid odors and flavors, PV, thiobarbituric acid reacting substances, anisidine value
Carbohydrates	Oxidized sugars and oligosaccharides		Oxygen consumption
AOXs	Oxidized vitamins, polymerized polyphenolics, quinones, ratio of oxidized/reduced form: Fe^{3+}/Fe^{2+} Cu^{2+}/Cu^+	Colorimetric assays coupling AOX with redox-sensitive reagent, HPLC (reverse and normal phase), HPLC-MS	Oxygen consumption, color change or bleaching, molecular size

such as polyacrylamide gel electrophoresis (PAGE) using surfactants such as sodium dodecyl sulfate (SDS) and, optionally, reducing agents to dissociate protein subunits (Huff-Lonergan and Lonergan 2005). SDS-PAGE can be also conducted by capillary gel electrophoresis (Bennett et al. 1994) and using gel permeation chromatography with strongly chaotropic mobile phases (urea, guanidine hydrochloride). With careful experimental design, changes in the extent of protein cross-linking resulting from posttranslational oxidative processes can be quantified. Native cross-linkages in proteins are important determinants of structure, which are usually distinguishable from process-driven cross-linking, often accompanied by denaturation, leading to structural scrambling. Alternatively, these changes may be detectable by changes in macroscopic properties, such as viscosity, solubility, or light scattering (Table 3.3).

Detection of site-specific cross-linking can be achieved with chromatography and mass spectrometry with recent advances involving protein interaction report (PIR) technology (Tang and Bruce 2010). If the specific nature and location of cross-linkages are important, then chemical methods for freezing the three-dimensional cross-linked structure using exogenous cross-linking agents, followed by enzymatic digestion and mass spectroscopic analysis, can be undertaken (Sinz 2006; Bitan

2006). In-depth proteomic analysis is necessary to identify digestive fragments produced from nonnative configurations of cross-linked proteins.

Di-tyrosine cross-links are specifically representative of oxidative stress and conveniently detected by fluorescence spectroscopy (Balasubramanian and Kanwar 2002). The elevation of di-tyrosine cross-linked proteins in the brains of Alzheimer's disease patients was detected by high performance liquid chromatography (HPLC) with electrochemical array detection (Hensley et al. 1998). Several oxidation products of tryptophan have been identified and synthesized for use as standards to support HPLC-based analysis with simple ultraviolet (UV) detection (Simat, Meyer, and Steinhart 1994). Taurine and carnosine are widely reported for their AOX activity (Jamilah et al. 2009), although less attention has been paid to the chemical elucidation of their oxidation products.

The production of carbonyl residues on proteins is typically measured by derivatization with 2,4-Dinitrophenylhydrazine (DNPH, Brady's reagent) and detection by UV (Ochs et al. 2010) or mass spectroscopy (MS) (Armenteros et al. 2009). Other sensing techniques for carbonyl detection include ESR and fluorescence spectroscopy with or without HPLC separation. The loss of sulfhydryl groups is routinely measured by 5,5-dithiobis(2-nitrobenzoate) (DTNB, Ellman's reagent) derivatization with recent improvements to the method reported (Nakagami, Ban, and Maruta 2010), while the loss of the tryptophan chromophore is conveniently detected by changes in fluorescence.

3.7.2 Analysis of Food Lipid Oxidation Products

Initial phases of lipid oxidation can be detected by measuring the peroxide value (PV), which quantifies the levels of peroxides and hydroperoxides formed at that stage. However, these products are metastable with respect to secondary oxidation products, so the levels follow a bell-shape trend as oxidation progresses (Figure 3.3). For the purpose of quantifying oxidation products that indicate extent or potential extent of oxidation, it is therefore recommended that chemically stable, secondary oxidation products of lipids are targeted, namely, aldehydes or carboxylic acids. Either the oxidized derivatives of fatty acids can be detected collectively by high-performance size-exclusion chromatography of the polar lipid fraction (Summo, Bilancia, and Caponio 2008), or the complex array of products arising from oxidative β-cleavage at alternative unsaturated carbons can be detected by Matrix-Assisted Laser Desorption/Ionisation Time Of Flight Liquid Chromatography with Mass Spectrograph (MALDI-TOF LC-MS) (Calvano et al. 2011). In addition, the standard practice of derivatizing fatty acids as methyl esters for GC analysis is also applicable to oxidized fatty acids (Cryle and De Voss 2007), achieving very high analytical sensitivity. The volatile secondary oxidation products of lipids are commonly analyzed by headspace gas chromatography using either FID or MS detection, which are also very sensitive analytical techniques (Olsen et al. 2005). Lipids are usually fractionated into polar and nonpolar chemical classes before analysis by HPLC using a range of possible detection principles. Oxidation products of longer chain triacyl glycerols are nonvolatile and can be characterized by normal phase HPLC with MS detection (Steenhorst-Slikkerveer et al. 2000).

Analysis of oxidation of lipids in human tissues has been extensively characterized and related to status of oxidative stress *in vivo* (Mateos and Bravo 2007) and particularly relevant to consumed forms of animal and fish flesh. Malondialdehyde is derived from oxidation of PUFAs, whereas the enzymatic oxidation of arachidonic acid found in membrane phospholipids yields a complex series of isoprostanes (Mateos and Bravo 2007) that is more relevant to living tissue. A range of chromatographic methods for analysis of malondialdehyde have been described as summarized by Mateos and Bravo (2007).

As lipids are highly susceptible to oxidation, technological strategies (and biological processes *in vivo*) are employed to inhibit oxidation by the use of AOXs. The products arising from the "sacrificial" oxidation of an AOX species are described below; however, the competitive chemistry of oxidation of lipids in the presence of an AOX is complex and dependent on the AOX and the conditions, with prooxidative effects also known to occur (Kolanowski, Jaworska, and Weissbrodt 2007). For example, if multiple substrates are available to react with peroxyl radicals formed by the addition of oxygen across a diene linkage, including itself (autoxidation), as can occur with carotenoids, then the oxygen-scavenging capacity of the AOX is attenuated. Furthermore, combinations of AOXs may elicit synergistic effects, such as the stabilization of sardine oil by α-tocopherol and rosemary extract (Kolanowski, Jaworska, and Weissbrodt 2007). Conversely, some AOXs with phenol substituents, such as apigenin and naringenin, can increase oxidation rates (Kolanowski, Jaworska, and Weissbrodt 2007) as was also the case for olive oil in the presence of β-carotene (Zeb and Murkovic 2011). Without systematic modeling of the competitive kinetics of *all* oxygen-dependent reactions on a per system basis, clearly a prohibitively challenging problem, it is clear that an approach for empirical evaluation of OP is required, one that is applicable to either an ingredient, mixture, or food system. Such an approach for measuring an index of OP is proposed below.

3.7.3 ANALYSIS OF FOOD CARBOHYDRATE OXIDATION PRODUCTS

Beyond simple sugars and oligosaccharides, the structural complexity of carbohydrates poses a significant analytical challenge even before oxidative changes are considered. Carbohydrates may also be present as glycan conjugates of proteins, lipids, and polyphenolics, but only the carbohydrate residue will be considered here. Carbohydrate ingredients are commonly added to processed foods to control flavor, texture, and other functional properties so that a range of molecular sizes of carbohydrates may be present if both endogenous and exogenous carbohydrates are taken into account. An excellent review of food carbohydrate analysis was authored by Molnar-Perl (2000). Typical oxidized forms of carbohydrates will contain oxidized forms of simple sugars in addition to polysaccharides with hydroxyaldehydes and hydroxycarboxylic acids at terminal glycans.

Significant progress has been made in carbohydrate analysis in recent years so that high-resolution chromatographic separation, coupled with mass spectrometry and bioinformatics data management, now permits evaluation of the glycome characteristics of clinical samples (Yamada and Kakehi 2011). Since 2003, carbohydrate separation technology was further improved by the development of capillary

(Lamari et al. 2002; Lamari, Kuhn, and Karamanos 2003) and microchip electrophoresis in combination with online derivatization using 1-phenyl-3-methyl-5-pyrazolone (PMP) (Honda, Suzuki, and Taga 2003). However, derivatization introduces an inconvenient delay in carbohydrate analysis by miniaturized microchip electrophoresis, and these devices, developed for clinical samples, employ electrochemical detection (Suzuki and Honda 2003). Otherwise, methods involving standard online electrophoretic (capillary and slab gels) and chromatographic techniques (HPLC, GC, paper chromatography) have been described (Wang and Fang 2004).

Apart from electrochemical (pulsed amperometric) detection (PAD) or the refractive index (Wang and Fang 2004) of underivatized carbohydrates (Cataldi, Campa, and De Benedetto 2000), detection usually requires either preseparation or postseparation derivatization, of which a broad range of molecular species can be used for chemical specificity and compatibility with the intended detection instrumentation (Gao et al. 2003; Sanz and Martinez-Castro 2007; Ruiz-Matute et al. 2011). Underivatized carbohydrates require short wavelength UV detection (190 or 210 nm) where optical interference from reagents and a sample matrix may be prohibitive. Alternatively, derivatization typically provides for longer wavelength detectability of products (Molnar-Perl 2000). For example, oxidized derivatives of laminaran (extracted from *Laminaria digitata*) were selectively detected as adducts of either 8-aminonaphthalene-1,3,6-trisulfonic acid (ANTS) for hydroxyaldehydes by polyacrylamide electrophoresis or using tyrosine *t*-butyl ester (TBT) for hydroxycarboxylic acids (Ovalle et al. 2001). The potential for selectivity on the basis of specific function groups of carbohydrates, for example, aldehydes or carboxylic acids, or chiral substituents provides for even further analytical specificity (Harvey 2011).

In the context of detecting molecular markers of carbohydrate oxidation, oxidized forms of small sugars are readily identified by mass spectroscopy or can be identified by oxygen-dependent accumulation. The carbohydrate composition of most foods has been characterized (Molnar-Perl 2000) but not necessarily the oxidation products, which can be expected to vary depending on the oxidation conditions. Compared to other food components, focusing on carbohydrates as chemical markers of oxidation is relatively more complicated and is probably best undertaken only where necessary for carbohydrate-rich foods.

3.7.4 ANALYSIS OF OXIDATION PRODUCTS OF ANTIOXIDANTS IN FOODS

The focus of investigation into the effects of natural and chemical AOXs in foods has been primarily to monitor the effectiveness of the AOX in protecting the susceptible substrate, usually the lipid, either by direct oxygen attack or by metal ion-mediated oxidation (e.g., myoglobins in meat) (Richards and Dettmann 2003). In this context, the oxidation products of the AOX are not usually considered. However, in order to account for the AOX activity of a particular AOX species, such as a vitamin, it may be necessary to quantify the oxidation products and metabolites. For example, vitamin E protects against lipid oxidation in pork (Trefan et al. 2011) by initially scavenging peroxide radicals (Figure 3.6). HPLC-based methods are able to detect vitamin E and its oxidation products: α-tocopherylquinone, epoxy-α-tocopherylquinones, and 8α-lipid-dioxy-α-tocopherones in human plasma (Yamauchi et al. 2002) with additional products detected by gas chromatography coupled with mass spectros-copy detection (GC-MS) (Liebler et al. 1996). The subsequent Pt- or Zn-catalyzed reduction of oxidized derivatives of vitamin E by online methods (Yamauchi et al. 2002) inferred the redox lability of the starting products.

Methods for analysis of oxidation products of ascorbic acid have been reviewed by Washko et al. (1992) who favored HPLC-based methods as being more reliable and less prone to interference compared with indirect colorimetric assays. The oxi-dized forms of ascorbic acid, semi-dehydroascorbic acid (minus 1 electron) and dehydroascorbic acid (minus 2 electrons), are reversibly formed, whereas the hydro-lytic product 2,3-diketogulonic acid is irreversible.

The polyphenolic class of AOXs, present in tea, grapes (also wine), and other plants, has been highly researched in terms of chemical characterization (Perez-Jimenez et al. 2010) and AOX properties (Halvorsen et al. 2002). The basic oxida-tion chemistry of monophenols and diphenols is to form diphenols and o-quinones, respectively. For the linearly conjugated carotenoids, oxidation products include dihy-dro and epoxy-carotenes and apo-carotenoids (apocarotenals, apocarotenones, etc.). Analysis of carotenoids in colored avian appendages and in red yeasts has been suc-cessfully characterized by HPLC using either UV or MS detection (Garcia-de Blas et al. 2011; Weber, Anke, and Davoli 2007). Oxidation products of β-carotene (5,8-epox-ide and 6-apo-carotenal) were also analyzed by reverse phase HPLC and identified by Atmospheric-Pressure Chemical Ionization (APCI-MS, Zeb and Murkovic 2011).

Liquid chromatography coupled with mass spectrometric detection (LC-MS) has provided for capture of complex polyphenolic fingerprints and resolution of chemi-cal classes including glycosidic linkages (Ajila et al. 2011). Condensation reactions between the flavonoids present in tea because of chemical and enzymatic oxidation lead to polymeric theaflavins and tannin oxidation products (Wang and Ho 2009; Tanaka, Matsuo, and Kouno 2010). The fingerprint-like characteristics of polyphe-nolics in wine lend this feature to use for correlation with wine quality (Mazerolles et al. 2010), cultivar, and vintage (Pazourek et al. 2005).

It is the chemical heterogeneity of oxidation products resulting from AOXs that reflects their inherent role as AOXs: that is, to scavenge and then chemically dis-pose of adventitious ROS. While oxidation products of AOXs are usually eliminated from the body, in a static food system, the oxidation product is available for further chemical attack until its capacity to scavenge ROS is exhausted, or alternatively, AOX-localized radicals accumulate and attack the substrate intended for protection. Thus, the efficacy of AOXs is dose-, time-, and condition-dependent, and this further supports the need for an empirical approach to measuring OP.

3.8 PROPOSED INDEX OF FOOD OXIDATION POTENTIAL

In order to work toward measuring OP, first, the oxidation chemistry of major food components, separately and in blended foods, must be considered. The oxidation pathways for a blended food may differ from the oxidative chemical pathway of the isolated protein, carbohydrate, or lipid component. Oxidation pathways of specific substrates are likely to be affected by the physical properties and processing method of the food or ingredient. Consider, for example, the comparatively diverse states of a cooked carrot, a low-fat yogurt, a carbonated beverage, an emulsified salad dressing, or a dry baked product. Furthermore, the progression of oxidation in a piece of intact meat will be different from that of its homogenate dispersed in water. Thus, the OP of the system requires experimental evaluation under the ingredient state or environmental condition that provides a useful practical model of the system.

The OP of food reflects the susceptibility of suitable representative molecules from chemical classes present in the given food to undergo oxidative chemistry as a result of specific stresses, such as processing, cooking, and storage. The ratio of non-oxidized to oxidized products reflects the inherent antioxidizing capacity of the food system at any point in time. OP should reflect the oxygen dependence of the yield of a specific oxidation product (e.g., R) with established recognition as an oxidized molecular form associated with a chemical class or food category, for example, lipid hydroperoxide. The purpose of this chapter was to describe the oxidation chemistry of major chemical classes of foods, and identify oxidation products that might be suitable as standards and describe their methods for analysis for use in calculating OP.

Practically, it is necessary to measure a change in concentration of product R (i.e., $\Delta[R]$), or preferably change of *initial rate* of R (i.e., ΔR), to avoid anomalies resulting from reactants that may be present in limiting concentrations. The change in ΔR should reflect experimentally controlled progressive oxidation. Let us say that a standard condition for measuring ΔR involves sample incubation at 40°C for 24 h as depicted by the reaction coordinate under conditions where the concentration of an oxidant (oxygen, in this case) is regulated (Figure 3.8). The magnitude of ΔR will depend on the concentration of available oxygen with enhancement (Figure

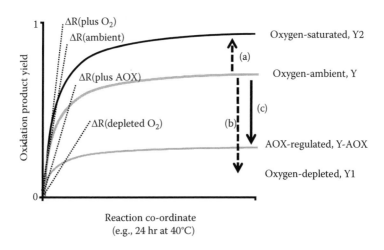

FIGURE 3.8 Schematic of proposed approach to measuring OP of food samples by determining change in rate of production (or depletion) of molecular species or surrogate property as a result of driving oxidation reaction to maximum (a), minimum (b), or AOX-modified extents (c).

3.8a), suppression (Figure 3.8b), or modulation (Figure 3.8c) of the oxidation rate as regulated by the concentration of oxygen or added AOX, respectively, leading to the following expected relationships: ΔR (plus O_2) > ΔR (ambient) > ΔR (plus AOX, ambient, or plus O_2) > ΔR (depleted O_2). Experimental determination of ΔR can be expressed as a series of ratios (of one or more chemical analytes or surrogate measures) that characterize the oxidation status and OP of the system as follows:

$$OP = \Delta R \text{ (plus } O_2)/\Delta R \text{ (ambient)} \tag{3.1}$$

$$OP_{max} = \Delta R \text{ (plus } O_2)/\Delta R \text{ (depleted } O_2) \tag{3.2}$$

$$OP_{mod} = 1 - [\Delta R \text{ (plus AOX)}/\Delta R \text{ (minus AOX)}] \tag{3.3}$$

Therefore, OP (Equation 3.1) characterizes the residual or inherent OP of the system with a value of 1 signifying exhausted and complete oxidation status of R, which cannot be further enhanced in the presence of excess oxygen, that is, ΔR (plus O_2) ~ ΔR (ambient). Usually, OP values would be >1 and increase to a maximum level under saturated oxygen conditions or for a low extent of oxidation of R under ambient conditions, leading to small values of ΔR (ambient). High values of OP signify the low endogenous AOX capacity of the system.

OP_{max} (Equation 3.2) represents the maximum potential for oxidation of the system with values of 1 to infinity increasing with increasing OP. An OP_{max} value of 1, that is, ΔR (plus O_2) ~ ΔR (depleted O_2), signifies that the system is highly stable and inert to oxidation.

OP_{mod} characterizes the OP of the system modified by an exogenous AOX and may be used to test and compare efficacy of AOX additives. Values of OP_{mod} scaled from 0 to 1 (Equation 3.3) can be adopted to indicate low to high efficacy of an added AOX in a given food system, reflected by increasing values of OP_{mod}. OP_{mod} can be conducted under either ambient or oxygen-saturated conditions to test the level of AOX required to stabilize the system under either status.

This approach seeks to link oxidation and oxidation suppression with a specific molecular species or class and enable the relative OP of different food chemical classes and food systems to be evaluated. In practical terms, it is envisaged that if it is not already in liquid form, a food sample would be dispersed to a minimum extent (say 50% w/w) to allow permeation of the gaseous oxidant (air or oxygen). The rate changes (ΔR, Figure 3.8) occurring after an incubation period under standardized conditions in a high, low, or modified (+AOX) oxidative environment would be measured by monitoring specific molecular species and/or a surrogate index of the system (Figure 3.9). The selection of suitable combinations of molecular markers and/or surrogate indices will be dependent on the particular food system with likely targets for respective chemical classes of food identified in Table 3.3 and discussed in this chapter. Over time, it is likely that the best analytes that offer useful dynamic ranges for characterizing the OP of particular foods and food ingredients will be identified

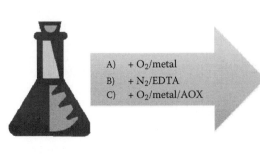

Measure changes in key molecular
markers of oxidation, e.g.
- Disulfide cross-links (proteins)
- Volatiles (lipids)
- Vitamin C or E oxidation (added AOX)
- Polyphenol polymerization
  (polyphenolics)

OR Changes in surrogate indices of
oxidation, e.g.
- Viscosity
- Molecular size
- Color
- Solubility

A)　+ O$_2$/metal
B)　+ N$_2$/EDTA
C)　+ O$_2$/metal/AOX

FIGURE 3.9 Practical aspects of measuring OP might involve a sample dispersed at 50% solids (or neat if already high water content) and incubation at 37°C for 24 h (or other standardized conditions). Alternative oxidation systems that might be adopted include Fenton reaction (Fe and hydrogen peroxide), UV irradiation, or enzyme-mediated.

and lead to a database of validated methods for shared use. The methods for analysis of oxidation products in foods are reviewed above and summarized in Table 3.3.

3.9 CONCLUSION

This chapter has aimed to review the chemistry of oxidation of food components and provide a general guide to the analytical methodology in current practice for detecting oxidized species, according to chemical class. Most importantly, by introducing the concept of OP and proposing a generic approach to its practical evaluation, we suggest that this information might find a use in (1) identifying the need for AOX protection and (2) demonstrating the comparative efficacy of preventing oxidation by different AOXs for specific food ingredients or systems.

REFERENCES

Aguedo, M., M. H. Ly, I. Belo, J. A. Teixeira, J. M. Belin, and Y. Wache. 2004. The use of enzymes and microorganisms for the production of aroma compounds from lipids. *Food Technol Biotechnol* 42: 327–336.
Ahern, T. J., and A. M. Klibanov. 1985. The mechanism of irreversible enzyme inactivation at 100-degrees-C. *Science* 228: 1280–1284.
Ajila, C. M., S. K. Brar, M. Verma, R. D. Tyagi, S. Godbout, and J. R. Valero. 2011. Extraction and analysis of polyphenols: Recent trends. *Crit Rev Biotechnol* 31: 227–249.
Armenteros, M., M. Heinonen, V. Illilainen, F. Toldra, and M. Estevez. 2009. Analysis of protein carbonyls in meat products by using the DNPH-method, fluorescence spectroscopy and liquid chromatography-electrospray ionisation-mass spectrometry (LC-ESI-MS). *Meat Sci* 83: 104–112.
Balasubramanian, D., and R. Kanwar. 2002. Molecular pathology of dityrosine cross-links in proteins: Structural and functional analysis of four proteins. *Mol Cel Biochem* 234: 27–38.
Bennett, L. E., W. N. Charman, D. B. Williams, and S. A. Charman. 1994. Analysis of bovine immunoglobulin-G by capillary gel-electrophoresis. *J Pharm Biomed Anal* 12: 1103–1108.

Bitan, G. 2006. Structural study of metastable amyloidogenic protein oligomers by photo-induced cross-linking of unmodified proteins. In *Amyloid, Prions, and Other Protein Aggregates, Pt C*, edited by I. Kheterpal and R. Wetzel, Academic Press, Waltham, MA, USA.

Borle, F., R. Sieber, and J. O. Bosset. 2001. Photo-oxidation and photoprotection of foods, with particular reference to dairy products—An update of a review article (1993–2000). *Sci Aliments* 21: 571–590.

Brewer, M. S. 2011. Natural antioxidants: Sources, compounds, mechanisms of action, and potential applications. *Comprehens Rev Food Sci Food Safety* 10: 221–247.

Cadwallader, K. R., and C. L. Howard. 1997. Analysis of aroma-active components in light-activated milk. *Abstr Pap Am Chem Soc* 214: 44–AGFD.

Calvano, C. D., I. D. van der Werf, F. Palmisano, and L. Sabbatini. 2011. Fingerprinting of egg and oil binders in painted artworks by matrix-assisted laser desorption ionization time-of-flight mass spectrometry analysis of lipid oxidation by-products. *Anal Bioanalyt Chem* 400: 2229–2240.

Cataldi, T. R. I., C. Campa, and G. E. De Benedetto. 2000. Carbohydrate analysis by high-performance anion-exchange chromatography with pulsed amperometric detection: The potential is still growing. *Fresenius J Analyt Chem* 368: 739–758.

Chaijan, M. 2008. Review: Lipid and myoglobin oxidation in muscle foods. *Songklanakarin J Food Sci Technol* 31: 47–53.

Chan, H. W. S. 1977. Photosensitized oxidation of unsaturated fatty-acid methyl-esters—Identification of different pathways. *J Am Oil Chem Soc* 54: 100–104.

Chia, Y. N., M. P. Latusek, and J. H. Holles. 2008. Catalytic wet oxidation of lactose. *Ind Eng Chem Res* 47: 4049–4055.

Choe, E., and D. B. Min. 2009. Mechanisms of antioxidants in the oxidation of foods. *Comprehens Rev Food Sci Food Safety* 8: 345–358.

Cilliers, J. J. L., and V. L. Singleton. 1991. Characterization of the products of nonenzymic autoxidative phenolic reactions in a caffeic acid model system. *J Agr Food Chem* 39: 1298–1303.

Couee, I., C. Sulmon, G. Gouesbet, and A. El Amrani. 2006. Involvement of soluble sugars in reactive oxygen species balance and responses to oxidative stress in plants. *J Exp Botany* 57: 449–459.

Cryle, M. J., and J. J. De Voss. 2007. Facile determination of the absolute stereochemistry of hydroxy fatty acids by GC: Application to the analysis of fatty acid oxidation by a P450(BM3) mutant. *Tetrahedron-Asymm* 18: 547–551.

Dalsgaard, T. K., D. Otzen, J. H. Nielsen, and L. B. Larsen. 2007. Changes in structures of milk proteins upon photo-oxidation. *J Agr Food Chem* 55: 10968–10976.

Davies, M. J. 2005. The oxidative environment and protein damage. *Biochim Biophys Acta-Proteins Proteomics* 1703: 93–109.

De Lederkremer, R. M., and C. Marino. 2003. Acids and other products of oxidation of sugars. *Adv Carbohydr Chem Biochem* 58: 199–306.

Deutsch, J. C., C. R. Santhoshkumar, K. L. Hassell, and J. F. Kolhouse. 1994. Variation in ascorbic-acid oxidation routes in H_2O_2 and cupric ion solution as determined by GC/MS. *Analyt Chem* 66: 345–350.

Devinat, G., S. Biasini, and M. Naudet. 1980. Sulfur-compounds in the rapeseed oils. *Rev Franc Corps Gras* 27: 229–236.

Dorantes-Alvarez, L., and A. Chiralt. 2000. Color of minimally processed fruits and vegetables as affected by some chemical and biochemical changes. In *Minimally Processed Fruits and Vegetables*, edited by S. M. Alzamora, M. S. Tapia and A. Lopez-Malo. Gaithersburg, MD: Aspen.

Estevez, M. 2011. Protein carbonyls in meat systems: A review. *Meat Sci* 89: 259–279.

Faustman, C., and R. G. Cassens. 1990. The biochemical basis for discoloration in fresh meat: A review. *J Muscle Foods* 1: 217–243.

Faustman, C., Q. Sun, R. Mancini, and S. P. Suman. 2010. Myoglobin and lipid oxidation interactions: Mechanistic bases and control. *Meat Sci* 86: 86–94.

Frankel, E. N. 1999. Food antioxidants and phytochemicals: Present and future perspectives. *Fett-Lipid* 101: 450–455.

Frankel, E. N. 2005. *Lipid Oxidation.* 2nd ed. Bridgewater, UK: The Oily Press.

Friedman, M. 1973. Displacement reactions III. Sulfhydryl-disulfide interchange and related equilibria. In *The Chemistry and Biochemistry of the Sulfhydryl Group in Amino Acids, Peptides and Proteins.* New York: Pergamon Press.

Gao, X. B., J. H. Yang, F. Huang, X. Wu, L. Li, and C. X. Sun. 2003. Progresses of derivatization techniques for analyses of carbohydrates. *Anal Lett* 36: 1281–1310.

Garcia-de Blas, E., R. Mateo, J. Vinuela, and C. Alonso-Alvarez. 2011. Identification of carotenoid pigments and their fatty acid esters in an avian integument combining HPLC-DAD and LC-MS analyses. *J Chromatog B-Analyt Technol Biomed Life Sci* 879: 341–348.

Gomez-Alonso, S., M. D. Salvador, and G. Fregapane. 2004. Evolution of the oxidation process in olive oil triacylglycerol under accelerated storage conditions (40–60 degrees C). *J Am Oil Chem Soc* 81: 177–184.

Hakansson, B., and M. Jagerstad. 1990. The effect of thermal inactivation of lipoxygenase on the stability of vitamin-e in wheat. *J Cereal Sci* 12: 177–185.

Halvorsen, B. L., K. Holte, M. C. W. Myhrstad, I. Barikmo, E. Hvattum, S. F. Remberg, A. B. Wold, K. Haffner, H. Baugerod, L. F. Andersen, J. O. Moskaug, D. R. Jacobs, and R. Blomhoff. 2002. A systematic screening of total antioxidants in dietary plants. *J Nutr* 132: 461–471.

Harvey, D. J. 2011. Derivatization of carbohydrates for analysis by chromatography; electrophoresis and mass spectrometry. *J Chromatogr B-Analyt Technol Biomed Life Sci* 879: 1196–1225.

Hedegaard, R. V., D. Kristensen, J. H. Nielsen, M. B. Frost, H. Ostdal, J. E. Hermansen, M. Kroger-Ohlen, and L. H. Skibsted. 2006. Comparison of descriptive sensory analysis and chemical analysis for oxidative changes in milk. *J Dairy Sci* 89: 495–504.

Hensley, K., M. L. Maidt, Z. Q. Yu, H. Sang, W. R. Markesbery, and R. A. Floyd. 1998. Electrochemical analysis of protein nitrotyrosine and dityrosine in the Alzheimer brain indicates region-specific accumulation. *J Neurosci* 18: 8126–8132.

Hidalgo, A., and A. Brandolini. 2010. Tocols stability during bread, water biscuit and pasta processing from wheat flours. *J Cereal Sci* 52: 254–259.

Holman, R. T., and O. C. Elmer. 1947. The rates of oxidation of unsaturated fatty acids and esters. *J Am Oil Chem Soc* 24: 127–129.

Honda, S., S. Suzuki, and A. Taga. 2003. Analysis of carbohydrates as 1-phenyl-3-methyl-5-pyrazolone derivatives by capillary/microchip electrophoresis and capillary electrochromatography. *J Pharm Biomed Anal* 30: 1689–1714.

Huff-Lonergan, E., and S. M. Lonergan. 2005. Mechanisms of water-holding capacity of meat: The role of postmortem biochemical and structural changes. *Meat Sci* 71: 194–204.

Jamilah, B., A. Mohamed, K. A. Abbas, R. A. Rahman, and R. Karim. 2009. A review on the effect of animal diets and presence of selected natural antioxidants on lipid oxidation of meat. *J Food Agr Env* 7: 76–81.

Kamal-Eldin, A., M. Makinen, A. M. Lampi, and A. Hopia. 2002. A multivariate study of alpha-tocopherol and hydroperoxide interaction during the oxidation of methyl linoleate. *Eur Food Res Technol* 214: 52–57.

Kanner, J. 1994. Oxidative processes in meat and meat-products—Quality implications. *Meat Sci* 36: 169–189.

Kolanowski, W., D. Jaworska, and J. Weissbrodt. 2007. Importance of instrumental and sensory analysis in the assessment of oxidative deterioration of omega-3 long-chain polyunsaturated fatty acid-rich foods. *J. Sci Food Agric* 87: 181–191.

Kosen, P. A. 1992. Disulfide bonds in proteins. In *Stability of Protein Pharmaceuticals. Part A. Chemical and Physical Pathways of Protein Degradation*, edited by T. Ahern and M. Manning. New York: Plenum Press.

Labuza, T. P. 1971. Kinetics of lipid oxidation in foods. *CRC Crit Rev Food Technol* 2: 355–405.

Lamari, F. N., X. M. Gioldassi, T. N. Mitropoulou, and N. K. Karamanos. 2002. Structure analysis of lipoglycans and lipoglycan-derived carbohydrates by capillary electrophoresis and mass spectrometry. *Biomed Chromatogr* 16: 116–126.

Lamari, F. N., R. Kuhn, and N. K. Karamanos. 2003. Derivatization of carbohydrates for chromatographic, electrophoretic and mass spectrometric structure analysis. *J Chromatogr B-Analyt Technol Biomed Life Sci* 793: 15–36.

Lea, C.H., and R. J. Ward. 1959. Relative anti-oxidant activities of the seven tocopherols. *J Sci Food Agr* 10: 537–548.

Lee, S. H., and I. A. Blair. 2000. Characterization of 4-oxo-2-nonenal as a novel product of lipid peroxidation. *Chem Res Toxicol* 13: 698–702.

Lichtenthaler, F. W., and S. Peters. 2004. Carbohydrates as green raw materials for the chemical industry. *Compt R Chimie* 7: 65–90.

Liebler, D. C., J. A. Burr, L. Philips, and A. J. L. Ham. 1996. Gas chromatography mass spectrometry analysis of vitamin E and its oxidation products. *Anal Biochem* 236: 27–34.

Lund, M. N., M. Heinonen, C. P. Baron, and M. Estevez. 2011. Protein oxidation in muscle foods: A review. *Mol Nutr Food Res* 55: 83–95.

Lundberg, W. O., and J. R. Chipault. 1947. The oxidation of methyl linoleate at various temperatures. *J Am Chem Soc* 69: 833–836.

Maischberger, T., T. H. Nguyen, P. Sukyai, R. Kittl, S. Riva, R. Ludwig, and D. Haltrich. 2008. Production of lactose-free galacto-oligosaccharide mixtures: Comparison of two cellobiose dehydrogenases for the selective oxidation of lactose to lactobionic acid. *Carbohydr Res* 343: 2140–2147.

Manning, M. C., K. Patel, and R. T. Borchardt. 1989. Stability of protein pharmaceuticals. *Pharm Res* 6: 903–918.

Mateos, R., and L. Bravo. 2007. Chromatographic and electrophoretic methods for the analysis of biomarkers of oxidative damage to macromolecules (DNA, lipids, and proteins). *J Separat Sci* 30: 175–191.

Mazerolles, G., S. Preys, C. Bouchut, E. Meudec, H. Fulcrand, J. M. Souquet, and V. Cheynier. 2010. Combination of several mass spectrometry ionization modes: A multiblock analysis for a rapid characterization of the red wine polyphenolic composition. *Analyt Chim Acta* 678: 195–202.

Mendes-Pinto, M. M. 2009. Carotenoid breakdown products the-norisoprenoids-in wine aroma. *Arch Biochem Biophys* 483: 236–245.

Miller, A. R. 1986. Oxidation of cell-wall polysaccharides by hydrogen-peroxide—A potential mechanism for cell-wall breakdown in plants. *Biochem Biophys Res Comm.* 141: 238–244.

Mitsumoto, M., R. N. Arnold, D. M. Schaefer, and R. G. Cassens. 1993. Dietary versus post-mortem supplementation of vitamin E on pigment and lipid stability in ground beef. *J Anim Sci* 71: 1812–1816.

Miyashita, K., M. Hirao, E. Nara, and T. Ota. 1995. Oxidative stability of triglycerides from orbital fat of tuna and soybean oil in an emulsion. *Fish Sci* 61: 273–275.

Molnar-Perl, I. 2000. Role of chromatography in the analysis of sugars, carboxylic acids and amino acids in food. *J Chromatogr A* 891: 1–32.

Mozhaev, V. V., and K. Martinek. 1982. Inactivation and reactivation of proteins (enzymes). *Enzyme Microb Technol* 4: 299–309.

Nakagami, Y., N. Ban, and K. Maruta. 2010. An improved method (TCEP-DTNB method) to determine serum sulfhydryl groups. *J Physiol Sci* 60: S197–S197.

Ochs, S. D., M. Fasciotti, R. P. Barreto, N. G. de Figueiredo, F. C. Albuquerque, M. Massa, I. Gabardo, and A. D. P. Netto. 2010. Optimization and comparison of HPLC and RRLC conditions for the analysis of carbonyl-DNPH derivatives. *Talanta* 81: 521–529.

Olsen, E., G. Vogt, D. Ekeberg, M. Sandbakk, J. Pettersen, and A. Nilsson. 2005. Analysis of the early stages of lipid oxidation in freeze-stored pork back fat and mechanically recovered poultry meat. *J Agr Food Chem* 53: 338–348.

Ostdal, H., M. J. Bjerrum, J. A. Pedersen, and H. J. Andersen. 2000. Lactoperoxidase-induced protein oxidation in milk. *J Agr Food Chem* 48: 3939–3944.

Ostdal, H., L. H. Skibsted, and H. J. Andersen. 1997. Formation of long-lived protein radicals in the reaction between H2O2-activated metmyoglobin and other proteins. *Free Radic Biol Med* 23: 754–761.

Ovalle, R., C. E. Soll, F. Lim, C. Flanagan, T. Rotunda, and P. N. Lipke. 2001. Systematic analysis of oxidative degradation of polysaccharides using PAGE and HPLC-MS. *Carbohydr Res* 330: 131–139.

Patras, A., N. P. Brunton, C. O'Donnell, and B. K. Tiwari. 2010. Effect of thermal processing on anthocyanin stability in foods: Mechanisms and kinetics of degradation. *Trends Food Sci Technol* 21: 3–11.

Pazourek, J., D. Gajdosova, M. Spanila, M. Farkova, K. Novotna, and J. Havel. 2005. Analysis of polyphenols in wines: Correlation between total polyphenolic content and antioxidant potential from photometric measurements—Prediction of cultivars and vintage from capillary zone electrophoresis fingerprints using artificial neural network. *J Chromatogr A* 1081: 48–54.

Perez-Jimenez, J., V. Neveu, F. Vos, and A. Scalbert. 2010. Systematic analysis of the content of 502 polyphenols in 452 foods and beverages: An application of the phenol-explorer database. *J Agr Food Chem* 58: 4959–4969.

Phillips, K. M., M. T. Tarrago-Trani, S. E. Gebhardt, J. Exler, K. Y. Patterson, D. B. Haytowitz, P. R. Pehrsson, and J. M. Holden. 2010. Stability of vitamin C in frozen raw fruit and vegetable homogenates. *J Food Compos Anal* 23: 253–259.

Podsedek, A. 2007. Natural antioxidants and antioxidant capacity of *Brassica* vegetables: A review. *LWT-Food Sci Technol* 40: 1.

Ponedel'kina, I. Y., E. A. Khaibrakhmanova, and V. N. Odinokov. 2010. Nitroxide-catalyzed selective oxidation of alcohols and polysaccharides. *Russian Chem Rev* 79: 63–75.

Porter, W. L. 1980. Recent trends in food applications of antioxidants. In *Autoxidation in Food and Biological Systems*, edited by M. Simic and M. Karel. New York: Plenum Press.

Purvis, A. C. 1997. The role of adaptive enzymes in carbohydrate oxidation by stressed and senescing plant tissues. *Hortscience* 32: 1165–1168.

Richards, A., C. Wijesundera, M. Palmer, and P. Salisbury. 2004. Regiospecific triacylglycerol composition of some cooking oils consumed in Australia. *Food Aust* 56: 365–372.

Richards, A., C. Wijesundera, and P. Salisbury. 2005. Evaluation of oxidative stability of canola oils by headspace analysis. *J Am Oil Chem Soc* 82: 869–874.

Richards, M. P., and M. A. Dettmann. 2003. Comparative analysis of different hemoglobins: Autoxidation, reaction with peroxide, and lipid oxidation. *J Agr Food Chem* 51: 3886–3891.

Ruiz-Matute, A. I., O. Hernandez-Hernandez, S. Rodriguez-Sanchez, M. L. Sanz, and I. Martinez-Castro. 2011. Derivatization of carbohydrates for GC and GC-MS analyses. *J Chromatogr B-Analyt Technol Biomed Life Sci* 879: 1226–1240.

Russo, M., G. Poggi, M. L. Navacchia, M. D'Angelantonio, and S. S. Emmi. 2006. OH radical oxidation of the sorbitylfurfural furanic ring to sugar derivatives induced by radiolysis in aerobic environment. *Res Chem Intermediat* 32: 153–170.

Sanz, M. L., and I. Martinez-Castro. 2007. Recent developments in sample preparation for chromatographic analysis of carbohydrates. *J Chromatogr A* 1153: 74–89.

Sayre, L. M., D. Lin, Q. Yuan, X. C. Zhu, and X. X. Tang. 2006. Protein adducts generated from products of lipid oxidation: Focus on HNE and ONE. *Drug Metab Rev* 38: 651–675.

Shingai, Y., A. Fujimoto, M. Nakamura, and T. Masuda. 2011. Structure and function of the oxidation products of polyphenols and identification of potent lipoxygenase inhibitors from FE-catalysed oxidation of resveratrol. *J Agr Food Chem* 59: 8180–8186.

Simat, T., K. Meyer, and H. Steinhart. 1994. Synthesis and analysis of oxidation and carbonyl condensation compounds of tryptophan. *J Chromatogr A* 661: 93–99.

Sinz, A. 2006. Chemical cross-linking and mass spectrometry to map three-dimensional protein structures and protein-protein interactions. *Mass Spectrom Rev* 25: 663–682.

Steenhorst-Slikkerveer, L., A. Louter, H. G. Janssen, and C. Bauer-Plank. 2000. Analysis of nonvolatile lipid oxidation products in vegetable oils by normal-phase high-performance liquid chromatography with mass spectrometric detection. *J Am Oil Chem Soc* 77: 837–845.

Summo, C., M. T. Bilancia, and F. Caponio. 2008. Assessment of the oxidative and hydrolytic degradation of the lipid fraction of mortadella by means of HPSEC analyses of polar compounds. *Meat Sci* 79: 722–726.

Suzuki, S., and S. Honda. 2003. Miniaturization in carbohydrate analysis. *Electrophoresis* 24: 3577–3582.

Talcott, S. T., C. H. Brenes, D. M. Pires, and D. Del Pozo-Insfran. 2003. Phytochemical stability and color retention of copigmented and processed muscadine grape juice. *J Agr Food Chem* 51: 957–963.

Talcott, S. T., and L. R. Howard. 1999. Phenolic autoxidation is responsible for color degradation in processed carrot puree. *J Agr Food Chem* 47: 2109–2115.

Tanaka, T., Y. Matsuo, and I. Kouno. 2010. Chemistry of secondary polyphenols produced during processing of tea and selected foods. *Int J Mol Sci* 11: 14–40.

Tang, X. T., and J. E. Bruce. 2010. A new cross-linking strategy: Protein interaction reporter (PIR) technology for protein-protein interaction studies. *Mol Biosyst* 6 (6): 939–947.

Thomsen, M. K., L. Lauridsen, L. H. Skibsted, and J. Risbo. 2005. Temperature effect on lactose crystallization, Maillard reactions, and lipid oxidation in whole milk powder. *J Agr Food Chem* 53: 7082–7090.

Tiwari, U., and E. Cummins. 2009. Nutritional importance and effect of processing on tocols in cereals. *Trends Food Sci Technol* 20: 511–520.

Tomas-Barberan, F. A., and J. C. Espin. 2001. Phenolic compounds and related enzymes as determinants of quality in fruits and vegetables. *J Sci Food Agr* 81: 853–876.

Trefan, L., L. Bunger, J. Bloom-Hansen, J. A. Rooke, B. Salmi, C. Larzul, C. Terlouw, and A. Doeschl-Wilson. 2011. Meta-analysis of the effects of dietary vitamin E supplementation on alpha-tocopherol concentration and lipid oxidation in pork. *Meat Sci* 87: 305–314.

van Aardt, M., S. E. Duncan, J. E. Marcy, T. E. Long, S. F. O'Keefe, and S. R. Nielsen-Sims. 2005. Effect of antioxidant (alpha-tocopherol and ascorbic acid) fortification on light-induced flavor of milk. *J Dairy Sci* 88: 872–880.

Verleyen, T., R. Verhe, A. Huyghebaert, K. Dewettinck, and W. De Greyt. 2001. Identification of alpha-tocopherol oxidation products in triolein at elevated temperatures. *J Agr Food Chem* 49: 1508–1511.

Volkin, D. B., and A. M. Klibanov. 1987. Thermal-destruction processes in proteins involving cystine residues. *J Biol Chem* 262: 2945–2950.

Wan, P. J. 1995. Accelerated stability tests. In *Methods to Assess Quality and Stability of Oils and Fat-Containing Foods*, edited by K. Warner and N. Eskin. Urbana, IL: American Oil Chemist Society Press.

Wang, Q. J., and Y. Z. Fang. 2004. Analysis of sugars in traditional Chinese drugs. *J Chromatogr B-Analyt Technol Biomed Life Sci* 812: 309–324.

Wang, Y., and C. T. Ho. 2009. Polyphenolic chemistry of tea and coffee: A century of progress. *J Agr Food Chem* 57: 8109–8114.

Warner, R. D., P. L. Greenwood, D. W. Pethick, and D. M. Ferguson. 2010. Genetic and environmental effects on meat quality. *Meat Sci* 86: 171–183.

Washko, P. W., R. W. Welch, K. R. Dhariwal, Y. H. Wang, and M. Levine. 1992. Ascorbic-acid and dehydroascorbic acid analyses in biological samples. *Anal Biochem* 204: 1–14.

Weber, R. W. S., H. Anke, and P. Davoli. 2007. Simple method for the extraction and reversed-phase high-performance liquid chromatographic analysis of carotenoid pigments from red yeasts (*Basidiomycota*, Fungi). *J Chromatogr A* 1145: 118–122.

Wijesundera, C., C. Ceccato, P. Watkins, P. Fagan, B. Fraser, N. Thienthong, and P. Perlmutter. 2008. Docosahexaenoic acid is more stable to oxidation when located at the sn-2 position of triacylglycerol compared to sn-1(3). *J Am Oil Chem Soc* 85: 543–548.

Wiking, L., and J. H. Nielsen. 2004. The influence of oxidation on proteolysis in raw milk. *J Dairy Res* 71: 196–200.

Yamada, K., and K. Kakehi. 2011. Recent advances in the analysis of carbohydrates for biomedical use. *J Pharm Biomed Anal* 55: 702–727.

Yamauchi, R., H. Noro, M. Shimoyamada, and K. Kato. 2002. Analysis of vitamin E and its oxidation products by HPLC with electrochemical detection. *Lipids* 37: 515–522.

Zale, S. E., and A. M. Klibanov. 1986. Why does ribonuclease irreversibly inactivate at high-temperatures? *Biochemistry* 25: 5432–5444.

Zeb, A., and M. Murkovic. 2011. Carotenoids and triacylglycerols interactions during thermal oxidation of refined olive oil. *Food Chem* 127: 1584–1593.

Zhang, Z. Q., X. Q. Pang, X. W. Duan, and Z. L. Ji. 2003. The anthocyanin degradation and anthocyanase activity during pericarp browning of lychee fruit. *Sci Agr Sin* 36: 945–949.

4 Mechanisms of Oxidation in Food Lipids

Gloria Márquez-Ruiz, Francisca Holgado, and Joaquín Velasco

CONTENTS

4.1 INTRODUCTION

Lipid oxidation is the cause of important deteriorative changes in chemical, sensory, and nutritional food properties. Moreover, lipid oxidation products have attracted a great deal of attention because of the wide variety of degenerative processes and diseases associated with oxidative stress, including cancer, atherosclerosis, and chronic inflammatory diseases. Food lipids are mainly triacylglycerols (TAGs), phospholipids, and sterols; the first two groups of compounds are constituted by fatty acyl groups such as the oxidizable substrates. TAGs are the major constituents of dietary lipids, accounting for more than 90% of food lipids and, thereby, the most important substrates contributing to oxidized dietary fats.

Lipids oxidize through a complex series of reactions producing myriad nonvolatile and volatile compounds. Despite the complexity of the oxidation process, the main reactions and variables involved in autoxidation, photoxidation, and enzymatic oxidation are well documented. However, identification and quantitation of oxidation compounds continue to be the subject of intensive investigations given the high number of compounds formed from each oxidizable substrate. In this chapter, the most important aspects of lipid oxidation mechanisms are briefly presented, noting the main differences found in oxidation of conjugated fatty acids and oxidation at high temperature. A summary of the general factors affecting lipid oxidation and those additionally involved in foods is included. Finally, some specific aspects of lipid oxidation in relevant foods are mentioned.

4.2 AUTOXIDATION

Oxidation of unsaturated lipids mainly proceeds by autoxidation through free radical chain reactions involving four steps: initiation, propagation, branching, and termination. Mechanisms and kinetics of lipid autoxidation have been extensively reviewed during the past decades by the most relevant researchers in the field (Grosch 1987; Pokorny 1987; Gardner 1989; Porter et al. 1995; Brimberg and Kamal-Eldin 2003; Frankel 2005; Kamal-Eldin and Min 2008; Schneider 2009).

4.2.1 MECHANISMS AND PRODUCTS FORMED

Initiation occurs by the loss of a hydrogen radical from an allylic position, and hence an alkyl radical is formed (Equation 4.1). Abstraction of hydrogen occurs in the presence of initiators, and it is the least known step of autoxidation. Hydroperoxides present as impurities; redox metals and exposure to light in the presence of a sensitizer produce radicals that act as initiators. In the propagation step, the alkyl radical reacts with oxygen at rates controlled by diffusion to form a peroxyl radical (Equation 4.2), which triggers the chain reaction by abstracting a hydrogen atom from another unsaturated lipid molecule and giving rise to a hydroperoxide as the primary oxidation product and a new alkyl radical that propagates the reaction chain (Equation 4.3). This latter step is slow and rate-limiting; therefore, hydrogen abstraction from unsaturated lipids becomes selective for the most weakly bound hydrogen (Frankel 2005). The susceptibility of lipids to oxidation thus depends on the availability of allylic hydrogens because the resulting allylic radicals are stabilized by resonance:

$$\text{Initiation: } RH \rightarrow R^\bullet + H^\bullet \tag{4.1}$$

$$\text{Propagation: } R^\bullet + O_2 \rightarrow ROO^\bullet \tag{4.2}$$

$$ROO^\bullet + RH \rightarrow ROOH + R^\bullet \tag{4.3}$$

$$\text{Branching: } ROOH \rightarrow RO^\bullet + HO^\bullet \text{ Monomolecular} \tag{4.4}$$

$$2\,ROOH \rightarrow ROO^\bullet + RO^\bullet + H_2O \text{ Bimolecular} \tag{4.5}$$

$$\text{Termination: } ROO^\bullet + ROO^\bullet \rightarrow ROOR + O_2 \tag{4.6}$$

$$R^\bullet + ROO^\bullet \rightarrow ROOR \tag{4.7}$$

$$R^\bullet + RO^\bullet \rightarrow ROR \tag{4.8}$$

$$R^\bullet + H^\bullet \rightarrow RH \tag{4.9}$$

$$RO^\bullet + H^\bullet \rightarrow ROH \tag{4.10}$$

$$ROO^\bullet + H^\bullet \rightarrow ROOH \tag{4.11}$$

$$R^\bullet + HO^\bullet \rightarrow ROH \tag{4.12}$$

Branching consists of hydroperoxide decomposition and hence leads to the increase in free radical concentration. Decomposition of hydroperoxides is first monomolecular (Equation 4.4) and becomes bimolecular (Equation 4.5) when the hydroperoxide concentration is high enough, this latter requiring lower activation energy. Finally, in the termination stage, radicals react between each other to yield relatively stable nonradical species (Equations 4.6 through 4.12). All stages of oxidation occur simultaneously in a complex series of sequential and overlapping reactions.

Formation of oxidation compounds is delayed by chain-breaking antioxidants, which act as hydrogen donors mainly reacting with the alkylperoxyl ($ROO^\bullet$) radicals.

4.2.1.1 Primary Oxidation Products: Hydroperoxides

In the propagation step, the resulting alkyl radical or pseudo allylic radical generated after hydrogen abstraction is stabilized by resonance, where the electronic density is accumulated at each end of the allylic system. As a result, oxygen attacks at each end of the allylic species. In the case of oleic acid, hydrogen abstraction occurs at the allylic carbon-8 and carbon-11 to give two delocalized three-carbon allylic radicals. The reaction with oxygen yields a mixture of four allylic hydroperoxides containing the hydroperoxy group on carbons 8, 9, 10, or 11. In polyunsaturated fatty acids

(PUFAs), that is, with two or more double bounds separated by a methylene group, hydrogen abstraction is more favored because there are methylene groups doubly activated by two adjacent double bonds. Thus, in linoleic acid, hydrogen abstraction takes place at the carbon-11 position, giving rise to a hybrid pentadienyl radical, effectively stabilized by resonance, which reacts with oxygen at the carbon-9 and carbon-13 positions to produce a mixture of two conjugated diene 9- and 13-hydroperoxides (Figure 4.1). In linolenic acid, with three double bonds, there are two *bis*-allylic methylene groups that act independently and are not activated by each other. Thus, two hydroperoxides form from each 1,4-pentadiene structure, that is, on one hand, the 9- and 13-hydroperoxides and, on the other, the 12- and 16-hydroperoxides.

The hydroperoxides formed from methyl oleate, linoleate, and linolenate have been well characterized and quantified (Table 4.1) (Frankel 2005). As the number of double bonds increases, more complex mixtures of hydroperoxides are formed, and less stable hydroperoxides result, which makes it difficult to analyze them quantitatively.

Hydroperoxides are unstable compounds and decompose into radicals (mainly alkoxyl and hydroxyl radicals) that follow different pathways to produce a great variety of secondary oxidation products. Hydroperoxides form and decompose simultaneously and constitute the most abundant compounds under low and moderate temperature conditions. When hydroperoxides are accumulated at relatively high levels, their decomposition becomes faster than their formation, and the overall oxidation rate increases exponentially. This is concomitant with the significant increase in secondary oxidation compounds, including the start of polymerization, complete depletion of naturally occurring antioxidants, and unequivocal detection of rancidity,

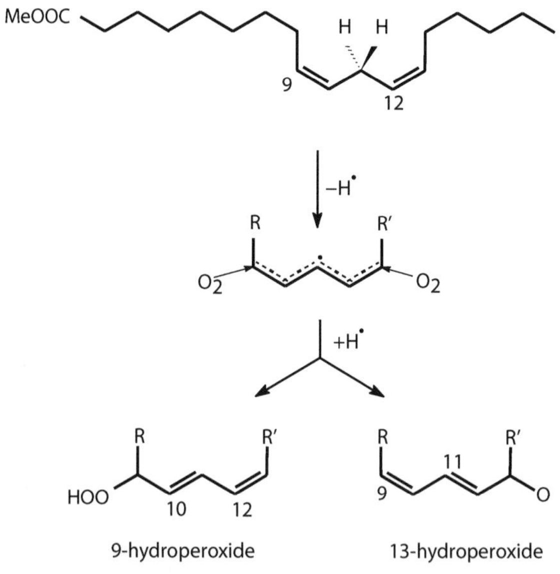

FIGURE 4.1   Formation of hydroperoxides from methyl linoleate.

TABLE 4.1
Hydroperoxides Formed from Autoxidation of Methyl Oleate, Linoleate, and Linolenate at 25°C

	(% of Total Hydroperoxides)						
	8-OOH	9-OOH	10-OOH	11-OOH	12-OOH	13-OOH	16-OOH
Me-oleate	26.4	24.2	22.8	26.6			
Me-linoleate		48.9				51.2	
Me-linolenate		30.6			10.1	10.8	48.6

thus denoting the end of the induction period (Márquez-Ruiz and Dobarganes 2005; Velasco et al. 2010). Nevertheless, rancidity appears during the induction period, much earlier than the complete depletion of antioxidants as a result of the presence of volatile lipid oxidation products causing off-flavors perceptible at extremely low concentrations, often at parts per billion levels.

4.2.1.2 Secondary Oxidation Products

Hydroperoxide decomposition and a great number of subsequent reactions give rise to a complex mixture of secondary oxidation products, which can be grouped according to molecular weight (MW) into

- volatile compounds, with MW lower than those of the original TAG, produced by alkoxyl radical breakdown
- oxidized monomers or compounds with MW similar to those of the original TAG bearing an oxygenated function in at least one of their fatty acyl groups
- polymerization compounds (dimers plus higher oligomers) formed through interaction of two or more TAG radicals and thus with MW higher than those of the original nonoxidized TAG.

4.2.1.2.1 Volatile Compounds

The most likely decomposition pathway of hydroperoxides is a homolytic cleavage of the hydroperoxide group to yield hydroxyl and alkoxyl radicals (Min and Boff 2002). Volatile products come from homolytic scission of the C–C bond in the β-position with respect to the oxygen of the alkoxyl radical. A multitude of volatile products are formed, including aldehydes, ketones, alcohols, alkanes, alkenes, etc. Flavor deterioration of food lipids is caused mainly by the presence of such volatile lipid oxidation products, which have an impact at extremely low concentrations. Figures 4.2 and 4.3 show formation of volatiles from the two conjugated diene 9- and 13-hydroperoxides in linoleic acyl of TAG. From 9-hydroperoxide, 3-nonenal and 2,4-decadienal are formed, and hexanal and pentane come from the 13-hydroperoxide. Concomitantly, TAG-bound short-chain compounds are formed.

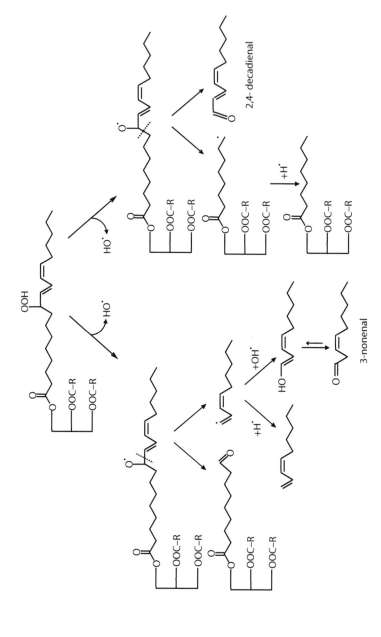

FIGURE 4.2 Reactions of β-scission of the diene 9-hydroperoxide in linoleyl acyl of TAGs involved in formation of volatile products.

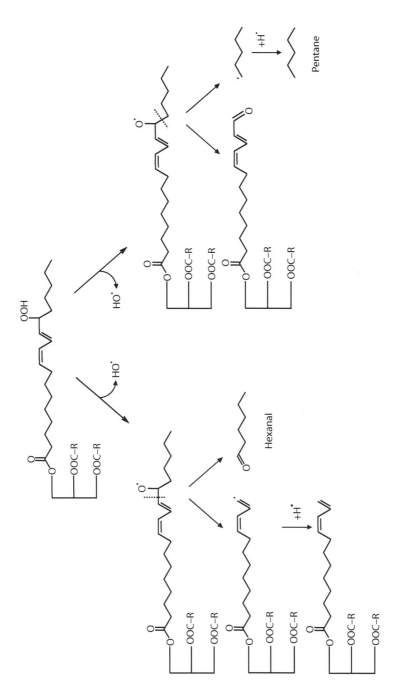

FIGURE 4.3 Reactions of β-scission of diene 13-hydroperoxide in linoleyl acyl of TAGs involved in formation of volatile products.

TABLE 4.2

Main Volatile Compounds Formed from Decomposition of Hydroperoxides from Methyl Oleate, Linoleate, and Linolenate at 25°C

	Oleate	Linoleate	Linolenate
Aldehydes	8:0	6:0	3:0
	9:0	7:1 (2t)	4:1 (2t)
	10:0	9:1 (3c)	6:1 (3c)
	10:1 (2t)	10:2 (2t 4c)	7:2 (2t 4c)
	11:1 (2t)		9:2 (3c 6t)
			10:3 (2t 4c 7c)
Hydrocarbons	7:0	5:0	2:0
	8:0	8:1 (2)	5:1 (2)
			8:2 (2,5)
Alcohols	7:0	5:0	2:0
	8:0	8:1 (2)	5:1 (2)
			8:2 (2,5)
Esters	7:0	8:0	8:0
	8:0	11:1 (9)	11:1 (9)
			14:2 (9,12)
ω-Oxo-esters	8:0	8:0	8:0
	9:0	10:1 (8)	10:1 (8)
	10:0	12:1 (9)	12:1 (9)
	10:1 (8)	13:2 (9,11)	13:2 (9,11)
	11:1 (9)		15:2 (9,12)
			16:3 (9,12,14)

Table 4.2 shows the major volatiles formed from oleic, linoleic, and linolenic acids (Frankel 2005).

4.2.1.2.2 Oxidized Monomers

The alkoxyl radical can participate in different reactions to produce compounds with oxygenated groups in at least one of the fatty acyl groups of the molecule, mainly, epoxy, keto, and hydroxy functions as well as short-chain n-oxo fatty acyl groups. These compounds are the most abundant secondary oxidation products formed at ambient or moderate temperature and those most relevant from the nutritional point of view because they are easily digested and absorbed (Dobarganes and Márquez-Ruiz 2003). Depending on the degree of unsaturation of the fatty acyl chain involved, more than one oxygenated function may be present in the same fatty acyl group, and more than one oxidized fatty acyl group may be present in one TAG molecule. Figure 4.4 illustrates formation of oxidized TAG monomers containing hydroxy and keto functions. Also, cholesterol oxides containing hydroxyl, keto, and epoxy functions have been identified (Figure 4.5).

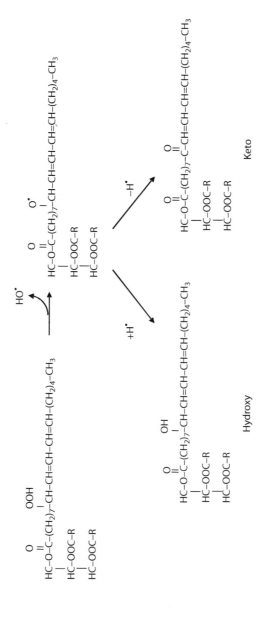

FIGURE 4.4 Formation of TAG secondary oxidation products containing hydroxy and keto functions.

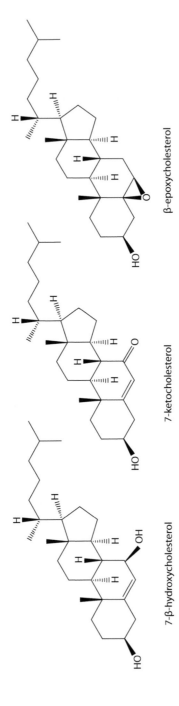

FIGURE 4.5   Formation of cholesterol secondary oxidation products containing hydroxy, keto, and epoxy functions.

4.2.1.2.3 Polymerization Compounds

The alkoxyl radicals also participate in condensation reactions to form polymerization compounds in significant amounts at the end of the induction period. As will be commented on later, polymers constitute the most abundant degradation compounds in used frying oils (Dobarganes 1998), but they also form, at ambient and moderate temperatures, being significant at the end of the induction period (Velasco et al. 2010). In oils rich in PUFAs or conjugated fatty acids, polymers can even be detected before the appearance of rancidity. Figure 4.6 shows the representative structures of TAG dimers and polymers linked by peroxide (C–O–O–C) or ether (C–O–C) linkages, which are those most normally found at ambient and moderate temperatures. The peroxy-linked dimers can be easily cleaved and produce volatile compounds or decompose to the ether-linked and carbon–carbon (C–C) linked dimers via the corresponding alkyl and alkoxyl radicals (Frankel 2005).

4.2.2 Oxidation of Conjugated Fatty Acids

Although the mechanism of autoxidation of methylene-interrupted fatty acid double bonds is well established, it has been suggested that the same mechanism is not likely to occur in conjugated fatty acid double bonds because high energy is previously required to separate double bonds from conjugation, which could explain why the formation of other compounds may be favored (Eulitz et al. 1999; Yurawecz et al. 2003; Brimberg and Kamal-Eldin 2003; Luna et al. 2007). Conjugated linoleic acid (CLA), normally a mixture of cis-9, trans-11, and trans-10, cis-12-octadecadienoic acid, is nowadays used as a supplement and added to dairy products because of its potential positive health effects. On the basis of the reaction products detected by gas chromatography–mass spectrometry, Yurawecz et al. reported that CLA underwent 1,2 and 1,4 cycloadditions with oxygen, which gave rise to dioxetane structures and endoperoxides leading to furan fatty acids, respectively. Other reactions, such as dimerization and polymerization, although not evaluated, were not ruled out by those authors. Even though Hämäläinen et al. (2002) reported that hydroperoxides are one type of primary oxidation products formed during autoxidation of CLA, this was found in the presence of unrealistic elevated contents (20 wt%) of α-tocopherol as hydrogen donor. Oxidation of CLA seems to proceed by the addition mechanism rather than by the hydrogen abstraction mechanism, suggesting that oligomeric peroxides are formed from the early events of lipid degradation (Brimberg and Kamal-Eldin 2003; Luna et al. 2007).

Figure 4.7 illustrates the results obtained by high-performance size-exclusion chromatography (HPSEC) that shows the time course of formation of nonvolatile compounds, that is, oxidized monomers, dimers, and oligomers for methyl linoleate (ML) and methyl conjugated linoleate (MCL) at 30°C (Luna et al. 2007). The typical oxidation profile was found for ML, that is, initial formation of oxidized monomers, mainly composed of hydroperoxides during early oxidation and the further acceleration of oxidation denoted by a significant rise in polymers (dimers plus oligomers) (Márquez-Ruiz and Dobarganes 2005; Márquez-Ruiz et al. 2007). As expected, accumulation of sufficient amounts of oxidized monomers led to the

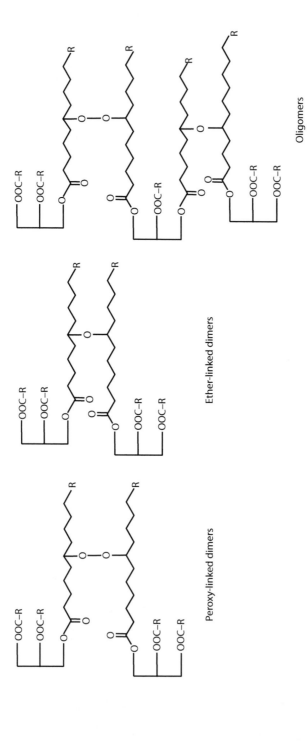

FIGURE 4.6 Representative structures of TAG dimers and oligomers linked by peroxide (C–O–O–C) or ether (C–O–C) linkages.

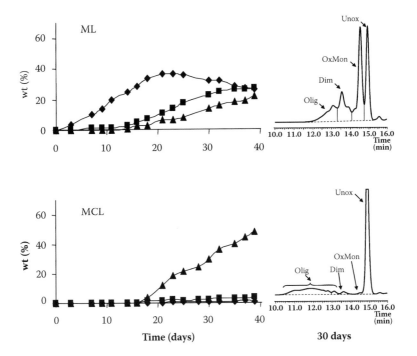

FIGURE 4.7 Time course of formation of oxidized monomers (♦), dimers (■), and oligo-mers (▲) by HPSEC analysis in methyl linoleate (ML) and methyl conjugated linoleate (MCL) during oxidation at 30°C.

formation of dimers, and likewise, oligomers did not build up until a notable increase in dimers had occurred. However, MCL samples showed a very different oxidation pattern; being oligomers, the first group of compounds formed, which continued to increase throughout the oxidation period without any significant parallel increase in oxidized monomers and up to levels markedly higher than those found in ML samples. These results show that formation of typical primary oxidation products, that is, hydroperoxides (included in the oxidized monomers peak), was negligible in the MCL samples. Further, the dimer formation was scarce, and the starting point of oxidation for these samples was characterized by the appearance of oligomers over a wide range of MW. The figure also illustrates the differences in the oxidation profiles at 30 days obtained in the HPSEC analysis. Peaks correspond to oligomers, dimers, oxidized monomers, and unoxidized monomers.

Figure 4.8 shows the time course of formation of the main volatile compounds in oils containing approximately 80% of either linoleic acid [safflower oil (SO)] or CLA [Tonalin™ oil (TO)]. Major volatiles found in TO were not those expected from theoretically stable hydroperoxides formed in CLA (García-Martínez et al. 2009). In SO, the volatile profile was close to that expected from the cleavage of the alkoxyl radicals formed from the hydroperoxides of autoxidized linoleic acid with the main volatile oxidation product being hexanal. Pentanal, t-2-heptanal, and

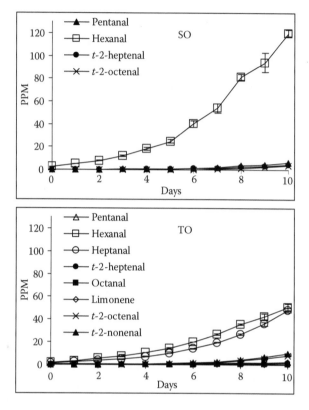

FIGURE 4.8 Time course of formation of main volatile compounds in SO (safflower oil) and TO (Tonalin™ oil) during oxidation at 30°C.

t-2-octenal were the other major volatiles formed during oxidation of SO and were also produced by decomposition of the most abundant linoleic acid hydroperoxides. However, the volatile profile of oxidized TO was characterized by the joint occurrence of two major volatile oxidation products, that is, hexanal and heptanal, and the latter compound was absent in oxidized SO. Another important difference was the presence of *t*-2-nonenal in TO while it was totally absent in SO. According to the hydroperoxide theory, formation of hexanal and pentanal is predictable from the expected major 13-hydroperoxides formed in both 9*c*, 11*t*-CLA and 10*t*, 12*c*-CLA, both isomers present in equal amounts in TO. In contrast, the presence of heptanal and *t*-2-nonenal, as well as that of other minor peaks, is not easily accounted for. An alternative route of formation for the oxidation of volatile compounds found in CLA could be based on the mechanisms proposed by Yurawecz et al. They suggested that CLA may undergo 1 or 2 cycloadditions with oxygen resulting in dioxetanes that would lead to volatile formation and proposed that heptanal would be a scission product of a 11,12-dioxetane, whereas 2-nonenal would result from the scissions of 9,10-dioxetane (Yurawecz et al. 2003).

4.2.3 OXIDATION AT HIGH TEMPERATURE: THERMOXIDATION

The chemistry of lipid oxidation at the high temperatures of food processes such as baking and frying is highly complex because both oxidative and thermal reactions are involved simultaneously. As temperature increases, the solubility of oxygen decreases drastically, although all the oxidation reactions are accelerated and formation of new compounds is very rapid. Mechanisms and the effect of variables involved in lipid oxidation during frying have been extensively reported (Dobarganes 1998; Dobarganes and Márquez-Ruiz 2006; Choe and Min 2007; Velasco et al. 2008; Sánchez-Muniz et al. 2008; Dobarganes et al. 2010; Márquez-Ruiz et al. 2010; Dobarganes et al. 2013).

Figure 4.9 summarizes the main groups of alteration compounds formed during frying. An example of a simplified structure is shown for each group of compounds.

Hydrolysis occurs as a result of the presence of moisture in the food. This involves breaking ester bonds and releasing free fatty acids and diacylglycerols. Additionally, because of the presence of air and exposure to high temperatures, oxidation and thermal alterations take place in the unsaturated fatty acids, leading to modified TAG with at least one of the three fatty acyl chains altered. To increase the complexity, the different reactions are interrelated. For example, free fatty acids originated by hydrolysis are oxidized more rapidly than in the original TAG. Although hydrolysis is one of the simplest reactions that occur during frying, inconsistent results on the variables promoting formation of free fatty acids have been obtained. For some authors, hydrolysis is the most important reaction during frying (Pokorny 1998), while in well-controlled frying operations of potatoes under many different conditions, hydrolytic products were minor compounds within the pool of degradation compounds, even though the substrate had a very high water content (Dobarganes and Márquez-Ruiz 2003).

Autoxidation at high temperatures proceeds by the same mechanisms outlined above, even though important differences are noted between oxidation at low or moderate and high temperatures.

- At low or moderate temperatures, formation of oxidation compounds during the induction period is slow; hydroperoxides are the major compounds formed, and their concentration increases until advanced stages of oxidation. Polymerization compounds only become significant in the accelerated stage of oxidation after the end of the induction period (Márquez-Ruiz and Dobarganes 2005; Velasco et al. 2010).
- At high temperatures, formation of new compounds is very rapid; the oxygen pressure is reduced, and consequently, the initiation reaction becomes more important and gives rise to an increase in the concentration of alkyl radicals ($R^\bullet$) with respect to alkylperoxyl radicals ($ROO^\bullet$). Besides, hydroperoxides decompose rapidly and are practically absent above 150°C, indicating that decomposition of hydroperoxides becomes faster than formation (Dobarganes 1998). As a result, polymeric compounds form from the very early stages of heating through termination reactions that mainly involve alkyl ($R^\bullet$) and alkoxyl ($RO^\bullet$) radicals. In addition, because of the low oxygen concentration, significant amounts of nonpolar TG dimers (C-C linkages) are also produced (Dobarganes and Márquez-Ruiz 2006).

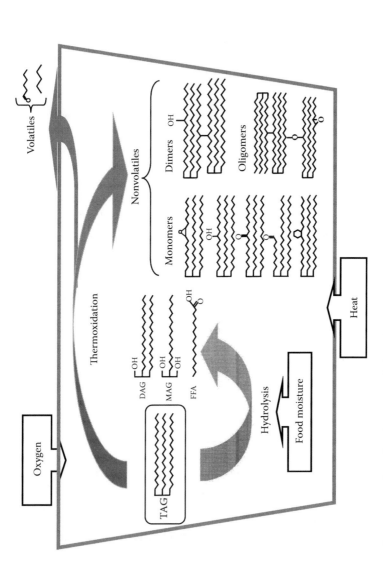

FIGURE 4.9 Schematic representation of main groups of alteration compounds formed during frying. Abbreviations: TAG, triacylglycerols; DAG, diacylglycerols; MAG, monoacylglycerols; and FFA, free fatty acids.

The main stable final products are TAG-oxidized monomers and polymers (dimers and oligomers) containing modified and nonmodified acyl groups (Figure 4.9). As already defined, oxidized monomers contain at least one of their fatty acyl groups oxidized, thus including TAG with different oxygenated functions, such as hydroxy, keto, epoxy, and others, as well as TAG with short-chain fatty acyl groups (Velasco et al. 2004, 2005). Monofunctional compounds containing hydroxy, keto, and epoxy functions constitute major groups within the fraction of oxidized TAG monomers (Marmesat et al. 2008). TAGs with short-chain fatty acyl groups mainly form through homolytic β-scission of alkoxyl radicals. Saturated fatty acyl chains of seven and eight carbon atoms, n-oxo saturated chains of eight and nine carbon atoms, known as core aldehydes, and the same aldehydes oxidized to carboxylic acids are the most abundant structures (Velasco et al. 2004, 2005). Polymers are the most specific and abundant compounds in used frying fats and are formed through interaction between TAG radicals. The main compounds are those containing carbon–carbon links or ether bonding, that is, carbon–oxygen–carbon links (Dobarganes and Márquez-Ruiz 2006). Mechanisms and reactions participating in the formation of nonpolar dimers have been studied by using fatty acid methyl esters subjected to high temperatures (between 200°C and 300°C) in the absence of air to inhibit oxidative reactions. Three main reactions have been proposed: (1) formation of dehydrodimers by combination of two allyl radicals, (2) formation of noncyclic dimers by intermolecular addition of the allyl radical to a double bond of an unsaturated molecule, and (3) formation of cyclic dimers by intramolecular addition of an intermediate dimeric radical to a double bond in the same molecule. When conjugated fatty acid methyl esters are present, thermal dimers are originated following the Diels–Alder reaction, that is, reaction between two molecules, one of them with a double bond acting as a dienophile and the other with a conjugated diene structure. The result is the formation of a cyclohexene tetrasubstituted compound (Dobarganes and Márquez-Ruiz 2006). The structure of polar dimers is still largely unknown because of the heterogeneity in this group of compounds. First, different oxygenated functions are likely to be present in oxidized monomers before dimer formation or generated by oxidation of nonpolar dimers. Second, more than one functional group can be present in the same dimeric molecule. Last, the oxygen may or may not be involved in the dimeric linkage. There is structural evidence of the presence of monohydroxy, dihydroxy, and keto groups in the C–C linked dimers of methyl linoleate at frying temperatures, together with the previously mentioned structures of nonpolar dimers. Definite structures for compounds with MW higher than dimers have not been reported. This is not strange, taking into account that much research remains to be done on structure elucidation and quantitation of simpler molecules, that is, oxidized monomers and dimers, which are intermediates in trimer and higher oligomer formation. Also, it has to be considered that the number of possibilities of different structures in trimer formation increases exponentially with respect to those compounds of lower MW as many different dimeric structures may be combined with many different monomeric structures. Nevertheless, the results reported so far indicate that the polymers formed are essentially dimers and trimers joined through C–C and C–O–C linkages.

Volatile compounds are formed simultaneously with the formation of short-chain fatty acids containing TAG by β-scission of alkoxyl radicals. Thus, the cleavage of a fatty acyl chain generates, on one hand, a glyceridic product and, on the other, compounds of low MW. Volatiles are removed to a large extent from the oil because of the effect of heating.

Formation of other groups of compounds present in used frying oils without extra oxygen, that is, Diels–Alder dimers, cyclic fatty acids, and positional and geometrical fatty acids, is explained by thermal reactions and not by radical interaction. They are minor compounds of nutritional interest and, paradoxically, are much better known than the major oxidation compounds because of their stability and low polarity.

4.2.4 MAIN FACTORS INVOLVED IN LIPID OXIDATION

The main factors include external factors, such as concentration of oxygen, temperature, and light, and intrinsic factors of lipids, namely, fatty acid composition, prooxidants, and antioxidants.

4.2.4.1 Oxygen

Because oxygen is an essential reactant to propagate autoxidation reactions, the absence of oxygen would prevent the oxidative alteration. Otherwise, geometrical and cyclic isomers, dimers, and oligomers—without extra oxygen—are the only degradation products formed provided that temperature is over 200°C (Gardner 1987). For example, formation of such compounds in substantial contents takes place in the deodorization step of the refining process of fats and oils (Gomes and Catalano 1988; Ruiz-Méndez et al. 1997).

When unlimited oxygen is available, the rate of oxidation is theoretically independent of the oxygen pressure, whereas, at lower oxygen concentrations, the oxidation rate is proportional to the oxygen pressure, that is, the lower the oxygen concentration, the larger the impact of a decrease in oxygen concentration on the rate of autoxidation. The surface area of lipids exposed to air has such an influence that when the surface-to-volume ratio is increased, a reduction in the oxygen pressure is less effective in decreasing the oxidation rate.

4.2.4.2 Temperature

The rate of oxidation increases exponentially with temperature. In addition, there is a strong interaction between temperature and oxygen because the oxygen solubility decreases as the temperature increases. Differences between oxidation at low or moderate and high temperatures have been described above.

4.2.4.3 Light

Light acts as a catalyst of hydrogen abstraction in the initiation step of autoxidation, influences the decomposition of hydroperoxides favoring formation of free radicals, and accelerates oxidation. This effect is different from that described below in the presence of photosensitizers, which gives rise to photoxidation.

4.2.4.4 Fatty Acid Composition

The degree of unsaturation is one of the most determining factors in the rate of lipid oxidation because of the different reactivity of unsaturated fatty acids. In mixtures, as occurs in nature, the oxidation rate of the most unsaturated fatty acid is determinant, and differences are much lower than expected from the results obtained in pure lipids oxidized separately (Bolland 1949). The position and geometrical configuration of double bonds and the length of the fatty acid chain also influence the susceptibility to oxidation (Sahasrabudhe and Farne 1964). Thus, it appears that *cis* fatty acids oxidize faster than their *trans* isomer counterparts. Not only fatty acid composition but also fatty acyl distribution in the different positions of the glycerol molecule (α and β) may exert a relevant influence on oxidation rate in TAG. In studies with synthetic TAG, Miyashita et al. (1990) reported that an unsaturated fatty acyl chain is more easily oxidized in the 2- than in the 1,3-TAG position. Finally, as expected from the basis of the lipid oxidation mechanisms, oxidation of saturated fatty acids can be considered virtually nonexistent at low or moderate temperatures.

4.2.4.5 Prooxidants

The most effective prooxidants are transition metals, such as copper and iron, which may be present as trace impurities or can even be added to fortify foods. Metal's prooxidant effects proceed by different mechanisms with the catalysis of the decomposition of hydroperoxides being the most relevant, followed by direct reaction with unoxidized substrate to produce alkyl radicals and activation of molecular oxygen to produce singlet oxygen and peroxide radicals (Schaich 1992; Kanner 2010). Free fatty acids, present in minor amounts in fats and oils, have also proven to act as prooxidants, and the effect is attributed to the carboxylic group (Miyashita and Takagi 1986).

4.2.4.6 Antioxidants

The inhibition of autoxidation by antioxidants is of the utmost importance in food lipids. Minor components naturally present in oils, such as tocopherols and polyphenols, exert an essential protective role against lipid oxidation. Also, synthetic antioxidants, such as propyl gallate, are efficient and commonly used. Antioxidants can act by different mechanisms, and the main one consists of interrupting the propagation chain of autoxidation by reacting with peroxyl radicals to produce less-reactive species. These are known as chain-breaking antioxidants and include phenolic antioxidants, such as tocopherols. The phenoxyl radicals produced are stabilized by resonance. Other protective mechanisms attributed to minor components of oil or food additives are chelation of metals (polyphenols, citric acid), reduction of hydroperoxides (ascorbic acid), and others. There are other chapters in this book dedicated to natural antioxidants and mechanisms of antioxidant activity.

4.3 ENZYMATIC OXIDATION

Lipoxygenases and other enzymes catalyze the oxidation of free PUFAs that are released from glycerides by the action of lipolytic enzymes; therefore, lipolytic hydrolysis is a necessary preliminary step (Wang and Hammond 2010). The

oxidation products are the same hydroperoxides produced in the autoxidation process, but the stereochemistry and relative proportions of hydroperoxides are different
because the reaction is stereospecific and regioselective. Only in unprocessed foods
or foods elaborated under mild conditions can oxidation be catalyzed by enzymes
that otherwise lose their activity in processed foods as a result of thermal degradation. Examples of enzymatic oxidation occurring in meat and fish products will be
commented on in other parts of this chapter.

4.4   PHOTOXIDATION

Hydroperoxides can also be formed by photoxidation, which is triggered by exposure
to light in the presence of oxygen and a sensitizer, such as different pigments present
in foods, mainly chlorophyll, hemoproteins, and riboflavin (Frankel 2005; see also
Section 2.2.3). Photosensitizers are activated by absorption of light, and the excited
species can act by two pathways. A type I sensitizer serves as a free-radical initiator and transfers electrons to lipids to form radicals that can react with oxygen. The
hydroperoxides produced are the same as those from the autoxidation process.

   The type II sensitizer interacts with oxygen by energy transfer to give nonradical
singlet oxygen, a very reactive species that reacts directly with unsaturated lipids by
a concerted "ene" addition mechanism (Figure 4.10). Singlet oxygen adds directly
to either end carbon of a double bond, which is shifted to an allylic position in the
trans configuration. Thus, the resulting hydroperoxides have an allylic *trans* double
bound.

   According to this mechanism, the hydroperoxide distribution is different from
autoxidation. Oleate produces a mixture of 9- and 10-hydroperoxides; linoleate a
mixture of 9-, 10-, 12-, and 13-hydroperoxides; and linolenate a mixture of 9-, 10-,
12-, 13-, 15-, and 16-hydroperoxides. With respect to linolenate, the 9-hydroperoxide
and the 13-hydroperoxide have conjugated double bonds and have the same structures as those formed by free radical autoxidation. However, the double bonds in the

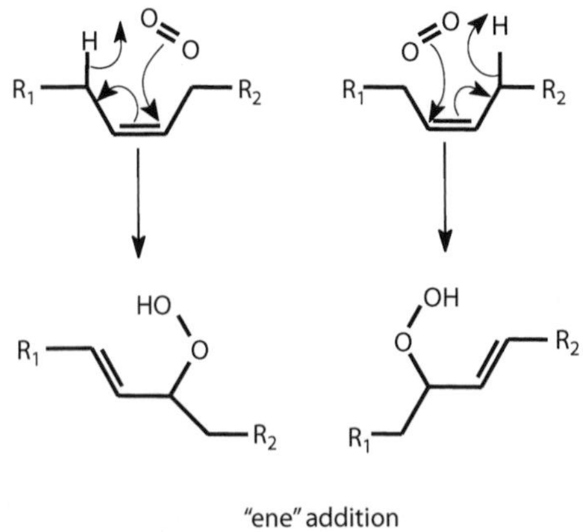

"ene" addition

FIGURE 4.10   Oxidation of oleate by singlet oxygen ("ene" addition mechanism).

10- and 12-hydroperoxide are not conjugated and therefore these hydroperoxides are unique to singlet oxidation. Once hydroperoxides are formed by photoxidation, the predominant mechanism is autoxidation (see also Chapter 2).

4.5 LIPID OXIDATION IN FOODS: ADDITIONAL FACTORS INVOLVED

4.5.1 FOOD STRUCTURE AND LIPID DISTRIBUTION

Foods are complex biological materials that contain a wide range of major and minor components. As a consequence of their composition and the method of preparation, the physical structure of foods and the state and distribution of lipids vary widely. Some foods are homogeneous, such as beverages or vegetable oils, with minor components dissolved or dispersed in water or in the oil, respectively. However, most foods are not homogeneous and thus contain distinct phases (Gordon 2010). Foods with lipids in a continuous phase normally present an oxidative behavior similar to the same lipids isolated from the food matrix. The critical parameters are the composition of fat and the surface area (Fritsch 1994).

One important factor influencing oxidation in foods where there is a noncontinuous lipid phase is the coexistence of a portion of the lipid phase that is hexane-extractable and usually called free or surface oil and a portion of the noncontinuous lipid phase wherein lipids are in droplets and whose extraction requires previous disruption of the matrix structure (Fritsch 1994). Therefore, the surface lipid fraction is the fraction more exposed to the air and more susceptible to oxidation. For most foods, this is true. For example, external oxidation (in the surface oil) might induce rancidity even if most lipids in food show an overall low oxidation level. This occurs in powdered infant formulas (Márquez-Ruiz et al. 2003; García-Martínez et al. 2010; Holgado 2011) as illustrated in Figure 4.11, which shows evolution of oxidation in the free and encapsulated oil fractions.

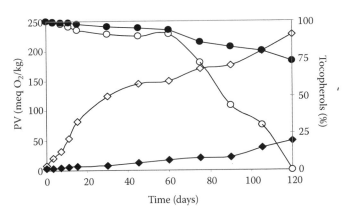

FIGURE 4.11 Evolution of oxidation in the free and encapsulated oil fractions of infant formula stored at ambient temperature. Free oil fraction: peroxide value ($\Diamond$) and tocopherols ($\bigcirc$); encapsulated oil fraction: peroxide value ($\blacklozenge$) and tocopherols ($\bullet$).

Even though free oil was only 3% of the total oil, its earlier oxidation led to the appearance of rancidity at 30 days. Otherwise, rancidity might not be detected until the oxidized encapsulated oil is released. In studies carried out in our laboratory on microencapsulated oils, which were obtained by the freeze-drying of oil-in-water emulsions, oxidation of the encapsulated fraction was unexpectedly faster than the oxidation of the free oil fraction. Differences in oxidation were so great that samples only showed clear rancidity (off-odor) when the matrix was disrupted with a mortar and pestle, allowing the oxidized fraction to be released. However, when the same oil was stripped of its natural antioxidants, oxidation of the free oil fraction was, as expected, faster than that of the encapsulated oil. These results indicate that the transport of oxygen through the solid matrix was the determinant step in the oxidation of the encapsulated stripped oil, but other factors played a decisive role in the relative oxidation rates of the two fractions in the sample containing the original oil (Márquez-Ruiz et al. 2003; Velasco et al. 2000, 2006, 2009a,b,c).

Moreover, evolution of oxidation in the noncontinuous or dispersed lipid phase may become very complex because lipid droplets are isolated from each other in the matrix, and consequently, different oxidation rates can occur in different droplets. As a result of the oxidation heterogeneity, encapsulated oil fractions of freeze-dried oil-in-water emulsions showed a much higher polymers-to-remaining-tocopherols ratio in the encapsulated oil fraction than that in the free oil fraction, indicating the coexistence in the former of oil globules at low oxidation stages and still protected by the presence of tocopherols and others devoid of antioxidants and well within the advanced oxidation stage (Márquez-Ruiz et al. 2003; Velasco et al. 2006, 2009a). This is illustrated in Figure 4.12 (Holgado 2011).

The molecular mobility of lipids is a function of the nature, composition, and state of the food and also of temperature and water activity. As an example, it is known that an increase in molecular mobility as a consequence of temperature or water activity results in the crystallization of lactose. Formation of lactose crystals breaks the food matrix structure giving rise to migration of lipids to the surface of

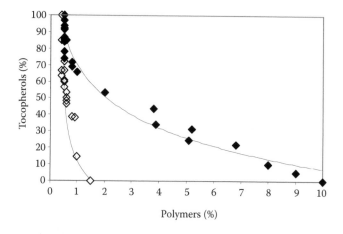

FIGURE 4.12 Tocopherols-to-polymers ratios in the free (hollow symbols) and encapsulated (solid symbols) oil fractions of dried microencapsulated oils during oxidation at 30°C.

the product and changing, therefore, the oxidative stability (Chuy and Labuza 1994). Other structural changes influencing lipid oxidation are related to water activity and are described below.

4.5.2 INTERACTIONS BETWEEN MATRIX COMPONENTS

The main reactions between food matrix components that may have relevant incidence on lipid oxidation are nonenzymatic browning or Maillard reactions.

Maillard reactions generally occur in foods with water activity in the range above the monolayer (0.3–0.7) and at temperatures over 50°C (Karel 1984; Eriksson 1987). Antioxidant properties of browning reaction products have long been known, but more recently, the interactions in the nonenzymatic browning produced as a consequence of lipid oxidation and the Maillard reaction have been examined (Zamora and Hidalgo 2005, 2011). Thus, the carbonyl compounds produced by lipid oxidation may compete with carbohydrate-derived carbonyls for amino compounds to produce carbonyl–amine reaction products. These aspects will be discussed elsewhere in this book.

Reactions between oxidized lipids and proteins may lead to loss of essential amino acids and hence impairment of nutritional value (Gardner 1979; Karel 1984; Eriksson 1987; Hidalgo et al. 1992; Genot et al. 2003; Schaich 2008). Hydrophobic interactions, radical reactions, and the formation of covalent compounds have been described (Hidalgo et al. 1992; Genot et al. 2003). Peroxyl radicals are very reactive with labile amino acids (tryptophane, histidine, cysteine, cystine, methionine, lysine, and tyrosine), undergoing decarboxylation, decarbonylation, and deamination. Methionine is oxidized to a sulfoxide, and combined cysteine is converted to cystine to form combined thiosulfinate. Imino Schiff bases are formed from the reaction of aldehydes and epoxides with amines, and Schiff bases polymerize by aldol condensation producing melanoidins, which, in turn, generate, by scission or dehydration, volatiles that affect food flavors. A great number of studies have been reported on model systems, but results obtained are difficult to extrapolate to foods, and it is poorly understood how these reactions proceed in foods at low water activity (Frankel 2005).

4.5.3 WATER ACTIVITY

The effect of water activity in foods has been extensively studied by Karel et al. (1967) and Labuza (1968, 1975). In general, the rate of lipid oxidation is low at water activities close to the water monolayer, which falls between 0.2 and 0.3 for most foods, because of a decrease in the catalytic effect of transition metals, quenching of free radicals, and singlet oxygen and/or retardation of hydroperoxide decomposition. However, the rate of lipid oxidation increases rapidly when the water activity is either decreased below or increased above the monolayer. Besides, moisture may lead to physical changes in the solid matrix of foods and affect the oil distribution and, consequently, the accessibility of oxygen to the oil. The glass transition theory can be used to explain the complex relationship between water content and lipid stability. The glass transition temperature is that at which amorphous components of food change from a glassy state to a rubbery state (Roos et al. 1996). When either moisture content or temperature increases, the food matrix changes from the glassy to the rubbery state. In the glassy state, the molecular mobility is very low, and the free volume is so reduced that diffusion of oxygen through the system is limited. In contrast, in the rubbery state, the molecular mobility is quite high, and the system is characterized by open structures. Because, in the glassy state, lipids remain encapsulated, there is a low free volume, and hence lipids are more stable to oxidation and formulations should be aimed at either bringing the food matrix into the glassy state or increasing its glass-transition temperature. As molecular mobility increases by the plasticizing effect of water or by temperature, crystallization of sugars and/or the so-called collapse may occur (Chuy and Labuza 1994). These physical changes result in the partial release of encapsulated lipids to the surface of the product, where they are more exposed to oxygen and undergo rapid oxidation (Shimada et al. 1991).

4.6 LIPID OXIDATION IN FOODS: INFLUENCE OF FOOD NATURE AND COMPOSITION

Apart from the variables affecting food lipid oxidation in general, some foods that are especially susceptible to oxidation show particular characteristics and specific components that influence mechanisms of lipid oxidation. Among such foods, those constituted by emulsions, fish and meat products, and processed foods are relevant.

4.6.1 FOOD EMULSIONS

Lipid oxidation in systems in which the fat or oil is dispersed as emulsion droplets is still poorly understood in spite of the large number of foods that consist either wholly or partially of emulsions or that have been in an emulsified form at some time during their production (Coupland and McClements 1996; Velasco et al. 2002; Decker et al. 2008; Skibsted 2010; Waraho et al. 2010). Two types of emulsions are common in foods: water-in-oil emulsions (butter, margarine) and, especially, oil-in-water emulsions (milk, mayonnaise, salad dressings, infant foods, sauces, beverages, cream, and soups). In oil-in-water emulsions, lipid droplets are dispersed in a continuous water phase, stabilized by proteins, phospholipids, or surfactants. Recently, certain food emulsions are showing uncontrolled oxidation problems, that is, functional dairy products enriched with ω-3 PUFAs or CLA to improve their beneficial health effects (Campbell et al. 2003; Kolanowski and Weißbrodt 2007; García-Martínez and Márquez-Ruiz 2009).

A number of additional variables that influence lipid oxidation in food emulsions are summarized as follows:

1. Characteristics (composition, location, concentration) and modifications (changes in electric charge, permeability, and others) of the emulsifier that constitutes the interface are among the most important factors involved in oxidation. The emulsifier can provide a protective barrier to the penetration and diffusion of radicals or molecules that initiate lipid oxidation (Frankel 2005). The electric charge of ionic emulsifiers influences greatly

the oxidation rate (Huang et al. 1996). Higher concentrations of an emulsifier can increase oxidative stability by causing tighter and thicker packing at the interface, hence becoming a more efficient barrier against diffusion of lipid oxidation initiators.

2. Partition of reactants and products between the interfacial region: oil and water phases resulting from their polarity and surface activity. Lesser polar molecules are mainly located in the oil phase, polar molecules in the water phase, and amphiphilic molecules in the interface. Orientation of molecules in this interfacial region affects the accessibility to oxygen of reactive species, such as peroxides, hydroxyl, and perhydroxyl radicals, which are soluble in water (Wedzicha 1988; Coupland and McClements 1996). The partition of scission products between the oil and water phases can have an important influence on sensorial perception in many food emulsions as aromatic compounds are perceived more intensely in the water phase (Sims 1994).

3. Interaction of lipids with other components of emulsions, which can act as prooxidants or antioxidants depending on their chemical properties. Carbohydrates can either protect from lipid oxidation by binding metals and scavenging radicals (Yamauchi et al. 1982; Sagone et al. 1983) or accelerate oxidation (Yamauchi et al. 1988). The effectiveness of proteins to delay the oxidation in emulsions depends on their conformation, interface composition, and partition between the interface and the water phase. Besides trapping free radicals, their antioxidant effect has been attributed to their capacity for formation of viscoelastic dense membranes that restrict the penetration or diffusion of initiators of oxidation inside the droplets (Tong et al. 2000). Proteins containing reducing sulfhydryl groups are particularly effective as antioxidants in milk, meat, and fish.

4. Effect of pH: The lipid oxidation rate is, in general, lower at high pHs and increases as the pH decreases, which may be attributed to solubilization of metal catalysts.

5. Metal catalysis: Hydrophilic metals are located toward the interface, and initiation of oxidation occurs in the lipid phase inside the interface (Schaich 1992). Therefore, chelating agents and reaction conditions that increase metal concentration in this site enhance their effectiveness. Charge of chelators and electrostatic environment that surround metals can affect their redox potential and other thermodynamic properties (Frankel 2005).

6. Antioxidants: In multiphase systems, antioxidants are distributed between the water phase, the oil phase, and the interfacial region, rich in emulsifiers, depending on their affinity and relative amounts. Lipophilic antioxidants are more effective in oil-in-water emulsions than are hydrophilic antioxidants, whereas the contrary effect occurs in bulk oils, which is known as the polar paradox. In oil-in-water emulsions, lipophilic antioxidants tend to be orientated in the oil–water interface and hence protect oil against oxidation, while hydrophilic antioxidants tend to dissolve and become diluted in the water phase (Porter 1980; Schwarz et al. 1996; Huang et al. 1996, 1997).

4.6.2 MEAT PRODUCTS

In meat, TAG, phospholipids, and cholesterol are the main substrates for lipid oxidation. Oxidation in phospholipids occurs earlier than in TAG because of the proximity of heme catalysts of mitochondria and microsomes. During processing and storage of meat products, cholesterol oxidation can be also accelerated by lipid radicals formed from unsaturated fatty acids in TAG and phospholipids (Faustman et al. 2010; Osada et al. 2000). Lipid stability depends on the composition of fatty acids and antioxidant content of each type of meat (i.e., beef is more stable than chicken) as well as on processing or presentation conditions. To limit oxygen so as to minimize lipid oxidation and microorganism growth, oxygen-impermeable packing is used (Brandon et al. 2009; Faustman et al. 2010). However, complete oxygen elimination is not recommended because a certain oxygen level is necessary to maintain oxymyoglobin content, responsible for the bright red color of meat that is considered very attractive to the consumer.

Heme-proteins play an important role in the mechanisms of lipid oxidation in meat products (Richards and Dettmann 2003; Ramanathan et al. 2009; Richards 2010; see also Section 2.2.2). Myoglobin and hemoglobin can be accelerators of lipid oxidation, and their effect is concentration-dependent. Oxidation of oxymyoglobin and myoglobin (red) to metmyoglobin (brown) decreases the meat quality, and this is enhanced by oxidized lipids, but the mechanism is unknown. In turn, myoglobin, oxymyoglobin, and hemoglobin are compounds more active than free metal ions in catalyzing decomposition of lipid hydroperoxides. In cooked meat, denaturation of proteins releasing iron induces lipid oxidation and the interaction of reactive aldehydes with amino groups. Moreover, the disruptions of cell membranes permit lipids to come in contact with catalysts. A rapid oxidation of phospholipids called "warmed-over flavor" also takes place during cooking, and carbonyl compounds formed give rise to characteristic and desirable flavors resulting from interactions with amino groups and phosphatidylethanolamine (Frankel 2005).

Muscle tissues have several types of lipid-soluble antioxidants (α-tocopherol, ubiquinone), water-soluble antioxidants (ascorbate), and enzymes with antioxidant activity (superoxide dismutase, catalase, glutathione peroxidase). To delay lipid oxidation, common strategies used are supplementation with vitamin E in animal diets, addition of sodium nitrite in cured meat, which also acts as an antimicrobial agent, and a combination of natural or synthetic antioxidants with synergists such as ascorbic acid. Recently, the inclusion of fish oil in diets to increase PUFA content in meat has led to undesirable effects, including poor oxidative stability and fishy flavors, which shows the need for more effective antioxidant combinations (Apple et al. 2009; Richards 2010).

4.6.3 FISH PRODUCTS

A large proportion (approximately 40%) of fish lipids are long-chain PUFAs ω-3, mainly eicosapentaenoic acid (C20:5) and docosahexaenoic acid (C22:6). Their beneficial health properties, particularly in cardiovascular diseases and atherosclerosis, are well demonstrated (Shahidi and Miraliakkbari 2004; Ruxton et al. 2007). However, their presence makes fish and fish products very susceptible substrates to oxidation, and the products formed can be potentially harmful and invalidate the positive health effects of their parent fatty acids, precisely affecting the same target organs (Dobarganes and Márquez-Ruiz 2003). Other negative consequences derived from lipid oxidation in fish include unacceptable organoleptic changes because of volatile formation, especially propanal, changes in texture and color resulting from interaction of oxidized lipids and fish proteins, and losses of essential nutrients and vitamins, especially vitamin E (Kulas et al. 2003). Volatile compounds from fish lipids have lower threshold values (parts per billion) than those derived from vegetable oils; they are readily detectable at very low levels of oxidation, and therefore, this is a specific problem in fishery products.

Lipid oxidation in fish muscle can be promoted by nonenzymatic processes, such as autoxidation and photosensitized oxidation (initiated by Fe-heme), or catalyzed by enzymes, such as lipoxygenase (present in the gills and fish tissues). Heme-proteins, transition metals, and lipoxygenases are the primary endogenous components involved in fish lipid oxidation in common with other muscle foods (Medina and Pazos 2010). In *in vivo* fish, there is a satisfactory balance between prooxidants (Fe-heme present in myoglobin and hemoglobin, Fe-no heme, nicotinamide adenine dinucleotide phosphate (NADP), ascorbate, ferritin, transferrin, and lipoxygenases) and antioxidants (superoxide dismutase, catalase, glutathione peroxidase and reductase, tocopherols, astaxanthin, ubiquinol, and vitamin C), but this is lost postmortem when hydrolysis and especially oxidation processes begin (Jacobsen et al. 2010).

During industrial processing and commercialization, temperature is normally kept below 18°C to avoid hydrolysis of TAG and phospholipids by lipases and phospholipases, respectively. Another parameter that is essential to be controlled is oxygen exposure during storage, normally by packaging with decreased oxygen using vacuum or modified atmospheres and materials impermeable to oxygen. As to the addition of antioxidants, it is nowadays preferred to use natural antioxidants from plant extracts (tocopherols, flavonoids, polyphenols) mixed with synergic compounds, such as radical scavengers (ascorbic acid and ascorbates) or metal chelators (ethylenediaminetetraacetic acid (EDTA), phosphates, carnosine). Finally, it is important to note that prevention of oxidation is of growing interest in fish products because many of the recently commercialized, ready-to-cook presentations, such as minced patties, are remarkably more susceptible to oxidation (Aubourg et al. 2005; Giménez et al. 2011).

4.6.4 PROCESSED FOODS

Processed foods are expected to be the most susceptible to lipid oxidation as a result of heat treatment, drying, fermentation, and other processes involved in their preparation and commercialization. A fundamental difference in the mechanisms of oxidation in processed foods versus natural, raw, or slightly treated foods is that enzymes are not active, and hence, autoxidation is the most important oxidation pathway. The main factors influencing lipid oxidation in processed foods are structural characteristics, lipid distribution, changes in water activity, and formation of nonenzymatic browning materials, all of them already commented on elsewhere in this chapter. In general, processed foods are composed of different phases, being the fat or oil in a noncontinuous or dispersed phase whose oxidative behavior is heterogeneous and difficult to predict (Fritsch 1994).

In those processed foods constituted by emulsions (milk products, sauces, creams, etc.), the main factors governing lipid oxidation are those derived from their emulsion nature as already discussed previously. Food powders are normally prepared from formulated emulsions, and hence, lipid oxidation is also affected by factors related with the interfacial phenomenon. Physical food structure, water activity, and particularly, lipid distribution are also important variables involved (Vignolles et al. 2007, 2009). Lipid-containing food powders obtained from drying natural emulsions include milk powders, dried eggs, or dehydrated soups and sauces. Others are obtained by drying formulated emulsions, such as infant formulas and microencapsulated oils (flavoring additives, pigments, microencapsulated fish oils, microencapsulated lipophilic vitamins, etc.). In the case of oils or lipophilic compounds, encapsulation is a strategy used to mask or preserve flavors and especially to protect them from oxidation (Velasco et al. 2003; Márquez-Ruiz et al. 2003; Madene et al. 2006; Drusch and Mannino 2009). Description of lipid oxidation mechanisms in microencapsulated oils was already included in Section 4.2.1.

Confectionery products (chocolate, coatings, fillings, caramels, toffees, etc.) show generally long shelf lives because they are made of high-stability saturated fats and oils (Talbot 2010). However, in cereal-based products, such as snacks and breakfast cereals, linoleic acid is the predominant fatty acid (approximately 50%–60% of total fatty acid composition in corn, barley, and wheat lipids), which makes them more susceptible to oxidation (Hall 2010).

Thermally processed foods (bakery and fried products) are more likely to develop lipid oxidation because both oxidative and thermal reactions are involved as discussed already. However, bakery products (breads, cakes, pastries, biscuits, cookies, and crackers) are mostly prepared with stable fats and oils that do not undergo relevant oxidation during baking (Cauvain and Young 2010). During storage, other sources of deterioration, such as staling, mold growth, softening, or toughening, occur usually earlier than lipid oxidation. Still, products with very low water activities (biscuits, cookies, and crackers) may become rancid during shelf life.

Deep-frying, one of the most common processes used for food preparation, is widely used by consumers and the food industry. Complex reactions are involved during lipid oxidation at high temperatures as already detailed in this chapter. Also, chemical reactions between main food constituents and between oxidation compounds and proteins or amino acids seem to be the most important pathways for formation of compounds responsible for color and flavor (Pokorny 1999). In fact, the smell and taste of the fried food are partly a result of oxidized compounds that are highly appreciated by consumers. The action of the main variables involved, either intrinsic (oil composition, minor compounds, and additives) or extrinsic (length of heating, temperature, and surface-to-oil volume ratio), as well as those related to the food being fried (oil absorption and lipid exchange) has been extensively studied in our laboratory (Jorge et al. 1996a,b; Dobarganes et al. 2000, 2010; Dobarganes and Márquez-Ruiz 2006; Velasco et al. 2008; Márquez-Ruiz et al. 2010). Results indicate that the effect of the variables depends on the type of frying, that is, continuous or discontinuous, and

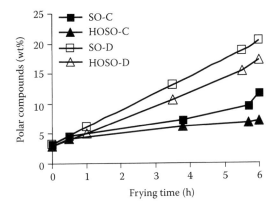

FIGURE 4.13 Formation of polar compounds in conventional and high-oleic sunflower oils during continuous (SO-C and HOSO-C, respectively) and discontinuous (SO-D and HOSO-D, respectively) frying at 175°C for 6 h.

demonstrate the primary importance of the continuous presence of food in the fryer and the addition of new oil to compensate for that removed by the fried product. In consequence, fried foods produced through the discontinuous frying process are those that can reach the highest degradation level. Figure 4.13 shows the large differences found in formation of polar compounds during continuous and discontinuous frying under similar conditions of temperature, initial surface-to-volume ratio, and total heating time in conventional and high-oleic sunflower oils (Jorge et al. 1996b).

Finally, it is important to remark that in processed foods oxidized under storage temperatures, rarely more than 4%–5% of TAG (approximately 100 meq O_2/kg fat) would be oxidized upon consumption because at these levels of oxidation, a rancid odor is clearly detectable and, therefore, the food objectionable. In contrast, in the case of frying fats, not only the present official regulations establish the limit of new compounds formed in as high as 25% (Firestone 1996), but even this level is often considerably surpassed in a significant number of oils and fats from fast food outlets. Because oil absorption is high (as much as 40% in the case of potato crisps), and the oil absorbed is not different from the frying oil in the fryer, most of the oxidized fats in foods are expected to come from fried products (Dobarganes and Márquez-Ruiz 2003).

ACKNOWLEDGMENTS

This work was funded by the Spanish Ministry of Science and Innovation (Project AGL2010-18307) and by the Autonomous Community of Madrid (Project ANALISYC-II S2009/AGR-1464).

REFERENCES

Apple, J.K., Maxwell, C.V., Galloway, D.L., Hamilton, C.R., and Yancey, J.W.S. 2009. Interactive effects of dietary source and slaughter weight in growing-finishing swine: II. Fatty acid composition of subcutaneous fat. *J Anim Sci* 87: 1423–1440.

Aubourg, S.P., Rodriguez, A., and Gallardo, J.M. 2005. Rancidity development during frozen storage of mackerel (*Scomber scombrus*): Effect of catching season and commercial presentation. *Eur J Lipid Sci Tech* 107: 316–323.

Bolland, J.L. 1949. Kinetics of olefin oxidation. *Quart Rev* 3: 1–21.

Brandon, K., Butler, F., Allen, P., and Beggan, M. 2009. The performance of several oxygen scavengers in varying oxygen environments at refrigerated temperatures: Implications for low-oxygen modified atmosphere packaging of meat. *Int J Food Sci Technol* 44: 188–196.

Brimberg, U.I. and Kamal-Eldin, A. 2003. On the kinetics of the autoxidation of fats: Substrates with conjugated double bonds. *Eur J Lipid Sci Tech* 105: 17–22.

Campbell, W., Drake, M.A., and Larick, D.K. 2003. The impact of fortification with conjugated linoleic acid (CLA) on the quality of fluid milk. *J Dairy Sci* 86: 43–51.

Cauvain, S.P. and Young, L.S. 2010. Chemical and physical deterioration of bakery products. In *Chemical Deterioration and Physical Instability of Food and Beverages*, edited by L.H. Skibsted, J. Risbo and M.L. Andersen, 381–412. Cambridge: Woodhead Publishing Limited.

Choe, E. and Min, D.B. 2007. Chemistry of deep-fat frying oils. *J Food Sci* 72: R77–R86.

Chuy, L.E. and Labuza, T.P. 1994. Caking and stickiness of dairy-based food powders as related to glass transition. *J Food Sci* 59: 43–46.

Coupland, J.N. and McClements, D.J. 1996. Lipid oxidation in food emulsions. *Trends Food Sci Technol* 7: 83–91.

Decker, E.A., Chaiyasit, W., Hu, M., Faraji, H., and McClements D.J. 2008. Lipid oxidation in food dispersions. In *Lipid Oxidation Pathways*, Volume 2, edited by A. Kamal-Eldin and D.B. Min, 273–289. Urbana, IL: AOCS Press.

Dobarganes, M.C. 1998. Formation and analysis of high molecular-weight compounds in frying fats and oils. *OCL-Oleagineux Corps Gras Lipides* 5: 41–47.

Dobarganes, M.C. and Márquez-Ruiz, G. 2003. Oxidized fats in foods. *Current Opin Clin Nutr* 6: 157–163.

Dobarganes, M.C. and Márquez Ruiz, G. 2006. Formation and analysis of oxidized monomeric, dimeric and higher oligomeric triglycerides. In *Deep Frying: Chemistry Nutrition and Practical Applications* (2nd edition), edited by M.D. Erickson, 87–110. Urbana, IL: AOCS Press.

Dobarganes, M.C., Márquez-Ruiz, G., Marmesat, S., and Velasco, J. 2010. Determination of oxidation compounds and oligomers by chromatographic techniques. In *Frying of Food: Oxidation, Nutrient and Non-nutrient Antioxidants, Biologically Active Compounds and High Temperatures* (2nd edition), edited by D. Boskou and I. Elmadfa, 152–174. London: Taylor and Francis.

Dobarganes, M.C., Márquez-Ruiz, G., Sébédio, J.L., and Christie, W.W. 2013. *Frying oils: Chemistry, Analysis and Nutritional Aspects*, edited by W.W. Christie. http://lipidlibrary.aocs. org/frying/frying.html. Urbana, IL: AOCS.

Dobarganes, M.C., Márquez-Ruiz, G., and Velasco, J. 2000. Interactions between fat and food during deep frying. *Eur J Lipid Sci Technol* 102: 521–528.

Drusch, S. and Mannino, S. 2009. Patent-based review on industrial approaches for the microencapsulation of oils rich in polyunsaturated fatty acids. *Trends Food Sci Technol* 20: 237–244.

Eriksson, C.E. 1987. Oxidation of lipids in food systems. In *Autoxidation of Unsaturated Lipids*, edited by H.W.-S. Chan, 207–231. London: Academic Press.

Eulitz, K., Yurawecz, M.P., and Ku, Y. 1999. The oxidation of conjugated linoleic acid. In *Advances in CLA Research*, Vol. 1, edited by M.P. Yurawecz, M.M. Mossoba, J.K.G. Kramer, M.W. Pariza and G.J. Nelson, 55–63. Champaign, IL: AOCS Press.

Faustman, C., Yin, S., and Tatiyaborwntham, N. 2010. Oxidation and protection of red meat. In *Oxidation in Foods and Beverages and Antioxidant Applications. Volume 2: Management in Different Food Sectors*, edited by E. Decker, R. Elias and D.J. McClements, 3–49. Cambridge: Woodhead Publishing Limited.

Firestone, D. 1996. Regulation of frying fats and oils. In *Deep Frying: Chemistry Nutrition and Practical Applications*, edited by E.G. Perkins and M.D. Erickson, 323–334. Urbana, IL: American Oil Chemists Society Press.

Frankel, E.N. 2005. *Lipid Oxidation*. Bridgwater, England: The Oily Press.

Fritsch, C.W. 1994. Lipid oxidation—The other dimensions. *INFORM* 5: 423–436.

García-Martínez, M.C., and Márquez-Ruiz, G. 2009. Lipid oxidation in functional dairy products. *Curr Nutr Food Sci* 5: 209–216.

García-Martínez, M.C., Márquez-Ruiz, G., Fontecha, J., and M. Gordon. 2009. Volatile oxidation compounds in a conjugated linoleic acid (CLA)-rich oil. *Food Chem* 113: 926–931.

García-Martínez, M.C., Rodriguez-Alcala, L.M., Marmesat, S., Alonso, L., Fontecha, J., and Márquez-Ruiz, G. 2010. Lipid stability in powdered infant formula stored at ambient temperatures. *Int J Food Sci Technol* 2337–2344.

Gardner, H.W. 1979. Lipid hydroperoxide reactivity with proteins and amino acids: A review. *J Agric Food Chem* 27: 220–229.

Gardner, H.W. 1987. Reaction of hydroperoxides—Products of low molecular weight. In *Autoxidation of Unsaturated Lipids*, edited by H.W.-S. Chan, 95–139. London: Academic Press.

Gardner, H.W. 1989. Oxygen radical chemistry of polyunsaturated fatty acids. *Free Radic Biol Med* 7: 65–86.

Genot, C., Meynier, A., and Riaublanc. A. 2003. Lipid oxidation in emulsions. In *Lipid Oxidation Pathways*, vol. 1, edited by A. Kamal- Eldin, 190–144. Urbana, IL: AOCS Press.

Giménez, B., Gómez-Guillén, M.C., Pérez-Mateos, M., Montero, P., and Márquez-Ruiz, G. 2011. Evaluation of lipid oxidation in horse mackerel patties covered with borage-containing film during frozen storage. *Food Chem* 124: 1393–1403.

Gomes, T. and Catalano, M. 1988. Caratteri di qualità degli oli alimentari. I trigliceridi ossidati. *Rev Ital Sostanze Grasse* 65: 125–127.

Gordon, M.H. 2010. Effects of food structure and ingredient interactions on antioxidant capacity. In *Oxidation in Foods and Beverages and Antioxidant Applications. Volume 1: Understanding Mechanisms of Oxidation and Antioxidant Activity*, edited by E. Decker, R. Elias and D.J. McClements, 321–331. Cambridge: Woodhead Publishing Limited.

Grosch, W. 1987. Reactions of hydroperoxides-products of low molecular weight. In *Autoxidation of Unsaturated Lipids*, edited by H.W.-S. Chan, 95–139. London: Academic Press.

Hall, C. 2010. Oxidation of cereals and snack products. In *Oxidation in Foods and Beverages and Antioxidant Applications. Volume 2: Management in Different Food Sectors*, edited by E. Decker, R. Elias and D.J. McClements, 369–390. Cambridge: Woodhead Publishing Limited.

Hämäläinen, T.I., Sundberg, S., Hase, T., and Hopia, A. 2002. Stereochemistry of the hydroperoxides formed during autoxidation of CLA methyl ester in the presence of α-tocopherol. *Lipids* 37: 533–540.

Hidalgo, F.J., Zamora, R., and Alaiz, M. 1992. Modifications produced in food proteins following interactions with oxidizing lipids. II. Mechanisms of oxidizing lipid-protein interactions. *Grasas Aceites* 43: 31–38.

Holgado, F. 2011. Lipid oxidation in microencapsulated oils: Effect of preparation conditions on model compounds and specific studies on foods. Ph.D. Dissertation, Universidad Autónoma de Madrid.

Huang, S.-W., Frankel, E.N., Aeschbach, R., and German, J.B. 1997. Partition of selected antioxidants in corn oil-water model systems. *J Agric Food Chem* 45: 1991–1994.

Huang, S.-W., Frankel, E.N., Schwarz, K., and German, B. 1996. Effect of pH on antioxidant activity of a-tocopherol and Trolox in oil-in-water emulsions. *J Agric Food Chem* 44: 2496–2502.

Jacobsen, C., Nielsen, H.H., Jorgensen, B., and Nielsen, J. 2010. Chemical processes responsible for quality deterioration in fish. In *Chemical Deterioration and Physical Instability of Food and Beverages,* edited by L.H. Skibsted, J. Risbo and M.L. Andersen, 439–465. Cambridge: Woodhead Publishing Limited.

Jorge, N., Márquez-Ruiz, G., Martín-Polvillo, M., Ruiz-Méndez, M.V., and Dobarganes, M.C. 1996a. Influence of dimethylpolysiloxane addition to edible oils: Dependence on the main variables of the frying process. *Grasas Aceites* 47: 14–19.

Jorge, N., Márquez-Ruiz, G., Martín-Polvillo, M., Ruiz-Méndez, M.V., and Dobarganes, M.C. 1996b. Influence dimethylpolyxilosane addition to frying oils: Performance of sunflower oils in discontinuous and continuous laboratory frying. *Grasas Aceites* 47: 20–25.

Kamal-Eldin, A. and Min, D.B. 2008. *Lipid Oxidation Pathways.* Urbana, IL: AOCS Press.

Kanner, J. 2010. Metals and food oxidation. In *Oxidation in Foods and Beverages and Antioxidant Applications. Volume 1: Understanding Mechanisms of Oxidation and Antioxidant Activity,* edited by E. Decker, R. Elias and D.J. McClements, 36–56. Cambridge: Woodhead Publishing Limited.

Karel, M. 1984. Chemical effects in food stored at room temperature. *J Chem Educ* 61: 335–339.

Karel, M., Labuza, T.P., and Maloney, J.F. 1967. Chemical changes in freeze-dried foods and model systems. *Cryobiology* 3: 288–296.

Kolanowski, W. and Weißbrodt, J. 2007. Sensory quality of dairy products fortified with fish oil. *Int Dairy J* 17: 1248–1253.

Kulas, E., Olsen, E., and Ackman, R.G. 2003. Oxidation of fish lipids and its inhibition with tocopherols. In *Lipid Oxidation Pathways*, vol. 1, edited by A. Kamal-Eldin, 190–144. Urbana, IL: AOCS Press.

Labuza, T.P. 1968. Sorption phenomena in foods. *Food Technol* 22: 15–24.

Labuza, T.P. 1975. Sorption phenomena in foods: Theoretical and practical aspects. In *Theory, Determination and Control of Physical Properties of Food Materials*, edited by C.K. Rha, 197. Dordrecht: Reidel.

Luna, P., De la Fuente, M.A., Salvador, D., and Márquez-Ruiz, G. 2007. Differences in oxidation kinetics between conjugated and non-conjugated methyl linoleate. *Lipids* 42: 1085–1092.

Madene, A., Jacquot, M., Scher, J., and Desobry, S. 2006. Flavour encapsulation and controlled release—A review. *Int J Food Sci Technol* 41: 1–21.

Marmesat, S., Velasco, J., and Dobarganes, M.C. 2008. Quantitative determination of epoxyacids, ketoacids and hydroxyacids formed in fats and oils at frying temperatures. *J Chromatogr A* 1211: 129–134.

Márquez-Ruiz, G. and Dobarganes, C. 2005. Analysis of non-volatile lipid oxidation compounds by high-performance size-exclusion chromatography. In *Analysis of Lipid Oxidation*, edited by A. Kamal-Eldin, 40–69. Urbana, IL: AOCS Press.

Márquez-Ruiz, G., Holgado, F., García-Martínez, M.C., and Dobarganes, M.C. 2007. A direct and fast method to monitor lipid oxidation progress in model fatty acid methyl esters by high-performance size-exclusion chromatography. *J Chromatogr A* 1165: 122–127.

Márquez-Ruiz, G., Ruiz-Méndez, M.V., Velasco, J., and Dobarganes, M.C. 2010. Preventing oxidation during frying of foods. In *Oxidation in Foods and Beverages and Antioxidant Applications. Volume 2: Management in Different Food Sectors*, edited by E. Decker, R. Elias and D.J. McClements, 239–273. Cambridge: Woodhead Publishing Limited.

Márquez-Ruiz, G., Velasco, J., and Dobarganes, C. 2003. Oxidation in dried microencapsulated oils. In *Lipid Oxidation Pathways*, edited by A. Kamal-Eldin, 245–264. Urbana, IL: AOCS Press.

Medina, I. and Pazos, M. 2010. Oxidation and protection of fish. In *Oxidation in Foods and Beverages and Antioxidant Applications. Volume 2: Management in Different Food Sectors*, edited by E. Decker, R. Elias and D.J. McClements, 91–120. Cambridge: Woodhead Publishing Limited.

Min, D.B. and Boff, J.M. 2002. Lipid oxidation of edible oil. In *Food Lipids: Chemistry, Nutrition and Biotechnology*, edited by C.C. Akoh and D.B. Min, 335–363. New York: Marcel Dekker.

Miyashita, K., Frankel, E.N., and Neff, W.E. 1990. Autoxidation of polyunsaturated triacylglycerols. III. Synthetic triacylglycerols containing linoleate and linolenate. *Lipids* 25: 48–53.

Miyashita, K. and Takagi, T. 1986. Study on the oxidative rate and prooxidant activity of free fatty acids. *J Am Oil Chem Soc* 63: 1380–1384.

Osada, K., Hoshina, S., Nakamura, S., and Sugano, M. 2000. Cholesterol oxidation in meat products and its regulation by supplementation of sodium nitrite and apple polyphenol before processing. *J Agric Food Chem* 41: 1893–1898.

Pokorny, J. 1987. Major factors affecting the autoxidation of lipids. In *Autoxidation of Unsaturated Lipids*, edited by H.W.-S. Chan, 141–205. London: Academic Press.

Pokorny, J. 1998. Substrate influence on the frying process. *Grasas Aceites* 49: 265–270.

Pokorny, J. 1999. Changes of nutrients at frying temperatures. In *Frying of Food*, edited by D. Boskou and I. Elmadf, 69–103. Lancaster, PA: Technomic Publishing Co.

Porter, N.A., Caldwell, S.E., and Mills, K.A. 1995. Mechanisms of free radical oxidation of unsaturated lipids. *Lipids* 30: 277–290.

Porter, W.L. 1980. Recent trends in food applications of antioxidants. In *Autoxidation in Foods and Biological Systems*, edited by M. Simic and G. Karel, 295–365. New York: Plenum Press.

Ramanathan, R., Konda, M.K.R., Mancini, R., and Faustman, C. 2009. Species-specific effects of sarcoplamic extracts on lipid oxidation *in vitro*. *J Food Sci* 74: c73–c77.

Richards, M.P. 2010. Heme proteins and oxidation in fresh and processed meats. In *Oxidation in Foods and Beverages and Antioxidant Applications. Volume 1: Understanding Mechanisms of Oxidation and Antioxidant Activity*, edited by E. Decker, R. Elias and D.J. McClements, 76–104. Cambridge: Woodhead Publishing Limited.

Richards, M.P. and Dettmann, M.A. 2003. Comparative analysis of different hemoglobins: Autoxidation, reaction with peroxide, and lipid oxidation. *J Agric Food Chem* 51: 3886–3891.

Roos, Y.H., Karel, M., and Kokini, J.L. 1996. Glass transitions in low moisture and frozen foods: Effects on shelf life and quality. *Food Technol* Nov: 95–108.

Ruiz-Méndez, M.V., Márquez-Ruiz, G., and Dobarganes, M.C. 1997. Relationships between quality of crude and refined edible oils based on quantitation of minor glyceridic compounds. *Food Chem* 60: 549–554.

Ruxton, C.H.S., Reed, S.C., Simpson, J.A., and Millington, K.J. 2007. The health benefits of omega-3 polyunsaturated fatty acids: A review of the evidence. *J Human Nutr Diet* 20: 275–285.

Sagone, A.L., Greenwald, J., Kraut, E.H., Bianchine, J., and Singh, D. 1983. Glucose: A role as a free radical scavenger in biological systems. *J Lab Clin Med* 101: 97–103.

Sahasrabudhe, M.R. and Farne, I.G. 1964. Effect of heat on triglycerides of corn oil. *J Am Oil Chem Soc* 41: 264–267.

Sánchez-Muniz, F.J., Bastida, S., Márquez-Ruiz, G., and Dobarganes, M.C. 2008. Effect of heating and frying on oil and food fatty acids. In *Fatty Acids in Foods and Their Health Implication,* edited by C.K. Chow, 511–543. Boca Raton: CRC Press.

Schaich, K.M. 1992. Metals and lipid oxidation. Contemporary issues. *Lipids* 27: 209–218.

Schaich, K.M. 2008. Co-oxidation of proteins by oxidizing lipids. In *Lipid Oxidation Pathways*. Volume 2, edited by A. Kamal-Eldin and D.B. Min, 181–272. Urbana, IL: AOCS Press.

Schneider, C. 2009. An update on products and mechanisms of lipid peroxidation. *Mol Nutr Food Res* 53: 315–321.

Schwarz, K., Frankel, E.N., and German, J.B. 1996. Partition behavior of antioxidative phenolic compounds in heterophasic systems. *Fett/Lipid* 98: 115–121.

Shahidi, F. and Miraliakkbari, H. 2004. Omega 3 (n-3) fatty acids in health and disease. *J Med Food*: 7:387.

Shimada, Y., Roos, Y., and Karel, M. 1991. Oxidation of methyl linoleate encapsulated in amorphous lactose-based food model. *J Agric Food Chem* 39: 637–641.

Sims, R.J. 1994. Oxidation of fats in food products. *INFORM* 5: 1020–1028.

Skibsted, L.H. 2010. Understanding oxidation processes in foods. In *Oxidation in Foods and Beverages and Antioxidant Applications. Volume 1: Understanding Mechanisms of Oxidation and Antioxidant Activity*, edited by E. Decker, R. Elias and D.J. McClements, 3–35. Cambridge: Woodhead Publishing Limited.

Talbot, G. 2010. Oxidation of confectionery products and biscuits. In *Oxidation in Foods and Beverages and Antioxidant Applications. Volume 2: Management in Different Food Sectors,* edited by E. Decker, R. Elias and D.J. McClements, 344–368. Cambridge: Woodhead Publishing Limited.

Tong, L.M., Sasaki, S., McClements, J.D., and Decker, E.A. 2000. Mechanisms of the antioxidant activity of a high molecular weight fraction of whey. *J Agric Food Chem* 48: 1473–1478.

Velasco, J., Dobarganes, C., Holgado, F., and Márquez-Ruiz, G. 2009b. A follow-up oxidation study in dried microencapsulated oils under the accelerated conditions of the Rancimat test. *Food Res Int* 42: 56–62.

Velasco, J., Dobarganes, M.C., and Márquez-Ruiz, G. 2000. Oxidation of free and encapsulated oil fractions in dried microencapsulated fish oils. *Grasas Aceites* 51: 439–446.

Velasco, J., Dobarganes, M.C., and Márquez-Ruiz, G. 2002. Lipid oxidation in heterophasic lipid systems: Oil-in-water emulsions. *Grasas Aceites* 53: 239–247.

Velasco, J., Dobarganes, M.C., and Márquez-Ruiz, G. 2003. Variables affecting lipid oxidation in dried microencapsulated oils. *Grasas Aceites* 54: 304–314.

Velasco, J., Dobarganes, M.C., and Márquez-Ruiz, G. 2010. Oxidative rancidity. In *Chemical Deterioration and Physical Instability of Food and Beverages*, edited by L.H. Skibsted, J. Risbo and M.L. Andersen, 1–33. Cambridge: Woodhead Publishing Limited.

Velasco, J., Holgado, F., Dobarganes, C., and Márquez-Ruiz, G. 2009a. Influence of relative humidity on oxidation of the free and encapsulated oil fractions in freeze-dried microencapsulated oils. *Food Res Int* 42: 1492–1500.

Velasco, J., Holgado, F., Dobarganes, C., and Márquez-Ruiz, G. 2009c. Antioxidant activity of added phenolic compounds in freeze-dried microencapsulated sunflower oil. *J Am Oil Chem Soc* 86: 445–452.

Velasco, J., Marmesat, S., Berdeaux, O., Márquez-Ruiz, G., and Dobarganes, M.C. 2004. Formation and evolution of monoepoxy fatty acids in thermoxidized olive and sunflower oils and quantitation in used frying oils from restaurants and fried food outlets. *J Agric Food Chem* 52: 4438–4443.

Velasco, J., Marmesat, S., Berdeaux, O., Márquez-Ruiz, G., and Dobarganes, M.C. 2005. Quantitation of short-chain glycerol-bound compounds in thermoxidized and used frying oils: A monitoring study during thermoxidation of olive and sunflower oils. *J Agric Food Chem* 53: 4006–4011.

Velasco, J., Marmesat, S., and Dobarganes, M.C. 2008. Chemistry of Frying. In *Deep Fat Frying of Foods*, edited by S. Sahin and G. Sumnu, 33–56. New York: Taylor and Francis.

Velasco, J., Marmesat, S., Dobarganes, C., and Márquez-Ruiz, G. 2006. Heterogeneous aspects of lipid oxidation in dried microencapsulated oils. *J Agric Food Chem* 54: 1722–1729.

Vignolles, M.L., Jeantet, R., Lopez, C., and Schuck, P. 2007. Free fat, surface fat and dairy powders: Interactions between process and product. A review. *Lait* 87: 187–236.

Vignolles, M.L., Lopez, C., Madec, M.N., Ehrhardt, J.J, Méjean, S., Schuck, P., and Jeantet, R. 2009. Fat properties during homogenization, spray-drying, and storage affect the physical properties of dairy powders. *J Dairy Sci* 92: 58–70.

Wang, T. and Hammond, E.G. 2010. Lipoxygenase and lipid oxidation in foods. In *Oxidation in Foods and Beverages and Antioxidant Applications. Volume 1: Understanding Mechanisms of Oxidation and Antioxidant Activity*, edited by E. Decker, R. Elias and D.J. McClements, 105–121. Cambridge: Woodhead Publishing Limited.

Waraho, T., Cardenia, V., Decaer, E.A., and McClements, D.J. 2010. Lipid oxidation in emulsified food products. In *Oxidation in Foods and Beverages and Antioxidant Applications. Volume 2: Management in Different Food Sectors*, edited by E. Decker, R. Elias and D.J. McClements, 306–343. Cambridge: Woodhead Publishing Limited.

Wedzicha, B.L. 1988. Distribution of low molecular weight additives in dispersed systems. In *Advances in Food Emulsions and Foams*, edited by E. Dickinson and G. Stainsby, 329–371. London: Elsevier Applied Science.

Yamauchi, R., Aoki, Y., Sugiura, T., Kato, K., and Yoshimitsu, U. 1982. Effect of sugars and sugar analogs on autoxidation of methyl linoleate and safflower oil. *Agric Biol Chem* 46: 2997–3002.

Yamauchi, R., Tatsumi, Y., Asano, M., Kato, K., and Yoshimitsu, U. 1988. Effects of metals, salts and fructose on the autoxidation of methyl linoleate in emulsions. *Agric Biol Chem* 52: 849–850.

Yurawecz, M.P., Delmonte, P., Vogel, T., and Kramer, J.K.G. 2003. Oxidation of conjugated linoleic acid: Initiators and simultaneous reactions: Theory and practice. In *Advances in CLA Research*, vol. 2, edited by J.L. Sébédio, W.W. Christie, and R. Adolf, 56–70. Champaign, IL: AOCS Press.

Zamora, R. and Hidalgo, F.J. 2005. Coordinate contribution of lipid oxidation and Maillard reaction to the nonenzymatic food browning. *Crit Rev Food Sci Nutr* 45: 49–59.

Zamora, R. and Hidalgo, F.J. 2011. The Maillard reaction and lipid oxidation. *Lipid Technol* 23: 59–62.

5 Protein Oxidation in Foods and Its Prevention

Caroline P. Baron

CONTENTS

5.1   INTRODUCTION

Reactive oxygen species (ROS), such as hydrogen peroxide, superoxide, hydroxyl radicals, peroxynitrite, singlet oxygen, alkoxyl, and peroxyl radicals, are formed in living cells as part of metabolic processes, such as electron transport systems, and as cell signaling molecules but can also be produced as a response to external stimuli, for example, irradiation, stress, and pollution. ROS are strong oxidants, which are able to modify cell constituents, including DNA, lipids, and proteins. In general, the living cell is able to deal with ROS using complex enzymatic and antioxidant defense and repair systems in order to control ROS and repair the damage caused by ROS. During aging, the metabolism is impaired, and enzymatic systems are less potent resulting in more ROS and in accumulation of oxidized DNA, lipids, and proteins, and this has been shown to result in the pathology of several diseases (Halliwell and Gutteridge 2007; Davies and Dean 2003).

ROS, which are present in biological systems, are also present in food and are mostly formed during food processing and storage. ROS in foods can be generated and accumulate depending on the food matrix composition, its structure, but also as a result of processing and storage conditions that contribute to the production of ROS. Oxidation of protein in foods has only received some attention in the last decade perhaps because of its complexity and the lack of appropriate analytical methods to measure protein oxidation but also because it results in changes in product quality that are not immediately perceived by consumers. In addition, proteins are very complex molecules organized in large structures, and oxidation may lead to a great number of modifications either on the protein side chains or on the protein backbone, including amino acid modifications, protein cleavage, and cross-linking. It is now accepted that food proteins oxidize and that even small modification at the protein's molecular level can have severe consequences for product quality and protein functionality but also nutritional implications with, for example, the loss of essential amino acids. Protein oxidation mechanisms are poorly understood probably because of the complexity of the target and of the reaction products. Nevertheless, some mechanisms have been put forward, and it is believed that protein oxidation mechanisms are very similar to lipid oxidation mechanisms.

The mechanisms responsible for the initiation of protein oxidation can be classified as direct oxidation of the protein with a direct attack of the radical species or hydrogen abstraction on the protein leading to a protein radical or anion. Indirect oxidation of protein refers to the interaction between protein and, for example, secondary lipid oxidation products, such as aldehydes or reducing sugars. The mechanisms involved in a direct free-radical attack on the protein oxidation are not clear, but it is generally assumed that free-radical species initiating lipid oxidation are also able to initiate protein oxidation. It is also believed that it follows the same scheme as lipid oxidation consisting of an initiation step with hydrogen abstraction or electron transfer, a propagation step with radical transfer/hydrogen abstraction from other biomolecules, and a termination mechanism step leading to dimerization. Radicals able to abstract a hydrogen atom from the protein or to transfer electron to protein leading to the formation of an initial radical on the protein side chain or backbone. It is so that electrophilic radicals will attack at electron-rich sites on the protein, and nucleophilic radicals will attack at electron-deficient sites on the protein. However, the initial radical can be formed at a different sites on the protein, not only depending on the attacking ROS but also depending largely upon the protein and its structures and also the protein environment, which, in food, is related to the food matrix and its structure. The initial radical can be a carbon-centered radical, an alkoxyl, a peroxyl radical, or a thiyl radical.

Even if protein oxidation is difficult to predict because of the complexity of the target and of the number of possible attacking species, it is not a stochastic process. In a model system, hydrogen abstraction on the protein backbone has been shown to take place at the alpha carbon and to lead to protein fragmentation. At the side chain, hydrogen atom abstraction is believed to take place on aliphatic side chains while an addition is expected to occur on aromatic side chains. Oxidation of proteins at the side chain often leads to protein carbonyls, alcohols, and peroxides. The amino acids, which are generally most susceptible to oxidation, are cysteine, tyrosine, phenylalanine, tryptophan, histidine, proline, arginine, lysine, and methionine. However, to date, a few products have been unambiguously identified in foods. In dairy products, methionine, tyrosine, and cysteine oxidation products, such as methionine sulfoxide, dityrosine,

TABLE 5.1

Selected Amino Acids and Their Oxidation Products as Well as Their Detection in Foods (Nonexhaustive List)

Amino Acid	Oxidation Products	Food	References
Cys	Disulfide, cystine, cysteic acid	Rapeseed flour, casein, and fishmeal	Anderson et al. 1975, Slump and Scheuder 1973
Met	Methionine sulfoxide, sulfone	Casein and fishmeal, milk, rapeseed flour	Slump and Scheuder 1973, Meltretter et al. 2008, Anderson et al. 1975
Tyr	Dityrosine	Dough, milk, cheese	Takasaki et al. 2005, Østdal et al. 1999, Balestrieri et al. 2002
Try	N-formylkynurenine	Milk, model system	Scheidegger et al. 2010, Kanner and Fennema 1987
Arg, Pro	γ-glutamic semialdehyde	Meat, meat products, fish	Armenteros et al. 2009, Timm-Heinrich et al. 2013
Lys	α-aminoadipic semialdehyde	Meat, meat products, fish	Armenteros et al. 2009, Eymard et al. 2012

and cysteic acid, respectively, have been detected (Alegria Toran et al. 1996; Østdal et al. 2000). In meat material, γ-glutamic semialdehyde (GGS) as well as α-aminoadipic semialdehyde (AAS) have been detected as oxidation products of arginine, proline, and lysine, respectively (Estevez et al. 2009). Some examples of amino acid oxidation products detected in food are presented in Table 5.1 (see also Chapter 3).

In general, formation of carbonyl compounds on amino acid side chains is well described as a result of metal-initiated protein oxidation, but other oxidative reactions can lead to the formation of protein carbonyl groups. The present chapter will report a present protein oxidation mechanism in food, evaluate protein oxidation during food processing and storage, and report strategies in order to prevent protein oxidation.

5.2 INITIATION OF PROTEIN OXIDATION IN FOODS

5.2.1 METALS

Transition metals and especially iron have been shown to play a central role in lipid oxidation and are also believed to be involved in the oxidation of proteins (Stadtman et al. 1990). Most proteins are able to chelate metals; some proteins have a specific iron or copper binding site, such as heme proteins, but more generally, protein can chelate metal when primary amine groups are present at their side chain with for example amino acids such as lysine and glutamine. The amount of free iron in food has been estimated to range from 1 up to 40 mg/kg depending on the food item with meat being in the highest and vegetables in the lowest range. It is therefore expected that iron either free or bound is significantly contributing to protein oxidation in food. In addition, metal-induced oxidation is particularly relevant in the presence of peroxides and especially hydrogen peroxide. Indeed, decomposition of hydrogen peroxide via Fenton chemistry leads to the formation of the hydroxyl radical ($\bullet$OH), which is a strong prooxidant able to oxidize all amino acids, although not all amino acids are reactive. Hydrogen peroxide is present in cells ranging from 0.01 to 0.1 μM and accumulates in muscle tissue postmortem (Harel and Kanner 1985) and has been reported to reach a concentration of up to 0.6 mM in biological tissues under ischemia (Halliwell and Gutteridge 2007). The level of hydrogen peroxide in muscle food *postmortem* is most likely low, but some processing conditions, which involve bleaching with hydrogen peroxide to whiten food and improve its color, may have a detrimental effect on protein oxidation, such as, for example, fish flesh (Jafarpour et al. 2008). In cheese production, hydrogen peroxide is sometimes added to whey to remove the colorant added in the cheese-making process (Kang et al. 2010). Hydrogen peroxide is added to food to improve not only its color but also its quality (e.g., the improvement of flour). However, this might enhance iron-initiated oxidation and promote Fenton chemistry leading to severe protein oxidation. Indeed, in whey protein, Munyua (1975) reported that hydrogen peroxide resulted in a decrease in the content of nonpolar amino acids, such as aspartic acid, threonine, glutamic acid, methionine, phenylalanine, histidine, lysine, tryptophan, and arginine. The author also reported that increasing concentrations of hydrogen peroxide increased the amount of whey protein denaturation. According to Stadtman and Levine (2003), the reaction takes place at the iron-binding site; the iron is released as ferric iron, and after deamination, a carbonyl group is formed on the protein side chain (Figure 5.1).

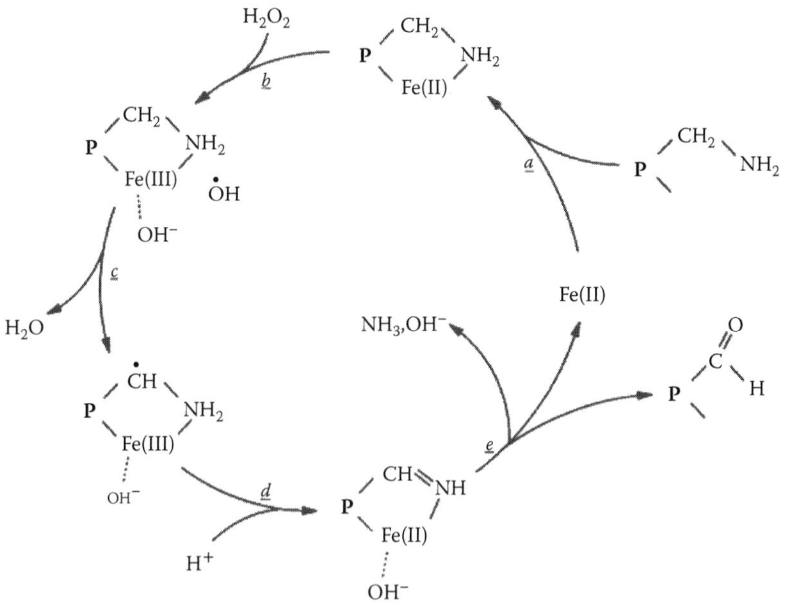

FIGURE 5.1 Iron-mediated protein oxidation. (With kind permission from Springer Science + Business Media: *Amino Acids*, Free radical-mediated oxidation of free amino acids and amino acid residues in proteins, 25, 2003, 207–218, Stadtman, E. R., and R. L. Levine.)

Investigations by Armenteros et al. (2009) in meat demonstrated the importance of metal-initiated protein oxidation with the detection of oxidation products of arginine and lysine side chains and the resulting formation of α-aminoadipic and β-glutamic semialdehydes. These oxidation products have been shown to be formed via metal-catalyzed oxidation but have so far only been detected in meat food. A study on Maillard reaction products in a milk-model system (Meltretter and Pischetsrieder 2007) showed the presence of the lysine oxidation product α-aminoadipic semialdehyde after the incubation of milk protein with lactose using matrix-assisted laser desorption ionization-time-of-flight mass spectrometer (MALDI-TOF-MS) and indicated that Maillard reactions could also significantly contribute to protein oxidation, but no mechanisms were put forward. However, it is believed that metal-catalyzed oxidation of protein is a predominant mechanism in food because of the abundance of transition metals, such as iron and copper, and because of the catalytic nature of these oxidative reactions.

5.2.2 Heme Proteins

Another mechanism involves heme proteins, such as peroxidases and pseudo-peroxidases, which, for example, include lactoperoxidase found in milk as well as myoglobin (Mb) and hemoglobin (Hb) found in muscle food. Heme proteins, with their heme iron center in the oxidation state III (in some cases, II), are activated in the presence of hydrogen peroxides or alkyl peroxides to hypervalent species. Compound I, a porphyrin radical cation and an iron (IV)-oxo ferryl species (also called perferryl species), is formed in a two-electron oxidation reaction and further autoreduced via an intramolecular electron transfer to compound II (iron (IV)-oxoferryl species, also called ferryl species) in a one-electron reduction mechanism (Figure 5.2). Compound II can autoreduce or is reduced back to its initial oxidation state by a series of antioxidants (Carlsen et al. 2005).

Compound I with its iron center in the oxidation state IV and with a radical on the heme protein has been shown to be able to oxidize a wide range of cellular compounds, including proteins. After intermolecular rearrangement of the initial radical on the globin (the identity of which is still a matter of controversy), the globin radical is able to be transferred to other proteins via an intermolecular radical transfer and to form long-lived secondary radicals (Irwin et al. 1999). It has been shown, for example, that horseradish peroxidase can generate a long-lived protein radical on bovine serum albumin (BSA), which is able to further transfer its odd electron to small antioxidative molecules, such as urate, leading to the speculation that radical transfer could be part of an antioxidant mechanism (Østdal et al. 2002). This mechanism is believed to be a common process in biological systems but is still poorly understood, especially whether this is part of an antioxidant or protective mechanism or whether this is ultimately resulting in further damage. This might occur readily in complex systems, such as foods, especially in the initiation and the propagation steps of free-radical damage to proteins. It has recently been shown in meat that the radical on the iron (IV)-oxo ferryl from myoglobin was rapidly transferred to myosin causing the generation of long-lived myosin radicals and formation of reversible and irreversible protein cross-linking between myosin molecules (Lund et al. 2008). The

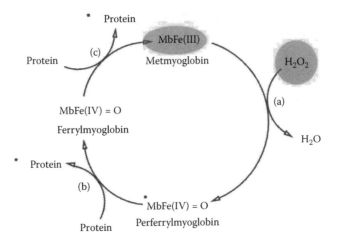

FIGURE 5.2 Heme protein-mediated oxidation with (a) activation of MbFe(III) by hydrogen peroxide to hypervalent species perferrylmyoglobin MbFe(IV) = O and ferrylmyoglobin MbFe(IV) = O. Subsequent reduction of MbFe(IV) = O (b) and MbFe(IV) = O (c) leads to initiation of the protein oxidation.

mechanisms have not been investigated very much, but radical transfer from heme protein to other proteins should probably receive more attention in relation to oxidation of food proteins (Østdal et al. 1999). Indeed, heme proteins are abundant in muscle foods with myoglobin being predominately present in meat and in dark fish muscle, while hemoglobin is usually present in fish and meat in small quantities. For example, a study performed on mackerel reported that hemoglobin ranged between 6 and 12 µmol/kg in a light muscle, while myoglobin reaches 120–150 µmol/kg in a muscle (Richards and Hultin 2002). An investigation of salted fish showed that hemoglobin peroxidase activity was persistent during fish ripening. This activity was postulated to be responsible for myosin cross-linking in the salted fish product (Christensen et al. 2011). In these studies, no mechanisms were proposed, but the significance of free-radical transfer as an initiating step in protein oxidation mediated by heme protein is a likely mechanism. In milk, it has been shown that lactoperoxidase can transfer a radical to other milk proteins, such as β-lactoglobulin, casein, and serum albumin and has been proposed to be a key element in the oxidation of milk proteins (Østdal et al. 2000). This suggests that this mechanism needs to be further investigated in a series of foods where heme proteins are abundant as this may affect food quality significantly.

5.2.3 LIGHT

Light-induced oxidation or photooxidation of protein has been extensively studied in biological system due to the fact that light has major damaging effects on cells and tissues (Pattison et al. 2011). The type I and type II mechanisms of photooxidation are believed to compete against each other depending on the conditions. They have not yet been unambiguously documented in food, but both are believed to occur, affecting both lipids and proteins. Type I involves the transfer of hydrogen atoms or electrons by interaction of the triplet excited state of the sensitizer with the target, and type II involves the generation of singlet oxygen by energy transfer from the excited triplet sensitizer to a ground state oxygen. Singlet oxygen is a strong oxidant that has been shown to be able to damage lipids, proteins, and DNA. In food, photooxidation of protein has been studied essentially in dairy products because they contain vitamin B2 or riboflavin, which is a photosensitizer (Dalsgaard et al. 2007). The content of riboflavin in milk has been estimated to reach approximately 180 µg/100 g milk (Kanno et al. 1991). Dalsgaard et al. (2007) also revealed that the milk proteins most susceptible to photooxidation were caseins probably because of their random coil structure. In contrast, the globular protein alpha lactalbumin, beta lactoglobulin, and lactoferrin were less susceptible to oxidative damage, and only their secondary structure was affected. In addition, photooxidation of milk protein has also been reported to effect yield in cheese production (Dalsgaard and Larsen 2009). One should also consider that some proteins may be able to absorb light themselves if they contain aromatic amino acid chains, such as Trp, Tyr, or Phe. However, the contribution of this effect to protein oxidation is probably limited due to the fact that they absorb at wavelengths below 300 nm. Also, some proteins contain chromophores at their active site, for example, the porphyrin ring of heme proteins, which are good photosensitizers and can be involved in protein damage. Indeed, a study by Silvester et al. (1997) showed that light-induced oxidation by porphyrins could initiate oxidation of BSA and generate a radical on serum albumin. It has been speculated that light might play a significant role in the radical transfer mechanism between heme proteins and food constituents. Protein oxidation in food containing porphyrin rings, such as meat and vegetables, because of the presence of myoglobin and chlorophyll, respectively, might need to be investigated more systematically. Lee et al. (2003) reported photooxidation of soy flour meal to be mediated by chromophore present in the flour. However, light-induced oxidation of proteins in food and its consequences for food quality have not been investigated thoroughly and deserve further attention because, along the production chain and during distribution and storage on the supermarket shelves, food items are often placed under light bulbs/tubes.

5.2.4 INDIRECT OXIDATION

Protein oxidation can be indirect when caused by the interaction between protein and lipid oxidation end products (ALEs) but also, to some extent, interaction between protein and advanced glycation end products (AGEs) as shown in Figure 5.3. The former reactions can take place between protein and secondary oxidation products of lipid oxidation, especially α-, β-unsaturated aldehydes, such as 4-hydroxynonenal (4-NHE) or trans-4-hydroxy-2-hexenal (HHE). These compounds are toxic and very reactive and can easily react with proteins or peptides. Amino groups on the side chains of proteins may subsequently generate Schiff bases via nucleophilic attack on the carbonyl groups of aldehydes. These reactions are reversible, but further rearrangements lead to the formation of irreversible adducts that, in general, result in the loss of a protein surface charge. In addition, α-, β-unsaturated aldehydes can undergo a Michael addition at the protein amino group side chain (Berlett and Stadtman

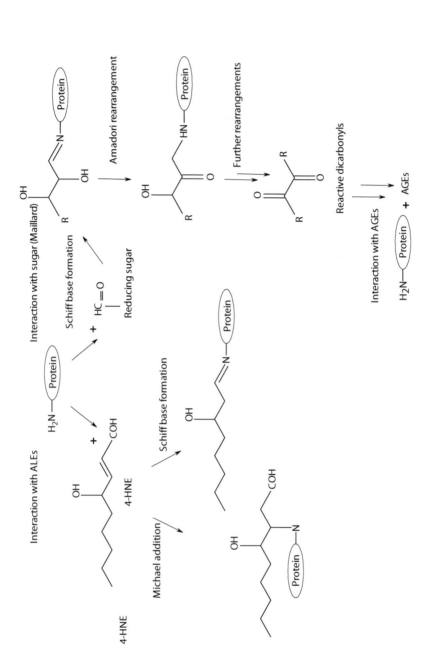

FIGURE 5.3 Carbonylation of protein via interaction of protein with advanced lipid oxidation end products (ALEs) and with reducing sugar leading to formation of advanced glycation end products (AGEs).

1997). During Maillard reaction, Schiff bases are formed between the aldehyde group of reducing sugars and amino groups of protein, and after subsequent rearrangements to Amadori products, and further rearrange through oxidation and degradation reaction, lead to AGEs. Interaction between AGEs and proteins results in formation of AGE–protein adducts, including carboxymethyllysine (CMLys), which was the first AGE to be identified in milk (Tauer et al. 1999).

CMLys has received a great deal of attention, is used as a marker of AGEs, and has been detected in a series of foods (Ames 2008). Strictly speaking, such interactions between sugar/lipid oxidation/degradation products and protein are not direct oxidation of the protein but often result in the addition of carbonyl groups to the protein via covalent binding between the AGE or ALE products. These interactions are important to consider not only in relation to protein functionality but also with respect to the potential toxicity of these protein/ALE and protein/AGE complexes and because of the accumulating evidence of their role in the pathologies of several diseases.

5.3 IMPACT OF PROTEIN OXIDATION ON FOOD QUALITY: PROCESSING AND STORAGE

During processing and storage, any exposure to light, metals, and temperature and interaction with ALEs and AGEs as well as any oxidants will result in the oxidation of proteins. The impact of food processing on protein oxidation has only been investigated to a minor extent, but more and more studies show that processing and storage conditions can induce protein oxidation and have consequences for food quality. Protein oxidation in food can affect food quality by inducing changes in protein hydrophobicity, charge, conformation, and solubility, as well as inactivation of enzymes, and can change protein susceptibility to proteolysis. Protein oxidation has often been associated with the loss in protein functionality, such as loss of emulsifying properties, loss of solubility, or loss of water-holding capacity, but these studies have mainly been performed in protein model systems (Decker et al. 1993; Srinivasan and Hultin 1995). In a meat model system, protein oxidation resulting in cross-linking of myosin has recently been revealed to decrease gel-forming ability and water-holding capacity (Ooizumi and Xiong 2004; Bertram et al. 2007). In meat, freeze–thawing cycles with pork have recently been shown to cause increased formation of protein carbonyls, loss of protein thiol groups, and formation of protein cross-linking (Xia et al. 2009). The same group (Xia et al. 2012) also compared thawing methods and demonstrated an increase in protein carbonyls in frozen meat content when compared to fresh meat irrespective of the defrosting method used. Cooking of beef has recently been reported to result in an increase in protein oxidation and Schiff base formation (Gatellier et al. 2010). Irradiation of meat has also been shown to increase protein carbonylation and affect texture by reducing tenderness (Rowe et al. 2004). A recent study by Estévez et al. (2011) showed that protein oxidation was more pronounced in minced meat products than in intact muscle. In surimi production, the mincing and washing of fish have also been shown to result in a significant increase in protein oxidation (Eymard et al. 2009). From all these studies, it is clear that processing conditions, such as mincing, freezing, cooking, irradiating, and washing, can induce protein oxidation in food and ultimately food quality.

In marinated herring production, protein oxidation was found to increase with ripening time (Andersen et al. 2007). Despite significant proteolysis of protein during marinated herring production, myosin cross-linking has been shown to correlate with the characteristic texture of salted herring, here highlighting a positive impact of protein oxidation on food product quality (Christensen et al. 2011). Indeed, in some products, protein oxidation might be desirable to obtain a characteristic of the product, such as a desired flavor or texture. In dairy products, ultra high temperature processing of milk was shown to induce a significant increase in the level of protein oxidation (Fenaille et al. 2005). A more recent investigation revealed that thermal processing affected milk protein carbonylation with the highest staining for protein oxidation obtained in powdered infant formula. They also demonstrated that α-lactalbumin was more susceptible to carbonylation than β-lactoglobulin. It was postulated that the spray-drying steps as well as the level of prooxidants were determinant in the oxidation of protein in powdered infant formula (Meyer et al. 2012). During mozzarella manufacturing, the level of protein carbonyl groups has been found to increase from raw milk to final product (Fedele and Bergamo 2001). Oxidation of milk proteins by ultraviolet (UV) or fluorescent light during production has also been shown to result in the formation of protein oxidation products, such as dityrosine, carbonyl groups, and N′-formylkynurenine, but also fragmentation and polymerization (Scheidegger et al. 2010).

Even if an increasing number of investigations revealed a correlation between processing conditions, protein oxidation, and food quality, more systematic investigations need to be performed to further assess the impact of processing on protein oxidation and its relation to food quality. In addition, this may reveal how, by controlling production conditions, the production of higher-quality products can be achieved. In addition, in some products, oxidation of protein might lead to the desired characteristic of the product. A better understanding of the mechanisms will probably lead to a better control of these reactions in foods.

As demonstrated for food processing conditions, food storage conditions can result in an increase in protein oxidation, and some conditions have been shown to promote protein oxidation. Exposure to light, temperature, metal, and high-oxygen-atmosphere packaging have been found to have a significant impact on the development of protein oxidation in food. Frozen storage or modified-atmosphere packaging in the presence of high oxygen in fish and meat has been shown to result in an increase in protein carbonyl groups, and vacuum packing has been shown to result in lower protein oxidation (Baron et al. 2007; Lund et al. 2007a). A correlation was found between protein carbonylation and water-holding capacity during frozen storage of pork, but it was also revealed that minced meat generated more protein oxidation products compared to intact muscle during frozen storage (Estévez et al. 2011). Protein oxidation during storage of meat and fish products has mainly been shown to be of consequence to the texture of the product. As observed for processing conditions, the storage conditions of milk and cheese exposed to fluorescent light cause an increased formation of protein oxidation products (Havemose et al. 2004). A study by Dalsgaard et al. (2012)

revealed that during storage of cheese, proteolysis seemed to enhance dityrosine formation but seemed to reduce the level of lipid oxidation products. This led to the speculation that dityrosine was involved in the termination of protein oxidative reactions. However, one should not forget that protein carbonyls as well as many protein oxidation products are reactive and are able to react further with other components in the food matrix. Indeed, in several matrices, protein carbonyl and semialdehyde contents have been shown to decrease with storage time. This might be a result of such reactions as Schiff base formation and further degradation into Stecker aldehydes, aldol condensation, or even further oxidation with for example AAS which was found to be further oxidized to α-aminoadipic acid (AAA) (Estévez 2011).

Another aspect that should not be neglected is the impact of protein oxidation directly on food enzymes or on their substrates by inactivating the enzyme or modifying the substrate's ability to interact and to be recognized by enzymes. This has been shown to be the case for calpains, which are involved in meat tenderization (Lametsch et al. 2008). In milk, oxidative degradation of casein has been shown to decrease its susceptibility to the rennet enzyme chymosin, resulting in a lower yield (Dalsgaard and Larsen 2009). Therefore, in food, any enzymatic reactions could be impaired directly or indirectly by protein oxidation. This can result in inactivation of the enzyme or accumulation of unfit substrate and can have severe consequences for food quality.

Nevertheless, all the above-mentioned studies have clearly shown that protein oxidation is unavoidable during processing and storage of food but that in order to minimize it, several strategies should be put forward. The existing strategies will be discussed further.

5.4 PREVENTION OF PROTEIN OXIDATION IN FOOD

In order to prevent protein oxidation in foods, several strategies could be employed. The first strategy consists of preventing exposure to conditions that promote protein oxidation. For example, reducing light exposure has been proposed during production of dairy products (Scheidegger et al. 2010). In meat, vacuum packing is known to prevent protein oxidation by removing oxygen in the packing; but, on the other hand, it is known to impart an unwanted color to meat products, resulting in consumer rejection. Other strategies consist of the addition of antioxidants to food, and two possibilities exists: (1) indirect addition of antioxidants by acting at the animal level, using a feeding regime and supplementation before the proteineous fraction is converted into food, or (2) direct addition to the food during processing and storage. Both strategies have been tested and will be discussed below on the basis of the existing literature.

5.4.1 ANTIOXIDANTS: FEEDING STRATEGIES

It is expected that the feeding regimen of animals might have an impact on the oxidative status of the animal products we eat, such as milk, fish, and meat. In a study investigating feeding regimens and protein and lipid oxidation in the rainbow trout, it was found that the oil type (fish oil versus vegetable oil) did not have a significant impact on the development of protein oxidation measured by protein carbonyl content as seen in Table 5.2 (Baron et al. 2009).

A similar study of beef supports these findings as no effect of feeding a high omega-3 diet on the development of protein oxidation was seen when compared to a conventional diet (Gatellier et al. 2010). However, while the level of unsaturation of the oil did not seem to affect the oxidation of protein, the quality of the oil used seemed to have an impact on the protein oxidation level in chicken meat (Wangang et al. 2011). Feeding chicks with oxidized vegetable oil had an impact on the level of protein carbonylation. Similarly, the level of antioxidant in the feed also impacted the development of protein oxidation. Santé-Lhoutellier et al. (2008) observed a lower level of protein carbonyls in lamb fed with pasture compared to lamb fed with concentrates, and this was found to correlate with the higher level of vitamin E in lamb fed with pasture. In fish, it was found that a diet containing carotenoid pigments and especially canthaxanthin was lowering the level of carbonylation in rainbow trout stored frozen for 22 months at –20°C as seen in Table 5.2 (Baron et al. 2009). As for milk, a study has shown that feeding with grass resulted in a higher concentration of antioxidants in the milk compared to milk from cows fed with corn, which resulted in less dityrosine (Havemose et al. 2006). Feeding strategies in dairy cows have been reported to help increase the content of urate in milk, which was shown to prevent dityrosine formation in milk (Østdal et al. 2008). It is therefore possible to control the extent of protein oxidation in some food by carefully selecting ingredients in the animal diet. In biology and medicine, several groups have investigated the impact of dietary antioxidants on the oxidative status, and it was found that a high level of antioxidants in the diet was associated with a reduced level of protein oxidation in plasma and a reduced risk of several types of diseases (Dragsted 2008; Griffiths 2002). Modification of the animal feed seemed to affect protein oxidation and ultimately food quality and should be considered as a good alternative in order to optimize food quality.

TABLE 5.2
Development of Protein Carbonyls in Fish

Carbonyls (nmol/mg)		Fish Oil	Vegetable Oil
T0	ATX	1.83a	1.83a
	CTX	1.66a	2.13a
	NOP	2.16a	2.21a
T22	ATX	5.26b	8.54c
	CTX	1.87a	1.76a
	NOP	4.24b	7.47c

Source: Reprinted with permission from Baron, C. P., et al., *J Agric Food Chem* 57: 4185–4194, 2009. Copyright 2009 American Chemical Society.

Note: Study conducted during storage at –20°C for 22 months with fish feed, either fish oil or vegetable oil, and with 200 ppm astaxanthin (ATX), canthaxanthin (CTX), or no pigment (NOP).

5.4.2 Antioxidants: Processing and Storage Strategies

Processing and storage conditions have been shown to impact significantly oxidation of protein in foods, and any conditions during processing and storage that will protect it from light, temperature, oxidizing species, etc. will contribute to a significant protection of the protein fraction. Alternatively, to prevent protein oxidation in food, it is possible to add antioxidants directly to the food either during processing or prior storage as it has been done for lipid oxidation for decades. Some antioxidants are able to effectively protect protein from oxidation, but the mechanisms are still unclear. Nevertheless, antioxidants effectively preventing lipid oxidation are expected to prevent protein oxidation to some extent by minimizing the formation of secondary lipid oxidation products, thereby preventing their interactions with proteins. In beef patties, a rosemary extract was found to protect protein from oxidation (Lund et al. 2007b), while in frankfurters, it has been shown to inhibit protein at low levels while higher levels resulted in a prooxidative effect, indicating that antioxidant and prooxidant balance depends on the product type and its characteristics as well as the concentration of antioxidant used (Estevez and Cava 2005). It is very difficult to describe the kinetics and mechanisms of the inhibition of protein oxidation by antioxidants in detail, and an overview of some of antioxidants tested in food matrices against protein is presented in Table 5.3. However, both phenolic compounds and

TABLE 5.3
Natural Antioxidant Tested in Food and Showing Either a Protective Effect (+), Lack of Protective Effect (–), or an Inconclusive Effect (+/–) on the Development of Protein Oxidation

Antioxidant	Concentration (ppm)	Food System	Effect	References
α-tocopherol	100 to 500	Whey protein isolate	(+)	Kong et al. 2012
Green tea extract	50 to 500	Whey	(–)	Jensen et al. 2011
AP/TC*	20/20 to 100/100	Whey	(–)	Jensen et al. 2011
Caffeic acid	100	Fish	(–/+)	Eymard et al. 2010
Spermine	400	Fish	(–/+)	Eymard et al. 2010
Black current extract	n/a	Pork patties	(+)	Jia et al. 2012
Rosemary-green tea	50 to 200	Pork patties	(–)	Haak et al. 2009
Rosemary essential oil	150, 300, 600	Frankfurters	(+/–)	Estevez and Cava 2005
Rosemary extract-AA/ citrate	n/a	Beef patties	(–)	Lund et al. 2007b
Mate leave extract	n/a	Italian sausage	(+)	Beal et al. 2011
White grape extract	500	Beef patties	(+)	Jøngberg et al. 2011
Canthaxanthin	200	Fish feed	(+)	Baron et al. 2003
Carrot juice	n/a	Sausages	(+)	Badr et al. 2011

Note: n/a, nonapplicable.

*AP/TC Ascorbyl palmitate/α-tocopherol.

carotenoids have been shown to have potential antioxidative activity on food protein, and some mechanisms have been put forward. Therefore, these two will be discussed in more detail.

5.4.3 Selected Examples

5.4.3.1 Phenolic Compounds

Plants are rich in phenolic compounds, which are secondary metabolites and have been shown to have good antioxidant properties against lipids. For example, extracts of green tea, avocado, berries, potato peels, and a number of seeds, fruits, and leaves from plants contain a unique blend of phenolic compounds, each of them with different antioxidant activities. The concentration and the activity of the compounds depend not only on the cultivar but also on the extraction method used to obtain the extracts. Phenolic antioxidants, however, often are divided into four groups including phenolic acids, flavonoids, diterpernes, and volatile oils, depending on the number and the arrangement of their ring structure (Brewer 2011). In rosemary extract, a very potent antioxidant, the most active compounds are carnosic acid and rosmaric acid, which are diterpenes. In addition, phenolic compounds have been tested in a selection of foods as additives because they are good alternatives to synthetic antioxidants. They have also been shown to exert some antioxidative protection of lipids and proteins in several food items, including meat, fish, dairy products, etc. Their antioxidative efficiency has been shown to be dependent on their structure and their concentration as well as the matrix itself. From a mechanistic point of view, phenolic compounds are good metal chelators and have good radical scavenging properties. In general, the antioxidant activities of phenolic compounds depend on the arrangement of hydroxyl substituents on the aromatic ring with the catechol structure, which are two adjacent hydroxyl substituents on the aromatic ring contributing to their strong chelating properties. The ability of phenolic compounds to prevent protein oxidation will inevitably lead to a reduction in oxidative damage on proteins because metals are good initiators of protein oxidation. However, one should also consider that proteins can be good metal chelators themselves, and, for example, whey protein isolates, soy isolate, and sodium caseinate (at a concentration of 10 mg/mL) have been reported to bind iron (185, 835, and 980 μmol/% of protein, respectively) (Faraji et al. 2004). Therefore, the antioxidant activity of phenolic compounds will also depend on the affinity of the iron for the different binding sites. As for their radical scavenging properties, oxidation of the phenol to quinone is taking place with the formation of a semi-quinone radical, which, depending on the other substitutions on the ring, is more or less stabilized by resonance (Brewer 2011). The mechanism involves either hydrogen atom transfer or single electron transfer. Further oxidation leads to the formation of quinones, which are relatively stable but, because of their electrophilic character, can react further. A recent study suggested that the quinones were able to react with protein thiol groups and form a stable protein quinine adduct. This reaction was reported to be part of a protective mechanism, defending protein from oxidation but, interestingly, was not preventing disulfide formation in a myofibrillar model system (Jøngberg et al. 2011). Several studies have showed inconsistency in the abilities

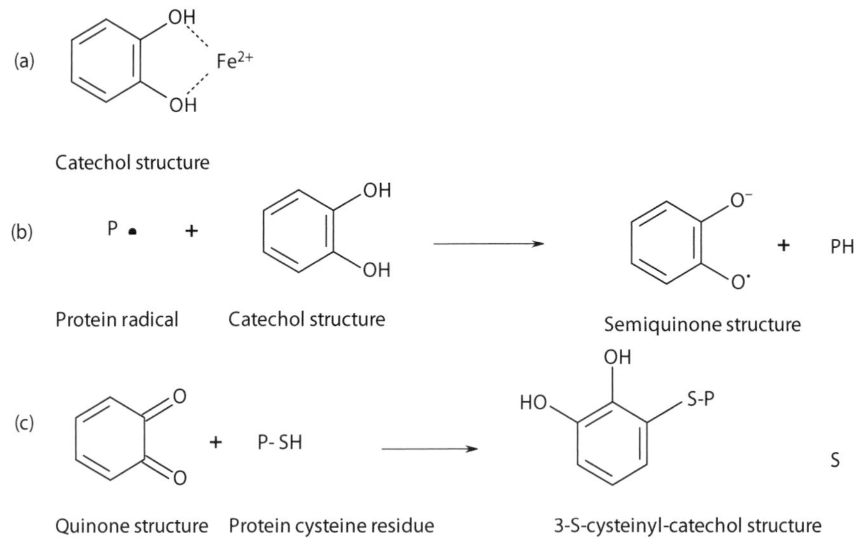

FIGURE 5.4 Phenol antioxidant activities toward proteins with (a) metal chelating, (b) radical scavenging, and (c) interaction with thiol groups.

of phenolic compounds to prevent protein oxidation in foods, which was ascribed to a dose-dependent effect of phenolic antioxidant activity. Indeed, a prooxidant effect of phenolic compounds has been reported at a low concentration in several foods and model systems (Frankel et al. 1997; Zhou and Elias 2012). It was postulated that the prooxidant activity of some phenolic compounds was a result of the amine oxidase activity of the quinone (Estevez 2011). It is also reported that under some conditions, phenolic compounds were able to generate hydrogen peroxide (Zhou and Elias 2012). Inconsistencies in the results on the antioxidative or prooxidative activity of phenolics could also be a result of different affinities between different phenols, metal iron, and proteins, highlighting the fact that interaction between the antioxidants and the target is of major importance as also reported by others (Dean et al. 1991). An overview of the proposed mechanisms by which phenolic compounds are able to inhibit protein oxidation is given in Figure 5.4.

5.4.3.2 Carotenoids

Another class of plant metabolites that has been shown to have promising impact on protein oxidation in food is the carotenoid pigment. Carotenoids are polyisoprenoid structures with 40 carbons in a long, conjugated, double-bond structure that sometimes has cyclization of the end of the polyenic chains. Carotenoids are good singlet oxygen quenchers as well as free radical scavengers. In several systems, carotenoids have been shown to be able to prevent lipid oxidation in food (Eunok and Min 2009). They have been shown to have good antioxidant activity in the body, preventing the development of several pathologies (Rao and Rao 2007). Recent studies showed that they are also able to prevent protein from oxidation both in feeding strategies and as additives added directly to the food products. Feed strategies in rainbow trout showed that fish fed with canthaxanthin was less oxidized compared to fish fed with no pigment or astaxanthin, irrespective of the oil type (Table 5.2). Similarly, in irradiated sausages, which had added carrot juice during production, less protein oxidation and higher sensory scores were obtained compared to samples without any carrot juice (Badr and Mahmoud 2011). This has been attributed to phenolic content, but carotenoids are also present and can significantly prevent protein oxidation. In surimi-type products, carrot fibers have been shown to be a good antioxidant, protecting proteins from oxidation (Karakaya and Aksun 2010). Further, in a study with fish feed, we were able to show that feed with added carotenoids was less susceptible to light-induced oxidation compared to feed not containing any carotenoids (Baron et al. 2003). In addition, the antioxidant activity of carotenoids *in vivo* has been demonstrated by many authors, but there is still a debate in the literature about the antioxidative activity of carotenoid pigments. This may be attributed to carotenoids interacting with other antioxidants as pointed out in a study by Zhang and Omaye (2000), highlighting that antioxidant activity cannot be evaluated by testing a single compound alone but that synergistic effects should be systematically evaluated as the interaction between antioxidants either sparing or compromising each other is important. Skibsted (2012) argues that carotenoids are playing a crucial role in membranes as they act as molecular wires across membranes and that their role protecting against protein oxidation should be further investigated. Indeed, close proximity of proteins and carotenoids in membranes has been reported as proteins have been accounted for maintaining the correct orientation of carotenoids in membranes to allow efficient energy transfer (Britton 1995). In addition, interaction between protein and carotenoid pigments should be investigated further because formation of carotenoprotein complexes leads to a change in the properties of carotenoids and may impact their antioxidant properties. Carotenoids are promising antioxidants for preventing protein oxidation, and more investigation should be performed to reveal their full potential as food protein antioxidants.

5.5 CONCLUSIONS

Oxidation of food proteins has been generating a lot of attention in the last 10–15 years. However, there is still a lot to reveal in relation to the impact of protein oxidation on food quality including functional properties, eating quality, nutritional value, and impact on human health. The difficulty resides in the fact that proteins are present together with a mixture of lipids, sugars, and other low molecular weight molecules, and the interaction between these multiple components and multiphasic systems, such as food, is difficult to assess. It is, however, clear that processing and storage conditions may be optimized in order to prevent oxidation of protein and ultimately result in products of higher quality. Elucidation of molecular modifications at the amino acid level and how they impact food properties needs to be investigated more systematically. With the development of new analytical methods, it is likely that a better understanding of protein modifications in food is impending. As for antioxidant strategies, classical lipid antioxidant strategy does not apply for protection of protein from oxidation. However, some antioxidants, such as phenolic compounds and carotenoid pigments, have shown a very promising effect on protein oxidation, and we are slowly unraveling the complex mechanisms by which they protect protein from oxidation.

ACKNOWLEDGMENTS

COST action CM1001 "Chemistry of nonenzymatic protein modification—modulation of protein structure and function" and especially the MC chair Tilman Grune. The National Food Institute, DTU, is greatly acknowledged for continuous support.

REFERENCES

Alegria Toran, A., R. Barbera, R. Farre, M. J. Lagarda, and J. C. Lopez. 1996. HPLC method for cyst(e)ine and methionine in infant formulas. *J Food Sci* 61: 1132–1135.

Ames, J. M. 2008. Determination of N-epsilon-(carboxymethyl) lysine in foods and related systems: Maillard reactions. *Recent Adv Food Biomed Sci* 1126: 20–24.

Andersen, E., M. L. Andersen, and C. P. Baron. 2007. Characterization of oxidative changes in salted herring (*Clupea harengus*) during ripening. *J Agric Food Chem* 55: 9545–9553.

Anderson, G. H., G. S. Li, J. D. Jones, and F. Bender. 1975. Effect of hydrogenated peroxides on the nutritional quality of rapeseed flourseed to weanling rat. *J Nutr* 105: 317–325.

Armenteros, M., M. Heinonen, V. Ollilainen, F. Toldrá, and M. Estévez. 2009. Analysis of protein carbonyls in meat products by using the DNPH-method, fluorescence spectroscopy and liquid chromatography–electrospray ionisation–mass spectrometry (LC–ESI–MS). *Meat Sci* 83: 104–112.

Badr, H., and K. A. Mahmoud. 2011. Antioxidant activity of carrot juice in gamma irradiated beef sausage during refrigerated and frozen storage. *Food Chem* 127: 1119–1130.

Balestrieri, M., M. S. Spagnuolo, L. Cigliano, G. Storti, L. Ferrara, P. Abrescia, and E. Fedele. 2002. Evaluation of oxidative damage in mozzarella cheese produced from bovine or water buffalo milk. *Food Chem* 77: 293–299.

Baron, C. P., L. Berner, and C. Jacobsen. 2003. Effect of astaxanthin and canthaxanthin on lipid and protein oxidation of fish feed exposed to UVA. *Free Radic Res* 37: 61.

Baron, C. P., I. V. H. Kjaersgard, F. Jessen, and C. Jacobsen. 2007. Protein and lipid oxidation during frozen storage of rainbow trout (*Oncorhynchus mykiss*). *J Agric Food Chem* 55: 8118–8125.

Baron, C. P., G. Hyldig, and C. Jacobsen. 2009. Does feed composition affect oxidation of rainbow trout (*Oncorhynchus mykiss*) during frozen storage? *J Agric Food Chem* 57: 4185–4194.

Beal, P., A. M. Faion, A. J. Cichoski, R. L. Cansian, A. T. Valduga, D. Oliveira, and D. de Valduga. 2011. Oxidative stability of fermented Italian-type sausages using mate leaves (*Ilex paraguariensis St. Hil*) extract as natural antioxidant. *Int J Food Sci Nutr* 62: 703–710.

Berlett, B. S., and E. R. Stadtman. 1997. Protein oxidation in aging, disease, and oxidative stress. *J Biol Chem* 272: 20313–20316.

Bertram, H. C., M. Kristensen, H. Østdal, and C. P. Baron. 2007. Does oxidation affect the water functionality of myofibrillar proteins? *J Agric Food Chem* 55: 2342–2348.

Brewer, M. S. 2011. Natural antioxidants: Sources, compounds, mechanisms of action, and potential applications. *Compr Rev Food Sci Food Safety* 10: 221–247.

Britton, G. 1995. Structure and properties of carotenoids in relation to function. *FASEB J* 9: 1551–1558.

Carlsen, C. U., J. K. S. Møller, and L. H. Skibsted. 2005. Heme-iron in lipid oxidation. *Coord Chem Rev* 249: 485–498.

Christensen, M., E. Andersen, L. Christensen, M. L. Andersen, and C. P. Baron. 2011. Textural and biochemical changes during ripening of old-fashioned salted herrings. *J Agric Food Chem* 91: 330–336.

Dalsgaard, T. K., and L. B. Larsen. 2009. Effect of photo-oxidation of major milk proteins on protein structure and hydrolysis by chymosin. *Int Dairy J* 19: 362–371.

Dalsgaard, T. K., D. Otzen, J. H. Nielsen, and L. B. Larsen. 2007. Changes in structures of milk proteins upon photo-oxidation. *J Agric Food Chem* 55: 10968–10976.

Dalsgaard, T. K., M. Bakman, M. Hammershøj, J. Sørensen, C. Nebel, R. Albrechtsen, L. Vognsen, and J. H. Nielsen. 2012. Light-induced protein and lipid oxidation in low-fat cheeses: Effect on degree of enzymatic hydrolysis. *Int J Dairy Technol* 65: 57–63.

Davies, M. J., and R. T. Dean. 2003. *Radical-mediated protein oxidation.* Oxford: Oxford Science Publications.

Dean, R. T., J. J. V. Hunt, A. J. Grant, Y. Yamamoto, and E. Niki. 1991. Free radical damage to proteins: The influence of the relative localization of radical generation, antioxidants, and target proteins. *Free Radic Biol Med* 11: 161–168.

Decker, E. A., Y. L. Xiong, J. T. Calvert, A. D. Crum, and S. P. Blanchard. 1993. Chemical, physical, and functional-properties of oxidized turkey white muscle myofibrillar proteins. *J Agric Food Chem* 41: 186–189.

Dragsted, L. O. 2008. Biomarkers of exposure to vitamins A, C, and E and their relation to lipid and protein oxidation markers. *Eur J Nur* 47: 3–18.

Estévez, M. 2011. Protein carbonyls in meat systems: A review. *Meat Sci* 89: 259–279.

Estevez, M., and R. Cava. 2005. Effectiveness of rosemary essential oil as an inhibitor of lipid and protein oxidation: Contradictory effects in different types of frankfurters. *Meat Sci* 72: 348–355.

Estévez, M., V. Ollilainen, and M. Heinonen. 2009. Analysis of protein oxidation markers α-aminoadipic and γ-glutamic semialdehydes in food proteins using liquid chromatography (LC)-electrospray ionization (ESI)-multistage tandem mass spectrometry (MS). *J Agric Food Chem* 57: 3901–3910.

Estévez, M., S. Ventanas, M. Heinonen, and E. Puolanne. 2011. Protein carbonylation and water-holding capacity of pork subjected to frozen storage: Effect of muscle type, premincing, and packaging. *J Anim Sci* 59: 5435–5443.

Eunok, C., and D. B. Min. 2009. Mechanisms of antioxidants in the oxidation of foods. *Compr Rev Food Sci Food Safety* 8: 345–358.

Eymard, S., C. P. Baron, and C. Jacobsen. 2009. Oxidation of lipid and protein in horse mackerel (*Trachurus trachurus*) mince and washed minces during processing and storage. *Food Chem* 114: 57–65.

Eymard, S., C. Jacobsen, and C. P. Baron. 2010. Assessment of washing with antioxidant on the oxidative stability of fatty fish mince during processing and storage. *J Agric Food Chem* 58: 6182–6189.

Faraji, H., D. J. McClements, and E. A. Decker. 2004. Role of continuous phase protein on the oxidative stability of fish oil-in-water emulsions. *J Agric Food Chem* 52: 4558–4564.

Fedele, E., and P. Bergamo. 2001. Protein and lipid oxidative stresses during cheese manufacture. *J Food Sci* 66: 932–935.

Fenaille, F., V. Parisod, J. C. Tabet, and P. A. Guy. 2005. Carbonylation of milk powder proteins as a consequence of processing conditions. *Proteomics* 5: 3097–3104.

Frankel, E., S. W. Huang, and R. Aeschbach. 1997. Antioxidant activity of green teas in different lipid systems. *J Am Oil Chem Soc* 74: 1309–1315.

Gatellier, P., A. Kondjoyan, S. Portanguen, and V. Santé-Lhoutellier. 2010. Effect of cooking on protein oxidation in n-3 polyunsaturated fatty acids enriched beef: Implication on nutritional quality. *Meat Sci* 85: 645–650.

Griffiths, H. R. 2002. The influence of diet on protein oxidation. *Nutr Res Rev* 15: 3–17.

Haak, L., K. Raes, and S. De Smet. 2009. Effect of plant phenolics, tocopherol and ascorbic acid on oxidative stability of pork patties. *J Sci Food Agric* 89: 1360–1365.

Halliwell, B., and J. M. C. Gutteridge. 2007. *Free radicals in biology and medicine.* Oxford: Oxford University Press.

Harel, S., and J. Kanner. 1985. Hydrogen peroxide generation in ground muscle tissue. *J Agric Food Chem* 33: 1186–1188.

Havemose, M. S., M. R. Weisbjerg, W. L. P. Bredie, and J. H. Nielsen. 2004. Influence of feeding different types of roughage on the oxidative stability of milk. *Int Dairy J* 14: 563–570.

Havemose, M. S., M. R. Weisbjerg, W. L. P. Bredie, H. D. Poulsen, and J. H. Nielsen. 2006. Oxidative stability of milk influenced by fatty acids, antioxidants, and copper derived from feed. *J Dairy Sci* 89: 1970–1980.

Irwin, J. A., H. Ostdal, and M. J. Davies. 1999. Myoglobin-induced oxidative damage: Evidence for radical transfer from oxidized myoglobin to other proteins and antioxidants. *Arch Biochem Biophys* 362: 94–104.

Jafarpour, A., F. Sherkat, B. Leonard, and E. M. Gorczyca. 2008. Colour improvement of common carp (*Cyprinus carpio*) fillets by hydrogen peroxide for surimi production. *Int J Food Sci Technol* 43: 1602–1609.

Jensen, B. M., J. Sørensen, G. Mortensen, M. B. Sørensen, and T. Dalsgaard. 2011. Effect of antioxidants on oxidation during the production of whey fat concentrate. *J Agric Food Chem* 59: 13012–13017.

Jia, N., B. Kong, Q. Liu, X. Diao, and X. Xia. 2012. Antioxidant activity of black currant (*Ribes nigrum L.*) extract and its inhibitory effect on lipid and protein oxidation of pork patties during chilled storage. *Meat Sci* 91: 533–539.

Jongberg, S., M. N. Lund, A. L. Waterhouse, and L. H. Skibsted. 2011. 4-Methylcatechol inhibits protein oxidation in meat but not disulfide formation. *J Agric Food Chem* 59: 10329–10335.

Kang, E. J., R. E. Campbell, E. Bastian, and M. A. Drake. 2010. Invited review: Annatto usage and bleaching in dairy foods. *J Dairy Sci* 93: 3891–3901.

Kanner, J. D., and O. Fennema. 1987. Photooxidation of tryptophan in the presence of riboflavin. *J Agric Food Chem* 35: 71–76.

Kanno, C., K. Shirahuji, and T. Hoshi. 1991. Simple method for separate determination of three flavins in bovine milk by high performance liquid chromatography. *J Food Sci* 56: 678–681.

Karakaya, B., and E. Tuğçe Aksun. 2010. The effect of different type of fibers (wheat, citrus and carrot fiber) on protein quality of crab leg analog paste and gel made from Alaska pollack (*Theragra chalcogramma*). Proceedings of the 40th annual WETA conference, 27, Turkey Izmir. Eds. Şükran Çaklı, S., U. Çelik, and C. Altınelataman.

Kong, B., Y. Sun, L. Jiang, Q. Liu, and X. Xia. 2012. The effectiveness of butylated hydroxyanisole and α-tocopherol in inhibiting oxidant-induced chemical and structural changes of whey protein. *Int J Dairy Technol* 65: 353–359.

Lametsch, R., S. Lonergan, and E. Huff-Lonergan. 2008. Disulfide bond within mu-calpain active site inhibits activity and autolysis. *Biochim Biophys Acta* 1784: 1215–1221.

Lund, M. N., R. Lametsch, M. S. Hviid, O. N. Jensen, and L. H. Skibsted. 2007a. High-oxygen packaging atmosphere influences protein oxidation and tenderness of porcine *longissimus dorsi* during chill storage. *Meat Sci* 77: 295–303.

Lund, M. N., M. S. Hviid, and L. H. Skibsted. 2007b. The combined effect of antioxidants and modified atmosphere packaging on protein and lipid oxidation in beef patties during chill storage. *Meat Sci* 76: 226–233.

Lund, M. N., C. Luxford, L. H. Skibsted, and M. J. Davies. 2008. Oxidation of myosin by heme proteins generates myosin radicals and protein cross-links. *Biochem J* 410: 565–574.

Lee, J. Y., S. Min, E. O. Choe, and D. B. Min. 2003. Formation of volatile compounds in soy flour by singlet oxygen oxidation during storage under light. *J Food Sci* 68: 1933–1937.

Meltretter, J., and M. Pischetsrieder. 2007. Application of mass spectrometry for the detection of glycation and oxidation products in milk proteins. *Ann N Y Acad Sci* 1126: 134–140.

Meyer, B., F. Baum, G. Vollmer, and M. Pischetsrieder. 2012. Distribution of protein oxidation products in the proteome of thermally processed milk. *J Agric Food Chem* 60: 7306–7311.

Munyua, J. K. 1975. Hydrogen peroxide alteration of whey protein in skim milk and whey protein solutions. *Milchwissenschaft* 30: 730–734.

Ooizumi, T., and Y. L. Xiong. 2004. Biochemical susceptibility of myosin in chicken myofibrils subjected to hydroxyl radical oxidizing systems. *J Agric Food Chem* 52: 4303–4307.

Østdal, H., H. J. Andersen, and M. J. Davies. 1999. Formation of long-lived radicals on proteins by radical transfer from heme enzymes—A common process? *Arch Biochemistry Biophys* 362: 105–112.

Østdal, H., M. J. Bjerrum, J. A. Pedersen, and H. J. Andersen. 2000. Lactoperoxidase-induced protein oxidation in milk. *J Agric Food Chem* 48: 3939–3944.

Østdal, H., M. J. Davies, and H. J. Andersen. 2002. Reaction between protein radicals and other biomolecules. *Free Radic Biol Med* 33: 201–209.

Østdal, H., M. R. Weisbjerg, L. H. Skibsted, and J. H. Nielsen. 2008. Protection against photo-oxidation of milk by high urate content. *Milchwissenschaft* 63: 119–122.

Pattison, D. I., A. S. Rahmanto, and M. J. Davies. 2011. Photo-oxidation of proteins. *Photochem Photobiol Sci* 11: 38–53.

Rao, A. V., and L. G. Rao. 2007. Carotenoids and human health. *Pharmacol Res* 55: 207–216.

Richards, M. P., and H. O. Hultin. 2002. Contributions of blood and blood components to lipid oxidation in fish muscle. *J Agric Food Chem* 50: 555–564.

Rowe, L. J., K. R. Maddock, S. M. Lonergan, and E. Huff-Lonergan. 2004. Influence of early postmortem protein oxidation on beef quality. *J Anim Sci* 82: 785–793.

Santé-Lhoutellier, V., E. Engel, and P. Gatellier. 2008. Assessment of the influence of diet on lamb meat oxidation. *Food Chem* 109: 573–579.

Scheidegger, D., R. P. Pecora, P. M. Radici, and S. C. Kivatinitz. 2010. Protein oxidative changes in whole and skim milk after ultraviolet or fluorescent light exposure. *J Dairy Sci* 93: 5101–5109.

Silvester, J. A., X. D. Wei, M. J. Davies, and G. S. Timmins. 1997. A study of photochemically-generated protein radical spin adducts on bovine serum albumin: The detection of genuine spin-trapping and artefactual, non-radical addition in the same molecule. *Redox Rep* 3: 225–232.

Skibsted, L. H. 2012. Carotenoids in antioxidant networks: Colorants or radical scavengers. *J Agric Food Chem* 60: 2409–2417.

Slump, P., and H. A. W. Schreuder. 1973. Oxidation of methionine and cystine in foods treated with hydrogen peroxide. *J Sci Food Agric* 24: 657–661.

Srinivasan, S., and H. O. Hultin. 1995. Hydroxyl radical modification of fish muscle proteins. *J Food Biochem* 18: 405–425.

Stadtman, E. R. 1990. Metal ion-catalyzed oxidation of proteins: Biochemical mechanism and biological consequences. *Free Radic Biol Med* 9: 315–325.

Stadtman, E. R., and R. L. Levine. 2003. Free radical-mediated oxidation of free amino acids and amino acid residues in proteins. *Amino Acids* 25: 207–218.

Takasaki, S., Y. Kato, M. Murata, S. Homma, and S. Kawakishi. 2005. Effects of peroxidase and hydrogen peroxide on the dityrosine formation and the mixing characteristics of wheat-flour dough. *Bios Biotechnol Biochem* 69: 1686–1692.

Tauer, A., K. Hasenkopf, T. Kislinger, I. Frey, and M. Pischetsrieder. 1999. Determination of N-epsilon-carboxymethyllysine in heated milk products by immunochemical methods. *Eur Food Res Technol* 209: 72–76.

Timm-Heinrich, M., S. Eymard, C. P. Baron, H. H. Nielsen, and C. Jacobsen. 2013. Oxidative changes during ice storage of rainbow trout (*Oncorhynchus mykiss*) fed different ratios of marine and vegetable feed ingredients. *Food Chem* 136: 1220–1230.

Wangang, Z., X. Shan, L. Eun Joo, and D. U. Ahn. 2011. Consumption of oxidized oil increases oxidative stress in broilers and affects the quality of breast meat. *J Agric Food Chem* 59: 969–974.

Xia, X., B. Kong, Q. Liu, and J. Liu. 2009. Physicochemical change and protein oxidation in porcine *longissimus dorsi* as influenced by different freeze–thaw cycles. *Meat Sci* 83: 239–245.

Xia, X., B. Kong, J. Liu, J. Q. Liu, and X. Diao. 2012. Influence of different thawing methods on physicochemical changes and protein oxidation of porcine longissimus muscle. *LWT - Food Sci Technol* 46: 280–286.

Zhang, P., and S. T. Omaye. 2000. Beta-carotene and protein oxidation: Effects of ascorbic acid and alpha-tocopherol. *Toxicol* 146: 37–47.

Zhou, L., and R. J. Elias. 2012. Factors influencing the antioxidant and pro-oxidant activity of polyphenols in oil-in-water emulsions. *J Agric Food Chem* 60: 2906–2915.

6 Use of Added Oxidants in Food Processing

Emanuela Zanardi

CONTENTS

6.1 INTRODUCTION

The gradual accumulation of oxygen that accompanied the evolution of photosynthetic organisms approximately 1.5 to 2 billion years ago was most significant in that an appropriate environment had been provided for the genesis of aerobic organisms. The transition from anaerobic to aerobic life required intense work of adaptation, in particular, genotypic adaptation (Porter and Wujek 1988). However, molecular oxygen is a paradoxical element of nature: It is a vital component of several biological reactions in which, stepwise, the enzymatically controlled oxidation of biomolecules is used to release energy and compounds essential for life; on the other hand, oxygen could be toxic to cells, and oxidative reactions are tightly controlled in biological systems (Kanner et al. 1987).

The reactivity of oxygen itself is rather poor, and many oxidation reactions in the cell are possible only because of the specific mechanisms of activation of molecular oxygen. The resulting activated oxygen species, called reactive oxygen species (ROS), are formed under physiological conditions during the reduction of oxygen to water, which proceeds by a series of single electron transfers, and have a high reactivity. ROS are either radicals or reactive nonradical compounds and are responsible for the toxic character of oxygen. ROS are also produced in the organism as part of the primary immune defense; phagocytic cells defend against foreign organisms by synthesizing large amount of ROS as a part of their killing mechanism. Besides its endogenous formation, the organism is also exposed to ROS from external sources: with the diet, many compounds of a prooxidant nature are delivered to the organism; an array of radicals are inhaled with cigarette smoke. Ozone, of which increasing levels are a result of air pollution, is a ROS that can oxidize lipids (see also Chapter 11). An imbalance between the generation and removal of ROS by the antioxidant defense systems may lead to chemical modifications of biologically relevant macromolecules, such as DNA, proteins, and lipids, which are possible pathobiochemical mechanisms involved in the initiation or progression phase of various diseases. Experimental data provide evidence that dietary antioxidants scavenge ROS, and epidemiological studies support the hypothesis that some dietary antioxidants may play a beneficial role in reducing the risk of several chronic disorders (Diplock et al. 1998). The role of ROS in the oxidative processes of lipids has been profusely studied, and mechanisms, products, and biological significance of lipid oxidation have received a great deal of attention in the literature by several reviews and books on this topic (see also Chapter 4).

Our food supply is safer and offers more variety today than it ever has in the past, and this can be largely attributed to the application of modern food technologies. Food processing preserves foods safely so that they can maintain high nutritional and sensory values during storage and achieve a wide distribution. After microbial spoilage, oxidation is the second most important cause of food spoilage, even in those products that might be considered low in oxidizable substrates. This has been known for a long time, and therefore, attention to the control of oxidative processes in foods has been one of the highest priorities of the food industry. The use of synthetic or natural antioxidants has been considered the tool in this fight against oxidation. However, because of the growing recognition that antioxidants are themselves important for the maintenance and optimization of health, the food industry is oriented to protect the antioxidant nutritional value of food by minimizing the amount and severity of processing operations. This is the basis of the "hurdle technology" concept, which has been driven in the last decades by consumer expectations of minimally processed and convenient food products; changes in product distribution practices; increased international food trade; emerging microbial pathogens; and increased interest, awareness, and scrutiny of food safety issues by consumers, the media, and activist groups.

In food, as well as in biological organisms, most of the research has been focused on lipid oxidation, and fats, oils, and lipid-based foods have received great interest in the last 50 years. However, the oxidation of food proteins is currently one of the most innovative research topics within food science.

Despite comprehensive reviews on the antioxidant systems to inhibit oxidation in food being widely available in the literature, with particular emphasis on the different antioxidant sources, mechanisms of action, preparation, regulation, changes, and application in food products, information on prooxidant systems is much more fragmented. To bridge this gap, the role of traditional and novel processing and preservation techniques in promoting the lipid and protein oxidation of food will be discussed in the present chapter. This is not meant to be completely comprehensive; rather, it will mainly address meats, which are the major area of research and interest of the author, and the current knowledge on the oxidation promoters in muscle food processing and preservation will be reviewed. The listed references cite extensive reviews and books that readers may consult if they are interested in more in-depth information in some specific areas.

6.2 FACTORS PROMOTING OXIDATION OF MEAT LIPIDS

6.2.1 ENDOGENOUS FACTORS

Lipid oxidation is one of the main causes of the deterioration of muscle foods. Oxidation initially occurs at the membrane level of the muscle cell in which the amounts of polyunsaturated fatty acids (PUFAs) of the phospholipid fraction are sufficient to allow the occurrence of oxidative reactions. Numerous findings support the hypothesis that phospholipids are the major contributors to oxidation and especially warmed-over flavor (WOF) in meats, while triglycerides play only a minor role (Toldrá 1998; Gandemer 1999).

The primary catalyst of lipid oxidation in skeletal muscle has been suggested to be iron. Transition metals, such as iron and copper, with their labile d-electron system, are well suited to catalyze redox reactions. They have a range of accessible oxidation states, which enables them to transfer electrons. There is evidence that transition metals may initiate lipid oxidation by hydrogen abstraction from a lipid molecule to yield a lipid radical. Moreover, they may interact directly with triplet oxygen to generate a superoxide radical or decompose lipid hydroperoxides; both mechanisms lead to the formation of more ROS and thus propagate the chain reaction (Kanner et al. 1987).

Whereas the amount of copper in muscle foods seems to be very low and mostly chelated to histidine dipeptides, such as carnosine, which prevent them catalyzing lipid oxidation, the level of iron is high, and the prooxidant activity of this metal has been widely documented.

Most of the iron in muscle foods occurs in heme proteins, myoglobin in particular. In fish muscle, where the blood may not be removed prior to processing, iron is bound to hemoglobin. Iron–protein complexes, such as ferritin and transferrin, are assigned to the storage and transport of non-heme iron. Considerable debate in the literature has focused on the relative contributions of heme and non-heme iron to lipid oxidation in meat (Baron and Andersen 2002; Carlsen et al. 2005). Both can function as prooxidants in model systems, but in muscle, the situation is much more complex, and the results are sometimes contradictory. Traditionally, meat lipid oxidation has been attributed to heme catalysts. The most probable mechanism of catalysis involves the formation of a coordinate complex between the heme group and the lipid hydroperoxide, followed by homolytic scission of the hydroperoxide to form free radicals. In this mechanism, there would be no change in the valence of heme iron. It has been also proven that myoglobin and hemoglobin are activated by hydrogen peroxide, producing a short-lived intermediate, a ferryl (Fe^{4+}) compound, which is able to initiate membrane lipid oxidation. Lipid and myoglobin oxidation often appear to be linked in meat, and the oxidation of one of the two leads to the formation of chemical species that can exacerbate oxidation of the other (Faustman et al. 2010). However, several studies provided evidence that non-heme iron is the major catalyst accelerating lipid oxidation in cooked meat. It seems that ferritin plays an important role in the process of muscle lipid oxidation being one of the main sources of free iron for this reaction (Shahidi 1994).

More recent studies have addressed residual hemoglobin in fish muscle. The iron released from trout hemoglobin during 2°C storage contributes little to hemoglobin-mediated lipid oxidation (Richards and Li 2004). However, lowering the pH within the range naturally occurring during postmortem storage of fish leads to the deoxygenation of hemoglobin; the increased deoxygenation could play a role in the observed increased prooxidant activity of hemoglobin as pH lowers (Richards et al. 2002; see also Chapters 2 and 4).

6.2.2 PRESLAUGHTER FACTORS

Animal nutrition plays an important role because of its regulatory effect on biological processes in muscle that are reflected in the quality of meat. Pasture-fed cattle produces meat with higher levels of *n-3* PUFA and conjugated linoleic acid (CLA) content than their counterparts fed with concentrate diets. Feeding concentrates containing linseed or fish oil results in important beneficial responses in the content of *n-3* PUFA and CLA in beef. However, dietary strategies to enhance the content of health-promoting fatty acids in beef and beef products may lead to increased susceptibility to oxidation, and high contents of antioxidants are necessary to help stabilize the effects of incorporating high levels of long-chain PUFA into meat (Scollan et al. 2006; Descalzo and Sancho 2008). A similar picture has been observed in pork; the several efforts made to increase the *n-3* PUFA concentration in pig tissues by dietary manipulation have always considered not only the oil source and the inclusion level of the pig diet but also the adequate supplementation with antioxidants (Raes et al. 2004; Haak et al. 2006). However, according to the findings of Rey et al. (2001), the inclusion of oils rich in linoleic fatty acids in pig diets modifies muscle fatty acid composition, but susceptibility to lipid oxidation does not appear to be increased with respect to that occurring in pigs given diets with no added fat. In the case of lamb meat, the incorporation of PUFA-rich oils in the diet of concentrate-fed animals has a deleterious effect on meat lipid stability during retail display, and the ratio of PUFA to vitamin E in muscle required to prevent loss of oxidative shelf life in lamb containing elevated levels of PUFA remains to be determined (Maloney et al. 2012). Species and conditions under which the animals are raised may indirectly affect lipid oxidation by contributing different levels of vitamin E and other natural antioxidants (Ponnampalam et al. 2001).

Lipid oxidative phenomena in muscle-based foods occur immediately after slaughter when the cellular mechanisms for controlling lipid oxidation no longer work. Nevertheless, events related to handling practices of live animals prior to slaughter, such as transport or type of stunning, may affect the lipid oxidative stability. There was evidence that 8-h road transport increased the thiobarbituric acid reactive substances (TBARS) values in the *longissimus dorsi* muscle of 6-month old lambs compared to nontransported animals (Zhong et al. 2011). Wang et al. (2009) showed that preslaughter exposure to heat, common in poultry production, increased muscle lipid and protein oxidation in broilers. Electrical stunning significantly increased lipid oxidation in light lamb meat 24 h post-slaughter compared to CO_2 stunning (Vergara et al. 2009). According to Linares et al. (2007), the CO_2 gas at stunning could delay the start of the oxidative process, and this could explain the results found at the initial time. However, the effect of CO_2 stunning depends on the gas concentration and exposure time. The results found by Bórnez et al. (2009) on suckling lamb meat 7 days postmortem suggest a negative relationship between lipid oxidation and the hypoxia level at the stunning time. In particular, the use of 80% CO_2 for 60 s was not enough to delay lipid oxidation compared to 90 s exposure time and to 90% CO_2 for both 60 and 90 s.

In the fish sector, recent research accounts for advanced slaughtering and chilling strategies. One such technology is flow ice (FI), which, when employed in the place of traditional flake ice, has shown many advantages, such as lower temperatures, faster cooling, lower physical damage to the product, and better heat exchange power. The FI system, including ozone (OFI), was tested by Ortiz et al. (2008) to extend the shelf life of farmed rainbow trout commercialized as a fresh product. The ozone presence has shown some profitable effects as leading to an extended shelf-life time by quality retention of several sensory parameters, but a slight prooxidant effect was observed in the fillets of trout slaughtered under OFI conditions compared to the ones slaughtered under FI conditions.

6.2.3 PROCESSING AND PRESERVATION TECHNIQUES

The formation of ROS is an inevitable consequence of the aerobic metabolism of animals, and oxidative reactions affecting muscle lipids take place *in vivo*. After slaughter, the *in vivo* antioxidant mechanisms partially collapse, and the exposure of muscle to oxygen and the biochemical changes occurring during the conversion of muscle to meat favor oxidation (Morrissey et al. 1998).

Besides their high degree of unsaturation, the susceptibility of muscle phospholipids to oxidation has also been attributed to their physical association with membranes and tissue catalysts of oxidation. Physical processes, such as chopping, grinding, mixing, emulsification, and cooking, disrupt the membranes and expose the phospholipids to oxygen, heme proteins, and metal ions, which catalyze their oxidation in raw and cooked meats. Moreover, the use of some ingredients and technologies in meat processing may have an impact on the extent of lipid oxidation.

6.2.3.1 Addition of Sodium Chloride

Sodium chloride (NaCl)—salt—has been employed since ancient times to preserve meat and is one of the most commonly used ingredients in processed meats. NaCl shows a number of effects on meat products—most of them desirable—which include imparting a salty taste, reduction of water activity, and, hence, the control of microbial spoilage, and facilitation of proteins to get dissolved. However, NaCl enhances the occurrence of oxidative processes (Ruiz 2007). It accelerates the oxidation of a triglyceride model system and induces rancidity in frozen, cooked, and cured meat, although some authors have not demonstrated such an effect in the long-processing dry-cured products (Andrés et al. 2004). The prooxidant effect of NaCl has been attributed to its ability to modify the distribution and reactivity of iron. NaCl releases iron from macromolecules in the cytosolic fraction of turkey muscle, and the displaced iron stimulates lipid oxidation (Kanner et al. 1991). Osinchak et al. (1992) found that NaCl induces oxidation through the ability of chloride ions to form an iron complex that is more catalytically active.

In the last decades, the addition of NaCl to foodstuffs has become a major issue for the processed food sector, in particular, the meat industry. Intake of dietary sodium has been linked to hypertension and, consequently, to increased risk of cardiovascular disease. Public health and regulatory authorities recommend reducing the use of NaCl in processing in order to decrease dietary sodium intake. Apart from lowering the level of NaCl added to products, there are a number of approaches to reducing the sodium content in processed meats, including using NaCl substitutes, using flavor enhancers, and optimizing the physical form of the salt so that it becomes more functional and bioavailable for taste (Desmond 2006). Calcium chloride used to partially replace NaCl in dry-fermented sausage promotes the formation of lipid oxidation compounds (Flores et al. 2005). The NaCl partial replacement by a mixture of potassium, magnesium, and calcium chlorides induces a significant increase in lipid oxidation in Italian salami (Zanardi et al. 2010).

The different salting methods of muscle foods affect the extent of lipid oxidation. Brine-salted and cold-smoked Atlantic salmon fillets show higher fatty acid oxidation than that observed in dry-salted and cold-smoked ones (Espe et al. 2001).

6.2.3.2 Mechanically Separated Meat and Restructured Meat

The mechanical separation of meat is a processing technique that provides functional proteins to be used in the preparation of a variety of further-processed meats. In the process of mechanical separation, used, in particular, in poultry slaughterhouses, meat is removed from the skeletal bone tissues by grinding the starting material (frames, necks, wings, etc.) and passing them through a sieve under high pressure. Most of the bones and cartilaginous materials are removed based on a differing resistance to shear (Froning and McKee 2010). In several countries, meat recovered from bones and carcass parts by mechanical procedures is generally considered of lower quality than manually recovered meat and has, therefore, been subjected to strict regulations concerning the use of the product as a binding agent or as a source of meat in minced-meat products (Froning and McKee 2010; Henckel et al. 2004). Mechanically separated poultry is widely used in further-processed poultry meat, such as patties, nuggets, turkey rolls, and soup mixes. Emulsified poultry products, such as frankfurters, are typically manufactured from chilled or frozen mechanically separated poultry meat.

Mechanically separated poultry is characterized by a paste-like consistency and high susceptibility to deteriorative changes that occur during storage. The stressful process and the compositional nature of the product contribute to its high oxidative potential. The mechanical separation of poultry meat increases the heme protein content by approximately three times that found in hand-deboned meat, and the increase is primarily a result of hemoglobin from the bone marrow. Hemoglobin presents significant color problems because it is easily oxidized and susceptible to heat denaturation during processing and storage. During the separation process, the meat is exposed to considerable air, which may accelerate the oxidation of heme pigments. This phenomenon is strictly linked to lipid oxidation, which, together with color instability, is the major problem with mechanically separated poultry (Dawson and Gartner 1983; see also Chapter 2).

The problem of lipid oxidation in meats has become even more important with the modern food formulation of restructured meat products, which characterize, in particular, the poultry meat sector and have contributed to an exceptional increase in the consumption of chicken and turkey meat over the last several decades. The poultry industry has been very accommodating to consumers' needs with the development of more ready-to-cook (RTC) and ready-to-eat (RTE) products. Consumers want foods that are easy to prepare, and restructured products fit into that category (Owens 2010).

Restructured meat products provide virtually unlimited versatility in shape, texture, and appearance to appeal to the consumer demand. The production of restructured meat products is a complex procedure involving several steps. They may be manufactured by taking small muscle particles that are produced by grinding, flaking, dicing, chopping, or slicing. These particles are then combined with a chilled brine, an appropriate binding material, and formed into a specific portion size and shape. Mechanically separated meat may be incorporated for its binding properties. Some products may be coated with a batter, breaded, precooked, and packaged for a subsequent reheating in a microwave oven, deep-fat fryer, or convection or conventional oven (Keeton and Osburn 2010). The various possibilities existing in each of the production steps not only enlarge the variety of these products but also increase the potential for problems if done incorrectly. A major concern in the production and distribution of these products is lipid oxidation, which starts with cooking and continues through frozen storage to produce off-flavors and off-odors (Owens 2010).

The effect of the use of mechanically separated turkey on the rate of lipid oxidation in chicken doner kebabs during storage was investigated by Kilic and Richards (2006). Mechanically separated turkey and a combination of mechanically separated turkey with sodium ascorbate (0.1%) included in the kebab accelerate lipid oxidation compared to a kebab manufactured with only chicken breast muscles. The antioxidant effect of ascorbate in the absence of mechanically separated turkey was converted to a prooxidant effect in the presence of mechanically separated turkey. This suggests that the excess of lipid hydroperoxides and iron complexes in mechanically separated turkey are activated as lipid oxidation catalysts by ascorbate to overwhelm the ability of ascorbate to inhibit lipid oxidation at lower concentrations of hemoglobin, iron, and peroxides. The addition of sodium nitrite (150 ppm) does not hinder lipid oxidation and color changes in mechanically separated meat of different origins during frozen storage (99 days at −18°C); only the addition of sodium nitrite (150 ppm) together with sodium erythorbate (500 ppm) seems effective in reducing the problem of lipid oxidation (Trinidade et al. 2008). Among the various polyphenolic classes from cranberry powder, flavonol aglycones are the most effective in inhibiting lipid oxidation in mechanically separated turkey meat (Lee et al. 2006).

The prooxidant effect of the inclusion of mechanically separated meat in the manufacture of meat products has not been confirmed by Trinidade et al. (2005). Based on their findings, the replacement of beef and pork with mechanically separated layer hen meat from 20% up to 100% does not affect the lipid oxidation in mortadella sausage. Nevertheless, because in this study the mechanically separated meat that had just been extracted was used, there may not have been enough time for the oxidation reactions to occur.

6.2.3.3 Freezing and Thawing

As global trade increases and the distance between producer and consumer expands, the need to freeze meat for transport has grown. The final temperature to which meat is frozen and stored determines the amount of unfrozen water that remains available for chemical reactions to proceed. The optimum temperature for the frozen storage of meat has been reported to be $-40°C$ as only a very small percentage of water is unfrozen at this value. The fraction of unfrozen water is important in terms of oxidation because chemical reactions that initiate primary lipid oxidation in the meat can occur during frozen storage. This phenomenon can lead to the formation of secondary lipid oxidation products upon thawing (Leygonie et al. 2012).

The detrimental effect of long-term freeze storage on the oxidative stability of pork was reported by Hansen et al. (2004). These authors followed the development of lipid oxidation during 6-day chill storage of chops from the *longissimus dorsi* muscle produced from the same pigs prior to and following 30 months of frozen storage. Lipid oxidation had the same initial value for fresh and prefrozen meat, but it developed more rapidly during chill storage in prefrozen chops. Multiple freeze–thaw cycles cause the destabilization of the muscle structure, leading to the redistribution of prooxidants and acceleration of lipid oxidation. In fish, lipid oxidation increases as the number of freeze–thaw cycles increases (Benjakul and Bauer 2001; Thanonkaew et al. 2006). The effect of length (0, 30, 75, and 90 days) and temperature ($-20°C$ and $-80°C$) of frozen storage on lipid oxidation of vacuum-packed beef was studied by Veira et al. (2009). TBARS values increased from 30 days of frozen storage, but statistical differences with respect to fresh meat only appeared after 90 days under frozen storage. No effect of freezing temperature was observed.

6.2.3.4 Irradiation

Irradiation of food and agricultural products, as part of the larger radiation-processing industry, is currently allowed by about 60 countries around the globe (Sommers and Fan 2006). Food irradiation is a well-known decontaminating technique able to increase food safety and shelf life, and its use, in combination with other methods of food preservation according to the hurdle technology approach, is gradually increasing worldwide. These effects are achieved by exposing food to gamma rays from radioactive nuclides, electrons from particle accelerators, or X-rays emitted by high-energy electron beams, all able to transfer energy to food material. The choice of a radiation source for a particular application depends on practical aspects, such as thickness and density of the food and irradiation dose to be applied (Cleland 2006). The maximum irradiation dose considered to be safe and wholesome is 10 kGy (SCF 2003).

Irradiation is efficient to disinfect fresh and durable agricultural commodities of quarantine pests because it is broadly effective against insects and mites (Follet and Griffin 2006), and it is promising to improve the safety, sensory properties, and shelf life of a wide variety of fresh and fresh-cut produce (Niemira and Fan 2006). As regards the meat, the irradiation processing is recognized as a safe and effective method among the existing technologies for meat decontamination (O'Bryan et al. 2008). It is well known to be able to reduce pathogenic microorganisms, thus increasing meat safety and controlling food-borne diseases (Ahn et al. 2006). However, irradiation has been shown to accelerate lipid oxidation because ionizing radiation generates hydroxyl radicals, a strong initiator of lipid oxidation. Irradiation-induced oxidative chemical changes are dose-dependent, and the presence of oxygen has a significant effect on the development of oxidation. Irradiation accelerates lipid oxidation only when meat is irradiated and stored under aerobic conditions, especially in cooked meat, whereas the treatment and storage under vacuum seem sufficient to curb lipid oxidation. This indicates that oxygen availability is more important for the development of lipid oxidation than irradiation (Ahn and Lee 2006). Irradiation treatment is reported to induce lipid oxidation in aerobically packaged raw lamb meat (Kanatt et al. 2006), chicken meat (Du et al. 2000), turkey breast (Nam and Ahn 2003), pork (Ahn et al. 1998, 2000), ground beef (Murano et al. 1998), and cooked pork sausage (Jo et al. 2003). Besides the reduction of the presence of oxygen, low temperatures and antioxidants are other alternatives to retard lipid oxidation. The lipid oxidation changes induced by irradiation are lower in frozen meat than those in refrigerated meat, probably because of the limited mobility of free radicals in the frozen state (Nam et al. 2002). Natural antioxidants, such as oregano and rosemary extracts, in beef burgers subjected to electron-beam irradiation with doses up to 7 kGy and stored frozen up to 90 days showed a great capacity to reduce lipid oxidation (da Trindade et al. 2009). Antioxidant combinations using sesamol, gallate, and α-tocopherol effectively reduced lipid oxidation and off-odor volatiles in pork patties treated with electron-beam irradiation up to 4.5 kGy (Nam and Ahn 2003).

Some studies have been devoted to the determination of cholesterol oxides, a group of compounds produced by the oxidation of cholesterol. The levels of cholesterol oxides in turkey meat irradiated at 3 kGy were similar to those in the untreated meat (Farkas et al. 2009); similar amounts of cholesterol oxides were observed in nonirradiated turkey, beef, and pork patties compared to the same samples irradiated at 4.5 kGy. Nevertheless, the treatment at a high radiation dose (8 kGy) increased the cholesterol oxidation of cured pork products compared to the nonirradiated ones (Zanardi et al. 2009). Similar to fatty acid oxidation, the packaging type affects the extent of cholesterol oxidation: The contents of cholesterol oxides are lower in vacuum-packaged meat than in aerobically packaged meat (Nam et al. 2001; Lee et al. 2001).

6.2.3.5 High Hydrostatic Pressure

The prospect of the use of high hydrostatic pressure as a food preservation method was first reported in 1899 when spoilage microorganisms in milk were observed to be reduced by high-pressure treatment. Some years later, it was shown that egg white coagulated under specific conditions of pressure and temperature establishing that, in addition to killing microorganisms, high pressure could modify the protein structure. Nevertheless, at that time, no attempts were made to introduce high pressure into food preservation and processing because of the technical difficulties associated with pressure-processing units and packaging materials (Ludikhuyze et al. 2001). In the last decades, high hydrostatic pressure has gained renewed interest because growing consumer demand for high-quality, fresh-like, and additive-free foods has stimulated research efforts in the area of nonthermal technologies. Besides its application in food preservation, this technology is able to create products with new and unique functional or quality properties and opens a wide area to develop novel foods with a high added value. A number of commercial high pressure-treated food products are currently available in Europe, the United States, and Japan, including plant-based products, such as fruits juices and jams, and meat- and fish-based products, such as hams, fish sausages, and oysters (Indrawati et al. 2003).

High hydrostatic pressure technology is based on the Pascal or isostatic principle: The hydrostatic pressure at a given point is the same in all directions, and pressure is transmitted uniformly through the pressure-transferring medium. Thus, the effects of pressure are independent of product size and geometry. A high hydrostatic pressure system is composed of a pressure vessel and a pressure-generation device. In operation, after all air is removed, a pressure-transmitting medium (water or oil) is pumped from a reservoir into the pressure vessel where the food is inserted. The two methods of treatment of foods in high-pressure vessels are in-container and bulk processing for solid and liquid foods, respectively. The effectiveness of a high-pressure treatment is influenced by various intrinsic and extrinsic factors. Treatment time, the pressurization or decompression rate, temperature, number of pulses, food composition, and the physiological states of the microorganisms to be inactivated are all factors that must be taken into account when optimizing pressure treatments for the production of safe and high-quality foods (Indrawati et al. 2003).

In general, high hydrostatic pressure offers the advantage of minimal deleterious effects on food quality. However, lipid oxidation of pressurized foods is a challenging field of study. It is well established that pressure processing makes the meat more susceptible to oxidation. Several studies have shown that high-pressure treatment at room temperature (20°C–40°C) decreases the oxidative stability of fish and white and red meat. However, the different meats apparently become significantly more unstable at different pressures: the pressures required to initiate lipid oxidation changes seem to be lower for beef (200 MPa) compared to pork (300 MPa), cod (400 MPa), and chicken (600 MPa). The catalytic effects of pressure were still seen in chicken when subjected to pressure at higher temperatures, but in beef, all of the samples, irrespective of pressure treatment from 0.1 up to 800 MPa, were of similar stability. Of the antioxidants studied, metal chelators are the most efficient, supporting the contention that iron ions released from insoluble complexes are of major importance in catalyzing lipid oxidation in pressure-treated muscle foods (Ma et al. 2007). There is also evidence that the effects of pressure may relate to changes in the integrity of the cell membrane. The oxidative stability of chicken breast muscles subjected to high-pressure treatment at 300, 400, 500, 600, 700, or 800 MPa for 5 or 10 min or to heat treatment (80°C for 10 min) and subsequent storage at 5°C was evaluated over a 2-week period by Orlien et al. (2000). Lipid oxidation in pressure-treated muscle depended to a high degree on the working pressure and less on the pressuring time. The treatment at 800 MPa for 10 min was found to enhance lipid oxidation to the same extent as the heat treatment. Pressure treatment at 600 and 700 MPa resulted in less oxidation. Chicken breast muscle exposed to pressure at or below 500 MPa showed no indication of rancidity, similar to what was found for untreated poultry meat during chilled storage; accordingly, 500 MPa is considered a critical value for pressure treatment of chicken meat. Analysis of non-heme iron in pressure-treated chicken meat revealed that the remarkable increase in lipid oxidation caused by high pressure above 500 MPa did not result from the release of iron ions. Furthermore, no influence of high-pressure treatment on the catalytic activity of metmyoglobin on lipid oxidation was observed, and it was concluded that the induction of lipid oxidation was probably related to membrane damage in the muscle. The addition of rosemary to pressure-processed minced chicken breast at 600 MPa for 10 min seems to be very efficient in protecting against oxidative deterioration (Bragagnolo et al. 2005). NaCl and mechanical processing have a greater prooxidant effect on pressurized minced chicken breast (300 and 500 MPa for 30 min at 20°C) compared to the cooked one (90°C for 15 min). These findings indicate that pressure and heat treatments differently alter the chicken-meat structure (Beltran et al. 2003).

6.2.3.6 Packaging

Nowadays, the packaging of food performs beyond conventional properties for protection against deteriorative effects and provides many functions for the product. The packaging contains the product, making transport easier; communicates to the consumer as a marketing tool; and provides consumers with ease of use and convenience.

More advanced forms of meat packaging were required as butchers' cutting and wrapping of meat in paper or waxed paper upon demand by the purchaser were replaced by store cutting and display of the packages in refrigerated, self-service display cases in the 1960s. Air-permeable and moisture-barrier polyvinyl chloride that stretches around polystyrene trays was developed for raw meat. Consumers began to associate the bright red color of prepackaged meat in air-permeable packaging with meat freshness because this was the color of the meat first seen on display in self-service cases. Overwrapping in air-permeable film is still used, but the meat industry is utilizing modified atmosphere packaging (MAP) technology more and more as case-ready packaging of raw meat becomes more widely adopted, especially in the United States. Case-ready or centralized packaging is the fabrication and packaging of consumer-sized retail items in a processing warehouse or other centralized non-retail location for transport and subsequent display in retail stores with minimal or no package manipulation of the individual package after removal from the shipping carton. Many of the case-ready systems incorporate MAP because the development in packaging materials, equipment, and processing has made MAP economically competitive and highly efficient in terms of shelf-life extension for meat (McMillin 2008).

MAP is the removal and replacement of the atmosphere surrounding the product by gas or mixtures of gases before sealing in vapor-barrier materials. Vacuum packaging is simply the removal of air prior to sealing the product in a barrier film. For meat, vacuum packaging is considered a form of MAP because muscle and microbial metabolism utilizes residual oxygen to produce carbon dioxide, and the net result is a modified atmosphere that achieves significant shelf-life extension. MAP is distinguished from vacuum packaging by the headspace that allows introduction of a much larger volume of gases to the package and by elimination of the physical pressure on the product that occurs with vacuum packaging (Sebranek and Houser 2006).

Applications of MAP systems for meat and poultry products include the use of carbon dioxide, oxygen, and nitrogen and their mixtures in a variety of ratios, depending on the product being packaged. Carbon dioxide is an effective antimicrobial agent; at least 20% of this gas is necessary to impact bacterial growth and extend shelf life. Carbon dioxide can be absorbed by meat because of its high solubility in muscle tissue, and a percentage higher than 30% can induce the collapse of the package. The main role of oxygen in the packaging of meat and poultry is the development and maintenance of the cherry-red color that is considered essential to the display of raw meat. The red oxymyoglobin pigment develops readily in normal atmospheric oxygen pressure, but an elevated oxygen concentration of 65% to 80% in MAP helps to form a deeper layer of oxymyoglobin pigment that will extend the time during which the color appears attractive. However, because oxygen also promotes the growth of rapidly proliferating aerobic microorganisms, oxygen in MAP systems for raw meat is usually combined with 20% to 25% carbon dioxide to achieve improved microbial control. Nitrogen is an inert gas with no direct effect on microbial growth; the low solubility of nitrogen is advantageous for use as a filler gas with carbon dioxide to prevent package collapse. Therefore, for retail display of raw meat, MAP may include a high level of oxygen (up to 80%) with carbon dioxide and sometimes nitrogen for balance.

Vacuum packaging of raw meat has typically been restricted to distribution of wholesale cuts because the dark purple color of meat is unacceptable for retail display (Sebranek and Houser 2006). Vacuum packaging improves the oxidative stability of meat, and anaerobic conditions reduce lipid and heme-pigment oxidation (Fernández-López et al. 2008). Lipid and protein oxidation of ostrich meat overwrapped in air-permeable film for 5 days at 4°C increased up to 275% and 30%, respectively, compared to vacuum packaging (Filgueras et al. 2010).

Although MAP of raw meat is designed primarily to preserve the bright red appearance of meat, increased lipid oxidation has been reported for raw meat stored at elevated oxygen concentrations. In the study by Formanek et al. (2001) involving beef patties overwrapped in air-permeable film and packed in three different MAP systems consisting of oxygen/carbon dioxide mixtures with 30%, 70%, and 80% oxygen, respectively, MAP provided the least protection against oxidative deterioration with the level of lipid oxidation increasing as the oxygen content of the gas mixture increased. The increase in lipid oxidation between 7 and 10 days storage at 4°C in the dark was significantly higher in minced beef packed in high oxygen (40%, 60%, and 80%) compared to low oxygen (20%) MAP systems (O'Grady et al. 2000). The oxidative stability of beef steaks stored under MAP with 0%, 10%, 20%, 50%, and 80% of oxygen at 4°C under fluorescent light for 15 days decreased with storage, and the rate was dependent on the level of oxygen used in the package. By day 9, TBARS values increased with increasing the oxygen level in MAP, although only the differences between steaks packed in 50% and 80% oxygen treatments on day 15 were significant (Zakrys et al. 2008). Similar findings were reported by Esmer et al. (2011) in the study of the effect of modified atmosphere gas composition, with 30%, 50%, and 70% oxygen, on lipid oxidation of minced beef. Therefore, an approach involving both high oxygen atmospheres and antioxidants seems necessary to improve the oxidative stability of raw meat packed in MAP systems. However, other researchers did not find any significant increase in lipid oxidation by the increased oxygen level in MAP. Kennedy et al. (2004) did not observe a significant difference between TBARS values from lamb packed under three different gas mixtures (O_2/CO_2/N_2 80:20:0, 60:20:20, and 60:40:0) and stored in a refrigerated, illuminated display cabinet up to day 9. According to the response surface models for predicting the effects of temperature, storage time, and modified atmosphere composition on lipid oxidation developed by Jakobsen and Bertelsen (2000), a reduction in oxygen concentration in the headspace from 80% to 55% did not have much influence on the lipid oxidation of MAP packaged beef. A further decrease in oxygen concentration below 55% was required to obtain reduced lipid oxidation in beef at 3°C. Moreover, a low temperature (below 4°C) almost prevented lipid oxidation, regardless of oxygen level, and when the temperature was raised, the oxygen level became more critical.

6.2.3.7 Functional Meat Products

Besides the dietary strategies on live animals previously mentioned, a modern approach to enhance the content of health-promoting fatty acids is the direct addition of oils to processed meat products. This approach is most promising for *n-3* fatty acids, which only need to be added at low levels to be nutritionally significant. An advantage of this approach is that the fatty acids can be encapsulated in delivery systems that inhibit oxidation without decreasing bioavailability (Decker and Park 2010).

In dry-fermented sausage, the partial substitution of pork back fat with vegetable oils (soy, linseed, olive) and fish oil is successful in reducing the content of saturated fatty acids and increasing the PUFA level. However, one of the potential problems derived from these modifications could be an acceleration of the oxidation processes as a result of the increment of unsaturated fatty acids, which are more prone to oxidation. Muguerza et al. (2004) observed a greater lipid oxidation in chorizo de Pamplona, a traditional Spanish dry-fermented sausage, manufactured with the inclusion of fish oil extracts compared to the traditional one. However, a significant reduction of lipid oxidation was detected in Greek sausages produced with a partial replacement of pork back fat with 20% olive oil, probably because of the antioxidant substances present in the virgin oil (Muguerza et al. 2003). Thus, when intervention strategies aimed at obtaining nutritional benefits in terms of fatty acid composition are adopted, antioxidant systems must also be used to minimize oxidative deterioration (Ansorena and Astiasaran 2007).

6.2.4 CULINARY COOKING PRACTICES

The use of fire to cook or smoke meat and the use of sunlight to dry meat are part of human survival and cultural practices. The benefits of heat in terms of safety and palatability are widely known; however, cooking can negatively affect meat quality as a result of the potential loss of some nutrients and formation of toxic compounds. Over the centuries, the media used to apply heat have changed, and nowadays, several cooking methods are available. Microwave treatment is one of the most often employed cooking methods at home and in restaurants and catering systems because of advantages, such as the high rate of heat transmission, savings in time and energy, cleanliness and ease of use.

The effect of household cooking methods on lipid oxidation has been investigated in some studies. Cooking induces a generalized increase in the formation of lipid oxidation products. However, the type of culinary practice (moist or dry heat), temperature of cooking medium, cooking time, heating rate, end-point temperature, and post-cooking rise are all parameters that strongly affect the course of lipid oxidation (Skibsted et al. 1998; Monahan 2000). Boiling in water, broiling under an electric grill, oven roasting, and microwaving increase fatty acid oxidation in different beef muscles, but only with the first two culinary practices is the increment statistically significant (Badiani et al. 2002). Pan-frying causes a significant increase of primary lipid oxidation products in minced beef but not in the secondary ones, probably because of the unsuitability of the assay to test them (Ferioli et al. 2010).

In relation to cholesterol oxidation, the increase in cholesterol oxidation products (COPs) as a consequence of heat treatment has been widely proved. Tai et al. (2000) overviewed the COP content in foods and concluded that most of the processed foods containing cholesterol are susceptible to forming COPs with heating being the main causative factor. Conchillo et al. (2003), analyzing the effect of grilling and roasting in chicken breast meat, found an increase of 4–4.5 times the total COPs with cooking, whereas a 16-fold increment was observed with microwave heating (Conchillo et al. 2005). In beef and chicken patties, the increase was 1.5–2.6 times with frying in olive oil (Echarte et al. 2003). Pan-frying with olive oil and soya oil also induced a mild increase in cholesterol oxidation in salmon; the highest levels of COPs were observed in roasted salmon (Echarte et al. 2001). The minimal effect of cooking techniques such as pan-frying on a stove or hotplate on cholesterol oxidation has been shown by other authors in hamburgers (Larkeson et al. 2000; Vincente and Torres 2007; Ferioli et al. 2008).

6.3 FACTORS PROMOTING OXIDATION OF MEAT PROTEINS

The oxidation of food proteins is currently one of the emerging research topics within food science, in particular, in the field of meat and meat products. Although several studies have been carried out on the denaturation and hydrolytic degradation of meat proteins after animal slaughter and during processing and storage, the oxidative damage of meat proteins and the consequences of this phenomenon on specific meat traits and global meat quality are still poorly understood. Carbonylation is generally recognized as one of the most remarkable chemical modifications in oxidized proteins. An excellent review of the current knowledge of the mechanisms and consequences of protein carbonylation in meat systems has been presented by Estevez (2011) at the 57th International Congress of Meat Science and Technology held in Ghent, Belgium.

The main prooxidant systems able to initiate meat protein carbonylation are similar to those of meat lipid oxidation. The carbonylation of meat proteins can be induced by ROS-generating systems, including transition metals, such as heme and non-heme iron and copper. Lipid-derived ROS are also initiators of protein carbonylation. Other factors may affect the oxidation of proteins and amino acids: light and irradiation are able to initiate protein oxidation (Garrison 1987; Rowe et al. 2004). The impact on protein oxidation of freezing and cooking of meat has recently been investigated. There is evidence that multiple freeze–thaw cycles cause porcine protein oxidation (Xia et al. 2009). Heat treatment (100°C for 30 min) clearly induces myofibrillar protein oxidation and, as a consequence, the formation of protein aggregates and the altered ability of proteins to build hydrogen and electrostatic bonds with water molecules. The positive correlation between protein oxidation and drip loss suggests that protein oxidation may alter the water-holding capacity of meat (Traore et al. 2012a,b; see also Chapter 5).

6.4　FINAL REMARKS

Factors promoting lipid oxidation in meats were the major emphasis of this chapter and were discussed in the light of the most recent findings. Lipid oxidation is normally not considered to be a limiting factor for the shelf life of raw meat as it occurs at a slower rate than microbial growth or discoloration. However, when systems that repress the other deteriorative mechanisms are adopted, lipid oxidation might limit the shelf life of meats. As lipid oxidation of meats is strongly influenced by formulation and some manufacturing steps may have a detrimental impact, it is very important in the industry to monitor the overall process so that oxidation of the products can be minimized. Moreover, the storage and culinary practices of the consumers must be taken into account because some of them have shown prooxidant properties.

REFERENCES

Ahn, D.U., and Lee, E.J. 2006. Mechanisms and prevention of quality changes in meat by irradiation, in *Food Irradiation Research and Technology*, C.H. Sommers and X. Fan (Eds.), pp. 127–142, Blackwell Publishing, Oxford.

Ahn, D.U., Olson, D.G., Ju, C., Chen, X., Wu, C., and Lee, J.I. 1998. Effect of muscle type, packaging, and irradiation on lipid oxidation, volatile production, and color in raw pork patties. *Meat Sci* 49: 27–39.

Ahn, D.U., Jo, C., Du, M., Olson, D.G., and Nam, K.C. 2000. Quality characteristics of pork patties irradiated and stored in different packaging and storage conditions. *Meat Sci* 56: 203–209.

Ahn, D.U., Lee, E.J., and Mendonca, A. 2006. Meat decontamination by irradiation, in *Advanced Technologies for Meat Processing*, L.M.L. Nollet and F. Toldrá (Eds.), pp. 155–191, CRC Press, Boca Raton, FL.

Andrés, A.I., Cava, R., Ventanas, J., Muriel, E., and Ruiz, J. 2004. Lipid oxidative changes throughout the ripening of dry-cured Iberian hams with different salt contents and processing conditions. *Food Chem* 84: 375–381.

Ansorena, D., and Astiasarán, I. 2007. Functional meat products, in *Handbook of Fermented Meat and Poultry*, F. Toldrá (Ed.), pp. 257–266, Blackwell Publishing, Oxford.

Badiani, A., Stipa, S., Bitossi, F., Gatta, P.P., Vignola, G., and Chizzolini, R. 2002. Lipid composition, retention and oxidation in fresh and completely trimmed beef muscles as affected by common culinary practices. *Meat Sci* 60: 169–186.

Baron, C.P., and Andersen, H.J. 2002. Myoglobin-induced lipid oxidation: A review. *J Agric Food Chem* 50: 3887–3897.

Beltran, E., Pla, R., Yuste, J., and Mor-Mur, M. 2003. Lipid oxidation of pressurized and cooked chicken: Role of sodium chloride and mechanical processing on TBARS and hexanal values. *Meat Sci* 64: 19–25.

Benjakul, S., and Bauer, F. 2001. Biochemical and physicochemical changes in catfish (*Silurus glanis* Linne) muscle as influenced by different freeze-thaw cycles. *Food Chem* 72: 207–217.

Bórnez, R., Linares, M.B., and Vergara, H. 2009. Microbial quality and lipid oxidation on Manchega breed suckling lamb meat: Effect of stunning method and modified atmosphere packaging. *Meat Sci* 83: 383–389.

Bragagnolo, N., Danielsen, B., and Skibsted, L.H. 2005. Effect of rosemary on lipid oxidation in pressure-processed, minced chicken breast during refrigerated storage and subsequent heat treatment. *Eur Food Res Technol* 221: 610–615.

Carlsen, C.U., Moller, J.K.S., and Skibsted, L.H. 2005. Heme-iron in lipid oxidation. *Coord Chem Rev* 249: 485–498.

Cleland, M.R. 2006. Advances in gamma ray, electron beam, and x-ray technologies for food irradiation, in *Food Irradiation Research and Technology*, C.H. Sommers and X. Fan (Eds.), pp. 11–55, Blackwell Publishing, Oxford.

Conchillo, A., Ansorena, D., and Astiasarán, I. 2003. The combined effect of cooking (grilling and roasting) and chilling storage (with and without air) on the lipid and cholesterol oxidation in chicken breast. *J Food Prot* 66: 840–846.

Conchillo, A., Ansorena, D., and Astiasarán, I. 2005. Use of microwave in chicken breast and application of different storage conditions: Consequences on oxidation. *Eur Food Res Technol* 221: 592–596.

da Trindade, R.A., Mancini, J., and Villavicencio, A. 2009. Effects of natural antioxidants on the lipid profile of electron beam-irradiated beef burgers. *Eur J Lipid Sci Tech* 111: 1161–1168.

Dawson, L.E., and Gartner, R. 1983. Lipid oxidation in mechanically deboned poultry. *Food Techn* July: 112–116.

Decker, E.A., and Park, Y. 2010. Healthier meat products as functional foods. *Meat Sci* 86: 49–55.

Descalzo, A.M., and Sancho, A.M. 2008. A review of natural antioxidants and their effects on oxidative status, odor and quality of fresh beef produced in Argentina. *Meat Sci* 79: 423–436.

Desmond, E. 2006. Reducing salt: A challenge for the meat industry. *Meat Sci* 74: 188–196.

Diplock, A.T., Charleux, J.L., Crozier-Willi, G., Kok, F.J., Rice-Evans, C., Roberfroid, M., Stahl, W., and Viña-Ribes, J. 1998. Functional food science and defence against reactive oxidative species. *Br J Nutr* 80: S77–S112.

Du, M., Ahn, D.U., Nam, K.C., and Sell, J.L. 2000. Influence of dietary conjugated linoleic acid on volatile profiles, color and lipid oxidation of irradiated raw chicken meat. *Meat Sci* 56: 387–395.

Echarte, M., Zulet, M.A., and Astiasarán, I. 2001. Oxidation process affecting fatty acids and cholesterol in fried and roasted salmon. *J Agric Food Chem* 49: 5662–5667.

Echarte, M., Ansorena, D., and Astiasarán, I. 2003. Consequences of microwave heating and frying on the lipid fraction of chicken and beef patties. *J Agric Food Chem* 51: 5941–5945.

Esmer, O.K., Irkin, R., Degirmencioglu, N., and Degirmencioglu, A. 2011. The effects of modified atmosphere gas composition on microbiological criteria, color and oxidation values of minced beef meat. *Meat Sci* 88: 221–226.

Espe, M., Nortvedt, R., Lie, Ø., and Hafsteinsson, H. 2001. Atlantic salmon (*Salmo salar*, L.) as raw material for the smoking industry. I: Effect of different salting methods on the oxidation of lipids. *Food Chem* 75: 411–416.

Estevez, M. 2011. Protein carbonyls in meat systems: A review. *Meat Sci* 89: 259–279.

Farkas, J., Andrassy, E., Mészáros, L., Polyák-Fehér Beczner, J., Gaál, O., Lebovics, V.K., and Lugasi, A. 2009. Part II: Effects of gamma irradiation on lipid and cholesterol oxidation in mechanically deboned turkey meat, in *Irradiation to Ensure the Safety and Quality of Prepared Meals*. Results of the Coordinated Research Project organised by the Joint FAO/IAEA Division of Nuclear Techniques in Food and Agriculture (2002–2006), pp. 95–102, Vienna: IAEA.

Faustman, C., Sun, Q., Mancini, R., and Suman, S.P. 2010. Myoglobin and lipid oxidation interactions: Mechanistic bases and control. *Meat Sci* 86: 86–94.

Ferioli, F., Caboni, M.F., and Dutta, P.C. 2008. Evaluation of cholesterol and lipid oxidation in raw and cooked minced beef stored in under oxygen-enriched atmosphere. *Meat Sci* 80: 681–685.

Ferioli, F., Dutta, P.C., and Caboni, M.F. 2010. Cholesterol and lipid oxidation in raw and pan-fried minced beef stored under aerobic packaging. *J Sci Food Agric* 90: 1050–1055.

Fernández-López, J., Sayas-Barberá, E., Muñoz, T., Sendra, E., Navarro, C., and Pérez-Alvarez, J.A. 2008. Effect of packaging conditions on shelf-life of ostrich steaks. *Meat Sci* 78: 143–152.

Filgueras, R.S., Gatellier, P., Aubry, L., Thomas, A., Bauchart, D., Durand, D., Zambiazi, R.C., and Santé-Lhoutellier, V. 2010. Colour, lipid and protein stability of Rhea Americana meat during air- and vacuum-packaged storage: Influence of muscle on oxidative processes. *Meat Sci* 86: 665–673.

Flores, M., Nieto, P., Ferrer J.M., and Flores, J. 2005. Effect of calcium chloride on the volatile pattern and sensory acceptance of dry-fermented sausages. *Eur Food Res Tech* 221: 624–630.

Follet, P.A., and Griffin, R.L. 2006. Irradiation as a phytosanitary treatment for fresh horticultural commodities: Research and regulations, in *Food Irradiation Research and Technology*, C.H. Sommers and X. Fan (Eds.), pp. 143–168, Blackwell Publishing, Oxford.

Formanek, Z., Kerry, J.P., Higgins, F.M., Buckley, D.J., Morrissey, P.A., and Farkas, J. 2001. Addition of synthetic and natural antioxidants to α-tocopheryl acetate supplemented beef patties: Effects of antioxidants and packaging on lipid oxidation. *Meat Sci* 58: 337–341.

Froning, G.W., and McKee, S.R. 2010. Mechanical separation of poultry meat and its use in products, in *Poultry Meat Processing*, C.M. Owens, C.Z. Alvarado, and A.R. Sams (Eds.), pp. 295–309, CRC Press, Boca Raton, FL.

Gandemer, G. 1999. Lipids and meat quality: Lipolysis, oxidation, Maillard reaction and flavour. *Sci Alim* 19: 439–458.

Garrison, W.M. 1987. Reaction mechanisms in the radiolysis of peptides, polypeptides, and proteins. *Chem Rev* 87: 381–398.

Haak, L., Raes, K., Smet, K., Claeys, E., Paelinck, H., and De Smet, S. 2006. Effect of dietary antioxidant and fatty acid supply on the oxidative stability of fresh and cooked pork. *Meat Sci* 74: 476–486.

Hansen, E., Juncher, D., Henckel, P., Karlsson, A., Bertlesen, G., and Skibsted, L.H. 2004. Oxidative stability of chilled pork chops following long term storage freeze storage. *Meat Sci* 68: 479–484.

Henckel, P., Vyberg, M., Thode, S., and Hermansen, S. 2004. Assessing the quality of mechanically and manually recovered chicken meat. *LWT-Food Sci Tech* 37: 593–601.

Indrawati, I., Van Loey, A., Smout, C., and Hendrickx, M. 2003. High hydrostatic pressure technology in food preservation, in *Food Preservation Techniques*, P. Zeuthen and L. Bøgh-Sørensen (Eds.), pp. 428–448, Woodhead Publishing, Cambridge.

Jakobsen, M., and Bertelsen, G. 2000. Colour stability and lipid oxidation of fresh beef: Development of a response surface model for predicting the effects of temperature, storage time, and modified atmosphere composition. *Meat Sci* 54: 49–57.

Jo, C., Ahn, H.J., Son, J.H., Lee, J.W., and Byun, M.W. 2003. Packaging and irradiation effect on lipid oxidation, color, residual nitrite content, and nitrosamine formation in cooked pork sausage. *Food Control* 14: 7–12.

Kanatt, S.R., Chander, R., and Sharma, A. 2006. Effect of radiation processing of lamb meat on its lipids. *Food Chem* 9: 80–86.

Kanner, J., German, J.B., and Kinsella, J.E. 1987. Initiation of lipid peroxidation in biological systems. *CRC Crit Rev Food Sci Nutr* 25: 317–364.

Kanner, J., Harel, H., and Jaffe, R. 1991. Lipid peroxidation of muscle foods as affected by NaCl. *J Agric Food Chem* 39: 1017–1021.

Keeton, J.T., and Osburn, W.N. 2010. Formed and emulsion products, in *Poultry Meat Processing*, C.M. Owens, C.Z. Alvarado, and A.R. Sams (Eds.), pp. 245–278, CRC Press, Boca Raton, FL.

Kennedy, C., Buckley, D.J., and Kerry, J.P. 2004. Display life of sheep meats retail packaged under atmospheres of various volumes and composition. *Meat Sci* 68: 649–658.

Kilic, B., and Richards, M.P. 2006. Lipid oxidation in poultry döner kebab: Pro-oxidative and anti-oxidative factors. *J Food Sci* 68: 686–689.

Larkeson, B., Dutta, P.C., and Hansson, I. 2000. Effects of frying and storage on cholesterol oxidation in minced meat products. *J Am Oil Chem Soc* 77: 675–680.

Lee, C.H., Reed, J.D., and Richards, M.P. 2006. Ability of various polyphenolic classes from cranberry to inhibit lipid oxidation in mechanically separated turkey and cooked ground pork. *J Muscle Foods* 17: 248–266.

Lee, J.I., Kang, S., Ahn, D.U., and Lee, M. 2001. Formation of cholesterol oxides in irradiated raw and cooked chicken meat during storage. *Poultry Sci* 80: 105–108.

Leygonie, C., Britz, T.J., and Hoffman, L.C. 2012. Impact of freezing and thawing on the quality of meat: Review. *Meat Sci* 91: 93–98.

Linares, M.B., Bórnez, R., and Vergara, H. 2007. Effect of different stunning systems on meat quality of light lamb. *Meat Sci* 76: 675–681.

Ludikhuyze, L., Van Loey, A., Indrawati, I., and Hendrickx, M. 2001. Combined high pressure thermal treatment of food, in *Thermal Technologies in Food Processing*, P. Richardson (Ed.), pp. 266–284, Woodhead Publishing, Cambridge.

Ma, H.J., Ledward, D.A., Zamri, A.I., Frazier, R.A., and Zhou, G.H. 2007. Effects of high pressure/thermal treatment on lipid oxidation in beef and chicken muscle. *Food Chem* 104: 1575–1579.

Maloney, A.P., Kennedy, C., Noci, F., Monahan, F.J., and Kerry, J.P. 2012. Lipid and colour stability of *M. longissimus* muscle from lambs fed camelina or linseed as oil or seeds. *Meat Sci* 92: 1–7.

McMillin, K.W. 2008. Where is MAP going? A review and future potential of modified atmosphere packaging for meat. *Meat Sci* 80: 43–65.

Monahan, F.J. 2000. Oxidation of lipids in muscle food: Fundamental and applied concerns, in *Antioxidants in Muscle Foods: Nutritional Strategies to Improve Quality*, E. Decker, C. Faustman, and C.J. Lopez-Bote (Eds.), pp. 3–23, John Wiley & Sons, New York.

Morrissey, P.A., Sheehy, P.J.A., Galvin, K., Kerry, J.P., and Buckley, D.J. 1998. Lipid stability in meat and meat products. *Meat Sci* 49: S73–S86.

Muguerza, E., Ansorena, D., Bloukas, J.G., and Astiasarán, I. 2003. Effect of fat level and partial replacement of pork backfat with olive oil on the lipid oxidation and volatile compounds of Greek dry fermented sausages. *J Food Sci* 68: 1531–1536.

Muguerza, E., Ansorena, D., and Astiasarán, I. 2004. Functional dry fermented sausages manufactured with high levels of n-3 fatty acids: Nutritional benefits and evaluation of oxidation. *J Sci Food Agric* 84: 1061–1068.

Murano, P.S., Murano, E.A., and Olson, D.G. 1998. Irradiated ground beef: Sensory and quality changes during storage under various packaging conditions. *J Food Sci* 63: 548–551.

Nam, K.C., and Ahn, D.U. 2003. Combination of aerobic and vacuum packaging to control lipid oxidation and off-odour volatiles of irradiated raw turkey breast. *Meat Sci* 63: 389–395.

Nam, K.C., Du, M., Jo, C., and Ahn, D.U. 2001. Cholesterol oxidation products in irradiated raw meat with different packaging and storage time. *Meat Sci* 58: 431–435.

Nam, K.C., Hur, S.J., Ismail, H., and Ahn, D.U. 2002. Lipid oxidation, volatiles, and color changes in irradiated turkey breast during frozen storage. *J Food Sci* 67: 2061–2066.

Niemira, B.A., and Fan, X. 2006. Low-dose irradiation of fresh and fresh-cut produce: Safety, sensory and shelf-life, in *Food Irradiation Research and Technology*, C.H. Sommers and X. Fan (Eds.), pp. 169–184, Blackwell Publishing, Oxford.

O'Bryan, C.A., Crandall, P.G., Ricke, S.C., and Olson, D.G. 2008. Impact of irradiation on the safety and quality of poultry and meat products: A review. *Crit Rev Food Sci Nutr* 48: 442–457.

O'Grady, M.N., Monahan, F.J., Burke, R.M., and Allen, P. 2000. The effect of oxygen level and exogenous α-tocopherol on the oxidative stability of minced beef in modified atmosphere packs. *Meat Sci* 55: 39–45.

Orlien, V., Hansen, E., and Skibsted, L.H. 2000. Lipid oxidation in high-pressure processed chicken breast muscle during chill storage: Critical working pressure in relation to oxidation mechanism. *Eur Food Res Technol* 211: 99–104.

Ortiz, J., Palma, O., González, N., and Aubourg, S.P. 2008. Lipid damage in farmed rainbow trout (*Oncorhynchus mykiss*) after slaughtering and chilled storage. *Eur J Lipid Sci Technol* 110: 1127–1135.

Osinchak, J.E., Hultin, H.O., Zajicek, O.T., Kelleher, S.D., and Huang, C. 1992. Effect of NaCl on catalysis of lipid oxidation by the soluble fraction of fish muscle. *Free Rad Biol Med* 12: 35–41.

Owens, C.M. 2010. Coated poultry products, in *Poultry Meat Processing*, C.M. Owens, C.Z. Alvarado, and A.R. Sams (Eds.), pp. 279–293, CRC Press, Boca Raton, FL.

Ponnampalam, E.N, Trout, G.R., Sinclair A.J., Egan, A.R., and Leury, B.J. 2001. Comparison of the color stability and lipid oxidative stability of fresh and vacuum packaged lamb muscle containing elevated omega-3 and omega-6 fatty acid levels from dietary manipulation. *Meat Sci* 58: 151–161.

Porter, N.A., and Wujek, D.G. 1988. The autoxidation of polyunsaturated lipids, in *Reactive Oxygen Species in Chemistry, Biology, and Medicine*, A. Quintanilha (Ed.), pp. 55–79, Plenum Press, New York.

Raes, K., De Smet, S., and Demeyer, D. 2004. Effect of dietary fatty acids on incorporation of long chain polyunsaturated fatty acids and conjugated linoleic acid in lamb, beef and pork meat: A review. *Anim Food Sci Technol* 113: 199–221.

Rey, A.I., López-Bote, C.J., Kerry, J.P., Lynch, P.B., Buckley, D.J., and Morrissey, P. 2001. Effects of dietary vegetable oil inclusion and composition on the susceptibility of pig meat to oxidation. *Anim Sci* 72: 457–463.

Richards, M.P., and Li, R. 2004. Effects of released iron, lipid peroxides, and ascorbate in trout haemoglobin-mediated lipid oxidation of washed cod muscle. *J Agric Food Chem* 52: 4323–4329.

Richards, M.P., Østdal, H., and Andersen, H.J. 2002. Deoxyhemoglobin-mediated lipid oxidation in washed fish muscle. *J Agric Food Chem* 50: 1278–1283.

Rowe, L.J., Maddock, K.R., Lonergan, S.M., and Huff-Lonergan, E. 2004. Influence of early postmortem protein oxidation on beef quality. *J Anim Sci* 82: 785–793.

Ruiz, J. 2007. Ingredients, in *Handbook of Fermented Meat and Poultry*, F. Toldrá (Ed.), pp. 59–76, Blackwell Publishing, Oxford.

SCF. 2003. Scientific Committee on Food of European Commission. Revision of the opinion of the Scientific Committee on Food on the irradiation of food, SCF/CS/NF/IRR/24 Final, 24 April 2003. http://ec.europa.eu/food/fs/sc/scf/out193_en.pdf (accessed December 27, 2011).

Scollan, N., Hocquette, J.F., Nuernberg, K., Dannenberger, D., Richardson, I., and Moloney, A. 2006. Innovation in beef production systems that enhance the nutritional and health value of beef lipids and their relationship with meat quality. *Meat Sci* 7: 17–33.

Sebranek, J.G., and Houser, T.A. 2006. Modified atmosphere packaging, in *Advanced Technologies for Meat Processing*, L.M.L. Nollet and F. Toldrá (Eds.), pp. 419–447, CRC Press, Boca Raton, FL.

Shahidi, F. 1994. Assessment of lipid oxidation and off-flavor development in meat and meat products, in *Flavor of Meat and Meat Products*, F. Shahidi (Ed.), pp. 247–266, Chapman & Hall, London.

Skibsted, L.H., Mikkelsen, A., and Bertelsen, G. 1998. Lipid-derived off-flavours in meat, in *Flavor of Meat, Meat Products and Seafoods*, F. Shahidi (Ed.), pp. 217–256, Blackie Academic and Professional, London.

Sommers, C.H., and Fan, X. 2006. *Food Irradiation Research and Technology*. Blackwell Publishing, Oxford.

Tai, C.Y., Chen, Y.C., and Chen, B.H. 2000. Analysis, formation and inhibition of cholesterol oxidation products in foods: An overview (part II). *J Food Drug Anal* 8: 1–15.

Thanonkaew, A., Benjakul, S., Visessanguan, W., and Decker, E.A. 2006. The effect of metal ions on lipid oxidation, colour and physicochemical properties of cuttlefish (*Sepia pharaonis*) subjected to multiple freeze-thaw cycles. *Food Chem* 95: 591–599.

Toldrá, F. 1998. Proteolysis and lipolysis in flavour development of dry-cured meat products. *Meat Sci* 49: S101–S110.

Traore, S., Aubry, I., Gatellier, P., Przybylski, W., Jaworska, D., Kajak-Siemaszko, K., and Santé-Lhoutellier, V. 2012a. Effect of heat treatment on protein oxidation in pig meat. *Meat Sci* 91: 14–21.

Traore, S., Aubry, I., Gatellier, P., Przybylski, W., Jaworska, D., Kajak-Siemaszko, K., and Santé-Lhoutellier, V. 2012b. Higher drip loss is associated with protein oxidation. *Meat Sci* 90: 917–924.

Trinidade, M.A., Contreras, C.J., and De Felicio, P.E. 2005. Mortadella sausage formulations with partial and total replacement of beef and pork backfat with mechanically separated meat from spent layer hens. *J Food Sci* 70: S236–S241.

Trinidade, M.A., Nunes, T.P., Contreras, C.J., and De Felicio, P.E. 2008. Estabilidade oxidativa e microbologica em carne de galinha mecanicamente separada e adicionada de antioxidants durante periodo de armazenamento a −18°C. *Cien Tecn Alim* 28: 160–168.

Veira, C., Diaz, M.T., Martinez, B., and García-Cachán, M.D. 2009. Effect of frozen storage conditions (temperature and length of storage) on microbiological and sensory quality of rustic crossbred beef at different states of ageing. *Meat Sci* 83: 398–404.

Vergara, H., Bórnez, R., and Linares, M.B. 2009. CO_2 stunning procedure on Manchego light lambs: Effect on meat quality. *Meat Sci* 83: 517–522.

Vincente, S.J.V., and Torres, E.A.F.S. 2007. Formation of four cholesterol oxidation products and loss of free lipids, cholesterol and water in beef hamburgers as a function of thermal processing. *Food Control* 18: 63–68.

Wang, R.R., Pan, X.J., and Peng, Z.Q. 2009. Effects of heat exposure on muscle oxidation and protein functionalities of pectoralis majors in broilers. *Poult Sci* 88: 1078–1084.

Xia, X., Kong, B., Liu, Q., and Liu, J. 2009. Physicochemical change and protein oxidation in porcine *longissimus dorsi* as influenced by different freeze-thaw cycles. *Meat Sci* 83: 239–245.

Zakrys, P.I., Hogan, S.A., O'Sullivan, M.G., Allen, P., and Kerry, J.P. 2008. Effects of oxygen concentration on the sensory evaluation and quality indicators of beef muscle packed under modified atmosphere. *Meat Sci* 79: 648–655.

Zanardi, E., Battaglia, A., Ghidini, S., Conter, M., Badiani, A., and Ianieri, A. 2009. Lipid oxidation of irradiated pork products. *LWT-Food Sci Tech* 42: 1301–1307.

Zanardi, E., Ghidini, S., Conter, M., and Ianieri, A. 2010. Mineral composition of Italian salami and effect of NaCl partial replacement on compositional, physico-chemical and sensory parameters. *Meat Sci* 86: 742–747.

Zhong, R.Z., Liu, H.W., Zhou, D.W., Sun, H.X., and Zhao, C.S. 2011. The effects of road transportation on physiological responses and meat quality in sheep differing in age. *J Anim Sci* 89: 3742–3751.

7 Effects of Oxidation on Sensory Characteristics of Food Components during Processing and Storage

Susan Brewer

CONTENTS

7.1 INTRODUCTION

Food quality is ultimately defined in terms of consumer acceptability: taste, aroma, and appearance. Oxidation, both autoxidative and enzymatic, can affect all three. While instrumental measures (pH; thiobarbituric acid reactive substance [TBARS] values; L^*, a^*, and b^* values; hexanal concentration; etc.) are useful, they are only indicators of sensory acceptability. Ultimately, the sensory characteristics must be correlated with the instrumental measures if the instrumental measures are to be used to accurately predict food quality.

There has been rapid growth in the demand for refrigerated and frozen products, particularly those that are precooked, ready-to-heat, or ready-to-eat (Hofstrand 2008). Because of the raw materials, ingredients, processing, and expected shelf life, these products are often susceptible to oxidative deterioration. Therefore, addressing the precipitating factors becomes a primary goal of the food industry in order to maintain quality and satisfy consumer expectations.

7.2 SENSORY EVALUATION

Sensory evaluation is used in the food industry to set standards (criteria, references), for quality control and quality assurance, for new product development, to assess the absolute characteristics (cream flavor) of a product, to assess the "degree of liking," and to assess the shelf life of a product. Characteristics amenable to sensory evaluation include taste, odor, and flavor (taste + odor), texture, appearance (color, wetness, etc.), preference, and difference (amount of difference of a defined parameter, such as pH, in order for a sensory panel to find a difference between two or more samples). The ultimate purpose of most types of sensory evaluation is to end up with some way to compare products: numbers (mean juiciness score, linear relationship between rancid odor and hexanal content, etc.), percentages (proportion of people in Texas who prefer brand X hot dogs versus those in Illinois who prefer brand X), or comparative statistics ("A is not statistically different from B, but both are different from C") is what we are usually after.

7.2.1 TASTE

Taste is one of the senses used to detect the chemical makeup of ingested food—that is, to establish its palatability, nutritional composition, and safety. It is a chemical sensation (Meilgaard et al. 1999). There are four basic tastes—sweet, salt, bitter, and sour—and four accessory tastes: unami (MSG, chemical), metallic, pungent (pepper-hot, menthol-cool, tannin-astringent; trigeminal stimulation), and alkaline (chalky). To be tasted, substances must be in solution, and the concentration must fall within the detection range of the human gustatory system. Factors that affect the ability of a substance to elicit a taste are generally those that affect the degree to which a substance is in solution and available to bind to the taste receptors. These include temperature, solution viscosity, solvent (water, oil, alcohol), and other compounds present.

7.2.2 ODOR

Odor is also a chemical sensation. Volatile odor molecules move through the nasal passages and dissolve in the mucus lining of the superior portion of the nasal cavity. They are then detected by olfactory receptors on the olfactory sensory neurons in the olfactory epithelium. There are thousands of odors that can be discriminated. Our sense of smell is our most acute sense. To be detected as an odor, a substance must be volatile under the conditions of evaluation. Factors important in determining odor are the threshold of the aroma in the air, the concentration in the food, the solubility in oil and water (and possibly other substances, such as alcohol), the partition coefficient between the air and the food, the temperature, the pH, and the viscosity of the food matrix. The partial pressure of the odor substance may be affected by other substances (solutes, gases) present in the product. Substances that are 100% solvated (water soluble) may not volatilize easily. The identified odor of a food may be a result of substances that are present in very small concentrations and/ or combinations of substances at varying levels. Detection thresholds are very low for some compounds.

7.2.3 FLAVOR

Flavor is a combination of taste, olfaction (smell), and other sensations, including those generated by mechanoreceptor and thermoreceptor sensory cells in the oral cavity. Taste sensory cells, located primarily on the tongue, respond principally to the water-soluble chemical stimuli present in food, whereas olfactory sensory cells respond to volatile (airborne) compounds. However, soluble and volatile compounds are often detected at the same time when food is introduced into the mouth. The minimum (threshold) concentrations of substances in solution or in air that result in taste or odor sensations vary dramatically from substance to substance.

7.2.4 COLOR

Food color plays a significant role in the perception of flavor intensity or taste attribute (sweetness, saltiness). It also plays a role in flavor identification (strawberry, banana) and acceptability of the food for consumption (overripe, spoiled). Judgment of flavor identity is often affected by changing the color of a food (whether appropriate, inappropriate, or absent) (Spence et al. 2010).

7.3 OXIDATION

Oxidation is one of the primary forms of deterioration affecting sensory quality of foods. It is a complex sequence of chemical changes that result from the interaction of oxygen with lipids, pigments, metal ions, polyphenols, or other components that can be initiated by enzymes, exposure to energy (cooking, light, irradiation), or exposure to transition metals or free radicals originating from a variety of sources. Once the process is initiated, the presence of oxygen completes and/or continues the process. Oxidation often has negative effects on the flavor, color, and texture of food products and can lower their nutritional value (Byrne et al. 2001). Vitamins such as alpha tocopherol, ascorbic acid, and beta-carotene lose their physiological activity once oxidized.

The extent of oxidation that occurs in a food product depends on the composition of the raw material, endogenous prooxidative (iron) and antioxidative (vitamin E) constituents, processing operations (heating), other ingredients, and the gas environment surrounding the product (Brewer 2011; Rojas and Brewer 2007). Intrinsic antioxidants contained in both plant and animal tissues, including tocopherols, carotenoids, carnosine, polyphenolic compounds, and antioxidant enzymes, are capable of controlling oxidative reactions; however, processing can significantly reduce their activity. In addition, several Maillard reaction products formed during cooking appear to have antioxidant activity. Ingredients, such as sodium chloride, added to many foods, can act as prooxidants (Cheng et al. 2007).

7.3.1 Lipid Oxidation

Lipids play diverse roles in nutrition and health in that they supply calories, essential fatty acids (linoleic acid, linolenic acid), act as fat-soluble vitamin (A, D, E, and K) carriers, increase the palatability of food, and confer a feeling of satiety. Acylglycerols (monoesters, diesters, and triesters of glycerol with fatty acids) constitute 99% of the lipids in depot fats in animals and plants. Food lipids are composed of fatty acids, which may be saturated or unsaturated (Figure 7.1). Many food raw materials (oils, plastic fats, lard) contain unsaturated fatty acids, which are extremely susceptible to quality deterioration, especially under oxidative stress. They may be part of the neutral triglyceride fraction (triacylglycerol) or part of the phospholipid fraction. The electron-deficient regions of the individual fatty acids (the oxygen atom of the carbonyl group [C=O]; unsaturated double bonds [C=C]) make them susceptible to attack by a variety of oxidizing and high-energy agents (Nawar 1996). Triglycerides are primarily straight chains of saturated fatty acids (16- to 18-carbon), while phospholipids can contain up to 15 times the amount of unsaturated fatty acids (C18:4, C20:4, C20:5, C22:5, C22:6) found in triglycerides. Polyunsaturated fatty

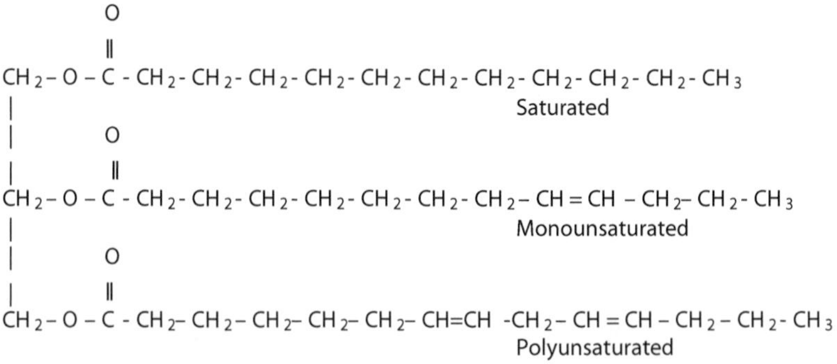

FIGURE 7.1 Triglyceride with saturated, monounsaturated, and polyunsaturated fatty acids.

acids are most susceptible to oxidation via formation of fatty acid radicals because the carbon–hydrogen bond dissociation energy is lower than that in monounsaturated or saturated fatty acids. Linoleic acid (18:2) is estimated to be 10–40 times more susceptible to oxidation than oleic acid (18:1) (Damodaran et al. 2008; Elmore et al. 1999).

When a hydrogen atom (H$^{\cdot}$) is extracted from an unsaturated fatty acid, forming an alkyl radical, lipid oxidation is initiated (Figure 7.2). This reaction is generally initiated by the presence of other radical compounds, by the decomposition of hydroperoxides, or by pigments that act as photosensitizers. The double bond (*cis*) of the alkyl radical then undergoes a positional shift (trans) and a location shift to produce a conjugated diene system. The alkyl radical can react with oxygen (O:O) to form a high-energy peroxyl radical (C–O$^{\cdot}$O$^{\cdot}$), which can go on to abstract a hydrogen atom from another unsaturated fatty acid, leaving behind a new, free alkyl radical and forming a hydroperoxide (–C–O$^{\cdot}$O$^{\cdot}$H; Figure 7.3). In this fashion, autoxidation propagates to and from one fatty acid to another (Fennema 2008). The primary products of lipid oxidation, hydroperoxides, are tasteless and odorless. However, in the presence of heat, metal ions, and/or light, they can decompose to compounds (aldehydes and carbonyls) that contribute off-odors and off-flavors. This chain reaction ultimately terminates when two radical species combine to form a nonradical or when an antioxidant inhibits the chain reaction by donating hydrogen atoms to radicals (Figure 7.4; Sroka and Cisowski 2003) (see also Chapter 4).

Gamma irradiation, ultraviolet A radiation (UVA, 400–320 nm), a pulsed electric field, microwaves, and ohmic processing of foods can produce superoxide radical anions. Water in the food absorbs radiation energy and undergoes radiolysis forming ionized water (H$_2$O$^{+\cdot}$) and excited water (H$_2$O*) (Choe and Min 2006). Electrons

$$R:H + O::O + Initiator \rightarrow R^{\cdot} + HOO^{\cdot}$$

$$R^{\cdot} + O::O \rightarrow ROO^{\cdot}$$

$$ROO^{\cdot} + R:H \rightarrow ROOH + R^{\cdot}$$

$$RO:OH \rightarrow RO^{\cdot} + HO^{\cdot}$$

$$R::R + {}^{\cdot}OH \rightarrow R:R-O^{\cdot}$$

$$R^{\cdot} + R^{\cdot} \rightarrow R:R$$

$$R^{\cdot} + ROO^{\cdot} \rightarrow ROOR$$

$$ROO^{\cdot} + ROO^{\cdot} \rightarrow ROOR + O_2$$

$$ROO^{\cdot} + AH \rightarrow ROOH + A^{\cdot}$$

$$ROO^{\cdot} + A^{\cdot} \rightarrow ROOA$$

FIGURE 7.2 Free radical oxidation mechanism.

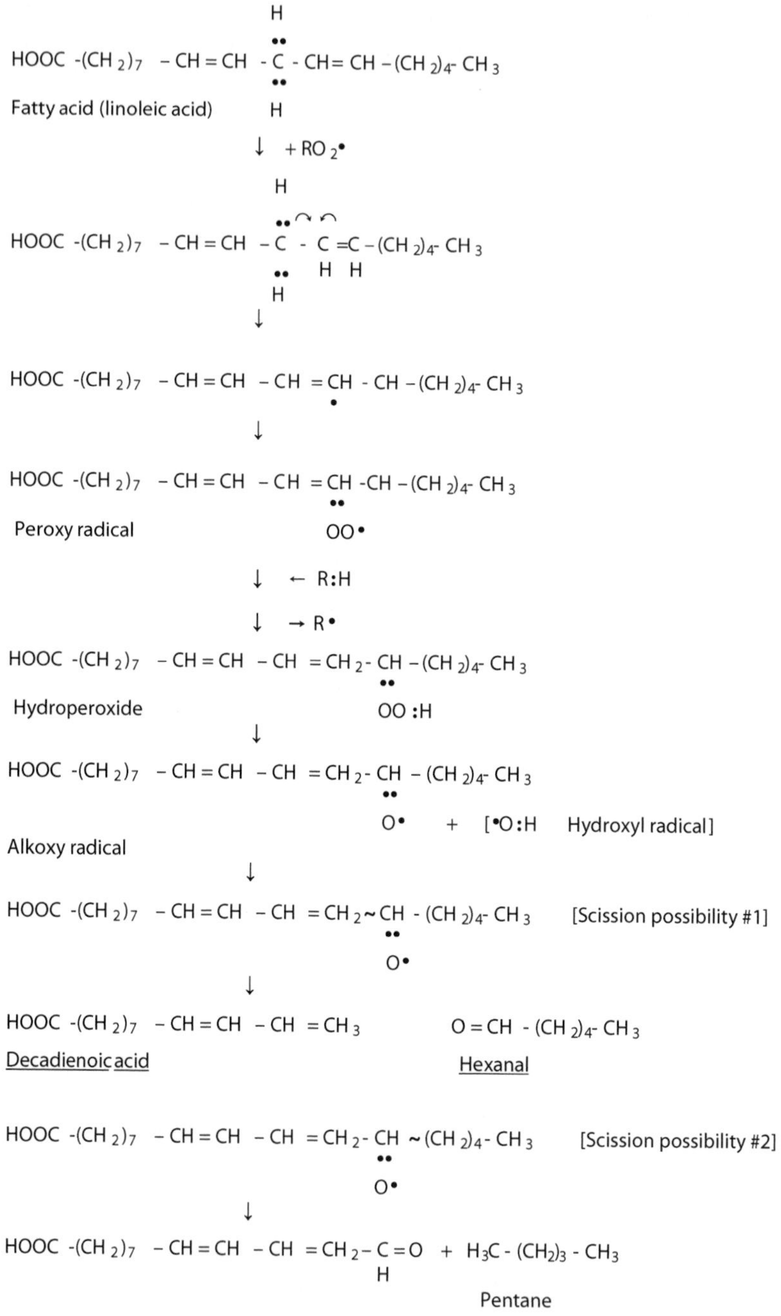

$$
\begin{array}{l}
\text{H} \\
\bullet\bullet \\
\text{HOOC -(CH}_2)_7 \ - \text{CH}=\text{CH} \ - \text{C} - \text{CH}=\text{CH} - (\text{CH}_2)_4\text{- CH}_3 \\
\bullet\bullet \\
\text{H}
\end{array}
$$

Fatty acid (linoleic acid)   H

$$\downarrow \ \ + \text{RO}_2{}^\bullet$$

$$
\begin{array}{l}
\text{H} \\
\bullet\bullet \frown \frown \\
\text{HOOC -(CH}_2)_7 \ - \text{CH}=\text{CH} \ - \text{C} - \text{C}=\text{C} - (\text{CH}_2)_4\text{- CH}_3 \\
\bullet\bullet \quad\quad \text{H} \ \text{H} \\
\text{H}
\end{array}
$$

$$\downarrow$$

$$
\text{HOOC -(CH}_2)_7 \ - \text{CH}=\text{CH} \ - \text{CH} = \text{CH} - \text{CH} - (\text{CH}_2)_4\text{- CH}_3
$$
•

$$\downarrow$$

$$
\text{HOOC -(CH}_2)_7 \ - \text{CH}=\text{CH} \ - \text{CH} = \text{CH} - \text{CH} - (\text{CH}_2)_4\text{- CH}_3
$$

Peroxy radical   OO •

$$\downarrow \ \ \leftarrow \text{R:H}$$

$$\downarrow \ \ \rightarrow \text{R}\bullet$$

$$
\text{HOOC -(CH}_2)_7 \ - \text{CH}=\text{CH} \ - \text{CH} = \text{CH}_2\text{- CH} - (\text{CH}_2)_4\text{- CH}_3
$$

Hydroperoxide   OO :H

$$\downarrow$$

$$
\text{HOOC -(CH}_2)_7 \ - \text{CH}=\text{CH} \ - \text{CH} = \text{CH}_2\text{- CH} - (\text{CH}_2)_4\text{- CH}_3
$$

                         O•   +   [•O:H   Hydroxyl radical]

Alkoxy radical

$$\downarrow$$

$$
\text{HOOC -(CH}_2)_7 \ - \text{CH}=\text{CH} \ - \text{CH} = \text{CH}_2 \sim \text{CH} - (\text{CH}_2)_4\text{- CH}_3 \quad \text{[Scission possibility \#1]}
$$

                        O•

$$\downarrow$$

$$
\text{HOOC -(CH}_2)_7 \ - \text{CH}=\text{CH} \ - \text{CH} = \text{CH}_3 \quad\quad O=\text{CH} - (\text{CH}_2)_4\text{- CH}_3
$$

<u>Decadienoic acid</u>   <u>Hexanal</u>

$$
\text{HOOC -(CH}_2)_7 \ - \text{CH}=\text{CH} \ - \text{CH} = \text{CH}_2\text{- CH} \sim (\text{CH}_2)_4\text{- CH}_3 \quad \text{[Scission possibility \#2]}
$$

                        O•

$$\downarrow$$

$$
\text{HOOC -(CH}_2)_7 \ - \text{CH}=\text{CH} \ - \text{CH} = \text{CH}_2\text{-C}=O \ + \ \text{H}_3\text{C} - (\text{CH}_2)_3 - \text{CH}_3
$$
H

                                 Pentane

FIGURE 7.3   Peroxidation of linoleic acid.

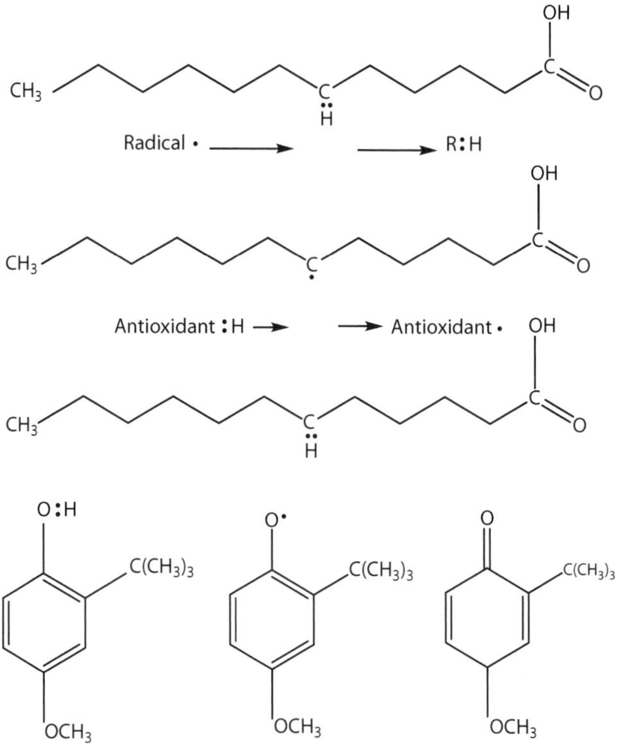

FIGURE 7.4 Antioxidant (BHA) donating H· to fatty acid radical and rearranging to a stable quinone.

surrounded by water molecules are powerful reducing agents. They can reduce triplet oxygen ($^3O_2$) to a superoxide anion:

$$2\ H_2O \rightarrow H_2O* + H_2O^{+\bullet} + e^-(aq)$$

$$^3O_2 + e^-(aq) \rightarrow O_2^{\cdot-}$$

Superoxide anion radicals can also be formed enzymatically from triplet oxygen. Xanthine oxidase acts on xanthine or hypoxanthine in the presence of molecular triplet oxygen to produce $O_2^{\cdot-}$ (Kellogg and Fridovich 1975):

$$\text{Xanthine} + 2\,^3O_2 \xrightarrow{\text{Xanthine Oxidase}} \text{Uric acid} + 2O_2^{\cdot-} + 2H^+$$

In addition, complexes containing iron, such as heme, can generate $O_2^{\cdot-}$ (Winterbourn 1990):

$$O_2 + \text{Heme}(Fe^{2+}) \rightarrow O_2^{\cdot-} + \text{Heme}(F^{3+})$$

Aldehydes, unsaturated alcohols, ketones, and lactones are some of the more important products of lipid oxidation as they have relatively low detection thresholds (Mottram 1998). A number of these compounds, their characteristic odors, and their detection thresholds are shown in Table 7.1. Carbonyls are considered the major compounds responsible for oxidized flavors. Undesirable odors resulting from oxidation are commonly described as stale, wet cardboard, painty, grassy, or rancid (Campo et al. 2006). Compounds that contribute to these odors include hexanal, pentanal, 2,3-octanedione, 2-octenal, and 2-4, decadiene (St. Angelo et al. 1990).

A variety of antioxidant substances are used to prevent or delay color, odor, and flavor deterioration in foods. Synthetic phenolic antioxidants (butylated hydroxyanisole, butylated hydroxytoluene, propyl gallate) effectively inhibit oxidation; chelating agents, such as ethylenediaminetetraacetic acid, can bind metals, reducing their contribution to the process (Hider et al. 2001). Some vitamins (ascorbic acid, α-tocopherol), many herbs and spices (rosemary, thyme, oregano, sage, basil, pepper, clove, cinnamon, nutmeg), and plant extracts (tea, grapeseed) contain antioxidant components as well (Brewer 2011; Figure 7.5). Natural phenolic antioxidants, like synthetics, can effectively scavenge free radicals, absorb light in the UV region

TABLE 7.1
Flavors and Aromas Produced in Foods as a Result of Lipid Oxidation

Compound	Flavors and Aromas	Odor Detection Threshold
Acetone	Sour, pungent	13–24 ppb
Butanoic acid	Rancid, cheesy	240 ppb
Propanoic acid	Pungent, rancid, soy	20 ppm
Methional	Potato-like	0.20 ppb
Pentanal	Pungent, malty	12–42 ppb
Hexanal	Green, grassy, tallowy	4.5–5 ppb
Heptanal	Green, oily, rancid	3.0 ppb
Octanal	Sweet, fatty, soapy	3.0 ppm
Octanoic acid	Sweaty, cheesy	0.86 ppb
Nonanal	Tallowy, waxy	1.0 ppb
Decanal	Rancid, burnt	0.1–2.0 ppb
Decenal	Soapy, tallowy	0.3–0.4 ppb
2-Nonenal	Paper	0.08–0.1 ppb
2-Hexenal	Rancid	17 ppb
2-Octenal	Fatty, nutty, green	3.0 ppb
2-Decenal	Green, pungent,	0.3–0.4 ppb
Deca-2,4-dienal	Fatty, fried potato, green	0.7 ppb
Nona-2,4-dienal	Green, grassy, fatty	0.01 ppb
2-Propanone	Livery	500 ppm
3-Penten-2-one	Fruity	1.50 ppb
3-Hydroxy-2-butanone	Rancid, beany, grassy	800 ppb
1-Octen-3-one	Mushroom-like	0.05 ppb

(continued)

TABLE 7.1 (Continued)

Flavors and Aromas Produced in Foods as a Result of Lipid Oxidation

Compound	Flavors and Aromas	Odor Detection Threshold
2,3-Octanedione	Oxidized fat or oil, fishy	na
Nonenone	Pungent	na
2-Heptanone	Soapy	140–3000 ppb
Delta-decalactone	Peach-like	100 ppb
Methanethiol	Rotten cabbage	0.002 ppm
Dimethyl disulfide	Onion, cabbage, putrid	1.85 ppm
Dimethyl trisulfide	Sulfur, fish, cabbage	0.005–0.01 ppm
3-Methyl-1H-indole	Mothball-like	5.6 ppb
2-Acetyl-1-pyrroline	Popcorn-like	0.10 ppb
3-Methylbutanal	Malty	0.32 ppb
3-Methylbutanoic acid	Sweaty	120–700 ppb
Phenylacetaldehyde	Honey-like	4 ppb

Sources: Fazzalari, F. A., 1978; Frankel, E. N., 1991; Shahidi, F, Wanasundara, P. K., 1992; Spanier, A. M. et al., 1992; Spanier and Miller 1993, 1996; Maruri, J. L., and Larick, D. K., 1992; Mottram and Grosch, 1982; Mottram, D. S., 1998; Kerler, J. and Grosch, W., 1996; Kao, J. W. et al., 1998; Kao, J. W. et al., 1998; Brewer, M. S. et al., 1999; Brewer, M. S. et al., 1999; Yong, J. et al., 2000; Min, D. B. and Boff, J. M., 2002; Min, D. B. et al., 2003; Rowe, D., 2002; Yang, A. et al., 2002; Mahrour, A. et al., 2003; Nam, K. C. and Ahn, D. U., 2003; Nam, K. et al., 2003; Vega, J. D. and Brewer, M. S., 1993; Acree, T. and Arn, H., 2004; Rochat, S. and Chaintreau, A., 2005; Obana, H. et al., 2006; Yancey, E. J. et al., 2006; Calkins, C. R. and Cuppett, S., 2006; Campo, M. M. et al., 2006; Lam, H. S. and Proctor, A., 2003; Cometto-Muñiz, J. E., and Abraham, M. H., 2010.

(100 to 400 nm), and chelate transition metals, thus stopping progressive autoxidative damage and production of off-odors or flavors.

7.3.2 PIGMENT OXIDATION

Pigment oxidation can precede lipid oxidation. Photoactivation of sensitizers, especially pigments, such as chlorophylls and porphyrins, can result in production of O_2^{-} (Buettner and Oberley 1980; Whang and Peng 1988; Haseloff et al. 1989). Heme iron can undergo several reactions involving the central iron atom (changing the oxidation state from Fe^{2+} to Fe^{3+}; binding oxygen or carbon monoxide) that alter meat color (Table 7.2).

7.4 MEAT

Color and appearance are the most important determiners of retail purchase decisions of red meat because consumers presume they are indicators of meat freshness and quality (Robbins et al. 2003; Brewer et al. 2002). Consumers can discriminate differences as small as 0.39a* value units (Zhu and Brewer 1999). Consumers presented with fresh pork loin chops ranging from pale (L* = 57, a* = 8.9) to dark pink

VV URE 7.5   Natural antioxidants.

(L^* = 38, a^* = 10.3) have no difficulty discriminating among colors (Brewer and McKeith 1999). Appearance acceptability was higher for the darker-colored pork. If pork color is not acceptable, consumers say they "definitely would not buy it" or "probably would not buy it" (Jensen et al. 2003).

7.4.1 MEAT FLAVOR

The initial fatty acid differences in meat from various sources make them more or less susceptible to lipid oxidation (Table 7.3). Species differences, livestock genetics, diet, and handling immediately before and after slaughter can have significant effects on the fatty acid composition of the muscle tissues and on the aroma volatiles generated (Maruri and Larick 1992; Fernandez et al. 1999; Elmore et al. 1999; Insausti et

TABLE 7.2
Myoglobin Forms and Characteristics

Pigment	Ligand	Bond	Conditions	State of Globin	State of Iron	Color
Deoxymyoglobin		Ionic	Very low oxygen tension (<5 mm Hg)	Native	Fe^{++}	Purple-red
Oxymyoglobin	$:O_2$	Covalent	High oxygen tension (70–80 mm Hg)	Native	Fe^{++}	Bright red
Metmyoglobin	$:O_2$	Ionic	Loss of electron, low oxygen tension (~10 mm Hg)	Native	Fe^{+++}	Brown
Globin myohemochromogen	H_2O	Covalent	Heating oxymyoglobin, myohemichromogen in a reducing environment	Denatured	Fe^{++}	Dull red-crimson
Globin myohemichromogen	H_2O	Ionic	Heating of myoglobin, oxymyoglobin, metmyoglobin, hemochromogen	Denatured	Fe^{+++}	Brown-gray
Carboxymyoglobin	CO:	Covalent	Preferentially bound (to O_2); not consumed in vacuum	Native	Fe^{++}	Bright red
Sulfmyoglobin	HS	Ionic	Reaction of H_2S and O_2 with myoglobin	Native	Fe^{++}	Green
Metsulfmyoglobin	HS	Covalent	Oxidation of sulfmyoglobin, loss of electron	Native	Fe^{+++}	Red
Choleglobin	OOH		H_2O_2 reaction with myoglobin or oxymyoglobin	Native	Fe^{++} or Fe^{+++}	Green

Source: Lawrie, R. A., in *Meat Science.* Pergamon Press, New York. pp. 152–172, 1991.

TABLE 7.3
Fatty Acid Composition (g/100 g) of Selected Foods

Product	Fat	16:0	18:0	16:1	18:1	18:2	18:3	20:5n-3	22:6n-3
Beef sirloin[a]	5.03	1.12	0.66	0.15	1.85	0.14	0.01	0.00	0.00
Beef frankfurter	29.57	0.15	6.48	1.22	12.43	1.01	0.18	0.00	0.00
80/20 ground beef	15.94	3.39	1.88	0.58	6.06	0.36	0.05	0.00	0.00
Lamb[b]	7.74	1.49	0.95	0.13	3.14	0.41	0.05	0.00	0.00
Pork loin	9.44	1.81	0.91	0.22	3.35	0.85	0.04	0.00	0.00
Pork sausage, cooked	28.36	5.80	?.89	0.78	11.28	3.29	0.00	0.00	0.00
Chicken[c]	4.51	0.87	0.32	0.18	1.30	0.74	0.04	0.00	0.00
Turkey[c]	0.74	0.11	0.07	0.02	0.11	0.13	0.00	0.00	0.00
Salmon, dry cooked	10.97	1.01	0.16	0.32	1.34	0.11	0.01	0.53	0.70
Tuna, in water	0.82	0.16	0.06	0.03	0.09	0.01	0.00	0.02	0.22
Flounder, dry cooked	1.53	0.23	0.06	0.07	0.17	0.01	0.02	0.05	0.26
Shrimp, steamed	1.08	0.14	0.10	0.06	0.11	0.02	0.01	0.17	0.14
Milk, 2% fat	1.98	0.56	0.24	0.03	0.47	0.07	0.01	0.00	0.00
Cottage cheese, 2%	2.45	0.44	0.20	0.03	0.41	0.06	0.01	0.00	0.00

Fatty Acid

Eggs, hard-boiled	10.61	2.35	0.83	0.31	3.73	1.19	0.04	0.01	0.04
Soybeans, boiled	8.97	0.95	0.32	0.03	1.96	4.67	0.60	0.00	0.00
Tofu	4.78	0.51	0.17	0.01	1.04	2.38	0.32	0.00	0.00
Black beans, boiled	0.54	0.13	0.01	–	0.05	0.13	0.11	0.00	0.00
Pinto beans, boiled	0.65	0.13	0.00	0.00	0.13	0.10	0.14	0.00	0.00
American cheese	31.25	9.10	3.80	1.03	7.51	0.61	0.38	0.00	0.00
Peanut butter	50.39	5.77	1.75	0.00	23.15	13.79	0.08	0.00	0.00
Walnuts, English	65.21	4.40	1.66	0.00	8.80	38.09	9.08	0.00	0.00
Oat bran, raw	7.01	1.13	0.07	0.01	2.37	2.62	0.12	0.00	0.00
Split peas, boiled	0.39	0.01	0.01	0.00	0.08	0.14	0.03	0.00	0.00

Source: USDA National Nutrient Database for Standard Reference, Release 20 2007, http://www.nal.usda.gov/fnic/foodcomp/cgi-bin.

[a] Beef, top sirloin, separable lean only, trimmed to 1/8 in. fat, select, raw; contains less than 0.5 g 4:0, 6:0, 8:0, and 10:0.

[b] Lamb, domestic, rib, separable lean only, trimmed to 1/4 in fat, choice, raw.

[c] Chicken, broilers or fryers, separable fat, raw; contains less than 0.5 g 4:0, 6:0, 8:0, and 10:0.

al. 2005; Janz et al. 2008). Makeup of the fat component in the diet of meat animals, particularly if it is high in polyunsaturated fatty acid content, can influence flavor and fat softness or can serve as the initial substrate for reactions that generate expected cooked flavors or off-flavors (oxidation) (Guo et al. 2006). Dietary vitamin E locates in the cell membrane in proximity to phospholipids, preventing development of free radicals in membranes *in vivo* and postmortem (Onibi et al. 2000). Feeding natural sources of vitamin E to finishing pigs has been shown to be more effective than artificial sources in reducing lipid oxidation of pork during subsequent storage and display (Boler et al. 2009). Yang et al. (2002) found that meat from pasture-fed cattle contained as much alpha-tocopherol as grain-fed cattle supplemented with 2500 IU vitamin E. It contained a higher percentage of linolenic acid and a lower percentage of linoleic acid, and was less prone to lipid oxidation and development of warmed-over flavor (WOF). Diet can also affect the color of the resultant meat. Vitamin E supplemented into swine diets can stabilize meat color and decrease fluid loss when fed at >200 mg/kg of diet during the finishing phase (Asghar et al. 1980; Cheah et al. 1995).

Processes such as aging and enhancement can have significant effects on beef and pork quality (Brewer et al. 2004; Wicklund et al. 2005; Brewer and Novakofski 2008; Stetzer et al. 2008). Aging and storage can increase fatty flavor and negative attributes, such as painty, cardboard, bitter, and sour tastes, which ultimately affects the characteristics of the cooked product (Spanier et al. 1997, 1998; Mottram 1998; Gorraiz et al. 2002; Bruce et al. 2005). Positive flavor compounds, such as 3-hydroxy-2-butanone, 2-pentyl furan, 2,3-octanedione, and 1-octene3-ol decrease, and negative compounds, such as pentanal, nonanal, and butanoic acid, which have detection thresholds as low as 1.0 ppb, increase with aging (Stetzer et al. 2008).

To determine detection thresholds of selected volatile organics known to be produced during the oxidation of food lipids, Vega and Brewer (1994) chose gelatin to simulate a complex, thermally sensitive food system and added pentanal, hexanal, t-2-hexenal, heptanal, t-2-octenal, and t,t,-2,4-decadienal to it. The detectable odor thresholds were positively correlated with viscosity and negatively correlated with temperature. Detectable odor thresholds ranged from 22 to 170 ppb and increased in the order of pentanal < hexanal < heptanal < t,t-2,4-decadienal < t-2-hexenal < t-2-octenal. In order to model an oxidizing meat system, Vega and Brewer (1995) added pentanal, hexanal, t-2-hexenal, t-2-heptanal, t-2-octenal, and t,t-2,4-decadienal individually to lean ground beef. The detectable odor threshold for pentanal was 2.67 ppm, for hexanal 5.87 ppm, for heptanal 0.23 ppm, for t-2-hexenal 7.87 ppm, for t-2-octenal 4.20 ppm, and for t,t-2,4-decadienal 0.47 ppm. Common terms used to describe the odor of meat containing these added compounds were rancid, painty, and herbal.

Oxidation of fatty acids to carbonyl compounds is a significant contributor to beef odor and off-odor. It can be affected by gas atmosphere during storage, cooking, and storage after cooking. Increases in carbonyls derived from lipid oxidation can contribute to off-flavors, decrease flavor identity, and increase metallic flavor (Yancey et al. 2005, 2006). Gas atmosphere surrounding meat during storage can also have significant effects on quality. It has been reported that a high-oxygen modified atmosphere packaging (MAP) (60% O_2/30% CO_2/10% N_2) environment during storage can result in beef flavor quality degradation accompanied by an increase in 2,3,3-trimethylpentane, 2,2,5-trimethylhexane, 3-octene, 3-methyl-2-heptene, 2-octene, and

2-propanone and a decrease in dimethyl sulfide (Insausti et al. 2002). Yamato et al. (1970) reported that heating (150°C) beef fat in N_2 produced ethanal, propanal, isobutanal, isopentanal, benzaldehyde, acetone, methyl ethyl ketone, methyl isobutyl ketone, glyoxal, and pyruvaldehyde and their 2,4-dinitrophenylhydrazones. Beef fat heated (200°C) in air produces hexanal, heptanal, 2-heptenal, octanal, 2-octenal, nonanal, 2-nonenal, 2-decenal, 2,4-decadienal, and 2-undecenal. The total long-chain carbonyl content was higher, and the oily odor and beef aroma were stronger in beef fat heated in air than that heated in N_2.

Cooking, refrigerating, or freezing and then reheating meat can result in WOF, which is generally attributed to lipid oxidation (O'Sullivan et al. 2003; Rhee et al. 2005). The phospholipid phosphatidylethanolamine has been implicated in the development of this unacceptable flavor defect (Igene and Pearson 1979). Using sensory evaluation, Kerler and Grosch (1996) determined that WOF results from a combination of a loss of desirable odorants (4-hydroxy-2,5-dimethyl-3(2H)-furanone and 3-hydroxy-4,5-dimethyl-2(5H)-furanone) and an increase in lipid peroxidation products (n-hexanal and trans-4,5-epoxy-(E)-2-decenal).

7.4.2 Meat Color

Myoglobin is a monomeric, globular protein, which serves to deliver and store oxygen in living cells. Meat color is a result of the concentration of heme pigments (myoglobin, hemoglobin), the condition of the central iron moiety (Fe^{2+} or Fe^{3+}), and the ligand bound to the iron. Oxygen can bind to heme iron only if it is in the ferrous state (Fe^{2+}). However, many other ligands (CN, NO, CO, and N_3) can bind to either the ferrous (Fe^{2+}) or ferric form (Fe^{3+}). The identity of the ligand, the oxidation state of the iron center, and the relative concentrations of the various forms determine the color of meat (Mancini and Hunt 2005; Table 7.1). In its native state, deoxymyoglobin, Fe^{+2} is bound to the porphyrin ring at four of its six coordination sites and to the apoprotein at the fifth. Deoxymyoglobin contains Fe^{2+}, lacks a sixth ligand, and is purple-red, the characteristic color of vacuum-packaged meat or myoglobin at low oxygen tension (O'Keefe and Hood 1981). Oxymyoglobin, which has a bright, cherry-red color, forms when deoxymyoglobin reversibly binds oxygen at the sixth ligand with Fe^{2+} in the reduced state (Mancini and Hunt 2005). However, when exposed to O_2 for an extended period, the central iron atom can lose an electron (oxidizing to Fe^{3+}), producing metmyoglobin (MetMb), which is gray-brown (Jayasingh et al. 2002). Metmyoglobin can be activated by H_2O_2, becoming a catalyst for lipid oxidation (Harel and Kanner 1988; Rhee and Ziprin 1987; see also Chapters 2 and 4).

Oxygen in the air is present in a sufficient amount (20%) to produce a bright red meat color and is often used in meat packaging at elevated levels (80%) to enhance the natural color. Common mixtures of gases for MAP include those containing carbon monoxide (0.4% CO/30% CO_2/69.6% N_2) and those containing high levels of oxygen (Sebranek et al. 2006). Because of the presence (or absence) of oxygen, these atmospheres can suppress or enhance lipid oxidation. The cherry-red carboxymyoglobin, formed when CO binds with myoglobin, produces a color that is visually identical to that produced by oxygen. The CO-based pigment is stable for a longer period of time than the oxygen-based pigment and is less likely to oxidize to metmyoglobin (Hunt et al. 2004). In addition to maintaining the red color of beef and pork, CO in MAP suppresses microbial growth without affecting flavor or overall acceptability (Wicklund et al. 2006; Stetzer et al. 2007; Jayasingh et al. 2001, 2002). Viana et al. (2005) found that pork loins in a 1% CO/99% CO_2 atmosphere had the highest consumer acceptance, and color remained acceptable after 20 days of storage (see also Chapters 2 and 5).

7.5 OILS

Oils are particularly susceptible to rancidity—oxidative and hydrolytic—because of the degree of unsaturation of the fatty acids (linoleic, linolenic) and because of the presence of oxidizing enzymes in the raw materials from which they are derived (soybeans, corn, canola). Which compound(s) are responsible for the oxidized aroma of soybean oil is unclear. Concentrations of oxidation-produced volatiles found in oxidized soybean oil, such as 2-heptanone, identified by GC have been shown to be below their flavor thresholds. Lee et al. (1995) reported that the simple sum of the intensities of the flavors of the volatiles accounted for less than half of the flavor intensity of the oxidized oil samples. The strong bitter taste in oxidized soybean oil has been attributed to the free fatty acid fraction. Usuki and Kaneda (1980) determined that the bitter taste is related to the presence of a carboxyl group, a hydroxyl group, and a double bond.

7.5.1 OIL FLAVOR

Undesirable odors, such as fruity, plastic, and waxy, are characteristic of higher oleic acid-containing oils. Triolein and trilinolein have been used to model higher oleic acid-containing oils. The predominant odors of heated triolein are fruity and plastic as well as acrid and grassy. Volatile compounds that produce these odors in heated triolein, in order of increasing concentration, are hexanal (grassy), octanal (fruity), (E)-2-decenal (plastic), nonanal (fruity), and (E)-2-undecenal (plastic). (E)-2-nonenal (plastic), pentanal (grassy), and hexanal (grassy) are produced in heated trilinolein. Neff et al. (2000) reported that the amount of volatiles produced and the intensity of the odors were lower in trilinolein than in triolein.

Lipase and lipoxygenase, enzymes present in oil seeds, help catalyze the reactions that ultimately result in the development of grassy, beany off-flavors in soy products through the oxidation of polyunsaturated fatty acids. Lipase releases the fatty acids from the glycerol of triacylglycerides, making them much more susceptible to oxidation. Lipoxygenase-mediated oxidation, in particular, has been implicated in off-flavor development in soybean products. Soybean seeds contain three lipoxygenase isozymes: lipoxygenase 1 (L-1), lipoxygenase 2 (L-2), and lipoxygenase 3 (L-3). All of these isozymes increase the level of carbonyl compounds and TBARS in aqueous extracts of whole soybean seeds with L-2 and L-3 activity being greater than that of L-1. A disproportionate level of free fatty acid hydroperoxides have been detected in water extracts of soybeans, which implies that lipase action precedes lipoxygenase-catalyzed lipid oxidation (Hildebrand and Kito 1984).

Freshly deodorized soybean oil has a characteristic nutty flavor, which may be a result of the glycerol esters themselves (Kao et al. 1998b). Flavor compounds resulting from hydroperoxide decomposition by lipoxygenase indicate that very little oxidation may be necessary to result in objectionable levels of off-flavor compounds (Wolf 1975). The compounds with the most odor in stale soybean oil are carbonyls, especially heptanal and cis-4-heptenal (Kao et al. 1998b).

There is a linear relationship between the logarithm of the concentration of methyl ketones, aldehydes, 2-enals, and trans,trans-2,4-dienals and the logarithm of the 2-heptanone concentration, giving an equal flavor intensity in a mineral oil/water system (Dixon and Hammond 1984). Flavor intensities of mixtures of carbonyls found in oxidized soybean oil are similar to those predicted from add-ing the intensities of the individual carbonyls (Dixon and Hammond 1984). A high temperature during soybean processing can inactivate lipoxygenase. While processing by grinding with hot water, dry heat-extrusion cooking, blanching, and grinding at low pH followed by cooking can inactivate lipoxygenase, and protein denaturation and loss of functionality may also occur. Alternatively, hex-ane-ethanol or hexane-2-propanol extraction of these flavor components, after they are formed, can reduce odors or flavors with little damage to the protein (Wolf 1975).

Lipoxygenase-free oil contains similar amounts of linoleic acid as oil from con-trol soybeans. After storage, lipoxygenase-free oil has lower peroxide values; how-ever, flavor and other measures of oxidative stability are unaffected (King et al. 1998). Lipoxygenase-free oil does contain higher levels of tocopherols, which may serve to slow oxidation.

Soybean oil can also undergo "flavor reversion," a type of light-induced oxidation (Kao et al. 1998a). The breakdown of furanoid fatty acids can produce 3-methyl-nonane-2,4-dione, which has an intense straw-like, fruity odor. However, whether 3-methylnonane-2,4-dione is responsible for flavor reversion in soybean oil is unclear because it is perceptible between 0.09 and 2.56 ppm in a mineral oil/water emulsion but at <0.80 ppb in soybean oil (Kao et al. 1998a). 2-Pentylfuran and its isomers appear to be some of the compounds responsible for flavor reversion in soybean oil. Both increase in the presence of light and chlorophyll. It has been suggested that the singlet oxygen oxidation mechanism of linolenic acid oxidation is responsible for the formation of 2-pentylfuran and its isomer, and chlorophyll removal will reduce reversion flavor formation (Min et al. 2003).

Major volatiles in good-quality olive oil that influence its sensory characteristics include hexanal, trans-2-hexenal, 1-hexanol, 3-methylbutan-1-ol, and hydroxytyrosol (Kiritsakis 1998). Tyrosol, caffeic acid, coumaric acid, and p-hydroxybenzoic acid are present in lesser-quality oils. Pentanal, hexanal, octanal, and nonanal are the major compounds formed in oxidized olive oil, but 2-pentenal and 2-heptenal are mainly responsible for the off-flavor.

7.5.2 Oil Processing for Stability

Deodorizing soybean oil preserves carotenoids and pigmentation and produces oils with an average of 0.25% free fatty acids (Soares et al. 2004). Removing oxygen (by nitrogen flushing) in the headspace of bottled soybean oil can also be used to increase the sensory quality during storage. Shelf life can be increased from 60 to

90, 120, and 180 days as the initial oxygen concentration is reduced from >15% to 7–9% to 5–6.5% and to <3%, respectively (Arruda et al. 2006).

Fatty acid composition can be modified and additives included to produce frying oils that are alternatives to hydrogenated fats containing trans isomers. Newer oil-processing techniques have been evaluated individually and in combination to increase the fry life of the oil and shelf life of foods. Brewer et al. (1999b) reported that after 15 days of oil use, low linolenic acid soybean oil and creamy partially hydrogenated soybean oil produced higher hexanal concentrations in French fries than did liquid low linolenic acid hydrogenated soybean oil and liquid partially hydrogenated soybean oil. Hexanal concentration was negatively correlated with overall odor quality and positively correlated with grassy, rancid, painty, and chemical odor. Based on rancid flavor intensity and hexanal concentration after storage, tortilla chips fried in expeller-pressed low linolenic acid soybean oil have been shown to be of significantly better sensory quality than chips fried in control soybean oil or expeller-pressed soybean oil (Warner 2009). Using total polar compounds as quality indicators of mid-oleic sunflower oil for frying tortilla chips, gamma tocopherol is more effective than alpha or delta tocopherols. Low linolenic acid soybean oil retains more tocopherols. Hexanal content and rancid odor intensity were highest in chips fried in the control and in oil containing only alpha-tocopherol. The most stable chips were fried in oil containing all three (alpha, gamma, and delta) tocopherols; however, the lowest hexanal concentration occurred when gamma and delta tocopherols were added at their highest concentrations (Warner and Moser 2009). Kiatrichart et al. (2003) showed that heated (~180°C) mid-oleic sunflower and canola oil samples contained 20% polymer after approximately 18 and 22 min of heating.

Oils have been filtered in an effort to remove oxidation products produced during frying. Daily filtration of frying oil can reduce off-flavor compound concentration. Magnesium silicate-filtered oil had lower nonanal concentrations after all oil use times than unfiltered and diatomaceous earth-filtered oil (Brewer et al. 1999a). Nonanal was well correlated with buttery and sweet odors of fries. t-2-octenal was moderately correlated with grassy, rancid, and painty odors and with overall odor quality, while hexanal, t-2-hexenal, heptanal, t-2-heptenal, and 2-pentylfuran were not correlated with sensory characteristics.

7.5.3 MODIFICATION FOR STABILITY

Genetic modifications have been made in soybeans in an effort to produce more oxidatively stable oils. Removing the lipoxygenase L2 isozyme from soybeans used to produce soymilk reduces beany, rancid, and oily flavor and aroma scores and increases dairy and cereal flavor and aroma scores. It has similar effects in soy flour. However, removal of the L1 and L3 isozymes does not improve sensory characteristics (Davies et al. 1987). Eliminating seed lipoxygenase isozymes 1, 2, and 3 reduces the amount of volatile off-flavor compounds in stored soybeans and soy products significantly but not completely, indicating that another enzyme may be responsible. Even when these enzymes are genetically eliminated, volatile compounds produced are similar to lipoxygenase-generated products of polyunsaturated fatty acids; oxygen is consumed; and typical lipoxygenase-inhibitory compounds, such as propyl gallate and nordihydroguaiaretic acid, reduce the generation of these flavor compounds (Iassonova et al. 2009).

In an effort to increase oil stability, especially under high-temperature (frying) conditions, fatty acid profiles have been genetically modified. Ultra-low-linoleic acid (1%) soybean oil is more oxidatively stable than low-linoleic acid (2.2%) soybean oil. Su et al. (2003) found that, initially, ultralow-linoleic acid oil had higher peroxide values and lower sensory scores than low-linoleic acid (2.2%) oil; however, these differences disappeared with storage. In terms of maintaining sensory quality, addition of an antioxidant (TBHQ) was more beneficial to ultralow-linoleic acid oil than to low-linoleic acid oil during high temperature storage (Su et al. 2003).

7.5.4 OILSEED-CONTAINING PRODUCTS

Oleic acid is the predominant fatty acid (44.8% and 64.2%, respectively) in peanut oil and virgin olive oil, making them more resistant to oxidation at frying temperature than other refined vegetable oils (sunflower and soybean oils). Virgin olive and peanut oils have been shown to have lower free fatty acids and p-anisidine values after frying peanuts in them. Peanuts fried in virgin olive oil and peanut oil have higher consumer acceptability scores than those fried in other oils (Ryan et al. 2008).

At room temperature (23°C), canola oil and meal are the least stable to oxidative rancidity during storage, while peanut oil and meal are the least stable to hydrolytic rancidity. At cooking temperature (65°C), soybean oil and canola are the least stable to oxidative rancidity, while peanut oil and meal are the least stable to hydrolytic rancidity. Screw press-extracted crude soybean oil appears to be more stable and acceptable than canola or peanut oils under typical storage conditions (Stevens et al. 1997). Sensory evaluation (of bread and salad dressing using these oils) indicated that flavor, odor intensity, acceptability, and overall preference may be of concern for screw press-extracted canola oil if used in an unrefined form.

Products other than oil produced from soybeans can have their own distinct flavor problems. A number of treatments have been developed to address these issues. The beany off-flavor of soybean protein preparations has been attributed to medium-chain aldehydes (such as hexanal). Addition of diaphorase can reduce the rate of hexanal oxidation (Takahashi et al. 1980). Enzymatic oxidation of aldehydes using aldehyde dehydrogenase can eliminate the beany off-flavor in soybean extract and soy milk. Incubation of soybean extracts with aldehyde oxidase can reduce the green, beany odors. Purified aldehyde oxidase (aldehyde oxygen oxidoreductase) can oxidize medium-chain aldehydes, such as hexanal and pentanal, to the corresponding acids using dissolved O_2 as the electron acceptor (Takahashi et al. 1979).

7.6 DAIRY PRODUCTS

Enriching dairy products with unsaturated fatty acids and conjugated linoleic acid can increase nutritional value; however, these fatty acids are susceptible to oxidation and off-flavor development. Compounds including 3-methyl-1H-indole (mothball-like), pentanal (fatty), heptanal (green), butanoic acid (cheesy), and delta-decalactone (peach-like) have been identified in butter enriched with these compounds. While photooxidation of conventional butter increases heptanal, (E)-2-octenal, and *trans*-4,5-epoxy-(E)-2-decenal compared to enriched butter, it has been suggested that the higher vitamin content in enriched samples may be protective as far as oxidation (Mallia et al. 2009).

Exposing milk products to light can result in oxidation and flavor change. If exposed to sufficient fluorescent lightning, dairy products, such as sour cream, can develop off-odor and flavor (sunlight taste) in a few hours. Larsen et al. (2009) reported that sour cream stored in white cups (low light barrier) became very rancid during 36 h of exposure to fluorescent light. Only cups with a high light barrier (incorporation of a black pigment into the packaging material) protected the sour cream flavor sufficiently. The flavor of ice cream can deteriorate as a result of photooxidation of the milk fat and generation of volatile aldehydes, particularly trans-2-decenal (Shiota et al. 2004). It has been suggested that milk with elevated levels of vaccenic acid and/or conjugated linoleic acid is more susceptible to light-induced lipid oxidation; however, sensory results have not born this out (Lynch et al. 2005).

Variation in atmosphere can produce significant differences in rancid flavor of milk stored and exposed to different wavelengths of light. Milk stored in N_2 has been shown to undergo the most sensory deterioration under orange and red filters, while that stored in air deteriorated most under noncolored filters. Based on gas chromatographic results, red, green, and amber filters offered better protection against photooxidation. Degradation of protoporphyrin and chlorophyllic compounds in N_2 was correlated with sensory characteristics related to photooxidation. Blocking visible and UV riboflavin excitation wavelengths reduces light oxidation flavor better than blocking only a single visible excitation wavelength plus all UV excitation wavelengths (Webster et al. 2009). Light exposure (400 and 570 nm) increases hexanal production in milk within 7 days. To protect milk from photooxidation, it must be protected from light in the entire visible region as well as that in the UV region (Intawiwat et al. 2010).

Processing milk with ultra-high temperature (UHT; 135°C–150°C) significantly improves the safety and storage stability; however, it can be detrimental to the sensory characteristics. Sensory changes of UHT milk during storage can be divided into three stages (Prasad 1990). During the first 2 weeks, the milk has a strong sulfury odor (cooked), which is determined by the concentration of free -SH groups and other volatile sulfur compounds. Between 2 weeks and 3 months, the product is acceptable, and this is the period during which most reactive -SH groups are oxidized but before nutty, metallic oxidized, stale, and other off-odors and flavors emerge. During the final 3 to 6 months, off-odors and flavors become more obvious until the milk becomes totally unacceptable at the end of 6 months.

7.7 VEGETABLES

7.7.1 Vegetable Color and Flavor

Vegetables undergo a series of reactions during the ripening process that alter the aroma or flavor, color, and texture. Postharvest yellowing of broccoli and other green vegetables as a result of chlorophyll degradation can be catalyzed by chlorophyllase, chlorophyll-degrading peroxidase, and Mg-dechelatase. The color change from blue-green to bright green to yellow-green resulting from chemical changes in chlorophyll is an indicator of ripeness and/or freshness to consumers.

Plant tissues contain a number of phenolic or polyphenolic molecules that act as antioxidants; however, enzymatic reactions that affect these molecules can result in the formation of melanins, which are brown in color (Falguera et al. 2010). Polyphenol oxidases, the enzymes that catalyze many of these reactions, are usually found in plant chloroplasts. They can be released during ripening or senescence or in response to tissue injury (Mayer 2006). Polyphenol oxidases are copper-containing enzymes that oxidize compounds that have two adjacent phenolic groups on them. These enzymes can use catechin, catechol, chlorogenic acid, caffeic acid, and gallic acid as substrates (Altunkaya and Gokmen 2008).

Catechol oxidase (catecholase) can catalyze the oxidation of an aromatic group with two adjacent phenols, a diphenol, forming two quinones. Cysteine is an effective inhibitor of this enzyme. Tyrosinase (monophenolase) adds one oxygen atom to a carbon atom adjacent to a phenolic group on an aromatic compound, converting it to a diphenol. The enzyme will then mediate catechol oxidase activity, which converts the molecule to one with two quinones (Sariri et al. 2009). Tyrosinases, first characterized in edible mushrooms, catalyze both the o-hydroxylation of monophenols and the subsequent oxidation of the resulting o-diphenols into reactive o-quinones, which evolve spontaneously to produce intermediates that associate to produce dark brown pigments (Halaouli et al. 2006).

During the process of tissue disintegration (peeling, cutting, chipping, grating), light-colored vegetable tissues brown quickly. Potatoes undergo this type of enzymatic oxidative degradation altering their color to an unacceptable gray-brown. Non-browning potatoes (without polyphenol oxidase) have a better odor than wild-type potatoes, even though the former exhibit a more intense vegetable odor (Llorent et al. 2010). Non-browning potatoes also maintain their odor quality for a longer period of time. Four months after the harvest of potatoes, lipoxygenase activity in whole potatoes increases. However, Petersen et al. (2003) reported that oxidation products of linoleic and linolenic acids that typically cause off-flavor in chill-stored potatoes actually decrease. Authors concluded that this off-flavor change was not a result of increases in lipoxygenase activity.

Acceptable cooked potato flavor is related to nonvolatile metabolites, including the major umami compounds (glutamate and aspartate and the 5′-nucleotides, GMP and AMP), glycoalkaloids, and sugars (Morris et al. 2007, 2010). Off-odors and off-flavors in boiled potatoes are strongly correlated to 2-pentenal, 2-hexenal, 2-heptenal, 2-pentylfuran, and 2-decenal (Blanda et al. 2003). Neither ascorbate nor citrate treatment after cooking prevents formation of off-flavors.

7.7.2 Processes to Stabilize Vegetable Color and Flavor

Heat treatment is one of the primary approaches to inactive enzymes that cause degradative changes in the sensory quality of fruits and vegetables during cold and frozen storage. Water blanching (90°C) decreases peroxidase activity and total phenolic content but, initially, has no effect on sensory characteristics (Goncalves et al. 2009).

Broccoli floret yellowing can be retarded by 2 days by exposure to hot air treatment (50°C for 2 h; Shigenaga et al. 2005). Authors suggest that hydrogen peroxide, which is generated by the heat treatment, might activate enzymes related to the ascorbate–glutathione cycle (dehydroascorbate reductase and glutathione reductase), which subsequently suppresses senescence. An ethylene inhibitor, 1-methylcyclopropene, delays senescence of broccoli by inhibiting 1-aminocyclopropane-1-carboxylate acid activity, thus delaying the peak activity of 1-aminocyclopropane-1-carboxylate acid C synthase activity. This delays yellowing and chlorophyll degradation (Gang et al. 2009). Exposing broccoli florets to ethanol vapor during cold, dark storage also suppresses chlorophyll catabolic enzyme activities (chlorophyllase, chlorophyll-degrading peroxidase, Mg-dechelatase), delaying yellowing of the vegetable (Fukasawa et al. 2010).

Inactivation or suppression of oxidative enzymes is one of the most effective mechanisms to reduce degradation during frozen storage of vegetables. Broccoli, cauliflower, Brussels sprouts, and potatoes that are frozen without preheating (blanching) discolor and develop off-flavors within 6 months. Preheating reduces peroxidase activity substantially (Kovacs 1979). Treating green vegetables (green peppers, broccoli, pea pods, green petiole cabbage) with a carbonate buffer solution (0.2–0.4N, pH 10) containing $MgCl_2$ (0.5%) by vacuum infiltration prior to cooking preserves green color and sensory quality during holding (50°C for 4 h) and cold storage (4°C for 14 days) (Lu and Chang 2000). Microwave treatment offers an alternative to steam- and water-blanching of fruits and vegetables; high-temperature, short-time treatment often results in minimal damage. Blanching corn prior to frozen storage reduces off-flavor development by limiting hexanal production resulting from lipoxygenase oxidization of unsaturated fatty acids, mainly linoleic (Lee 1981). Microwave blanching of broccoli reduces ascorbic acid content and peroxidase activity. Some peroxidase regeneration does occur during frozen storage (Brewer et al. 1995). However, after 4 weeks of frozen storage, microwave-blanched broccoli retains color and sensory characteristics similar to steam-blanched broccoli.

Exposure to UV light can also delay color change. UVB is more effective than UVA in delaying yellowing and chlorophyll degradation of broccoli florets during cold storage (Aimlaor et al. 2009). Irradiation (3 kGy) can extend shelf life (microbial and odor) for up to 14 days (4°C). The process is preservative but does not change the color, firmness, or other quality characteristics of broccoli (Gomes et al. 2008).

Discoloration of avocado flesh, primarily as a result of the activity of polyphenol oxidase, can be prevented by treatment with a combination of sodium bisulfite and ascorbic acid without causing any flavor change. High-acid avocado purees stored at freezing temperatures retain their flavor and texture for more than a year (Ahmed and Barmore 1978). Better color is retained when avocado puree is microwave-processed; however, flavor loss is substantial. The combination of microwaves (30 s), reduced pH (5.5), and the addition of avocado leaves (1%) to the puree has been shown to minimize development of lipid oxidation volatiles and flavor loss and results in a product with characteristic avocado flavor (Guzman-Geronimo et al. 2008).

Heat treatments (blanching) significantly reduce the degradation of phenolic substances in potatoes (Begic-Akagic and Pilizot 2010). Potato polyphenol oxidase exhibits a time-related decline in activity following treatment at 43°C with high-pressure CO_2 (58 atm) (Chen et al. 1992). Citric acid, ascorbic acid, and potassium bisulfate also effectively inhibit enzymatic browning.

Nonenzymatic oxidation occurs during the processing of potatoes into potato flakes. Ascorbic acid, phenolic compounds, and carotenoids, the primary endogenous compounds that prevent oxidation in potatoes, decrease by 95%, 82%, and 27%, respectively (Gosset et al. 2008). For this reason, exogenous antioxidants are necessary to maintain sensory quality during storage. During storage of potato flakes, off-flavors appear at various points. Linoleic acid-derived oxylipins predominate (Laine et al. 2006). In descending order, they are hexanal, hydroxyl-, oxo-, hydroperoxy-, and divinyl ether polyunsaturated fatty acids.

Modification of the storage atmosphere to preserve fresh fruits and vegetables reduces respiration rate, reduces oxidative tissue damage, reduces chlorophyll and chlorophyll degradation, and reduces ethylene-mediated phenomena and aroma biosynthesis likely to be responsible for off-flavor (Beaudry 1999). Yellowing of broccoli is minimal at 2.5°C regardless of O_2 concentration. Broccoli odor and flavor are best in samples stored in 0.5% or 1% O_2. However, 0.25% O_2 or less impairs both. Visible low-O_2 injury develops at 0.1% O_2. Addition of CO_2 at 10% also retards yellowing; however, it can induce formation of off-odors, which disappear upon cooking. Pretreating broccoli with 0.06 nL/L of sorbitol followed by holding in packaging that allows CO_2 to accumulate above the recommended 5%–10% decreases chlorophyll degradation and ethanol and acetaldehyde accumulation (DeEll et al. 2006). These compounds are often considered to be responsible for off-odor and off-flavor development. Sensory properties of broccoli packaged and stored in low-density polyethylene (5% O_2/7% CO_2) for 4 days at 10°C with an ethylene absorber has sensory characteristics similar to fresh broccoli (Jacobsson et al. 2004).

In a very low oxygen/carbon dioxide (1.1% O_2/3% CO_2) or anaerobic environment, Brassica vegetables generate methanethiol, dimethyl sulfide, and dimethyl disulfide from S-methyl-methionine because of C-S lyase degradation of sulfur-containing compounds (Dipentima et al. 1995). Dan et al. (1999) reported that methanethiol appears to be the primary compound responsible for the off-flavor of these vegetables.

Avocados are rich in oleic, palmitic, linoleic, and palmitoleic acids (up to 30%) located primarily in the mesocarp. Oxidative rancidity of these fatty acids can be minimized by packaging the processed product under inert atmosphere, use of antioxidants, and storage at low temperature (Ahmed and Barmore 1978).

Controlled temperature in conjunction with controlled atmosphere can have significant effects on oxidation in vegetables. Vacuum cooling of mushrooms stored at 5°C increases superoxide dismutase, catalase, peroxidase, and polyphenoloxidase and activity while it decreases malondialdehyde levels and superoxide anion generation slightly (Fei et al. 2007). Mushrooms stored in modified atmospheres without oxygen or in a 20%–50% oxygen environment have poorer sensory quality than those stored in a higher oxygen environment because of chilling and physiological injury (Tao et al. 2011). These injuries increase malondialdehyde and superoxide anion and browning to some degree. An 80% oxygen environment enhances activity of the antioxidant system. The antioxidant enzyme system, including superoxide dismutase, catalase, peroxidase, and polyphenol oxidase, is activated to scavenge reactive oxygen species and to reduce injury during the initial storage period. However, it does induce senescence. Storage in 80% O_2 delays senescence and decreases post-harvest quality loss (Tao et al. 2011). Superatmospheric oxygen concentrations can also prevent enzymatic browning by polyphenol oxidase (Gomez at al. 2006).

Many vegetables, including mushrooms, are dried to enhance their shelf life. The speed and temperature at which water is removed have major effects on enzymatic activity, texture, flavor, and odor. The drying method can have varying effects on sensory characteristics. Giri and Prasad (2009) reported that freeze-drying produces mushrooms with sensory characteristics (appearance, color, and overall acceptability) equal to those of microwave-vacuum dried mushrooms and higher than air-dried products.

Alternatively, activating systems that break down the products of oxidation can be effective. Three-stage hypobaric storage of green asparagus increases the activities of superoxide dismutase and catalase activities; decreases malondialdehyde, super-oxide anion $\left(O_2^{\cdot-}\right)$, and hydrogen peroxide (H_2O_2) accumulation; and delays surface color degeneration and the increase in peroxidase activity (Li et al. 2008).

7.8 FRUITS

7.8.1 FRUIT COLOR AND FLAVOR

Color change in fruits is primarily a result of enzymatic browning reactions. In fruit, polyphenol oxidase (catechol oxidase) and peroxidase are both located in the meso-carp. Polyphenol oxidase, primarily in the membrane fraction in a latent state, is an indicator of surface browning potential in fresh-cut fruit (peaches; Gonzalez-Buesa et al. 2011). Peroxidase activity occurs in the soluble fraction (Jimenez-Atienzar et al. 2007). Mechanical damage to light-colored fruits (peaches, apples, bananas) initiates polyphenoloxidase-catalyzed oxidation of the naturally occurring pheno-lic compounds to quinones, which polymerize forming brown pigments (Luh and Phithakpol 1972).

Polyphenol oxidase activity is influenced by pH and temperature. Above 60°C, the natural pH of peach tissue plus 0.08% w/w ascorbic acid will control this browning reaction (Zhou et al. 2008; Torralles et al. 2010). Browning in fresh juice can generally be avoided by low temperature storage. However, some soft-fleshed fruits, such as peaches and bananas, are subject to chilling injury (storage at 0°C for 28 days), which results in internal browning and flesh wooliness in the intact fruit. Preconditioning at 12°C for 6 days prior to 0°C storage can alleviate chilling injury in peaches (Yan et al. 2010).

Damaging (cutting) apple tissue increases polyphenol oxidase activity, resulting in browning. The optimal substrate for polyphenol oxidase activity is catechol; the optimum pH is 6.5. After injury and storage at higher temperatures, an increase in 5-hydroxymethylfurfural content indicates nonenzymatic browning as well (Queiroz et al. 2011). Direct application of sodium metabisulfite (10 mM) to cut apples packed in polyvinyl chloride (PVC) film can preserve the original visual color for up to 7 days (5°C; Cortez-Vega et al. 2008). In apple juice, gallic, protocatechuic, and cin-namic acids make significant contributions to flavor. Cinnamic acid is hydrolyzed during storage at 40°C, resulting in some flavor loss (Querioz et al. 2011).

7.8.2 Processes to Stabilize Fruit Color and Flavor

Because it is an enzyme, polyphenol oxidase can be inactivated by treatments that denature proteins: heat, extremes of pH, and high ionic strength solutions. Therefore, blanching (immersion, steam, microwave), acidification, salt dips, and sugar packs can significantly reduce the problem.

Oxygen content of the environment also affects enzymatic browning. Peaches stored for up to 92 days in $5\%CO_2 + 5\%O_2$ and $10\%CO_2 + 5\%O_2$ have lower polyphenol oxidase and peroxidase activities, exhibit less enzymatic browning, exhibit delayed senescence, have better quality, and have no off-flavor compared to those stored in air (ShiPing et al. 2002). Argon enrichment of an air atmosphere ($3\%O_2/97\%Ar$) is more inhibitory to polyphenol oxidase-induced enzymatic browning than nitrogen enrichment of an air atmosphere ($3\%O_2/97\%N_2$; O'Beirne et al. 2011).

Polyphenol oxidase (in apple juice and slices) can be inactivated by UVC light exposure via protein aggregation. UVC light-exposed apples are equivalent, from a sensory standpoint, to freshly cut apples (Manzocco et al. 2009). However, naturally occurring phenols can undergo photooxidation. Combining ultrasound and ascorbic acid inactivates monophenolase, diphenolase, and peroxidase in freshly cut apples (JiHyun and Deog 2010). Polyphenol oxidase can be reduced to <5% when banana puree is blanched (7 min) and then subjected to high hydrostatic pressure (689 MPa, 10 min; Palou et al. 1999).

7.9 GRAIN PRODUCTS

Cooked rice from freshly harvested rice is stickier than that from aged rice and is generally not preferred from a sensory standpoint (Horincar et al. 2009). Changes occurring during storage result in physicochemical and physiological changes, which have been attributed to changes in the cell wall and protein, interaction between proteins and breakdown products of lipid oxidation, and starch–protein interactions. While they may seem bland, grain flavors are actually quite complex. More than a dozen different aromas and flavors have been identified in rice by descriptive sensory analysis. More than 200 volatile compounds have been separated. One compound, 2-acetyl-1-pyrroline (popcorn aroma), has been confirmed to contribute a characteristic rice aroma (Champagne 2008). In addition, it is the only volatile compound for which the relationship between concentration and sensory intensity has been established. Concentration reduction of this compound compromises sensory quality of rice. Octanal (fatty) and 2-nonenal (rancid) are also major contributors to milled rice aroma.

Volatile compounds produced by oxidation of the major unsaturated fatty acids of rice bran lipid that develop during storage of milled rice are potential contributors to stale or rancid flavor. 2-Nonenal, octanal, and hexanal increase during storage. The aroma intensities of hexanal and 2-pentylfuran change by a larger factor than do those of heptanal, 2-nonenal, 3-penten-2-one, and octanal during early storage. Hexanal and 2-pentylfuran have the greatest effect on aroma change at the beginning of storage, whereas 2-nonenal has the greatest effect on aroma change during later storage (Lam and Proctor 2003).

Flavor compounds are an important factor in the taste acceptability of commercial breads. Compounds generated in breads depend on the raw materials and on the fermentation process. Wheat flour (not whole grain) can be divided into two types: unbleached flour (bread flour) and bleached flour. The primary difference between the two is the processing. Freshly ground wheat has a yellow color because of the presence of xanthophylls (carotenoids) and poor dough-forming characteristics (Black 2006). Flour is oxidized either naturally (by O_2) by holding it for a sufficient period of time or by subjecting it to bleaching and maturing agents (calcium peroxide). For unbleached flour to bleach naturally, it must be held for up to 40 days in a cold environment to prevent development of rancidity. If held at high temperatures, the lipids oxidize and the resultant flour tastes stale. Flours can be chemically oxidized to whiten them and improve their dough-forming ability. Chemically oxidizing flour alters the ability of the gluten proteins to form disulfide bonds, enabling the flour to form stronger, more elastic dough.

In polished-wheat-flour breads, 2-methylpropanol (iso-butanol) and 2-phenylethanol (beta-phenyl-ethyl-alcohol) are favorable flavor compounds (Maeda et al. 2009). Fresh wheat bread has a higher concentration of the fermentation products 2,3-butanedione and 3-hydroxy-2-butanone and the Strecker aldehydes 2- and 3-methylbutanal, which contribute dough and bran aromas and flavors (Jensen et al. 2011). Bread stored 2 to 3 weeks has a dusty aroma and flavor and a bitter taste, which appear to be related to the formation of secondary lipid oxidation products together with decreasing levels of Maillard reaction compounds. The sourdough method increases the proportions of acids and aldehydes in the crust but decreases the proportion of alcohols and methoxybenzenes.

Wheat germ or endosperm found in whole grain flour contains approximately 10 g lipid/100 g wheat germ. A large proportion of these fatty acids are polyunsaturated and highly susceptible to oxidative rancidity, limiting the storage stability of this flour. Major compounds contributing to the off-flavor of stale wheat germ are n-hexanal, 2-n-pentyl furan, (E,E)-3,5-octadien-2-one, (E,E)-2,4-decadienal, and 6,10-dimethyl-(E)-5,9-undecadien-2-one (El-Saharty et al. 1998).

Among the 26 odor-active volatiles identified in rye flour, 1-octen-3-one (mushroom-like), methional (cooked potato), and (E)-2-nonenal (fatty, green) have the highest flavor dilution (FD) factors (Kirchoff and Schieberle 2002). During fermentation, 3-methylbutanol, acetic acid, and 2,3-butanedione increase, while (E,E)-2,4-decadienal and 2-methylbutanal decrease. Additional compounds are generated during the fermentation process of making sourdough bread. Twenty-two flavor compounds have been identified in the FD factor range of 128 to 2048 (Kirchoff and Schieberle 2001). Contributors to the overall crumb flavor include 3-methylbutanal (malty), (E)-2-nonenal (green, fatty), (E,E)-2,4-decadienal (fatty, waxy), hexanal (green), acetic acid (sour, pungent), phenylacetaldehyde (honey-like), methional (boiled potato-like), vanillin (vanilla-like), 2,3-butanedione (buttery), 3-hydroxy-4,5-dimethyl-2(5H)-furanone (spicy), and 2- and 3-methylbutanoic acid (sweaty). The relative proportions of these compounds determine whether the bread has an acceptable flavor.

Corn products also undergo oxidative changes that affect aroma or flavor quality. As storage time (up to 23 weeks) of corn masa increases, lipid oxidation increases;

increasing the storage temperature (from 15°C to 55°C) decreases the time required to reach the rancid flavor thresholds (Vidal-Quintanar et al. 2003). Total carbonyls of extrusion-cooked, maize-based snack products increase as storage temperature increases (from 25°C to 40°C). Storage at 40°C reduces the sensory acceptance of the product (Lasekan et al. 1996). Storing (12 weeks) corn flakes at ambient (23°C) and elevated temperatures (45°C) results in an increase in the total number of aroma compounds ranging from 9 to 46 with FD factors of 1 to 900 (Kim et al. 2001).

Cereal grains (wheat flour, corn meal) can be irradiated (up to 7 kGy) to reduce insect and microbial attack during storage. Irradiation is a form of high energy, which could potentially initiate oxidative changes. It appears to have no effect on oxidative quality of the flours; however, it can negatively impact viscoelastic and organoleptic properties (daSilva et al. 2010).

7.10   FINAL REMARKS

Oxidation is a primary form of deterioration in foods that affects sensory quality. It often has negative effects on the flavor, color, and texture of food products and can lower their nutritional value. Vitamins, such as alpha tocopherols, ascorbic acid, and beta-carotene, lose their physiological activity once oxidized. Chemical changes may result from the interaction of oxygen with lipids, pigments, metal ions, polyphenols, or other components, can be initiated by enzymes, exposure to energy, or the presence of or exposure to transition metals or free radicals originating from a variety of sources. Once initiated, the presence of oxygen completes and/or continues the oxidation process.

The extent of oxidation that occurs in a food product depends on the raw material composition, endogenous prooxidative (iron) and antioxidative (vitamin E) constituents, processing operations, other ingredients, the gas environment surrounding the product, and subsequent storage conditions. Intrinsic antioxidants contained in both plant and animal tissues, including tocopherols, carotenoids, carnosine, polyphenolic compounds, and antioxidant enzymes, are capable of controlling oxidative reactions; however, processing can significantly reduce their activity.

The primary forms of oxidation affecting animal-food products are hydrolytic and autoxidative of lipids. Light exposure and oxygen both play significant roles as does the heating process (cooking, pasteurization). These types of oxidation result primarily in the generation of volatile aldehydes and ketones, which contribute stale, rancid off-flavors particularly when these products are stored in an oxygen-containing environment. Oxidation of myoglobin in meat, wherein the central iron moiety of the molecules is converted from the Fe^{2+} to the Fe^{3+} state, results in the color change from red/purple to brown. While this is a normal consequence of cooking, this color change in fresh meat is unacceptable to consumers because it implies that the meat is no longer fresh.

Oilseeds contain lipoxygenase, which catalyzes oxidation of a significant quantity of unsaturated fatty acids. This enzyme is generally inactivated by heat treating (toasting) the oilseeds before the oil is extracted. Even so, because of the highly unsaturated nature of oilseed lipids, autoxidation is likely to occur at some point during storage and in foods manufactured using these oils as ingredients. Storage in low-oxygen environments under cool, dark conditions can slow but not eliminate these changes. Antioxidants are often used to extend the shelf life of oils and of foods containing them.

The primary form of oxidation in plant tissues (fruits and vegetables) is enzymatic browning catalyzed by polyphenol oxidase. This enzyme catalyzes the addition of oxygen to phenolic compounds. Continued reactions (tyrosinase, polymerization) result in the formation of brown pigment, especially in light-colored fruits and vegetables (apples, potatoes). These reactions can be prevented using various pretreatments (ascorbic acid dip, sodium metabisulfite) or by mild heat treatment (blanching), which inactivates the enzyme. Vegetables also contain lipoxygenase, which can catalyze oxidative degradation of the lipids, resulting in off-flavor formation in frozen vegetables. Heat treatment is the primary approach for maintaining both color and flavor quality in these vegetables.

REFERENCES

Acree, T., and Arn, H. 2004. Flavornet and human odor space. http://www.flavornet.org, Datu Inc.

Ahmed, E. M., and Barmore, C. R. 1978. Quality of processed avocado products. *Am Chem Soc* 176: *AGFD 48*.

Aimlaor, S., Yamauchi, N., Takino, S., and Shigyo, M. 2009. Effect of UV-A and UV-B irradiation on broccoli (*Brassica oleracea* L. Italica group) floret yellowing during storage. *Postharvest Biol Technol* 54: 177–179.

Altunkaya, A., and Gökmen, V. 2008. Effect of various inhibitors on enzymatic browning, antioxidant activity and total phenol content of fresh lettuce (*Lactuca sativa*). *Food Chem* 107: 1173–1179.

Arruda, C. S., Garcez, W. S., Barrera-Arellano, D., and Block, J. M. 2006. Industrial trial to evaluate the effect of oxygen concentration on overall quality of refined, bleached, and deodorized soybean oil in PET bottles. *J Am Oil Chem Soc* 83: 797–802.

Asghar, A., and Pearson, A. M. 1980. Influence of ante- and post-mortem treatments on muscle composition and meat quality. *Adv Food Res* 26: 53–61.

Beaudry, R. M. 1999. Effect of O_2 and CO_2 partial pressure on selected phenomena affecting fruit and vegetable quality. *Postharvest Biol Technol* 15: 293–303.

Begic-Akagic, A., and Pilizota, V. 2010. Prevention of enzymatic browning in recent potato varieties. *Radovi Poljoprivrednog Fakulteta Univerziteta u Sarajevu* 60: 187–200.

Black, M. 2006. In *The Encyclopedia of Seeds: Science, Technology and Uses*. Eds. Bewley, J. D. and Halmer, P. CABI Publishing, Wallingford.

Blanda, G., Cerretani, L., Comandini, P., Toschi, T. G., and Lercker, G. 2003. Investigation of off-odour and off-flavour development in boiled potatoes. *Food Chem* 118: 283–290.

Boler, D. D., Gabriel, S. R., Yang, H., Balsbaugh, R., Mahan, D. C., Brewer, M. S., McKeith, F. K., and Killefer, J. 2009. Effect of different dietary levels of natural-source vitamin E in grow-finish pigs on pork quality and shelf life. *Meat Sci* 83: 723–740.

Brewer, M. S. 2011. Natural antioxidants: A review. 2011. *Comp Rev Food Safety Technol* 10: 221–247.

Brewer, M. S., and McKeith, F. K. 1999. Consumer-rated quality characteristics as related to purchase intent of fresh pork. *J Food Sci* 64: 171–174.

Brewer, M. S., and Novakofski, J. E. 2008. Consumer quality evaluation of aging of beef. *J Food Sci* 73: S78–S82.

Brewer, M. S., Begum, S., and Bozeman, A. 1995. Microwave and conventional blanching effects on chemical, sensory, and color characteristics of frozen broccoli. *J Food Qual* 18: 479–493.

Brewer, M. S., Vega, J. D., and Perkins, E. G. 1999a. Filter aid removal of selected flavor significant compounds: Effect on sensory characteristics of French fries. *J Food Lipids* 5: 63–74.

Brewer, M. S., Vega, J. D., and Perkins, E. G. 1999b. Volatile compounds and sensory characteristics of frying fats. *J Food Lipids* 6: 47–61.

Brewer, M. S., Jensen, J., Prestat, C., Zhu, L. G., and McKeith, F. K. 2002. Visual acceptability and consumer purchase intent of pumped pork loin roasts. *J Muscle Foods* 13: 53–68.

Brewer, M. S., Ryan, K., Jensen, J., Prestat, C., Zhu, L. G., Sosnicki, A., Field, B., Hankes, R., and McKeith, F. K. 2004. Enhancement effects on quality characteristics of pork derived from pigs of various commercial genetic backgrounds. *J Food Sci* 69: 5–10.

Bruce, H. L., Beilken, S. L., and Leppard, P. 2005. Textural descriptions of cooked steaks from bovine M. longissimus thoracis et lumborum from different production and ageing regimes. *J Food Sci* 70: S309–S316.

Buettner, G. R., and Oberley, L. W. 1980. The apparent production of superoxide and hydroxyl radicals by hematoporphyrin and light as seen by spin-trapping. *FEBS Lett* 121: 161–164.

Byrne, D. V., Bredie ,W. L. P., Bak, L. S., Bertelsen, G., Martens, H., and Martens, M. 2001. Sensory and chemical analysis of cooked porcine meat patties in relation to warmed-over flavour and pre-slaughter stress. *Meat Sci* 59: 229–249.

Calkins, C. R., and Cuppett, S. 2006. Volatile compounds in beef and their contribution to off-flavors. *Final Report to the National Cattlemens Beef Association.* Centennial, CO.

Campo, M. M., Nute, G. R., Hughes, S. I., Enser, M., Wood, J. D., and Richardson, R. I. 2006. Flavour perception of oxidation in beef. *Meat Sci* 72: 303–311.

Champagne, E. T. 2008. Rice aroma and flavor: a literature review. *Cereal Chem* 85: 445–454.

Cheah, K. S., Cheah, A. M., and Krausgrill, D. I. 1995. Effect of dietary supplementation of vitamin E on pig meat quality. *Meat Sci* 39: 255–264.

Chen, J. S., Balaban, M. O., Wei, C. I., Marshall, M. R., and Hsu, W. Y. 1992. Inactivation of polyphenol oxidase by high-pressure carbon dioxide. *J Agric Food Chem* 40: 2345–2349.

Cheng, J. H., Wang, S. T., and Ockerman, H. W. 2007. Lipid oxidation and color change of salted pork patties. *Meat Sci* 75: 71–77.

Choe, E., and Min, D. B. 2006. Chem. and reactions of reactive oxygen species in foods. *Crit. Rev. Food Sci Nutr* 46: 1–22.

Cometto-Muñiz, J. E., and Abraham, M. H. 2010. Structure–activity relationships on the odor detectability of homologous carboxylic acids by humans. *Exp Brain Res* 207: 75–84.

Cortez-Vega, W. R., Becerra-Prado, A. M., Soares, J. M., and Fonseca, G. G. 2008. Effect of L-ascorbic acid and sodium metabisulfite in the inhibition of the enzymatic browning of minimally processed apple. *Int J Agric Res* 3: 196–201.

Damodaran, S., Parkin, K. L., and Fennema, O. R. 2008. *Fennema's Food Chemistry*, 4th ed. CRC Press, Boca Raton, FL.

Dan, K., Nagata, M., and Yamashita, I. 1999. Mechanism of off-flavor production in Brassica vegetables under anaerobic conditions. *Jpn Agric Res Quart* 33: 109–114.

daSilva, R. C., Pino, L. M., Spoto, M. H. F., and D'Arce, M. A. B. R. 2010. Oxidative and sensorial stability of radiated wheat and corn flour. *Cienc Tecnol Aliment* 30: 406–413.

Davies, C. S., Nielsen, S. S., and Nielsen, N. C. 1987. Flavor improvement of soybean preparations by genetic removal of lipoxygenase-2. *J Am Oil Chem Soc* 64: 1428–1433.

DeEll, J. R., Toivonen, P. M. A., Cornut, F., Roger, C., and Vigneault, C. 2006. Addition of sorbitol with KMnO4 improves broccoli quality retention in modified atmosphere packages. *J Food Qual* 29: 65–75.

Dipentima, J. H., Rios, J. J., Clemente, A., and Olias, J. M. 1995. Biogenesis of off-odor in broccoli storage under low-oxygen atmosphere. *J Agric and Food Chem* 43: 1310–1313.

Dixon, M. D., and Hammond, E. G. 1984. The flavor intensity of some carbonyl compounds important in oxidized fats. *J Am Oil Chem Soc* 61: 1452–1456.

Elmore, S., Mottram, D. S., Enser, M., and Wood, J. D. 1999. Effect of the polyunsaturated fatty acid composition of beef muscle on the profile of aroma volatiles. *J Agric Food Chem* 47: 1619–1625.

El-Saharty, Y. S., El-Zeany, B. A., and Berger, R. G. 1998. Volatile flavour and key off-flavour compounds of over-stored wheat germ. *Adv Food Sci* 20: 198–202.

Falguera, V., Pagan, J., and Ibarz, A. 2010. A kinetic model describing melanin formation by means of mushroom tyrosinase. *Food Res Int* 43: 66–69.

Fazzalari, F. A. 1978. Compilation of odor and taste threshold data. Ed. Fazzalari, F. A. *Am. Soc. Testing Materials Data Series. DS 48A.*

Fei, T., Min, Z., and Qing, Y. H. 2007. Effect of vacuum cooling on physiological changes in the antioxidant system of mushroom under different storage conditions. *J Food Eng* 79: 1302–1309.

Fennema, O. 2008. In *Fennema's Food Chemistry* 4th ed. Eds. Damodaran, S., Parkin, K. L., Fennema, O. CRC Press, Boca Raton, FL.

Fernandez, X., Monin, G., Talmont, A., Mourot, J., and Lebret, B. 1999. Influence of intra-muscular fat content on the quality of pig meat–1. Composition of the lipid fraction and sensory characteristic of m. longissimus lumborum. *Meat Sci* 53: 59–65.

Frankel, E. N. 1991. Review. Recent advances in lipid oxidation. *J Sci Food Agric* 54: 495–511.

Fukasawa, A., Suzuki, Y., Terai, H., and Yamauchi, N. 2010. Effects of postharvest ethanol vapor treatment on activities and gene expression of chlorophyll catabolic enzymes in broccoli florets. *Postharvest Biol Technol* 55: 97–102.

Gang, M., Wang, R., Wang, C. R., Kato, M., Yamawaki, K., Qin, F. F., and Xu, H. L. 2009. Effect of 1-methylcyclopropene on expression of genes for ethylene biosynthesis enzymes and ethylene receptors in post-harvest broccoli. *Plant Growth Reg* 57(3): 223–232.

Giri, S. K., and Prasad, S. 2009. Quality and moisture sorption characteristics of microwave-vacuum, air and freeze-dried button mushroom (*Agaricus bisporus*). *J Food Proc Pres* 33: 237–251.

Gomes, C., da Silva, P., Chimbombi, E., Kim, J., Castell-Perez, E., and Moreira, R. G. 2008. Electron-beam irradiation of fresh broccoli heads (*Brassica oleracea* L. *italica*). *LWT— Food Sci Technol* 41: 1828–1833.

Gomez, P. A., Geysen, S., Verlinden, B. E., Artes, F., and Nicolai, B. M. 2006. Modelling the effect of superatmospheric oxygen concentrations on in vitro mushroom PPO activity. *J Sci Food and Agric* 86: 2387–2394.

Goncalves, E. A., Pinheiro, J., Alegria, C., Abreu, M., Brandao, T. R. S., and Silva, C. L. M. 2009. Degradation kinetics of peroxidase enzyme, phenolic content, and physical and sensorial characteristics in broccoli (*Brassica oleracea* L. ssp Italica) during blanching. *J Agric Food Chem* 57: 5370–5375.

Gonzalez-Buesa, J., Arias, E., Salvador, M. L., Oria, R., and Ferrer-Mairal, A. 2011. Suitability for minimal processing of non-melting clingstone peaches. *Int J Food Sci Technol* 46: 819–826.

Gorraiz, C., Beriain, M. J., Chasco, J., and Insausti, K. 2002. Effect of ageing time on volatile compounds, odor, and flavor of cooked beef from Pirenaica and Friesian bulls and heifers. *J Food Sci* 67: 916–922.

Gosset, V., Goebel, C., Laine, G., Delaplace, P., Du Jardin, P., Feussner, I., and Fauconnier, M. L. 2008. The role of oxylipins and antioxidants on off-flavor precursor formation during potato flake processing. *J Agric Food Chem* 56: 11285–11292.

Guo, Q., Richert, B. T., Burgess, J. R., Webel, D. M., Orr, D. E., and Blair, M. 2006. Effects of dietary vitamin E and fat supplementation on pork quality. *J Anim Sci* 84: 3089–3099.

Guzman-Geronimo, R. I., Lopez, M. G., and Dorantes-Alvarez, L. 2008. Microwave process-ing of avocado: Volatile flavor profiling and olfactometry. *Innov Food Sci Emerg Technol* 9: 501–506.

Halaouli, S., Asther, M., Sigoillot, J. C., Hamdi, M., and Lomascolo, A. 2006. Fungal tyrosinases: new prospects in molecular characteristics, bioengineering and biotechnological applications. *J Appl Microbiol* 100: 219–232.

Harel, S. and Kanner, J. 1988. Muscle membranal lipid peroxidation initiated by H_2O_2-activated metmyoglobin. *J Agric Food Chem* 33: 1188–1192.

Haseloff, R. F., Ebert, B., and Roeder, B. 1989. Generation of free radicals by photoexcitation of pheophorbide a, haematoporphyrin and protoporphyrin. *J PhotoChem Photobiol B*: *Biol* 3: 593–602.

Hider, R. C., Liu, Z. D., and Khodr, H. H. 2001. Metal chelation of polyphenols. *Methods Enzymol* 335: 190–203.

Hildebrand, D. F., and Kito, M. 1984. Role of lipoxygenases in soybean seed protein quality. *J Agric Food Chem* 32: 815–819.

Hofstrand, D. 2008. Domestic perspectives on food versus fuel. Agric. Marketing Resource Center. Available at www.agmrc.org. Accessed February 2010.

Horincar, S., Baston, O., and Pricop, E. 2009. Studies regarding the effect of storing rice at low temperatures upon the sensory qualities of cooked rice. *Ann Food Sci Technol* 10: 486–488.

Hunt, M. C., Mancini, R. A., Hachmeister, K. A., Kropf, D. H., Merriman, M., Delduca, G., and Milliken, G. (2004). Carbon monoxide in modified atmosphere packaging affects color, shelf life, and microorganisms of beef steaks and ground beef. *J Food Sci* 69: C45–C52.

Iassonova, D. R., Johnson, L. A., Hammond, E. G., and Beattie, S. E. 2009. Evidence of an enzymatic source of off flavors in "lipoxygenase-null" soybeans. *J Am Oil Chem Soc* 86: 59–64.

Igene, J. O. and Pearson, A. M. 1979. Role of phospholipids and triglycerides in warmed-over flavor development in meat model systems. *J Food Sci* 44: 1285–1290.

Insausti, K., Beriain, M. J., Gorraiz, C., and Purroy, A. 2002. Volatile compounds of raw beef from 5 local Spanish cattle breeds stored under modified atmosphere. *J Food Sci* 67: 1580–1589.

Insausti, K., Goni, V., Petri, E., Gorraiz, C., and Beriain, M. J. 2005. Effect of weight at slaughter on the volatile compounds of cooked beef from Spanish cattle breeds. *Meat Sci* 70: 83–90.

Intawiwat, N., Pettersen, M. K., Rukke, E. O., Meier, M. A., Vogt, G., Dahl, A. V., Skaret, J., Keller, D., and Wold, J. P. 2010. Effect of different colored filters on photo-oxidation in pasteurized milk. *J Dairy Sci* 93: 1372–1382.

Jacobsson, A., Nielsen, T., Sjoholm, I., and Wendin, K. 2004. Influence of packaging material and storage condition on the sensory quality of broccoli. *J Food Qual Pref* 15: 301–310.

Janz, J. A. M., Morel, P. C. H., Purchas, R. W., Corrigan, V. K., Cumarasamy, S., Wilkinson, B. H. P., and Hendriks, W. H. 2008. The influence of diets supplemented with conjugated linoleic acid, selenium, and vitamin E, with or without animal protein, on the quality of pork from female pigs. *J Anim Sci* 86: 1402–1408.

Jayasingh, P., Cornforth, D. P., Carpenter, C. E., and Whittier, D. 2001. Evaluation of carbon monoxide treatment in modified atmosphere packaging or vacuum packaging to increase color stability of fresh beef. *Meat Sci* 59: 317–324.

Jayasingh, P., Cornforth, D. P., Brennand, C. P., Carpenter, C. E., and Whittier, D. R. 2002. Sensory evaluation of ground beef stored in high-oxygen modified atmosphere. *J Food Sci* 67: 3493–3496.

Jensen, J., Robbins, K., Ryan, K., Homco-Ryan, C., McKeith, F. K., and Brewer, M. S. 2003. Enhancement solution effects on color, sensory and shelf life characteristics of enhanced pork in retail display. *J Food Qual* 26: 271–283.

Jensen, S., Oestdal, H., Skibsted, L. H., Larsen, E., and Thybo, A. K. 2011. Chemical changes in wheat pan bread during storage and how it affects the sensory perception of aroma, flavour, and taste. *J Cereal Sci* 5: 259–268.

JiHyun, J., and Deog, M. K. 2010. Inhibition of polyphenol oxidase and peroxidase activities on fresh-cut apple by simultaneous treatment of ultrasound and ascorbic acid. *Food Chem* 124: 444–449.

Jimenez-Atienzar, M., Pedreno, M. A., Caballero, N., Cabanes, J., and Garcia-Carmona, F. 2007. Characterization of polyphenol oxidase and peroxidase from peach mesocarp (*Prunus persica* L. cv. Babygold). *J Sci Food Agric* 87: 1682–1690.

Kao, J. W., Wu, X., Hammond, E. G., and White, P. J. 1998a. The impact of furanoid fatty acids and 3-methylnonane-2,4-dione on the flavor of oxidized soybean oil. *J Am Oil Chem Soc* 75: 831–835.

Kao, J. W., Hammond, E. G., and White, P. J. 1998b. Volatile compounds produced during deodorization of soybean oil and their flavor significance. *J Am Oil Chem Soc* 75: 1103–1107.

Kellogg, E. W., and Fridovich, I. 1975. Superoxide, hydrogen peroxide, and singlet oxygen in lipid peroxidation by a xanthine oxidase system. *J Biol Chem* 250: 8812–8817.

Kiatrichart, S., Brewer, M. S., Cadwallader, K. R., and Artz, W. G. 2003. Pan frying stability of NUSUN oil, a mid-oleic sunflower oil. *J Am Oil Chem Soc* 80: 479–483.

Kim, Y.-S., Cassens, J., Dickmann, R., and Reineccius, G. 2001. Gas chromatography-olfactometry of static headspace for the analysis of flavor change in corn flakes during storage. *Food Sci Biotech* 10: 261–266.

King, J. M., Svendsen, L. K., Fehr, W. R., Narvel, J. M., and White, P. J. 1998. Oxidative and flavor stability of oil from lipoxygenase-free soybeans. *J Am Oil Chem Soc* 75: 1121–1126.

Kirchhoff, E., and Schieberle, P. 2001. Determination of key aroma compounds in the crumb of a three-stage sourdough rye bread by stable isotope dilution assays and sensory studies. *J Agric Food Chem* 49: 4304–4311.

Kirchhoff, E., and Schieberle, P. 2002. Quantitation of odor-active compounds in rye flour and rye sourdough using stable isotope dilution assays. *J Agric Food Chem* 50: 5378–5385.

Kiritsakis, A. K. 1998. Flavor components of olive oil—A review. *J Am Oil Chem Soc JAOCS* 75: 673–681.

Kovacs, O. 1979. Peroxidase activity in quick-frozen vegetables. *Huetoeipar* 26: 100–108.

Laine, G., Gobel, C., Du Jardin, P., Feussner, I., and Fauconnier, M. L. 2006. Study of precursors responsible for off-flavor formation during storage of potato flakes. *J Agric Food Chem* 54: 5445–5452.

Lam, H. S., and Proctor, A. 2003. Milled rice oxidation volatiles and odor development. *J Food Sci* 68: 2676–2681.

Larsen, H., Geiner Tellefsen, S. B., and Dahl, A. V. 2009. Quality of sour cream packaged in cups with different light barrier properties measured by fluorescence spectroscopy and sensory analysis. *J Food Sci* 74: S345–S350.

Lasekan, O. O., Lasekan, W., Idowu, M. A., and Ojo, O. A. 1996. Effect of extrusion cooking conditions on the nutritional value, storage stability and sensory characteristics of a maize-based snack food. *J Cereal Sci* 24: 79–85.

Lawrie, R. A. 1991. The storage and preservation of meat. *Meat Science*. Pergamon Press, New York, 152–172.

Lee, I., Fatemi, S. H., Hammond, E. G., and White, P. J. 1995. Quantitation of flavor volatiles in oxidized soybean oil by dynamic headspace analysis. *J Am Oil Chem Soc* 72: 539–546.

Lee, Y. C. 1981. Lipoxygenase and off-flavor development in some frozen foods. *Korean J Food Sci Technol* 13: 53–56.

Li, W. X., Zhang, M., and Wang, S. J. 2008. Effect of three-stage hypobaric storage on membrane lipid peroxidation and activities of defense enzyme in green asparagus. *LWT—Food Sci Technol* 41: 2175–2181.

Lu, Y.-L., and Chang, P.-Y. 2000. Prevention of discoloration of cooked green vegetables during storage. *Taiwanese J Agric Chem Food Sci* 38: 490–497.

Luh, B. S., and Phithakpol, B. 1972. Characteristics of polyphenoloxidase related to browning in cling peaches. *J Food Sci* 37: 264–268.

Lynch, J. M., Lock, A. L., Dwyer, D. A., Noorbaksh, R., Barbano, D. M., and Bauman, D. E. 2005. Flavor and stability of pasteurized milk with elevated levels of conjugated linoleic acid and vaccenic acid. *J Dairy Sci* 88: 489–498.

Maeda, T., Kim, J. H., Ubukata, Y., and Morita, N. 2009. Analysis of volatile compounds in polished-graded wheat flour bread using headspace sorptive extraction. *Eur Food Res Technol* 228: 457–465.

Mahrour, A., Caillet, S., Nketsia-Tabiri, J., and Lacroix, M. 2003. The antioxidant effect of natural substances on lipids during irradiation of chicken legs. *J Am Oil Chem Soc* 80: 679–684.

Mallia, S., Escher, F., Dubois, S., Schieberle, P., and Schlichtherle-Cerny, H. 2009. Characterization and quantification of odor-active compounds in unsaturated fatty acid/conjugated linoleic acid (UFA/CLA)-enriched butter and in conventional butter during storage and induced oxidation. *J Agric Food Chem* 57(16): 7464–7472.

Mancini, R. A., and Hunt, M. C. 2005. Current research in meat color: A review. *Meat Sci* 71: 100–121.

Manzocco, L., Quarta, B., and Dri, A. 2009. Polyphenoloxidase inactivation by light exposure in model systems and apple derivatives. *Innov Food Sci Emerg Technol* 10: 506–511.

Maruri, J. L., and Larick, D. K. 1992. Volatile concentration and flavor of beef as influenced by diet. *J Food Sci* 57: 1275–1281.

Mayer, A. M. 2006. Polyphenol oxidases in plants and fungi: Going places? A review. *Phytochem* 67: 2318–2331.

Meilgaard, M., Civille, G. V., and Carr, B. T. 1999. *Sensory Evaluation Techniques*. 3rd ed. CRC Press, Boca Raton, FL.

Min, D. B., and Boff, J. M. 2002. Chemistry and reactions of singlet oxygen in foods. *Comp Rev Food Sci Food Safety* 1: 58–61.

Min, D. B., Callison, A. L., and Lee, H. O. 2003. Singlet oxygen oxidation for 2-pentylfuran and 2-pentenylfuran formation in soybean oil. *J Food Sci* 68: 1175–1178.

Morris, W. L., Ross, H. A., Ducreux, L. J. M., Bradshaw, J. E., Bryan, G. J., and Taylor, M. A. 2007. Umami compounds are a determinant of the flavor of potato (*Solanum tuberosum* L.) *J Agric Food Chem* 55: 9627–9633.

Morris, W. L., Wayne, L., Shepherd, T., Verrall, S. R., McNicol, J. W., and Taylor, M. A. 2010. Relationships between volatile and non-volatile metabolites and attributes of processed potato flavor. *Phytochem* 71: 1765–1773.

Mottram, D. S. 1998. Flavor formation in meat and meat products: A review. *Food Chem* 62: 415–424.

Mottram, D. S., Edwards, R. A., and MacFie, H. J. H. 1982. A comparison of the flavor volatiles from cooked beef and pork meat systems. *J Sci Food Agric* 33: 934–944.

Nam, K. C., and Ahn, D. U. 2003. Use of antioxidants to reduce lipid oxidation and off-odor volatiles of irradiated pork homogenates and patties. *Meat Sci* 63: 1–8.

Nam, K. C., Min, B. R., Yan, H., Lee, E. J., Mendonca, A., Wesley, I., and Ahn, D. U. 2003. Effect of dietary vitamin E and irradiation on lipid oxidation, color, and volatiles of fresh and previously frozen turkey breast patties. *Meat Sci* 65: 513–521.

Nawar, W. F. 1996. Lipids. In *Food Chemistry*. 3rd ed. Ed. Fennema, O. Marcel Dekker, New York, pp. 225–320.

Neff, W. E., Warner, K., and Byrdwell, W. C. 2000. Odor significance of undesirable degradation compounds in heated triolein and trilinolein. *J Am Oil Chem Soc* 77: 1303–1313.

Obana, H., Furuta, M., and Tanaka, Y. 2006. Detection of 2-alkylcyclobutanones in irradiated meat, poultry and egg after cooking. *J Health Sci* 52: 375–382.

O'Beirne, D., Murphy, E., and Eidhin, D. N. 2011. Effects of argon enriched low-oxygen atmospheres and of high-oxygen atmospheres on the kinetics of polyphenoloxidase (PPO). *J Food Sci* 76: E73–E77.

O'Keefe, M., and Hood, D. E. 1981. Anoxic storage of fresh beef. I. Nitrogen and carbon dioxide storage atmospheres. *Meat Sci* 5: 561–589.

Onibi, G. E., Scaife, J. R., Murray, I., and Fowler, V. R. 2000. Supplementary α-tocopherol acetate in full-fat rapeseed-based diets for pigs: Effect on performance, plasma enzymes and meat drip loss. *J Sci Food Agric* 80: 1617–1624.

O'Sullivan, M. G., Byrne, D. V., Jensen, M. T., Andersen, H. J., and Vestergaard, J. 2003. A comparison of warmed-over flavor in pork by sensory analysis, GC/MS and the electronic nose. *Meat Sci* 65: 1125–1138.

Palou, E., Lopez-Malo, A., Barbosa-Canovas, G. V., Welti-Chanes, J., and Swanson, B. G. 1999. Polyphenoloxidase activity and color of blanched and high hydrostatic pressure treated banana puree. *J Food Sci* 64: 42–45.

Petersen, M. A., Poll, L., and Larsen, L. M. 2003. Changes in flavor-affecting aroma compounds during potato storage are not associated with lipoxygenase activity. *Am J Potato Res* 80: 397–402.

Prasad, S. K. 1990. The sensory characteristics of heat-treated milks, with special reference to UHT processing. Index to Theses Accepted for Higher Degrees by the Universities of Great Britain and Ireland and the Council for National Academic Awards, 39: 443.

Queiroz, C., daSilva, A. J. R., Lopes, M. L. M., Fialho, E., and Valente-Mesquita, V. L. 2011. Polyphenol oxidase activity, phenolic acid composition and browning in cashew apple (*Anacardium occidentale*, L.) after processing. *Food Chem* 125: 128–132.

Rhee, K. S., and Ziprin, Y. A. 1987. Lipid oxidation in retail beef, pork, and chicken muscle as affected by concentrations of heme pigments and nonheme iron and microsomal enzymic lipid peroxidation activity. *J Food Biochem* 11: 1–15.

Rhee, K. S., Anderson, L. M., and Sams, A. R. 2005. Comparison of flavor changes in cooked-refrigerated beef, pork and chicken meat patties. *Meat Sci* 71: 392–396.

Robbins, K., Jensen, J., Ryan, K. J., Homco-Ryan, C., McKeith, F. K., and Brewer, M. S. 2003. Consumer attitudes towards beef and acceptability of enhanced beef. *Meat Sci* 65: 721–729.

Rochat, S., and Chaintreau, A. 2005. Carbonyl odorants contributing to the in-oven roast beef top note. *J Agric Food Chem* 53: 9578–9585.

Rojas, M. C., and Brewer, M. S. 2007. Effect of natural antioxidants on oxidative stability of cooked, refrigerated beef and pork. *J Food Sci* 72: S282–S288.

Rowe, D. 2002. High impact aroma chemicals. Part 2: The good, the bad, and the ugly. *Perfumer Flavorist* 27: 24–29.

Ryan, L. C., Mestrallet, M. G., Nepote, V., Conci, S., and Grosso, N. R. 2008. Composition, stability and acceptability of different vegetable oils used for frying peanuts. *Int J Food Sci Technol* 43: 193–199.

Sariri, R., Aghaghaziani, F., and Sajedi, R. H. 2009. Inhibition of mushroom tyrosinase by aliphatic alcohols. *Biosci Biotechnol Res Asia* 6: 489–496.

Sebranek, J. G., Hunt, M. C., Cornforth, D. P., and Brewer, M. S. 2006. Perspectives—Carbon monoxide packaging of fresh meat. *Food Technol* 60: 184.

Shahidi, F., and Wanasundara, P. K. 1992. Phenolic antioxidants. *Crit Rev Food Sci Nut* 32: 67–103.

Shigenaga, T., Yamauchi, N., Funamoto, Y., and Shigyo, M. 2005. Effects of heat treatment on an ascorbate-glutathione cycle in stored broccoli (*Brassica oleracea* L.) florets. *Postharvest Biol Technol* 38: 152–159.

Shiota, M., Takahashi, N., Konishi, H., and Yoshioka, T. 2004. Impact of oxidized off-flavor of ice cream prepared from milk fat. *J Am Oil Chem Soc* 81: 455–460.

ShiPing, T., Yong, X., AiLi, J., and Yi, W. 2002. Changes in enzymatic activity and quality attributes of late-mature peaches in response to controlled atmosphere conditions. *Agric Sci China* 1: 207–212.

Soares, M., Ribeiro, A. P. B., Goncalves, L. A. G., Fernades, G. B., and Bolini, H. M. A. 2004. Sensory acceptance of soybean oil deodorized and degummed by ultrafiltration. *Bol Centro Pesquisa Process Aliment* 22: 283–294.

Spanier, A. M., McMillin, K. W., and Miller, J. A. 1990. Enzyme activity levels in beef: Effect of postmortem ageing and end point cooking temperature. *J Food Sci* 55: 318–322, 326.

Spanier, A. M. and Miller, J. A. 1993. Role of proteins and peptides in meat flavor. *Food Flavor and Safety: Molecular Analysis and Design*, ACS Symposium series No. 528, eds A. M. Spanier, H. Okai and M. Tamura. ACS Books, Washington, D.C., 78–97.

Spanier, A. M. and Miller, J. A. 1996. Effect of temperature on the quality of muscle food. *J. Muscle Foods*, 7: 355–375.

Spanier, A. M., Vercellotti, J. R., and James, J. R. C. 1992. Correlation of sensory, instrumental and chemical attributes of beef as influenced by meat structure and oxygen exclusion. *J Food Sci* 57: 10–15.

Spence, C., Levitan, C. A., Shankar, M. U., and Zampini, M. 2010. Does food color influence taste and flavor perception in humans? *Chemosens Percept* 3: 68–84.

Sroka, Z., and Cisowski, W. 2003. Hydrogen peroxide scavenging, antioxidant and anti-radical activity of some phenolic acids. *Food Chem Toxicol* 41: 753–758.

Stephens, S. D., Watkins, B. A., and Nielsen, S. S. 1997. Storage stability of screwpress-extracted oils and residual meals from CELSS candidate oilseed crops. *Adv Space Res* 20: 1879–1889.

Stetzer, A. J., Wicklund, R., Tucker, E., Paulson, D., McFarlane, B., Lockhorn, G., and Brewer, M. S. 2007. Effect of carbon monoxide and high oxygen modified packaging (MAP) on quality characteristics of beef strip steaks. *J Muscle Foods* 18: 56–66.

Stetzer, A. J., Cadwallader, K., Singh, T. K., McKeith, F. K., and Brewer, M. S. 2008. Effect of enhancement and ageing on flavor and volatile compounds in various beef muscles. *Meat Sci* 79: 13–19.

St. Angelo, A. J., Crippen, K. L., Dupuy, H. P., and James, C. Jr. 1990. Chemical and sensory studies of antioxidant-treated beef. *J Food Sci* 55: 1501–1505, 1539.

Su, C. P., Gupta, M., and White, P. 2003. Oxidative and flavor stabilities of soybean oils with low- and ultra-low-linolenic acid composition. *J Am Oil Chem Soc* 80: 171–176.

Takahashi, N., Sasaki, R., and Chiba, H. 1979. Enzymatic improvement of food flavor. IV. Oxidation of aldehydes in soybean extracts by aldehyde oxidase. *Agric Biol Chem* 43: 2557–2561.

Takahashi, N., Kitabatake, N., Sasaki, R., and Chiba, H. 1980. Enzymatic improvement of food flavor. V. Oxidation of aldehydes in soybean extracts by an NAD+-regenerating system made up of aldehyde dehydrogenase and diaphorase. *Agric Biol Chem* 44: 1669–1670.

Tao, W. C., Ping, C. Y., Nout, M. J. R., Guo, S. B., and Liu, L. 2011. Effect of modified atmosphere packaging (MAP) with low and superatmospheric oxygen on the quality and antioxidant enzyme system of golden needle mushrooms (*Flammulina velutipes*) during postharvest storage. *Europ Food Res Technol* 232: 851–860.

Toralles, R. P., Vendruscolo, J. L., Vendruscolo, C. T., del Pino, F. A. B., and Antunes, P. L. 2010. Control of peach polyphenoloxidase by the interaction of pH, temperature and ascorbic acid concentration. *Braz J Food Technol* 13: 120–127.

Usuki, R., and Kaneda, T. 1980. Bitter taste of oxidized fatty acids. *Agric Biol Chem* 44: 2477–2481.

Vega, J. and Brewer, M. S. 1993. Absolute odor threshold determinations of selected organic compounds at selected temperatures in a gelatin model system. IFT, July 11–14, Chicago, IL.

Vega, J. D., and Brewer, M. S. 1994. Detectable odor thresholds of selected lipid oxidation compounds at various temperatures in a gelatin model system. *J Food Lipids* 1: 229–244.

Vega, J. D., and Brewer, M. S. 1995. Detectable odor thresholds of selected lipid oxidation compounds in a meat model system. *J Food Sci* 60: 592–595.

Viana, E. S., Gomide, L. A. M., and Vanetti, M. C. D. 2005. Effect of modified atmospheres on microbiological, color and sensory properties of refrigerated pork. *Meat Sci* 71: 696–705.

Vidal-Quintanar, R. L., Love, M. H., Love, J. A., White, P. J., and Johnson, L. A. 2003. Lipid-autoxidation-limited shelf-life of nixtamalized instant corn masa. *J Food Lipids* 10: 153–163.

Warner, K. 2009. Oxidative and flavor stability of tortilla chips fried in expeller pressed low linolenic acid soybean oil. *J Food Lipids* 16: 133–147.

Warner, K., and Moser, J. 2009. Frying stability of purified mid-oleic sunflower oil triacylglycerols with added pure tocopherols and tocopherol mixtures. *J Am Oil Chem Soc* 86: 1199–1207.

Webster, J. B., Duncan, S. E., Marcy, J. E., and O'Keefe, S. F. 2009. Controlling light oxidation flavor in milk by blocking riboflavin excitation wavelengths by interference. *J Food Sci* 74: S390–S398.

Whang, K., and Peng, I. C. 1988. Electron paramagnetic resonance studies of the effectiveness of myoglobin and its derivatives as photosensitizers in singlet oxygen generation. *J Food Sci* 53: 1863–1865, 1893.

Wicklund, S. E., Homco-Ryan, C., Ryan, K. J., McKeith, F. K., McFarlane, B. J., and Brewer, M. S. 2005. Aging and enhancement effects on quality characteristics of beef strip steaks. *J Food Sci* 70: S242–S248.

Wicklund, R., Stetzer, A. J., Tucker, E., Paulson, D., McFarlane, B., Lockhorn, G., and Brewer, M. S. 2006. Effect of carbon monoxide and high oxygen modified packaging (MAP) on phosphate enhanced case-ready pork chops. *Meat Sci* 74: 704–709.

Winterbourn, C. C. 1990. Oxidative reactions of hemoglobin. *Methods Enzymol* 186: 265–272.

Wolf, W. J. 1975. Lipoxygenase and flavor of soybean protein products. *J Agric Food Chem* 23: 136–141, 136–141.

Yamato, T., Kurata, T., Kato, H., and Fujimaki, M. 1970. Volatile carbonyl compounds from heated beef fat. *Agric Biol Chem* 34: 88–94.

Yan, D., MeiLi, Y., HongJie, X., HuaTao, D., Yan, P. J., Feng, X., and Hua, Z. Y. 2010. Effects of low temperature conditioning on chilling injury and quality of cold-stored juicy peach fruit. *Trans Chin Soc Agric Eng* 26: 334–338.

Yancey, E. J., Dikeman, M. E., Hachmeister, K. A., Chambers, E. IV, and Milliken, G. A. 2006. Flavor characterization of top blade, top sirloin, and tenderloin steaks as affected by pH, maturity, and marbling. *J Anim Sci* 83: 2618–2623.

Yancey, E. J., Grobbel, J. P., Dikeman, M. E., Smith, J. S., Hachmeister, K. A., Chambers, E. C. IV, Gadgil, P., Milliken, G. A., and Dressler, E. A. 2006. Effects of total iron, myoglobin, hemoglobin, and lipid oxidation of uncooked muscles on livery flavor development and volatiles of cooked beef steaks. *Meat Sci* 73: 680–686.

Yang, A., Brewster, M. J., Beilken, S. L., Lanari, M. C., Taylor, D. G., and Tume, R. K. 2002. Warmed-over flavor and lipid stability of beef: Effects of prior nutrition. *J Food Sci* 67: 3309–3313.

Yong, J., Hun, K., Sung, Y. P. W., Seong, S. Y., and Young, J. Y. 2000. Identification of irradiation-induced volatile flavor compounds in chicken. *J Korean Soc Food Sci Nutr* 29: 1050–1056.

Zhou, J. Q., Zhao, G. Y., Zhang, P. Q., and Bai, Y. H. 2008. Color stability of fresh peach juice prepared by heating at high pressure during storage. *Modern Food Sci Technol* 24: 548–551.

Zhu, L. G., and Brewer, M. S. 1999. Relationship between instrumental and visual color in a raw, fresh beef and chicken model system. *J Muscle Foods* 10: 131–146.

8 Effects of Oxidation on the Nutritive and Health-Promoting Value of Food Components

Rosario Zamora, Rosa M. Delgado, and Francisco J. Hidalgo

CONTENTS

8.1   INTRODUCTION

Foods contain a number of chemical substances, traditionally named nutrients, which are necessary for the maintenance, growth, and health of people. These nutrients can come from either various food sources or can be added to foods, and they reach the cells of the body where they perform essential functions. Altogether, the functions of these nutrients ensure good health, and they also have a role in disease prevention.

The number of these substances is high, but they can be classified into a relatively limited number of groups: carbohydrates, acyl lipids, amino acids and their polymers, terpenoids, phenolic compounds, and vitamins (Table 8.1). In addition, specific sulfur compounds and certain indoles have also been suggested as having health-promoting value, and they are also included in Table 8.1.

When a food is oxidized, many of these substances can be modified, and their nutritive and health-promoting values are expected to change. However, these changes will depend on the reversibility of the oxidative process, the ability of the

TABLE 8.1

Food Components with Nutritive or Health-Promoting Effects

Group	Component	Selected Functions	Selected Sources	References
Carbohydrates	Saccharides (mono-, di- ...)	Source of energy	Bread, cereal products, starchy vegetables	Ensminger et al. 1995
	Oligosaccharides	Prebiotic effect	Chicory, Jerusalem artichoke, garlic	Goffin et al. 2011
	β-Glucans	Lowering blood cholesterol, reduction of postprandial glycemic response	Oat, barley	EFSA 2010a; EFSA 2011a
Acyl lipids	Triacylglycerols	Source of energy and essential fatty acids, absorption of fat-soluble vitamins	Vegetable oils, butter	Ensminger et al. 1995; EFSA 2011b
	ω-3 fatty acids	Visual development of infants, cardiac function	Fish, shellfish	EFSA 2009a; EFSA 2010b
	Linoleic acid	Reduction of blood cholesterol	Vegetable oils	EFSA 2009b
	α-Linolenic acid	Brain and nerve tissue development, reduction of blood cholesterol concentration	Flaxseed, fish	EFSA 2011c; EFSA 2009c
	Conjugated acids	Health-promoting effects	Vegetable oils, dairy products, meats	Hennessy et al. 2011
	Phosphatidylcholine (source of choline)	Lipid metabolism, liver function, homocysteine metabolism	Eggs, liver, wheat germ, soybean	EFSA 2011d
Amino acid derivatives	Amino acids and proteins	Maintenance and growth of tissues, regulatory functions	Meats, fish, poultry, eggs, cheese	EFSA 2008a; EFSA 2010c; EFSA 2011e
	Peptides	Hypotensive	Milk, macroalgae, potato, sweet potato	Fitzgerald et al. 2011; Mills et al. 2011

(continued)

TABLE 8.1 (Continued)
Food Components with Nutritive or Health-Promoting Effects

Group	Component	Selected Functions	Selected Sources	References
Terpenoids	Tocopherols and tocotrienols	Protection of DNA, proteins, and lipids from oxidative damage	Grains	EFSA 2010d
	Carotenoids	Antioxidants	Vegetables, fruits	Lu et al. 2011; Yuan et al. 2011
	Sterols	Lowering of LDL cholesterol	Wheat germ, vegetable oils	EFSA 2008b; EFSA 2008c
Phenolics	Flavonoids and nonflavonoids	Prevention of cardiovascular disease and cancer	Fruits and vegetables	Crozier et al. 2009; Shimizu et al. 2011; Smoliga et al. 2011
Other vitamins	Vitamin C	Reduction of tiredness and fatigue, normal psychological functions, regeneration of the reduced form of vitamin E	Oranges, grapefruit, strawberries	EFSA 2010e
	Riboflavin	Normal metabolism of iron, maintenance of normal skin and mucous membranes, normal vision, protection of DNA, proteins and lipids from oxidative damage	Milk, egg, almonds, spinach	EFSA 2010f
	Thiamine	Maintenance of normal neurological development, normal psychological functions, carbohydrate metabolism	Rice, lentils, peas, pork	EFSA 2011f; EFSA 2010g; EFSA 2010h
	Vitamin B_6	Protein and glycogen metabolism, function of the nervous system, red blood cell formation, function of the immune system, regulation of hormonal activity, reduction of tiredness and fatigue	Banana, salmon, chicken, spinach	EFSA 2009d; EFSA 2010i

Folate	Normal psychological functions, reduction of tiredness and fatigue, contribution to normal amino acid synthesis	Orange, spinach, asparagus, lentils, garbanzo beans	EFSA 2010j
Vitamin B_{12}	Red blood cell formation, cell division, energy-yielding metabolism, function of the immune system, normal neurological and psychological function, normal homocysteine metabolism, reduction of tiredness and fatigue	Clams, mussels, crab, salmon, beef	EFSA 2009e; EFSA 2010k
Biotin	Energy-yielding metabolism, macronutrient metabolism, maintenance of skin and mucous membranes, maintenance of normal hair, maintenance of normal function of nervous system, normal psychological function	Egg yolk, liver, yeast, salmon	EFSA 2009f; EFSA 2010l
Niacin	Reduction of tiredness and fatigue, normal psychological functions	Poultry, meat, tuna, salmon, cereals	EFSA 2010m
Vitamin D	Normal growth and development of bones in children and adolescents, maintenance of normal bones	Salmon, mackerel, sardines	EFSA 2008d; EFSA 2009g
Other compounds	Indole-3-carbinol	Decrease risk of cancer	Broccoli, Brussels sprouts, cabbage	Jeffery and Araya 2009; Marconett et al. 2010
	S-Allylcysteine	Decrease of blood pressure	Garlic	Ried et al. 2010

organism to absorb the modified substance, and the metabolism of this new substance. In addition, some food components are more stable than others, and the
changes produced as a consequence of the oxidation will depend on the food composition. Furthermore, some oxidative changes produce the formation of off-flavors
and color changes in the food, which will have as a consequence the rejection of the
food by the consumer.

This chapter will review our present knowledge of the changes produced in these
main food components as a consequence of oxidation and how these changes influence their nutritive and health-promoting values.

8.2 EFFECT OF OXIDATION ON NUTRITIVE AND HEALTH-PROMOTING EFFECTS OF CARBOHYDRATES

8.2.1 CARBOHYDRATE OXIDATION

Carbohydrates are quite stable to oxidation, and foods usually contain many other
components that are expected to be oxidized before carbohydrates. However, the
radicals formed in these other components are able to react with carbohydrates, producing the formation of carbonyl compounds (Spiteller 2008). The reaction pathway
for the carbohydrate degradation produced by lipid peroxyl radicals is collected in
Figure 8.1.

In the first step of the reaction, the C–H bond of the secondary alcoholic group
is cleaved to generate a carbon-centered radical. This radical adds oxygen instantly
to produce a peroxyl radical. This new radical can either release the hydrogen peroxyl radical to produce oxo derivatives of sugars or suffer an electronic rearrangement to fractionate the carbohydrate carbon chain and produce an aldehyde and
a new carbon-centered radical. This new radical may finally add oxygen and an
abstract hydrogen radical to produce an acid and oxygen peroxide after hydrolysis (Thornalley et al. 1984). Different monocarbonyl and dicarbonyl compounds are
produced in these reactions, depending on the site of attack by the lipid peroxyl

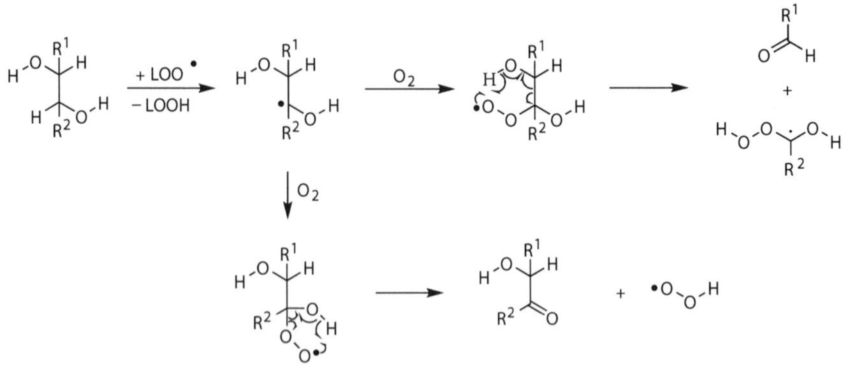

FIGURE 8.1   Carbohydrate oxidation pathways.

radical, the carbohydrate involved, and the fractionation or not of the carbohydrate molecule. Analogous reactive carbonyl compounds are also formed in foods during Maillard and caramelization reactions. In fact, 1,2-dicarbonyl compounds are common constituents in many food products (Arena et al. 2011; Hellwig et al. 2010; Mahar et al. 2010; see also Section 3.8).

8.2.2 Effect of Carbohydrate Oxidation on Nutritive and Health-Promoting Effects

Carbohydrates supply food energy and also fiber and oligosaccharides with potential health-promoting effects (Braegger et al. 2011; Broekaert et al. 2011; Nair et al. 2010; Torres et al. 2010). Because of their stability against oxidation in relation to other food components, the effect of oxidation in relation to their health-promoting effects has been scarcely studied. On the contrary, the effect of dicarbonyl compounds produced either as a consequence of carbohydrate oxidation or as a consequence of the Maillard reaction is better known. Thus, reactive dicarbonyl compounds have been described as cytotoxic, mutagenic, carcinogenic, and prooxidant. However, other studies have also suggested bactericidal, antiviral, antiparasitic, and antitumorigenic activities for these compounds (White 2009). Nevertheless, dicarbonyl compounds are very reactive and react very easily with terminal groups of amino acid residues to produce stable protein-bound amino acid derivatives, usually known as advanced glycation end products of the Maillard reaction (Henle 2005). The extent to which dietary advanced glycation end products are absorbed by the gastrointestinal tract and their possible role in the onset and promotion of disease are unclear at present (Thornalley 2007), although different studies have suggested that they do not seem to be a risk to human health (Ames 2007). On the other hand, other recent studies have suggested that reduction of advanced glycation end products in normal diets may lower oxidant stress or inflammation and restore levels of AGE receptor-1, an antioxidant, in healthy and aging subjects and in chronic kidney disease patients (Vlassara et al. 2009). In addition, reduced intake of dietary advanced glycation end products, combined with intensive glycemic control, may help to prevent the onset and progression of diabetes complications (Hsu and Zimmer 2010).

8.3 EFFECT OF OXIDATION ON NUTRITIVE AND HEALTH-PROMOTING EFFECTS OF ACYL LIPIDS

8.3.1 Acyl Lipid Oxidation

Differently than carbohydrates, acyl lipid constituents having one or more allyl groups within the fatty acid molecule are readily oxidized. This process, usually named lipid peroxidation, produces numerous volatile and nonvolatile compounds. Because some of these volatiles are exceptionally odorous compounds, lipid peroxidation is detected even in foods with unsaturated acyl lipids present as minor constituents or in foods in which only a small portion of lipids was subjected to oxidation. For this reason, lipid peroxidation has been a constant concern for the food industry in the last century. On the other hand, some volatile compounds produced as a consequence of lipid oxidation at a level below their off-flavor threshold values contribute to the pleasant aroma of many fruits and vegetables, fried products, and the rounding-off of the aroma of many fatty or oil-containing foods, for example.

The mechanisms of oxidation of food lipids have been long studied, and they are discussed in Chapter 4 of this volume. Therefore, they will not be discussed here in detail. Briefly, oxidation proceeds by a sequential, free-radical, chain-reaction mechanism in which lipid hydroperoxides are produced. The latter decomposition of these primary products of lipid oxidation initiates a cascade of reactions in which numerous secondary and tertiary products of lipid oxidation are formed. These are usually long- or short-chain oxygenated compounds having mainly one or two hydroxyl, keto, or epoxy functions, which may be conjugated with carbon–carbon double bonds.

In addition to acyl lipids having one or more allyl groups within the fatty acid molecule, acyl lipids can also have conjugated carbon–carbon double bonds, such as in the case of conjugated linoleic acid. These conjugated acyl lipids are much less common than nonconjugated acyl lipids. However, the interest in these acids rose exponentially when an isomeric mixture of conjugated linoleic acid was discovered to have anticancer properties (Ha et al. 1987). Nevertheless, despite the wide interest in conjugated linoleic acid and the large number of scientific articles published, little is known about the oxidation reactions of these conjugated acids (Pajunen and Kamal-Eldin 2008). The mechanisms involved remain controversial, and some authors have suggested that hydroperoxides are only minor products in the oxidation of conjugated linoleic oil. In fact, major volatiles obtained in the oxidation of conjugated linoleic acid were not those expected from the theoretically stable hydroperoxides formed in conjugated linoleic acid and could, in part, derive from dioxetanes coming from 1,2-cycloadditions of conjugated linoleic acid with oxygen (García-Martínez et al. 2009).

A special group of acyl lipids are phospholipids. Phospholipid peroxidation is receiving considerable attention in biology and medicine because specific oxidative modifications of these lipids seem to be critical to a number of cellular functions, disease states, and responses to oxidative stresses (Feige et al. 2010; Sparvero et al. 2010). In food, phospholipid fatty acids have been suggested as the major contributors to the development of oxidative rancidity in meat as a result of their higher content of polyunsaturated fatty acids in comparison to triacylglycerols (Hamilton 1995). This oxidation results in the formation of the corresponding hydroperoxides, which can be latter degraded (Evstigneeva 1993). The action of phospholipases and the reaction of the secondary oxidation products of acyl chains with the primary amino groups of amino phospholipids are also usually produced. In fact, these latter reactions have been suggested as playing a role in the antioxidant activity of amino phospholipids (Hidalgo et al. 2005).

Among the pool of compounds formed as a consequence of acyl lipid oxidation, the formation of long- and short-chain reactive carbonyls should be emphasized (Guillén and Goicoechea 2008). These compounds react with the surrounding reactive groups of amino acids and proteins to produce carbonyl-amine reaction products, also named advanced lipoxidation end products. In fact, these compounds should be considered as the last step of the lipid oxidation process because they are unavoidably formed when the lipid oxidation is produced in the presence of amino compounds (Hidalgo and Zamora 2002). There are many kinds of compounds produced in these reactions (Schaich 2008), and many of these compounds are very similar to those formed in the Maillard reaction. In fact, lipid oxidation and Maillard reactions are so interrelated that they should be considered simultaneously to understand the products of the Maillard reaction in the presence of lipids and vice versa (Zamora and Hidalgo 2005).

8.3.2 EFFECT OF ACYL LIPID OXIDATION ON NUTRITIVE AND HEALTH-PROMOTING EFFECTS

Acyl lipids have important nutritive functions in the body, including providing food energy and essential fatty acids, they are carriers of fat-soluble vitamins and participate in body structure and regulatory functions. In addition, certain kinds of acyl lipids have been suggested as having specific health-promoting effects. Thus, ω-3 fatty acids and α-linolenic acid have been suggested as having cardiovascular benefits (Sala-Vila and Ros 2011). Conjugated linoleic and linolenic acids have also been suggested to have many health-promoting properties (Benjamin and Spener 2009; Bougnoux et al. 2010; Hennessy et al. 2011). Finally, choline is considered an essential nutrient for public health (Zeisel and da Costa 2009).

These health-promoting effects are changed as a consequence of oxidation. Different studies have suggested that lipid oxidation products have detrimental effects on human health, including depletion of antioxidants, an increase in lipid peroxidation, impairment of glucose tolerance, and alterations of thyroid hormone homeostasis (Chao et al. 2007; Cohn 2002; Eder et al. 2002; Kanner 2007; Izaki et al. 1984; Liu and Huang 1996). On the other hand, ingestion of oxidized fats influences lipid metabolism, and a large number of feeding studies with experimental animals have demonstrated that oxidized fats, compared with fresh fats, cause a reduction in the concentration of triacylglycerols and cholesterol in liver and plasma (Ringseis and Eder 2011). This lipid-lowering action indicates that oxidized fats may be beneficial during states where lipid metabolism is disturbed (Ringseis and Eder 2011). Thus, oxidized fat has been suggested as useful in the prevention of the development of alcoholic fatty liver (Ringseis et al. 2007) and to activate peroxisome proliferator-activated receptor α in the liver and the vasculature and to inhibit atherosclerotic plaque development in the low-density lipoprotein receptor deficient mouse model of atherosclerosis (Kämmerer et al. 2011). All these data seem to suggest that oxidized fats are a mixture of chemically distinct substances, some of which exhibit potent regulatory activity on lipid metabolism (Ringseis and Eder 2011). These substances remain uncharacterized.

Among the different acyl lipids, ω-3 fatty acids are highly susceptible to oxidation. Therefore, they are expected to be oxidized with preference to other acyl lipids. This susceptibility to be oxidized has been suggested as related to a decrease in their beneficial health effects (Turner et al. 2006). Something similar can also occur in conjugated fatty acids (García-Martínez et al. 2009), although additional studies are needed.

There is concern that advanced lipoxidation end products (the products between the reactive carbonyls produced as a consequence of the oxidation of acyl chains and the amino groups of amino acids and proteins) may induce damage in the gastrointestinal tract, affecting gut health, or enter the body and promote vascular inflammation and tissue damage. However, at present, there is no direct evidence that these compounds are a source of damage in the intestines or that they are transported into the circulation and cause pathology (Baynes 2007). In fact, the proteolysis is inhibited in these modified proteins (Zamora and Hidalgo 2001), which will limit their absorption (Baynes 2007).

8.4 EFFECT OF OXIDATION ON NUTRITIVE AND HEALTH-PROMOTING EFFECTS OF AMINO ACIDS AND PROTEINS

8.4.1 Amino Acid and Protein Oxidation

Oxidation of amino acids and amino acid side chains in proteins can be either reversible, if oxidation is produced under mild conditions, or irreversible. It usually produces changes in amino acid side chains. In addition, proteins may also suffer changes in their hydrophobicity, conformation, and solubility; their susceptibility to proteolytic enzymes may be altered; and they can also undergo fragmentation (Lund et al. 2011; Schey and Finley 2000; Törnvall 2010; Xu and Chance 2007). Protein oxidation has been discussed in Chapter 5 of this volume, and it will not be described here in detail. Only the most significant changes related to nutritive and health-promoting effects will be briefly commented.

Because of the ease of oxidation of sulfur centers, the side chains of methionine and cysteine are expected to be the main oxidation sites within proteins under mild oxidative conditions. In addition, histidine, tryptophan, and tyrosine are also relatively susceptible to oxidation (Davies 2005; Li et al. 1995). Under more extreme conditions, protein carbonyls are formed, especially in lysine, arginine, proline, and threonine residues. The most commonly reported modifications resulting from amino acid side chain oxidations are given in Figure 8.2.

Protein carbonylation can also be produced by the Michael addition of one of the nucleophilic groups of amino acid side chains to the carbon–carbon double bonds of lipid oxidation products (Hidalgo and Zamora 2000; Zamora et al. 1999). These changes are usually reversible, different from the irreversible carbonyl-amine reaction products between oxidized lipids and amino acid side chains commented on in Section 3.1.

8.4.2 Effect of Amino Acid and Protein Oxidation on Nutritive and Health-Promoting Effects

Optimal dietary protein intake will provide all of the 20 amino acids (indispensable, conditionally indispensable, and dispensable amino acids) in the correct proportions to meet the body's needs for metabolic functions, including intestinal integrity

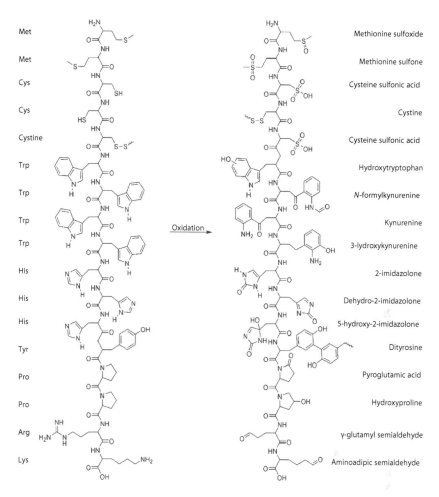

FIGURE 8.2   Oxidation of amino acid side chains.

(Wang et al. 2009), modulation of gene expression (Palii et al. 2009), protein synthesis (Lewis and Bayley 1995; Suryawan et al. 2009), regulation of cellular signaling pathways (Flynn et al. 2009; Rhoads and Wu 2009), and being key precursors for syntheses of hormones and low-molecular weight nitrogenous substances with each having enormous biological importance (Wu 2009). In addition, the nutritional quality of food proteins is also influenced by digestibility, a measure of the dietary intake, which is made available to the body after digestion and absorption (Elango et al. 2009; Moughan 2005).

Protein oxidation causes reduced meat tenderness and juiciness (Lund et al. 2007; Rowe et al. 2004), development of off-flavor in milk (Havemose et al. 2006), and overall eating quality in frozen and processed fish (Baron et al. 2007; Eymard et al. 2009). In addition, as discussed in the previous section, protein oxidation causes protein cross-linking and amino acid side-chain modification. Both changes are major causes of a lesser nutritional value of oxidized proteins. Thus, protein polymerization and aggregation have been related to the decreased proteolytic susceptibility of skeletal muscle myofibrillar proteins subjected to chemical oxidation (Morzel et al. 2006). In addition, oxidative damage to proteins from pork reduces their susceptibility to digestive enzymes (Santé-Lhoutellier et al. 2007). Furthermore, protein oxidation causes the destruction of some indispensable amino acids, including histidine, lysine, methionine, and tryptophan. On the other hand, restriction of some essential amino acids, such as methionine, has been lately related to increases in lifespan (McCarty et al. 2009).

8.5 EFFECT OF OXIDATION ON NUTRITIVE AND HEALTH-PROMOTING EFFECTS OF TERPENOIDS

Food contains many terpenoid compounds, including tocopherols and tocotrienols, carotenoids, and sterols. The effect of oxidation on the nutritive and health-promoting effects of these groups of compounds will be discussed in this section.

8.5.1 Effect of Oxidation on Nutritive and Health-Promoting Effects of Tocopherols and Tocotrienols

8.5.1.1 Tocopherol and Tocotrienol Oxidation

Tocopherols and tocotrienols, usually named as vitamin E, are a family of eight molecules of related structure. The four tocopherols consist of a chromanol ring with different substitution pattern of methyl groups at positions 5, 7, and 8, and a 16-carbon saturated phytyl residue as a side chain (Figure 8.3). Tocotrienols have the same substitution pattern on the chromanol ring but with an unsaturated isoprenoid side chain with 16 atom carbons and three double bonds (Figure 8.3). Tocopherols and tocotrienols are all-powerful antioxidants in foods and edible oils, although α-tocopherol is chemically and biologically the most active (Kamal-Eldin et al. 2008; Schneider 2005).

The antioxidative function of tocopherols and tocotrienols is a consequence of their ability to react with fatty acid peroxy radicals, the primary products of lipid peroxidation, and to intercept the chain reaction. In fact, α-tocopherol reacts with peroxyl radicals extremely quickly, and it is turned into a fairly stable radical (Burton and Ingold 1981). Under normal circumstances, it will only react with another radical to form stable, nonradical products. Some of the products of tocopherols and tocotrienols with peroxyl radicals are collected in Figure 8.3. Among the different tocopherols and tocotrienols, α-tocopherol is the most active form of vitamin E from a chemical point of view because of the substitution pattern of methyl groups on the chromanol ring. This substitution pattern makes the hydrogen of the C-6 hydroxy group especially active (Burton and Ingold 1981).

In addition to reacting with peroxyl radicals, tocopherols are readily oxidized by air, although they are stable to heat in the absence of air (Ottaway 2010). The formation of quinones and epoxy quinones analogous to those shown in Figure 8.3 has been described in different systems (Kamal-Eldin et al. 2008).

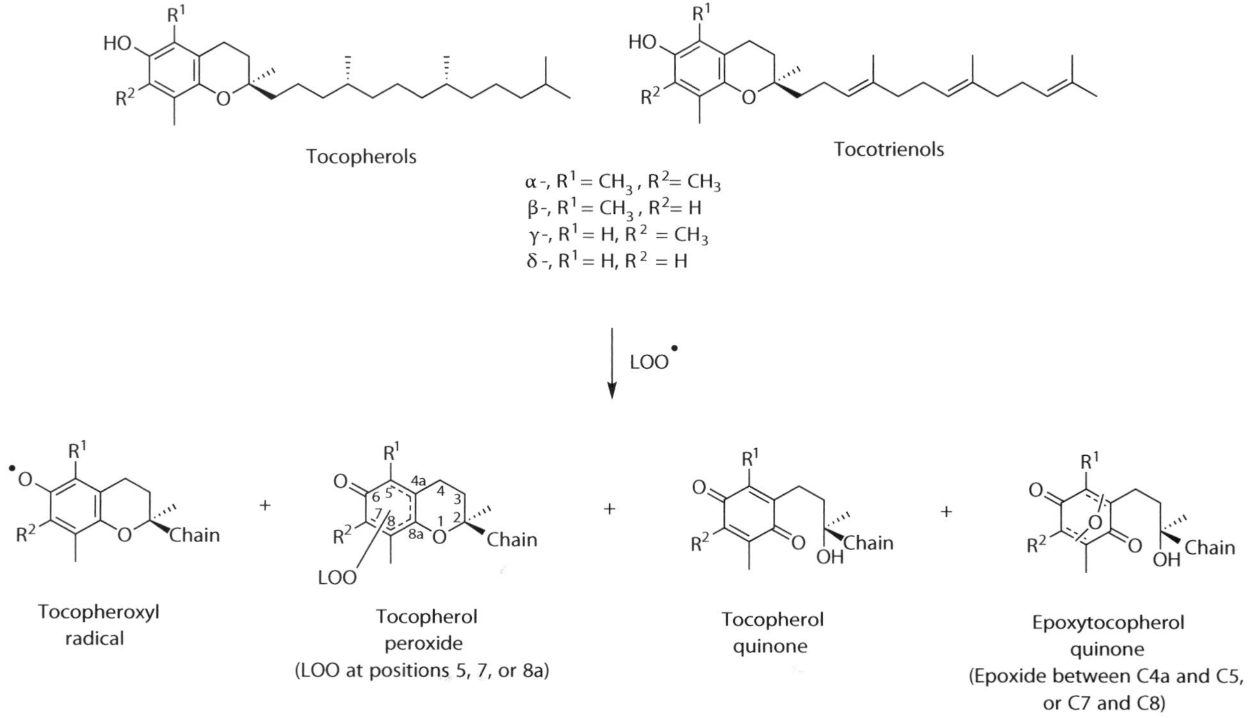

FIGURE 8.3 Oxidation of tocopherols and tocotrienols.

8.5.1.2   Effect of Tocopherol and Tocotrienol Oxidation on Nutritive and Health-Promoting Effects

As antioxidants, tocopherols and tocotrienols protect DNA, proteins, and lipids from oxidative damage (EFSA 2010d; Hamre 2011). However, it is, at present, unclear whether dietary supplementation with vitamin E has an additional beneficial outcome on human health (Clarke et al. 2008; Schneider 2005). Results from intervention trials relying on relatively high doses of a single isomer of vitamin E have been inconsistent (Schneider 2005).

Tocopherol oxidation produces oxidized products and results in the loss of antioxidant activity (Jung and Min 1992). In fact, some of these products act as prooxidants in lipids, and the more the oxidized tocopherols in the lipids are, the more the oxidation of lipids occurs (Choe and Min 2006). Prooxidant activity of tocopherol might be related to chain transfer reactions by the tocopheroxyl radical leading to the abstraction of a hydrogen atom from *bis*-allylic methylene groups of fatty acid molecules and/or hydroperoxides, an auto-initiation reaction between α-tocopherol with hydroperoxide leading to alkoxyl radical formation and reactions of the oxidation products of tocopherol (Kamal-Eldin et al. 2008).

8.5.2   Effect of Oxidation on Nutritive and Health-Promoting Effects of Carotenoids

8.5.2.1   Carotenoid Oxidation

Carotenoids are tetraterpenes characterized by a conjugated system of double bonds with delocalized π-electrons (Boon et al. 2010). They include carotenes (β-carotene and lycopene, among others), which are polyene hydrocarbons, and xanthophylls (lutein, zeaxanthin, capsanthin, canthaxanthin, astaxanthin, and violaxanthin, among others), which are more polar carotenoids with oxygen functions at one or both ends of the molecule. The conjugated polyene chain makes these compounds susceptible to degradation by a number of agents, including oxygen.

Reaction of carotenoids with atmospheric oxygen has been found to occur with relative ease, especially in systems consisting of purified carotenoids in organic solvents where more than 20 oxidation products were identified (Boon et al. 2010). This reaction involves free radicals, and the process results first in the production of epoxides, carbonyl compounds, and uncharacterized oligomers, followed by further oxidation reactions of these compounds to produce secondary short-chain carbonyl compounds, carbon dioxide, and carboxylic acids (Mordi et al. 1993). In addition, heat, light exposure, and singlet oxygen also produce carotenoid oxidation and degradation.

Although the oxidation of carotenoids occurs in the absence of other oxidizable substrates, it is generally enhanced by the presence of free-radical generators or unsaturated fatty acids where a coupled oxidation occurs (Kamal-Eldin 2008). The long conjugated double bond system of carotenoids makes them excellent substrates for radical attack. For example, peroxyl and alkoxyl radicals react with carotenoids at much higher rates than with unsaturated fatty acids (Weber and Grosch 1976). The addition of these lipid-derived radicals results in new carbon-centered radicals that are stabilized by resonance (Everets et al. 1995) and that may reversibly trap oxygen to form reactive peroxyl radicals (Liebler and McClure 1996). Among the different carotenoids, xanthophylls containing oxygenated functions seem to be more effective as peroxyl radical scavengers than β-carotene and lycopene (Woodall et al. 1997).

8.5.2.2 Effect of Carotenoid Oxidation on Nutritive and Health-Promoting Effects

Carotenoids are recognized as playing an important role in the prevention of human diseases and maintaining good health (Lu et al. 2011; Yuan et al. 2011). On the other hand, intervention trials of supplemental β-carotene indicated that supplements of this carotenoid are of little or no value in preventing cardiovascular disease and the major cancers occurring in well-nourished populations, and actually increased, rather than reduced, lung cancer in smokers (Mayne 1996). These results indicate the complexity of the health contribution of phytochemicals, and their dependence on the test situation and the level of other compounds, such as other antioxidants, that may synergize the carotenoids or even protect them against oxidative degradation (Kamal-Eldin 2008).

Carotenoids are believed to play a role as antioxidative substances both *in vivo* and *in vitro*. Therefore, their oxidation will destroy this ability. In addition, carotenoids have also been shown to have prooxidant effects. Thus, Burton and Ingold (1984) showed that β-carotene acted as an effective antioxidant at low oxygen pressure (~2% oxygen), its activity decreased with increased oxygen concentration (~20% oxygen), and it became a prooxidant at high oxygen pressure (~100% oxygen). Furthermore, the fact that carotenoids can easily absorb light or heat energies and get excited to higher energy states may also be involved in their prooxidant effects (Kamal-Eldin 2008).

The *in vivo* formation of toxic metabolites as a consequence of β-carotene oxidation has been suggested as a possible cause of the effects of high supplementation of this carotenoid on increased lung cancer risk in heavy smokers and asbestos-exposed workers (Rietjens et al. 2002). These metabolites might structurally resemble retinal and affect retinoid signaling. Diminishing of retinoid signaling, resulting from the suppression of RARβ gene expression, a tumor suppressor, and overexpression of activator protein-1 would be a mechanism to enhance tumorigenesis (Wang et al. 1999).

8.5.3 EFFECT OF OXIDATION ON NUTRITIVE AND HEALTH-PROMOTING EFFECTS OF STEROLS

8.5.3.1 Sterol Oxidation

Sterols are major components of the unsaponifiable fraction of lipids: cholesterol in animal lipids and a wide range of phytosterols in vegetable oils and fats (Kamal-Eldin and Lampi 2008). The basic skeleton is similar for cholesterol and the major sterols: They have a steroid nucleus and a hydroxyl group in C-3 (Figure 8.4). Because of the presence of a double bond between C5 and C6, sterols can undergo oxidative

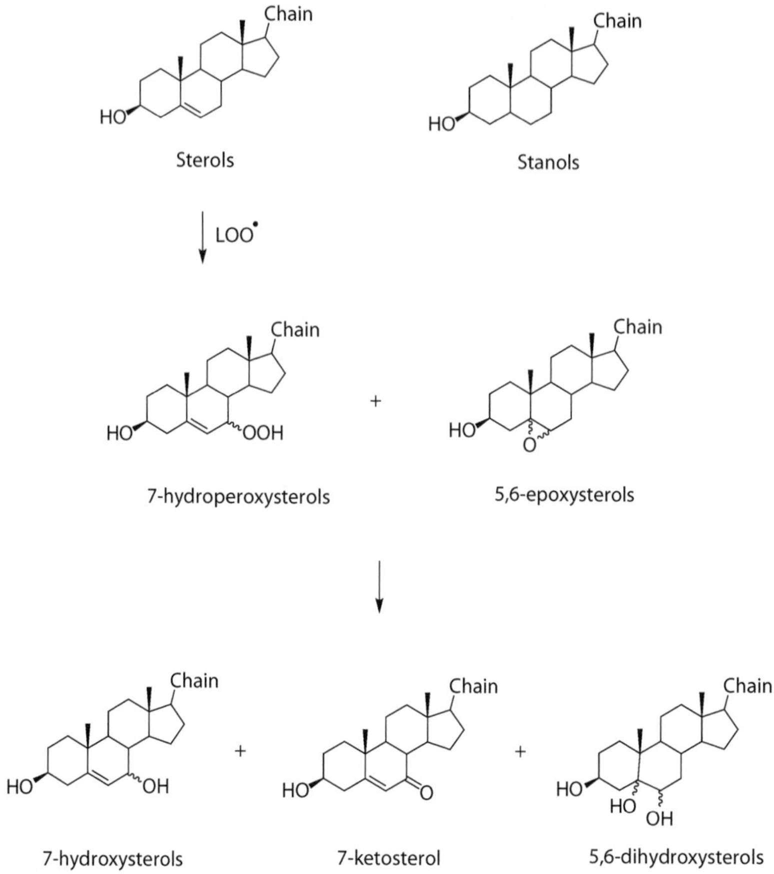

FIGURE 8.4 Oxidation of sterols.

processes (Hovenkamp et al. 2008). In contrast, plant stanols do not have this double bond and are more stable to oxidation (Soupas et al. 2004). Sterols differ in the substitutions in the ring and/or the side chains.

Sterols are susceptible to oxidation. This oxidation can involve reactive oxygen and free-radical species or physical processes, such as heating or radiation. Under these conditions, common steroid (ring) oxidation products are hydroxyl-, keto-, epoxy-, and dihydroxy-derivatives (Otaegui-Arrazola et al. 2010). Side-chain oxidation is believed to be mainly a result of enzymatic reactions (Hovenkamp et al. 2008). Chemical structures for major oxysterols are collected in Figure 8.4.

Accumulating experimental evidence suggests that autoxidation of sterols follows a free-radical mechanism (Kamal-Eldin and Lampi 2008). The major primary autoxidation products of cholesterol are 5,6-epoxysterols and 7-hydroperoxysterols, which are lately converted into 5,6-dihydroxysterols, 7-hydroxysterols, and 7-ketosterol.

8.5.3.2   Effect of Sterol Oxidation on Nutritive and Health-Promoting Effects

Cholesterol is an essential component of cells and organisms. However, dietary cholesterol has been related to cardiovascular disease risk, although dietary cholesterol raises blood cholesterol in only one-third of people (Constance 2009), and the dynamics of cholesterol homeostasis and of development of cardiovascular heart disease are extremely complex and multifactorial (Jones 2009). Because of their structural similarity to cholesterol, phytosterols reduce cholesterol absorption from the gut and plasma cholesterol levels, which may produce health-promoting effects (Marangoni and Poli 2010).

Oxidation of sterols produces changes in these health effects. Oxysterols are incorporated in plasma and tissues through a diet containing oxidized sterols, although some compounds, such as 7-hydroxysterols, seem to be better absorbed than others, such as 7-ketosterols (Grandgirard et al. 2004). In addition, oxysterols are also produced in the liver, where phytosterols and cholesterol are oxidized enzymatically and nonenzymatically.

Cholesterol oxidation products are associated with the initiation and progression of major chronic diseases, including atherosclerosis, neurodegenerative processes, diabetes, and kidney failure, among others (Sottero et al. 2009). The implication of phytosterol oxidation products in atherosclerosis, neurodegenerative processes, and other chronic diseases are still unknown (Otaegui-Arrazola et al. 2010). However, they have been associated with cytotoxic and proapoptotic effects (Hovenkamp et al. 2008).

Although sterols oxidized in the ring are implicated in toxic effects, those oxidized enzymatically in the side chain play important biological roles, including cholesterol homeostasis (Gill et al. 2008; Hovenkamp et al. 2008; Otegui-Arrazola et al. 2010; Ryan et al. 2009).

8.6   EFFECT OF OXIDATION ON NUTRITIVE AND HEALTH-PROMOTING EFFECTS OF FLAVONOIDS AND OTHER PHENOLIC COMPOUNDS

Phenolics are a large group of compounds (more than 8000 phenolic compounds have been reported) characterized by having at least one aromatic ring with one or more hydroxyl groups attached. They are widely dispersed throughout the plant kingdom, and many occur in food. Phenolics range from simple, low molecular weight, single aromatic-ring compounds to the large and complex tannins and derived polyphenols. They can be classified by the number and arrangement of their carbon atoms and are commonly found conjugated to sugars and organic acids (Crozier et al. 2009). General structures for most common groups of phenolic compounds are given in Figure 8.5.

Phenolics occurring naturally can be classified into two big groups: flavonoids and nonflavonoids. Flavonoids are a large family of compounds that have a common chemical structure with two aromatic rings connected by a three-carbon bridge. Flavonoids may be further divided into subclasses depending on the substituents

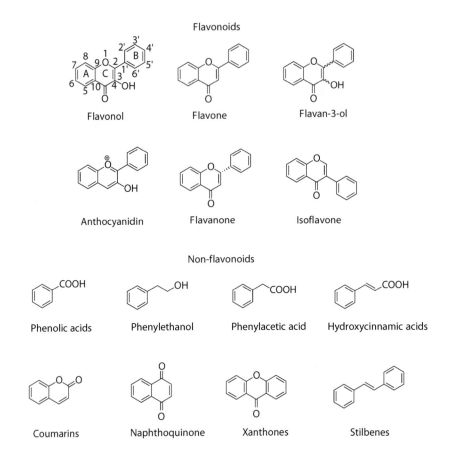

FIGURE 8.5 Chemical structures of the backbones of main dietary phenolic groups.

on the rings. The main subclasses of dietary flavonoids are anthocyanidins, flavanols, flavanones, flavonols, flavones, and isoflavones (Figure 8.5). In addition,
there are also other minor components of a diet with the structure of flavonoids.
The basic flavonoid skeleton can have numerous substituents, including sugar molecules. Hydroxyl groups are usually present at the 4'-, 5-, and 7-positions. The main
nonflavonoids of dietary significance are phenolic acids, hydroxycinnamates, and
stilbenes.

8.6.1 PHENOLIC COMPOUND OXIDATION

Phenolic compounds can be oxidized both enzymatically and nonenzymatically.
Enzymatic oxidation involves hydroxylation to the *ortho*-position adjacent to an
existing hydroxyl group of the phenolic substrate (monophenol oxidase activity)
and oxidation of *ortho*-dihydroxybenzenes to *ortho*-benzoquinones (diphenol oxidase activity) (Oliveira et al. 2011). The nonenzymatic oxidation process is favored

in polyphenols containing an *ortho*-dihydroxybenzene moiety (catechol ring) or a 1,2,3-trihydroxybenzene moiety (a galloyl group) (Li et al. 2008). These substrates are sequentially oxidized to semiquinone radicals and benzoquinones. The presence of transition metal ions seems to be necessary for this oxidation at least in wines (Waterhouse and Laurie 2006). The quinones formed in the oxidation are unstable and may undergo further reactions. Quinones can spontaneously combine with nucleophilic compounds (including some phenols, thiols, and amines) because of their electrophilic character (Oliveira et al. 2011). In addition, the produced adducts may form new dihydroxybenzene moieties through keto-enol tautomerism (Li et al. 2008). Moreover, these dimers or polymers are much more easily oxidized than the initial phenols, and the oxidation of these products results in an acceleration of the polymerization process (Oliveira et al. 2011). Additionally, the formed quinones can oxidize other phenolic compounds at the same time that they are reduced (Crozier et al. 2009).

Phenolic compounds are antioxidants. Therefore, they are able to scavenge free radicals. Their antioxidant activity is dependent on the balance between the electron-donating effect of substituents and the steric crowding around the phenolic hydroxyl groups, which is related to the position of the substituents (Choe and Min 2009). Phenolic compounds can donate hydrogen to peroxy radicals and semiquinone radicals are produced. As commented previously, these radicals are then converted into quinones, which may suffer further reactions.

8.6.2 Effect of Phenolic Compound Oxidation on Nutritive and Health-Promoting Effects

The current interest in dietary polyphenols has been driven primarily by epidemiological studies that suggest diets rich in these phytochemicals are beneficial to human health (Wang et al. 2011a). These beneficial effects have been considered traditionally related to the potent free radical-scavenging properties exhibited by phenolic compounds *in vitro*. Nevertheless, only a small percentage of dietary phenolic compounds reaches the tissues, and very little of this absorbed material retains the structure found in the plant (Crozier et al. 2009). In fact, most dietary phenolics are modified during absorption from the small intestine with the formation of the glucuronide, methyl, and sulfate metabolites, and in the large intestine, breakdown to phenolic acid and nonphenolic catabolites occurs. Therefore, the compounds that reach cells and tissues are chemically and biologically distinct from their dietary form.

As described in the previous section, phenolic compound oxidation is a really complex process in which many different products can be formed depending on the food composition. In addition, transformation and/or absorption of these oxidized products are mostly unknown. Therefore, very little is known of the health effects of oxidized phenolics. Although most of the beneficial effects associated with the ingestion of unmodified phenolics are expected to change, both positive and negative effects have been described as a consequence of this oxidation. Thus, for example, tea fermentation produces oxidation and conversion of simple flavonoids into more complex molecules, which was parallel to a decrease in the antioxidant capacity of the tea (Kim et al. 2011). This decrease in phenolic content is likely related to the higher goitrogenic or antithyroidal potential of unfractionated green tea extract than black tea extract (Chandra et al. 2011) or the higher safety of black tea as compared to green tea (Wang et al. 2010). In addition, black tea consumption was inversely associated with Parkinson's disease risk, and green tea drinking was unrelated to Parkinson's disease risk (Tan et al. 2008). On the contrary, a meta-analysis has shown that black tea does not have any protective role against coronary artery disease, but a tentative association of green tea consumption with a reduced risk of coronary artery disease was found (Wang et al. 2011b).

8.7 EFFECT OF OXIDATION ON NUTRITIVE AND HEALTH-PROMOTING EFFECTS OF OTHER VITAMINS

Vitamins comprise a diverse group of organic compounds that are nutritionally essential micronutrients. Because of their diversity, their chemical stabilities are also very variable. The chemical composition of food can strongly influence the stability of vitamins. Oxidizing agents directly degrade ascorbic acid, folate, vitamin A, carotenoids, and vitamin E and may indirectly affect other vitamins (Gregory 2008). The effect of oxidation on the health-promoting effects of some of them was discussed in previous sections. Those not discussed in the previous sections will be covered here.

8.7.1 Effect of Oxidation on Nutritive and Health-Promoting Effects of Ascorbic Acid

L-ascorbic acid (vitamin C) is a carbohydrate-like compound whose acidic and reducing properties are contributed by the 2,3-enediol moiety (see Figure 3.7). This vitamin plays an essential role in the reduction of tiredness and fatigue, the normal psychological functions, and the regeneration of the reduced form of vitamin E (EFSA 2010e). Oxidation of ascorbic acid is a quite complex process in which more than 50 low molecular weight products have been identified (Bradshaw et al. 2011; Gregory 2008). One of the first steps of the oxidation may involve the formation of L-dehydroascorbic acid, which still retains vitamin C activity. However, the opening of the lactone ring irreversibly destroys vitamin C activity.

8.7.2 Effect of Oxidation on Nutritive and Health-Promoting Effects of Thiamin

Thiamin is a substituted pyrimidine linked through a methylene bridge to a substituted thiazole (Figure 8.6). This vitamin contributes to the maintenance of normal neurological development and function, normal psychological functions, and carbohydrate and energy-yielding metabolism (EFSA 2010g,h, 2011f). Thiamin is oxidized under air to form the corresponding disulfide derivative (Dwivedi and Arnold 1973). This conversion involves the opening of the thiazole ring. More vigorous

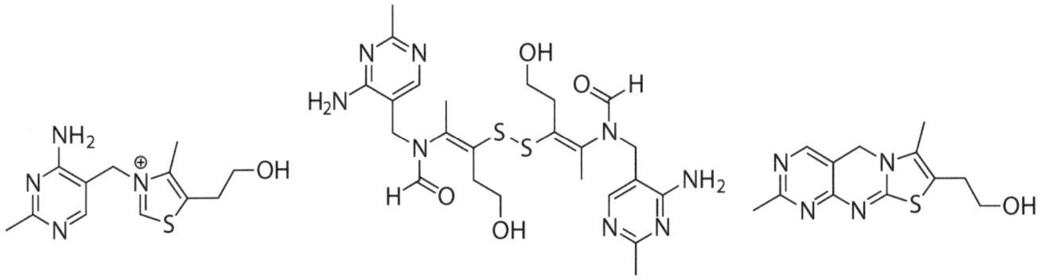

FIGURE 8.6   Chemical structures of thiamine and its oxidation products.

oxidation produces the fluorescent compound thiochrome (Figure 8.6). Differently from the formation of the disulfide, formation of thiochrome is usually considered an irreversible reaction, although the reduction of the thiochrome to thiamin by benzaldehyde has been described (Dwivedi and Arnold 1973). The conversion of thiamin into thiamin disulfide does not seem to affect the thiamin activity (Gregory 2008).

8.7.3   EFFECT OF OXIDATION ON NUTRITIVE AND HEALTH-PROMOTING EFFECTS OF RIBOFLAVIN

Riboflavin, formerly known as vitamin B_2, is the generic term for the group of compounds that exhibit the biological activity of riboflavin (Figure 8.7). Riboflavin plays a role in the normal energy-yielding metabolism, in the normal metabolism of iron, in the maintenance of normal skin and mucous membranes, in normal vision, in normal red blood cells, in reduction of tiredness and fatigue, in the normal function of the nervous system, and in the protection of DNA, proteins, and lipids from oxidative damage (EFSA 2010f). The chemical behavior of riboflavin and other flavins is complex because they can exist in several oxidation states as well as in multiple ionic forms: the native (fully oxidized) yellow flavoquinone, the flavosemiquinone (red or blue depending on pH), and the colorless flavohydroquinone (Rivlin 2001). The typical mechanism of degradation of riboflavin is a photochemical that yields two biologically inactive products, lumiflavin and lumichrome (Figure 8.7), and an array of free radicals (Woodcock et al. 1982). These radicals are able to degrade other food components. The extent to which photochemical degradation of riboflavin is responsible for photosensitized oxidation reactions in foods has not been quantitatively determined, although this process assuredly contributes significantly (Gregory 2008).

8.7.4   EFFECT OF OXIDATION ON NUTRITIVE AND HEALTH-PROMOTING EFFECTS OF VITAMIN B_6

Vitamin B_6 is a generic term for the group of 2-methyl-3-hydroxy-5-hydroxymethyl-pyridines having the vitamin activity of pyridoxine. The various forms of vitamin B_6 differ according to the nature of the substituent at the 4-position: an alcohol

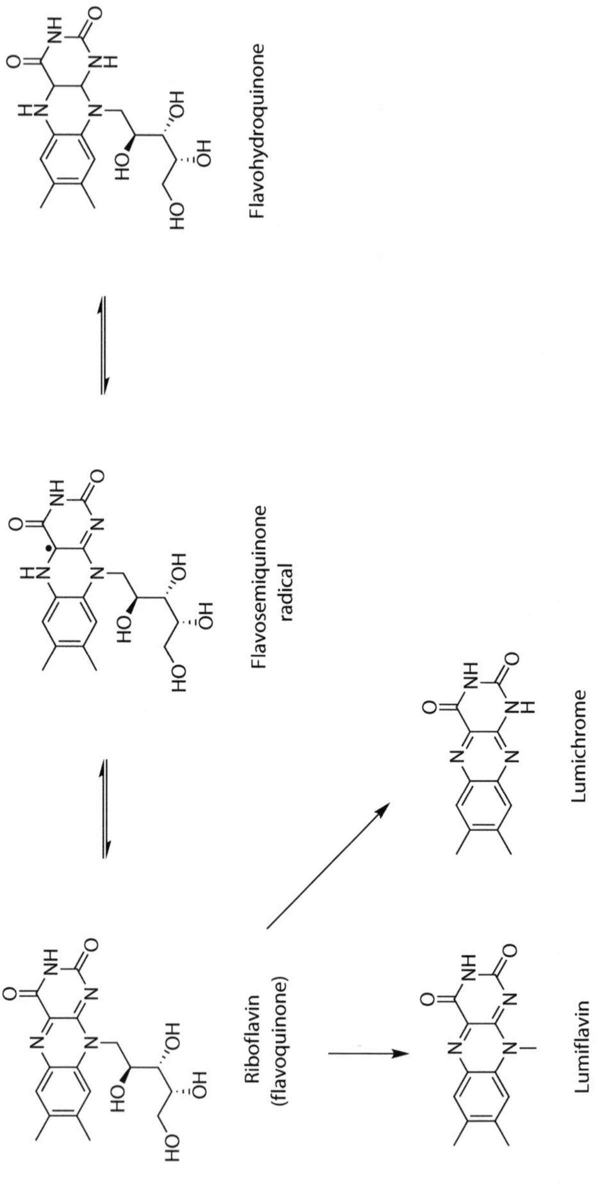

FIGURE 8.7 Chemical structures of riboflavin and its oxidation products.

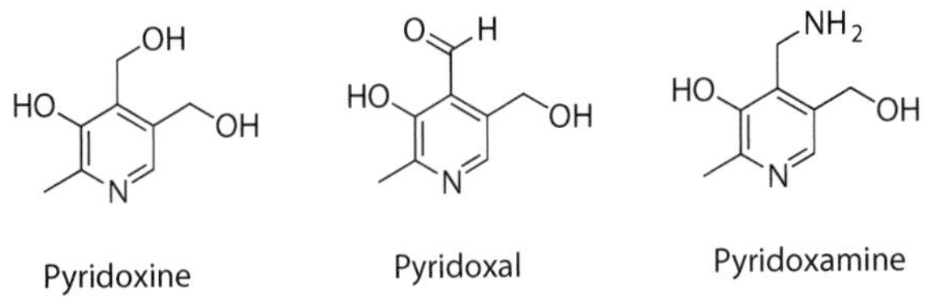

FIGURE 8.8 Chemical structures of vitamin B_6.

(pyridoxine), an aldehyde (pyridoxal), or an amine (pyridoxamine) (Figure 8.8). Vitamin B_6 participates in many functions, including protein and glycogen metabolism, the function of the nervous system, red blood cell formation, the function of the immune system, regulation of hormonal activity, contribution to normal homocysteine metabolism, normal energy-yielding metabolism, normal psychological functions, and reduction of tiredness and fatigue (EFSA 2009d, 2010i). All vitamin B_6 compounds are susceptible to light-induced degradation. Exposure of vitamin B_6 to light causes formation of the nutritionally inactive derivative 4-pyridoxic acid from both pyridoxal and pyridoxamine (Reiber 1972; Saidi and Warthesen 1983). Vitamin B_6 can also be converted to biologically inactive compounds by reactions with free radicals. Its reaction with hydroxyl radicals produces the biologically inactive 6-hydroxypyridoxine (Tadera et al. 1988).

8.7.5 EFFECT OF OXIDATION ON NUTRITIVE AND HEALTH-PROMOTING EFFECTS OF FOLATE

The generic term "folate" refers to the class of pteridine derivatives having a chemical structure and nutritional activity similar to that of folic acid. Folic acid exists naturally only in trace quantities. The majority of naturally occurring forms of folate are polyglutamyl species of tetrahydrofolates. Small amounts of dihydrofolates also occur naturally (Figure 8.9). All folates, regardless of the oxidation state of the pteridine ring, the substituents in N5 or N10, or the polyglutamyl chain length, exhibit vitamin activity. On the contrary, the L isomeric form of glutamic acid and the S configuration of C6 in tetrahydrofolates are needed to exhibit vitamin activity (Gregory 2008). Folates play a significant role in normal psychological functions, reduction of tiredness and fatigue, and contribution to normal amino acid synthesis (EFSA 2010j). All folates are subjected to oxidative degradation and produce nutritionally inactive products, such as p-aminobenzoylglutamate and a pterin, although some tetrahydrofolates can be oxidized and retain partial nutritional activity (Gregory 2008). The predominant degradation product of 5-methyltetrahydrofolate in some foods seems to be 4α-hydroxy-5-methyltetrahydrofolate (Gregory 2008). Oxidative degradation of 10-formyltetrahydrofolate can occur either by oxidation of the pteridine moiety to yield 10-formyldihydrofolate or 10-formylfolate or by oxidative cleavage to form a pterin and N-formyl-p-aminobenzoylglutamate. Both 10-formyldihydrofolate and 10-formylfolate retain nutritional activity while the cleavage products do not (Gregory 2008).

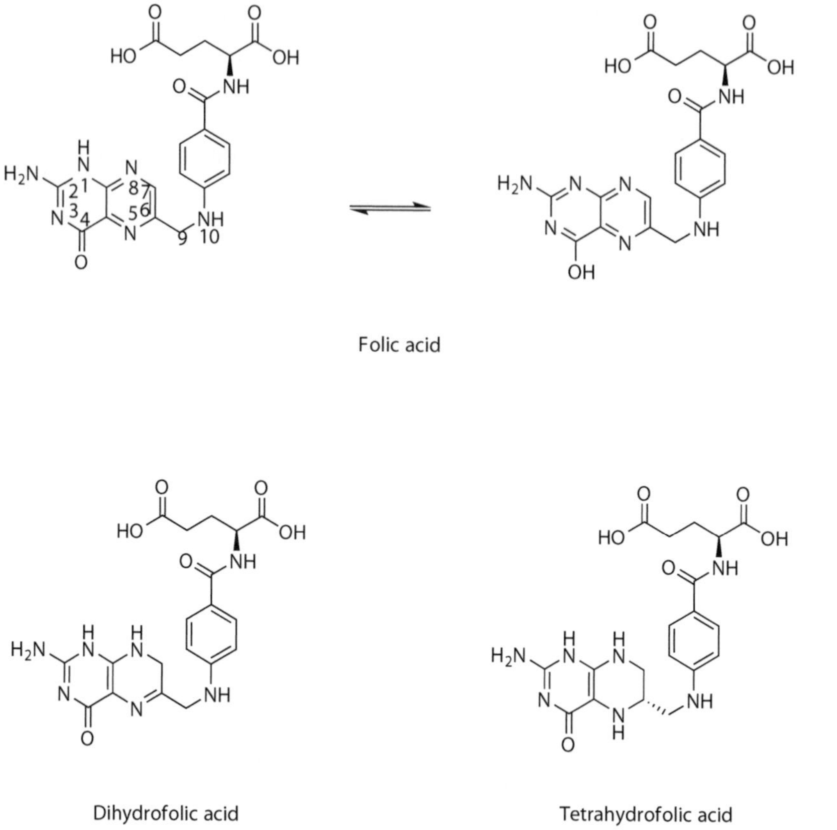

Folic acid

Dihydrofolic acid

Tetrahydrofolic acid

FIGURE 8.9 Chemical structures of folates.

8.7.6   EFFECT OF OXIDATION ON NUTRITIVE AND HEALTH-PROMOTING EFFECTS OF BIOTIN

Biotin is a bicyclic structure having carbamide and thioether groups (Figure 8.10). The two naturally occurring forms of biotin are free D-biotin and biocytin (ε-*N*-biotinyl-L-lysine) (Gregory 2008). The ring system of biotin can exist in eight possible stereoisomers, but only one of them (D-biotin) is the natural, biologically active form. Biotin plays a significant role in the energy-yielding metabolism, the macronutrient metabolism, the maintenance of skin and mucous membranes, the maintenance of normal hair, and the maintenance of the normal function of the nervous system and normal psychological function (EFSA 2009f, 2010l). Biotin is very stable to heat, light, and oxygen. However, strong oxidizing conditions can oxidize the sulfur atom to form biologically inactive biotin sulfoxide or sulfone (Gregory 2008).

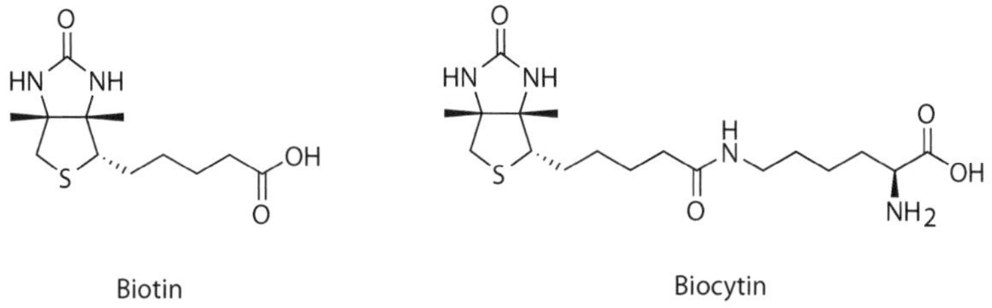

Biotin   Biocytin

FIGURE 8.10   Chemical structures of biotin and biocytin.

8.7.7   EFFECT OF OXIDATION ON NUTRITIVE AND HEALTH-PROMOTING EFFECTS OF VITAMIN B$_{12}$

Vitamin B$_{12}$ is the generic term for the group of compounds (cobalamins) having vitamin activity similar to cyanocobalamin. These compounds are corrinoids, tetra-pyrrole structures in which a cobalt atom is coordinated to the four pyrrole nitrogens. The fifth coordinate covalent bond to Co is with a nitrogen of the dimethylbenzimid-azole moiety, and the sixth position may be occupied by cyanide (cyanocobalamin), a hydroxyl group (hydroxocobalamin), a methyl group (methylcobalamin), water (aquocobalamin), glutathione (glutathionylcobalamin), a 5′-deoxyadenosyl group (5′-deoxyadenosylcobalamin), or other ligands, such as nitrite, ammonia, or sulfite (Figure 8.11). Approximately 20 naturally occurring analogs of vitamin B$_{12}$ have been identified, but not all of them have vitamin activity (Gregory 2008). Vitamin B$_{12}$ plays an important role in red blood cell formation, cell division, energy-yielding metabolism, the function of the immune system, normal neurological and psycho-logical function, normal homocysteine metabolism, and the reduction of tiredness

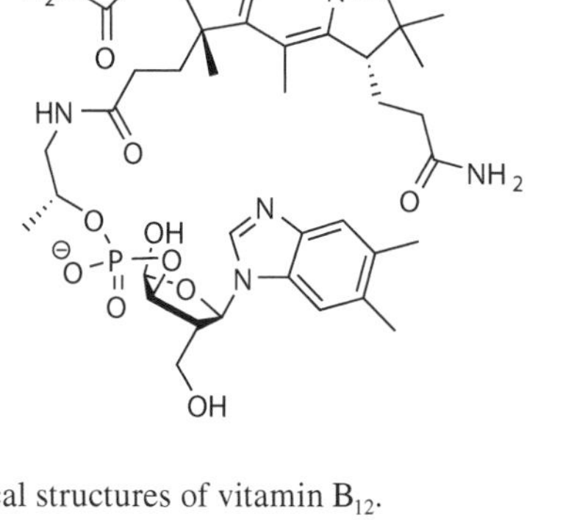

FIGURE 8.11   Chemical structures of vitamin B$_{12}$.

and fatigue (EFSA 2009e, 2010k). Photochemical degradation of vitamin B_{12} yields aquocobalamin, which has no influence on vitamin activity (Gregory 2008).

8.8 EFFECT OF OXIDATION ON NUTRITIVE AND HEALTH-PROMOTING EFFECTS OF OTHER FOOD COMPONENTS

Many other food components have also been described as playing a health-promoting role. However, the effect that oxidation of these compounds has on their health-promoting effects is lesser known. One example is indole-3-carbinol that is derived from the hydrolysis of glucobrassicin, a compound present in cruciferous vegetables, including broccoli, Brussels sprouts, and cabbage. This compound has been shown to alter estrogen metabolism, to cause cell cycle arrest and apoptosis of cancer cells, and in animals, to decrease the risk of cancer (Jeffery and Araya 2009; Marconett et al. 2010). Radicals can oxidize indole-3-methanol to yield the corresponding indolyl radical cation, which is later converted into the *N–N* linked dimer. Further oxidations can convert this dimer into a carbonyl derivative (Goyal et al. 2001). The effect that such changes can produce in the health-promoting effects of indole-3-methanol is not known at present.

Other compounds with suggested health-promoting effects are *S*-allylcysteine and other organosulfur compounds present in garlic. *S*-Allylcysteine is considered to produce health benefits, including protection against cardiovascular diseases, improvement of immune function, and anti-cancer effects (Powolny and Singh 2008). *S*-Allylcysteine oxidation produces bis(2-propenyl)disulfide, *S*-(2-propenyl) 2-propene-1-sulfinothioate (allicin), *S*-(2-propenyl) 2-propene-1-sulfonothioate, and 2-oxopropanoic acid (Freeman and Huang 1994), and some of these compounds have been related to the health benefits of garlic (Rana et al. 2011). In addition, the use of aged garlic, which might have suffered some kind of oxidation, has been suggested to treat patients with uncontrolled hypertension (Ried et al. 2010).

Finally, the oxidation mechanisms of some other health promoting nutrients (such as isothiocyanates or lipoic acid, for example) and how this oxidation affects their biological effects are still very poorly understood.

8.9 CONCLUDING REMARKS AND FUTURE RESEARCH NEEDS

Foods are very complex mixtures of substances that are present to very different proportions and that have very different properties and stabilities. In addition, there are interactions among the different food components that can both promote or protect those components from oxidative processes and that will influence the oxidative processes of the other food components. Furthermore, both natural and artificial antioxidants are routinely added to many food products to increase their stability and to avoid the formation of the off-flavors that produce the rejection of the food by the consumer.

Our present knowledge indicates that most food components are susceptible to oxidation, but some components will be oxidized more easily than others. However, more research is needed to know to what extent one component will be destroyed when other components are present.

Oxidative processes are complex, and usually only the most stable components have been isolated and characterized. In addition, these studies are usually carried out in simplified systems in which only a limited number of components are present. Therefore, oxidative pathways of many food components in complex mixtures are still poorly understood. Furthermore, the reaction of many oxidized products with other food components needs to be further explored.

Although oxidation of food components may be considered detrimental in many cases from a nutritive point of view, the reversibility of the oxidation reaction and the nutritional characteristics of the formed products also play a very important role in the health properties of food that has suffered an oxidative process. Furthermore, a mild oxidation may improve or, at least, it may not affect the nutritive properties of some food components. Moreover, the role of oxidation on the nutritive and health-promoting effects of many other food components is still very poorly understood.

Nowadays, new compounds with potential nutritive and health-promoting effects are becoming common food components. However, because of the antioxidative characteristics of many of them, they are easily oxidized. In this chapter, many examples of the changes of the nutritive and health-promoting properties of food components have been collected. Therefore, the effect of oxidation on the nutritive and health-promoting effects of these new components should be routinely studied as a part of their characterization.

REFERENCES

Ames, J. M. 2007. Evidence against dietary advanced glycation endproducts being a risk to human health. *Mol Nutr Food Res* 51: 1085–1090.

Arena, E., G. Ballistreri, F. Tomaselli, and B. Fallico. 2011. Survey of 1,2-dicarbonyl compounds in commercial honey of different floral origin. *J Food Sci* 76: C1203–C1210.

Baron, C. P., I. V. H. Kjaergard, F. Jessen, and C. Jacobsen. 2007. Protein and lipid oxidation during frozen storage of rainbow trout (*Oncorhynchus mykiss*). *J Agric Food Chem* 55: 8118–8125.

Baynes, J. W. 2007. Dietary ALEs are a risk to human health – NOT! *Mol Nutr Food Res* 51: 1102–1106.

Benjamin, S., and F. Spener. 2009. Conjugated linoleic acids as functional food: An insight into their health benefits. *Nutr Metab* 6: 36.

Boon, C. S., D. J. McClements, J. Weiss, and E. A. Decker. 2010. Factors influencing the chemical stability of carotenoids in foods. *Crit Rev Food Sci Nutr* 50: 515–532.

Bougnoux, P., N. Hajjaji, K. Maheo, C. Couet, and S. Chevalier. 2010. Fatty acids and breast cancer: Sensitization to treatments and prevention of metastatic re-growth. *Prog Lipid Res* 49: 76–86.

Bradshaw, M. P., C. Barril, A. C. Clark, P. D. Prenzler, and G. R. Scollary. 2011. Ascorbic acid: A review of its chemistry and reactivity in relation to a wine environment. *Crit Rev Food Sci Nutr* 51: 479–498.

Braegger, C., A. Chmielewska, T. Decsi, S. Kolacek, W. Mihatsch, L. Moreno, M. Piescik, J. Puntis, R. Shamir, H. Szajewska, D. Turck, and J. van Goudoever. 2011. Supplementation of infant formula with probiotics and/or prebiotics: A systematic review and comment by the ESPGHAN Committee on nutrition. *J Pediatr Gastr Nutr* 52: 238–250.

Broekaert, W. F., C. M. Courtin, K. Verbeke, T. van de Wiele, W. Vertraete, and J. A. Delcour. 2011. *Crit Rev Food Sci Nutr* 51: 178–194.

Burton, G. W., and K. U. Ingold. 1981. Autoxidation of biological molecules. 1. The antioxidant activity of vitamin E and related chain-breaking phenolic antioxidants *in vivo*. *J Am Chem Soc* 103: 6472–6477.

Burton, G. W., and K. U. Ingold. 1984. β-Carotene: An unusual type of antioxidant. *Science* 224: 569–573.

Chandra, A. K., N. De, and S. R. Choudhury. 2011. Effect of different doses of un-fractionated green and black tea extracts on thyroid physiology. *Hum Exp Toxicol* 30: 884–896.

Chao, P. M., H. L. Huang, C. H. Liao, S. T. Huang, and C. J. Huang. 2007. A high oxidized frying oil content diet is less adipogenic, but induces glucose intolerance in rodents. *Br J Nutr* 98: 63–71.

Choe, E., and D. B. Min. 2006. Mechanisms and factors for edible oil oxidation. *Comp Rev Food Sci Food Safety* 5: 169–186.

Choe, E., and D. B. Min. 2009. Mechanisms of antioxidants in the oxidation of foods. *Comp Rev Food Sci Food Saf* 8: 345–358.

Clarke, M. W., J. R. Burnett, and K. D. Croft. 2008. Vitamin E in human health and disease. *Crit Rev Clin Lab Sci* 45: 417–450.

Cohn, J. S. 2002. Oxidized fat in the diet, postprandial lipaemia and cardiovascular disease. *Curr Opin Lipidology* 13: 19–24.

Constance, C. 2009. The good and the bad: What researchers have learned about dietary cholesterol, lipid management and cardiovascular disease risk since the Harvard Egg Study. *Int J Clin Pract* 63: 9–14.

Crozier, A., I. B. Jaganath, and M. N. Clifford. 2009. Dietary phenolics: Chemistry, bioavailability and effects on health. *Nat Prod Rep* 26: 1001–1043.

Davies, M. J. 2005. The oxidative environment and protein damage. *Biochim Biophys Acta* 1703: 93–109.

Dwivedi, B. K., and R. G. Arnold. 1973. Chemistry of thiamine degradation in food products and model systems: A review. *J Agric Food Chem* 21: 54–60.

Eder, K., P. Skufca, and C. Brandsch. 2002. Thermally oxidized dietary fats increase plasma thyroxine concentrations in rats irrespective of the vitamin E and selenium supply. *J Nutr* 132: 1275–1281.

EFSA Panel on Dietetic Products, Nutrition and Allergies (NDA). 2008a. Scientific substantiation of a health claim related to animal protein and bone growth pursuant to Article 14 of Regulation (EC) No 1924/2006. *EFSA J* 858: 1–10.

EFSA Panel on Dietetic Products, Nutrition and Allergies (NDA). 2008b. Scientific substantiation of a health claim related to plant sterols and lower/reduced blood cholesterol and reduced risk of (coronary) heart disease pursuant to Article 14 of Regulation (EC) No 1924/2006. *EFSA J* 781: 1–12.

EFSA Panel on Dietetic Products, Nutrition and Allergies (NDA). 2008c. Scientific substantiation of a health claim related to plant stanol esters and lower/reduced blood cholesterol and reduced risk of (coronary) heart disease pursuant to Article 14 of Regulation (EC) No 1924/2006. *EFSA J* 825: 1–13.

EFSA Panel on Dietetic Products, Nutrition and Allergies (NDA). 2008d. Scientific substantiation of a health claim related to vitamin D and bone growth pursuant to Article 14 of Regulation (EC) No 1924/2006. *EFSA J* 827: 1–10.

EFSA Panel on Dietetic Products, Nutrition and Allergies (NDA). 2009a. Scientific substantiation of a health claim related to docosahexaenoic acid (DHA) and arachidonic acid (ARA) and visual development pursuant to Article 14 of Regulation (EC) No 1924/2006. *EFSA J* 941: 1–14.

EFSA Panel on Dietetic Products, Nutrition and Allergies (NDA). 2009b. Scientific opinion on the substantiation of health claims related to linoleic acid and maintenance of normal blood cholesterol concentrations (ID 489) pursuant to Article 13(1) of Regulation (EC) No 1924/2006. *EFSA J* 7: 1276.

EFSA Panel on Dietetic Products, Nutrition and Allergies (NDA). 2009c. Opinion on the substantiation of health claims related to alpha-linolenic acid and maintenance of normal blood cholesterol concentrations (ID 493) and maintenance of normal blood pressure (ID 625) pursuant to Article 13(1) of Regulation (EC) No 1924/2006. *EFSA J* 7: 1252.

EFSA Panel on Dietetic Products, Nutrition and Allergies (NDA). 2009d. Scientific opinion on the substantiation of health claims related to vitamin B6 and protein and glycogen metabolism (ID 65, 70, 71), function of the nervous system (ID 66), red blood cell formation (ID 67, 72, 186), function of the immune system (ID 68), regulation of hormonal activity (ID 69) and mental performance (ID 185) pursuant to Article 13(1) of Regulation (EC) No 1924/2006. *EFSA J* 7: 1225.

EFSA Panel on Dietetic Products, Nutrition and Allergies (NDA). 2009e. Scientific opinion on the substantiation of health claims related to vitamin B12 and red blood cell formation (ID 92, 101), cell division (ID 93), energy-yielding metabolism (ID 99, 190) and function of the immune system (ID 107) pursuant to Article 13(1) of Regulation (EC) No 1924/2006. *EFSA J* 7: 1223.

EFSA Panel on Dietetic Products, Nutrition and Allergies (NDA). 2009f. Scientific opinion on the substantiation of health claims related to biotin and energy-yielding metabolism (ID 114, 117), macronutrient metabolism (ID 113, 114, 117), maintenance of skin and mucous membranes (ID 115), maintenance of hair (ID 118, 2876) and function of the nervous system (ID 116) pursuant to Article 13(1) of Regulation (EC) No 1924/2006. *EFSA J* 7: 1223.

EFSA Panel on Dietetic Products, Nutrition and Allergies (NDA). 2009g. Scientific opinion on the substantiation of health claims related to calcium and vitamin D and maintenance of bone (ID 350) pursuant to Article 13(1) of Regulation (EC) No 1924/2006. *EFSA J* 7: 1272.

EFSA Panel on Dietetic Products, Nutrition and Allergies (NDA). 2010a. Scientific opinion on the substantiation of a health claim related to oat beta-glucan and lowering blood cholesterol and reduced risk of (coronary) heart disease pursuant to Article 14 of Regulation (EC) No 1924/2006. *EFSA J* 8: 1885.

EFSA Panel on Dietetic Products, Nutrition and Allergies (NDA). 2010b. Scientific opinion on the substantiation of health claims related to eicopentaenoic acid (EPA), docosahexaenoic acid (DHA), docosapentaenoic acid (DPA) and maintenance of normal cardiac function (ID 504, 506, 516, 527, 538, 703, 1128, 1317, 1324, 1325), maintenance of normal blood glucose concentrations (ID 566), maintenance of normal blood pressure (ID 506, 516, 703, 1317, 1324), maintenance of normal blood HDL-cholesterol concentrations (ID 506), maintenance of normal (fasting) blood concentrations of triglycerides (ID 506, 527, 538, 1317, 1324, 1325), maintenance of normal blood LDL cholesterol concentrations (ID 527, 538, 1317, 1325, 4689), protection of the skin from photooxidative (UV-induced) damage (ID 530), improved absorption of EPA and DHA (ID 522, 523), contribution to the normal function of the immune system by decreasing the levels of eicosanoids, arachidonic acid-derived mediators and pro-inflammatory cytokines (ID 520, 2914), and "immunomodulating agent" (4690) pursuant to Article 13(1) of Regulation (EC) No 1924/2006. *EFSA J* 8: 1796.

EFSA Panel on Dietetic Products, Nutrition and Allergies (NDA). 2010c. Scientific opinion on the substantiation of health claims related to protein and increase in satiety leading to a reduction in energy intake (ID 414, 616, 730), contribution to the maintenance or achievement of a normal body weight (ID 414, 616, 730), maintenance of normal bone (ID 416) and growth or maintenance of muscle mass (ID 415, 417, 593, 594, 595, 715) pursuant to Article 13(1) of Regulation (EC) No 1924/2006. *EFSA J* 8: 1811.

EFSA Panel on Dietetic Products, Nutrition and Allergies (NDA). 2010d. Scientific opinion on the substantiation of health claims related to vitamin E and protection of DNA, proteins and lipids from oxidative damage (ID 160, 162, 1947), maintenance of normal function of the immune system (ID 161, 163), maintenance of normal bone (ID 164), maintenance of normal teeth (ID 164), maintenance of normal hair (ID 164), maintenance of normal skin (ID 164), maintenance of normal nails (ID 164), maintenance of normal cardiac function (ID 166), maintenance of normal vision by protection of the lens of the eye (ID 167), contribution to normal cognitive function (ID 182, 183), regeneration of the reduced form of vitamin C (ID 203), maintenance of normal blood circulation (ID 216) and maintenance of normal a scalp (ID 2873) pursuant to Article 13(1) of Regulation (EC) No 1924/2006. *EFSA J* 8: 1816.

EFSA Panel on Dietetic Products, Nutrition and Allergies (NDA). 2010e. Scientific opinion on the substantiation of health claims related to vitamin C and reduction of tiredness and fatigue (ID 139, 2622), contribution to normal psychological functions (ID 140), regeneration of the reduced form of vitamin E (ID 202), contribution to normal energy-yielding metabolism (ID 1334, 3196), maintenance of the normal function of the immune system (ID 4321), and protection of DNA, proteins and lipids from oxidative damage (ID 3331) pursuant to Article 13(1) of Regulation (EC) No 1924/2006. *EFSA J* 8: 1815.

EFSA Panel on Dietetic Products, Nutrition and Allergies (NDA). 2010f. Scientific opinion on the substantiation of health claims related to riboflavin (vitamin B2) and contribution to normal energy-yielding metabolism (ID 29, 35, 36, 42), contribution to normal metabolism of iron (ID 30, 37), maintenance of normal skin and mucous membranes (ID 31, 33), contribution to normal psychological functions (ID 32), maintenance of normal bone (ID 33), maintenance of normal teeth (ID 33), maintenance of normal hair (ID 33), maintenance of normal nails (ID 33), maintenance of normal vision (ID 39), maintenance of normal red blood cells (ID 40), reduction of tiredness and fatigue (ID 41), protection of DNA, proteins and lipids from oxidative damage (ID 207), and maintenance of the normal function of the nervous system (ID 213) pursuant to Article 13(1) of Regulation (EC) No 1924/2006. *EFSA J* 8: 1814.

EFSA Panel on Dietetic Products, Nutrition and Allergies (NDA). 2010g. Scientific opinion on the substantiation of health claims related to thiamin and reduction of tiredness and fatigue (ID 23) and contribution to normal psychological functions (ID 205) pursuant to Article 13(1) of Regulation (EC) No 1924/2006. *EFSA J* 8: 1755.

EFSA Panel on Dietetic Products, Nutrition and Allergies (NDA). 2010h. Scientific opinion on the substantiation of a health claim related to thiamine and carbohydrate and energy-yielding metabolism pursuant to Article 14 of Regulation (EC) No 1924/2006. *EFSA J* 8: 1690.

EFSA Panel on Dietetic Products, Nutrition and Allergies (NDA). 2010i. Scientific opinion on the substantiation of health claims related to vitamin B6 and contribution to normal homocysteine metabolism (ID 73, 76, 199), maintenance of normal bone (ID 74), maintenance of normal teeth (ID 74), maintenance of normal hair (ID 74), maintenance of normal skin (ID 74), maintenance of normal nails (ID 74), contribution to normal energy-yielding metabolism (ID75, 214), contribution to normal psychological functions (ID 77), reduction of tiredness and fatigue (ID 78), and contribution to normal cysteine synthesis (ID 4283) pursuant to Article 13(1) of Regulation (EC) No 1924/2006. *EFSA J* 8: 1759.

EFSA Panel on Dietetic Products, Nutrition and Allergies (NDA). 2010j. Scientific opinion on the substantiation of health claims related to folate and contribution to normal psychological functions (ID 81, 85, 86, 88), maintenance of normal vision (ID 83, 87), reduction of tiredness and fatigue (ID 84), cell division (ID 195, 2881) and contribution to normal amino acid synthesis (ID 195, 2881) pursuant to Article 13(1) of Regulation (EC) No 1924/2006. *EFSA J* 8: 1760.

EFSA Panel on Dietetic Products, Nutrition and Allergies (NDA). 2010k. Scientific opinion on the substantiation of health claims related to vitamin B12 and contribution to normal neurological and psychological functions (ID 95, 97, 98, 100, 102, 109), contribution to normal homocysteine metabolism (ID 96, 103, 106), maintenance of normal bone (ID 104), maintenance of normal teeth (ID 104), maintenance of normal hair (ID 104), maintenance of normal skin (ID 104), maintenance of normal nails (ID 104), reduction of tiredness and fatigue (ID 108), and cell division (ID 212) pursuant to Article 13(1) of Regulation (EC) No 1924/2006. *EFSA J* 8: 1756.

EFSA Panel on Dietetic Products, Nutrition and Allergies (NDA). 2010l. Scientific opinion on the substantiation of health claims related to biotin and maintenance of normal skin and mucous membranes (ID 121), maintenance of normal hair (ID 121), maintenance of normal bone (ID 121), maintenance of normal teeth (ID 121), maintenance of normal nails (ID 121, 2877), reduction of tiredness and fatigue (ID 119), contribution to normal psychological functions (ID 120) and contribution to normal macronutrient metabolism (ID 4661) pursuant to Article 13(1) of Regulation (EC) No 1924/2006. *EFSA J* 8: 1728.

EFSA Panel on Dietetic Products, Nutrition and Allergies (NDA). 2010m. Scientific opinion on the substantiation of health claims related to niacin and reduction of tiredness and fatigue (ID 47), contribution to normal energy-yielding metabolism (ID 51), contribution to normal psychological functions (ID 55), maintenance of normal blood flow (ID 211), and maintenance of normal skin and mucous membranes (ID 4700) pursuant to Article 13(1) of Regulation (EC) No 1924/2006. *EFSA J* 8: 1757.

EFSA Panel on Dietetic Products, Nutrition and Allergies (NDA). 2011a. Scientific opinion on the substantiation of health claims related to beta-glucans from oats and barley and maintenance of normal blood LDL-cholesterol concentrations (ID 1236, 1299), increase in satiety leading to a reduction in energy intake (ID 851, 852), reduction of post-prandial glycaemic responses (ID 821, 824), and "digestive function" (ID 850) pursuant to Article 13(1) of Regulation (EC) No 1924/2006. *EFSA J* 9: 2207.

EFSA Panel on Dietetic Products, Nutrition and Allergies (NDA). 2011b. Scientific opinion on the substantiation of health claims related to fats and "function of the cell membrane" (ID 622, 2900, 2911) and normal absorption of fat-soluble vitamins (ID 670, 2902) pursuant to Article 13(1) of Regulation (EC) No 1924/2006. *EFSA J* 9: 2220.

EFSA Panel on Dietetic Products, Nutrition and Allergies (NDA). 2011c. Scientific opinion on the substantiation of a health claim related to alpha-linolenic acid and contribution to brain and tissue development pursuant to Article 14 of Regulation (EC) No 1924/2006. *EFSA J* 9: 2130.

EFSA Panel on Dietetic Products, Nutrition and Allergies (NDA). 2011d. Scientific opinion on the substantiation of health claims related to choline and contribution to normal lipid metabolism (ID 3186), maintenance of normal liver function (ID1501), contribution to normal homocysteine metabolism (ID 3090), maintenance of normal neurological function (ID 1502), contribution to normal cognitive function (ID 1502), and brain and neurological development (ID 1503) pursuant to Article 13(1) of Regulation (EC) No 1924/2006. *EFSA J* 9: 2056.

EFSA Panel on Dietetic Products, Nutrition and Allergies (NDA). 2011e. Scientific opinion on the substantiation of health claims related to L-tyrosine and contribution to normal synthesis of catecholamines (ID 1928), increased attention (ID 440, 1672, 1930), and contribution to normal muscle function (ID 1929) pursuant to Article 13(1) of Regulation (EC) No 1924/2006. *EFSA J* 9: 2056.

EFSA Panel on Dietetic Products, Nutrition and Allergies (NDA). 2011f. Scientific opinion on the substantiation of a health claim related to thiamin and maintenance of normal neurological development and function pursuant to Article 14 of Regulation (EC) No 1924/2006. *EFSA J* 9: 1980.

Elango, E., R. O. Ball, and P. B. Pencharz. 2009. Amino acid requirements in humans: With a special emphasis on the metabolic availability of amino acids. *Amino Acids* 37: 19–27.

Ensminger, A. H., M. E. Ensminger, J. E. Konlande, and J. R. K. Robson. 1995. *The Concise Encyclopedia of Foods & Nutrition*. Boca Raton, FL: CRC Press.

Everets, S. A., S. C. Kundu, S. Maddix, and R. L. Willson. 1995. Mechanisms of free radical scavenging by the nutritional antioxidant β-carotene. *Biochem Soc Trans* 23: 230S–233S.

Evstigneeva, R. 1993. Chemical stability. In *Phospholipids Handbook*, ed. G. Cevc, 323–333. New York: Marcel Dekker.

Eymard, S., C. P. Barn, and C. Jacobsen. 2009. Oxidation of lipid and protein in horse mackerel (*Trachurus trachurus*) mince and washed minces during processing and storage. *Food Chem* 114: 57–65.

Feige, E., I. Mendel, J. George, N. Yacov, and D. Harats. 2010. Modified phospholipids as anti-inflammatory compounds. *Curr Opin Lipidol* 21: 525–529.

Fitzgerald, C., E. Gallagher, D. Tasdemir, and M. Hayes. 2011. Heart health peptides from macroalgae and their potential use in functional foods. *J Agric Food Chem* 59: 6829–6836.

Flynn, N. E., J. G. Bird, and A. S. Guthrie. 2009. Glucocorticoid regulation of amino acid and polyamine metabolism in the small intestine. *Amino Acids* 37: 123–129.

Freeman, F., and B. G. Huang. 1994. Garlic chemistry. Nitric oxide oxidation of *S*-(2-propenyl) cysteine and (+)-*S*-2-(propenyl)-L-cysteine sulfoxide. *J Org Chem* 59: 3227–3229.

García-Martínez, M. C., G. Márquez-Ruiz, J. Fontecha, and M. H. Gordon. 2009. Volatile oxidation compounds in a conjugated linoleic acid-rich oil. *Food Chem* 113: 926–931.

Gill, S., R. Chow, and A. J. Brown. 2008. Sterol regulators of cholesterol homeostasis and beyond: The oxysterol hypothesis revisited and revised. *Prog Lipid Res* 47: 391–404.

Goffin, D., N. Delzenne, C. Blecker, E. Hanon, C. Deroanne, and M. Paquot. 2011. Will isomalto-oligosaccharides, a well-established functional food in Asia, break through the European and American market? The status of knowledge on these prebiotics. *Crit Rev Food Sci Nutr* 51: 394–409.

Goyal, R. N., A. Kumar, and P. Gupta. 2001. Oxidation chemistry of indole-3-methanol. *J Chem Soc, Perkin Trans* 2: 618–623.

Grandgirard, A., L. Martine, P. Juaneda, and C. Cordelet. 2004. Sitistanetriol is not formed *in vivo* from sitosterol in the rat. *Reprod Nutr Dev* 44: 609–616.

Gregory III, J. F. 2008. Vitamins. In *Fennema's Food Chemistry*, 4th ed., ed. S. Damodaran, K. L. Parkin, and O. R. Fennema, 439–521. Boca Raton, FL: CRC Press.

Guillén, M. D., and E. Goicoechea. 2008. Toxic oxygenated alpha,beta-unsaturated aldehydes and their study in foods: A review. *Crit Rev Food Sci Nutr* 48: 119–136.

Ha, Y. L., N. K. Grimm, and M. W. Pariza. 1987. Anticarcinogens from fried ground beef: Heat-altered derivatives of linoleic acid. *Carcinogenesis* 8: 1881–1887.

Hamilton, R. J. 1995. *Developments in Oils and Fats*. London: Blackie Academic & Professional.

Hamre, K. 2011. Metabolism, interactions, requirements and functions of vitamin E in fish. *Aquac Nutr* 17: 98–115.

Havemose, M. S., M. R. Weisbjerg, W. L. P. Bredie, H. D. Poulsen, and J. H. Nielsen. 2006. Oxidative stability of milk influenced by fatty acids, antioxidants, and copper derived from feed. *J Dairy Sci* 89: 1970–1980.

Hellwig, M., J. Degen, and T. Henle. 2010. 3-Deoxygalactosone, a "new" 1,2-dicarbonyl compounds in milk products. *J Agric Food Chem* 58: 10752–10760.

Henle, T. 2005. Protein-bound advanced glycation endproducts (AGEs) as bioactive amino acids in foods. *Amino Acids* 29: 313–322.

Hennessy, A. A., R. P. Ross, R. Devery, and C. Stanton. 2011. The health promoting properties of the conjugated isomers of alpha-linoleic acid. *Lipids* 46: 105–119.

Hidalgo, F. J., and R. Zamora. 2000. Modification of bovine serum albumin structure following reaction with 4,5(*E*)-epoxy-2(*E*)-heptenal. *Chem Res Toxicol* 13: 501–508.

Hidalgo, F. J., and R. Zamora. 2002. Methyl linoleate oxidation in the presence of bovine serum albumin. *J Agric Food Chem* 50: 5463–5467.

Hidalgo, F. J., F. Nogales, and R. Zamora. 2005. Changes produced in the antioxidative activity of phospholipids as a consequence of their oxidation. *J Agric Food Chem* 53: 659–662.

Hovenkamp, E., I. Demonty, J. Plat, D. Lütjohann, R. P. Mensink, and E. A. Trautwein. 2008. Biological effects of oxidized phytosterols: A review of the current knowledge. *Prog Lipid Res* 47: 37–49.

Hsu, D., and V. Zimmer. 2010. Canadian Diabetes Association National Nutrition Committee Technical Review: Advanced glycation end-products in diabetes management. *Can J Diabetes* 34: 136–140.

Izaki, Y., S. Yoshikawa, and M. Uchiyama. 1984. Effect of ingestion of thermally oxidized frying oil on peroxidative criteria in rats. *Lipids* 19: 324–331.

Jeffery, E. H., and M. Araya. 2009. Physiological effects of broccoli consumption. *Phytochem Rev* 8: 283–298.

Jones, P. J. H. 2009. Dietary cholesterol and the risk of cardiovascular disease in patients: A review of the Harvard Egg Study and other data. *Int J Clin Pract* 63: 1–8.

Jung, M. Y., and D. B. Min. 1992. Effects of oxidized α-, γ- and δ-tocopherols on the oxidative stability of purified soybean oil. *Food Chem* 45: 183–187.

Kamal-Eldin, A. 2008. Carotenoids and lipid oxidation reactions. In *Lipid Oxidation Pathways*, vol. 2, eds. A. Kamal-Eldin and D. B. Min, 143–180. Urbana, IL: AOCS Press.

Kamal-Eldin, A., and A. M. Lampi. 2008. Oxidation of cholesterol and phytosterols. In *Lipid Oxidation Pathways*, vol. 2, eds. A. Kamal-Eldin and D. B. Min, 111–126. Urbana, IL: AOCS Press.

Kamal-Eldin, A., H. J. Kim, L. Tavadyan, and D. Min. 2008. Tocopherol concentrations and antioxidant efficacy. In *Lipid Oxidation Pathways*, vol. 2, eds. A. Kamal-Eldin and D. B. Min, 127–141. Urbana, IL: AOCS Press.

Kämmerer, I., R. Ringseis, and K. Eder. 2011. Feeding a thermally oxidised fat inhibits atherosclerotic plaque formation in the aortic root of LDL receptor-deficient mice. *Br J Nutr* 105: 190–199.

Kanner, J. 2007. Dietary advanced lipid oxidation endproducts are risk factors to human health. *Mol Nutr Food Res* 51: 1094–1101.

Kim, Y., K. L. Goodner, J. D. Park, J. Choi, and S. T. Talcott. 2011. Changes in antioxidant phytochemicals and volatile composition of *Camillia sinensis* by oxidation during tea fermentation. *Food Chem* 129: 1331–1342.

Lewis, A. J., and H. S. Bayley. 1995. Amino acid availability. In *Bioavailability of Nutrients for Animals: Amino Acids, Minerals and Vitamins*, eds. C. B. Ammerman, D. H. Baker, and A. J. Lewis, 35–65. San Diego, CA: Academic Press.

Li, H., A. Guo, and H. Wang. 2008. Mechanisms of oxidative browning of wine. *Food Chem* 108: 1–13.

Li, S., C. Schöneich, and R. T. Borchardt. 1995. Chemical instability of protein pharmaceuticals: Mechanisms of oxidation and strategies for stabilization. *Biotechnol Bioeng* 18: 490–500.

Liebler, D. C., and T. D. McClure. 1996. Antioxidant reactions of β-carotene: Identification of carotenoid radical adducts. *Chem Res Toxicol* 9: 8–11.

Liu, J. F., and C. J. Huang. 1996. Dietary oxidized frying oil enhances tissue α-tocopherol depletion and radioisotope tracer excretion in vitamin E-deficient rats. *J Nutr* 126: 2227–2235.

Lu, R., H. X. Dan, R. Q. Wu, W. X. Meng, N. Liu, X. Jin, M. Zhou, X. Zeng, G. Zhou, and Q. M. Chen. 2011. Lycopene: Features and potential significance in the oral cancer and precancerous lesions. *J Oral Pathol Med* 40: 361–368.

Lund, M. N., R. Lametsch, M. S. Hviid, O. N. Jensen, and L. H. Skibsted. 2007. High-oxygen atmosphere packaging influences protein oxidation and tenderness of porcine *longissimus dorsi* during chill storage. *Meat Sci* 77: 295–303.

Lund, M. N., M. Heinonen, C. P. Baron, and M. Estévez. 2011. Protein oxidation in muscle foods: A review. *Mol Nutr Food Res* 55: 83–95.

Mahar, K. P., M. Y. Khuhawar, T. G. Kazi, K. Abbasi, and A. H. Channer. 2010. Quantitative analysis of glyoxal, methyl glyoxal and dimethyl glyoxal from foods, beverages and wines using HPLC and 4-nitro-1,2-phenylenediamine as derivatizing reagent. *Asian J Chem* 22: 6983–6990.

Marangoni, F., and A. Poli. 2010. Phytosterols and cardiovascular health. *Pharmacol Res* 61: 193–199.

Marconett, C. N., S. N. Sundar, K. M. Poindexter, T. R. Stueve, L. F. Bjeldanes, and G. L. Firestone. 2010. Indole-3-carbinol triggers aryl hydrocarbon receptor-dependent estrogen receptor (ER)α protein degradation in breast cancer cells disrupting an ERα-GATA3 transcriptional cross-regulatory loop. *Mol Biol Cell* 21: 1166–1177.

Mayne, S. T. 1996. Beta-carotene, carotenoids, and disease prevention in humans. *FASEB J* 10: 690–701.

McCarty, M. F., J. Barroso-Aranda, and F. Contreras. 2009. The low-methionine content of vegan diets may make methionine restriction feasible as a life extension strategy. *Med Hypotheses* 72: 125–128.

Mills, S., R. P. Ross, C. Hill, G. F. Fitzgerald, and C. Stanton. 2011. Milk intelligence: Mining milk for bioactive substances associated with human health. *Int Dairy J* 21: 377–401.

Mordi, R., J. C. Walton, G. W. Burton, L. Hughes, K. U. Ingold, D. A. Lindsay, and D. J. Moffatt. 1993. Oxidative degradation of beta-carotene and beta-apo-8′-carotenal. *Tetrahedron* 19: 911–928.

Morzel, M., P. Gatellier, T. Sayd, M. Renerre, and E. Laville. 2006. Chemical oxidation decreases proteolytic susceptibility of skeletal muscle myofibrillar proteins. *Meat Sci* 73: 536–543.

Moughan, P. J. 2005. Dietary protein quality in humans—An overview. *J AOAC Int* 88: 874–876.

Nair, K. K., S. Kharb, and D. K. Thompkinson. 2010. Inulin dietary fiber with functional and health attributes. A review. *Food Rev Int* 26: 189–203.

Oliveira, C. M., A. C. S. Ferreira, V. de Freitas, and A. M. S. Silva. 2011. Oxidation mechanisms occurring in wines. *Food Res Int* 44: 1115–1126.

Otaegui-Arrazola, A., M. Menéndez-Carreño, D. Ansorena, and I. Astiasarán. 2010. Oxysterols: A world to explore. *Food Chem Toxicol* 48: 3289–3303.

Ottaway, P. B. 2010. Stability of vitamins during food processing and storage. In *Chemical Deterioration and Physical Instability of Food and Beverages*, eds. L. H. Skibsted, J. Risbo, and M. L. Andersen, 539–560. Cambridge: Woodhead Publishing.

Pajunen, T. I., and A. Kamal-Eldin. 2008. Oxidation of conjugated linoleic acid. In *Lipid Oxidation Pathways*, vol. 2, eds. A. Kamal-Eldin and D. B. Min, 77–110. Urbana, IL: AOCS Press.

Palii, S. S., C. E. Kays, C. Deval, A. Bruhat, P. Fafournoux, and M. S. Kilberg. 2009. Specificity of amino acid regulated gene expression: Analysis of genes subjected to either complete or single amino acid deprivation. *Amino Acids* 37: 79–88.

Powolny, A. A., and S. V. Singh. 2008. Multitargeted prevention and therapy of cancer by diallyl trisulfide and related Allium vegetable-derived organosulfur compounds. *Cancer Lett* 269: 305–314.

Rana, S. V., R. Pal, K. Vaiphei, S. K. Sharma, and R. P. Ola. 2011. Garlic in health and disease. *Nutr Res Rev* 24: 60–71.

Reiber, H. 1972. Photochemical reactions of vitamin B_6 compounds, isolation and properties of products. *Biochim Biophys Acta* 279: 310–315.

Rhoads, J. M., and G. Wu. 2009. Glutamine, arginine, and leucine signaling in the intestine. *Amino Acids* 37: 111–122.

Ried, K., O. R. Frank, and N. P. Stocks. 2010. Aged garlic extract lowers blood pressure in patients with treated but uncontrolled hypertension: A randomized controlled trial. *Maturitas* 67: 144–150.

Rietjens, I. M. C. M., M. G. Boersma, L. de Haan, B. Spenkelink, H. M. Awad, N. H. P. Cnubben, J. J. van Zanden, H. van der Woude, G. M. Alink, and J. H. Koeman. 2002. The pro-oxidant chemistry of the natural antioxidants vitamin C, vitamin E, carotenoids and flavonoids. *Environ Toxicol Pharmacol* 11: 321–333.

Ringseis, R., and K. Eder. 2011. Regulation of genes involved in lipid metabolism by dietary oxidized fat. *Mol Nutr Food Res* 55: 109–121.

Ringseis, R., A. Muschick, and K. Eder. 2007. Dietary oxidized fat prevents ethanol-induced triacylglycerol accumulation and increases expression of PPARα target genes in rat liver. *J Nutr* 137: 77–83.

Rivlin, R. S. 2001. Rivoflavin. In *Present Knowledge in Nutrition*, 8th ed., eds. B. B. Bowman and R. M. Russell, 191–198. Washington, DC: ILSI Press.

Rowe, L. J., K. R. Maddock, S. M. Lonergan, and E. Huff-Lonergan. 2004. Oxidative environments decrease tenderization of beef steaks through inactivation of μ-calpain. *J Anim Sci* 82: 3254–3266.

Ryan, E., F. O. McCarthy, A. R. Maguire, and N. M. O'Brien. 2009. Phytosterol oxidation products: Their formation, occurrence, and biological effects. *Food Rev Int* 25: 157–174.

Sala-Vila, A., and E. Ros. 2011. Mounting evidence that increased consumption of alpha-linolenic acid, the vegetable n–3 fatty acid, may benefit cardiovascular health. *Clin Lipidol* 6: 365–369.

Saidi, B., and J. J. Warthesen. 1983. Influence of pH and light on the kinetics of vitamin B_6 degradation. *J Agric Food Chem* 31: 876–880.

Santé-Lhoutellier, V., L. Aubry, and P. Gatellier. 2007. Effect of oxidation on *in vitro* digestibility of skeletal muscle myofibrillar proteins. *J Agric Food Chem* 55: 5343–5348.

Schaich, K. M. 2008. Co-oxidation of proteins by oxidizing lipids. In *Lipid Oxidation Pathways*, vol. 2, eds. A. Kamal-Eldin and D. B. Min, 181–272. Urbana, IL: AOCS Press.

Schey, K. L., and E. L. Finley. 2000. Identification of peptide oxidation by tandem mass spectrometry. *Acc Chem Res* 33: 299–306.

Schneider, C. 2005. Chemistry and biology of vitamin E. *Mol Nutr Food Res* 49: 7–30.

Shimizu, M., S. Adachi, M. Masuda, O. Kozawa, and H. Moriwaki. 2011. Cancer chemoprevention with green tea catechins by targeting receptor tyrosine kinases. *Mol Nutr Food Res* 55: 832–843.

Smoliga, J. M., J. A. Baur, and H. A. Hausenblas. 2011. Resverastrol and health—A comprehensive review of human clinical trials. *Mol Nutr Food Res* 55: 1129–1141.

Sottero, B., P. Gamba, S. Gargiulo, G. Leonarduzzi, and G. Poli. 2009. Cholesterol oxidation products and disease: An emerging topic of interest in medicinal chemistry. *Curr Med Chem* 16: 685–705.

Soupas, L., L. Juntuned, A. M. Lampi, and V. Piironen. 2004. Effects of sterol structure, temperature, and lipid medium on phytosterol oxidation. *J Agric Food Chem* 52: 6485–6491.

Sparvero, L. J., A. A. Amoscato, P. M. Kochanek, B. R. Pitt, V. E. Kagan, and H. Bayir. 2010. Mass-spectrometry based oxidative lipidomics and lipid imaging: Applications in traumatic brain injury. *J Neurochem* 115: 1322–1336.

Spiteller, G. 2008. Peroxyl radicals are essential reagents in the oxidation steps of the Maillard reaction leading to generation of advanced glycation end products. *Ann N Y Acad Sci* 1126: 128–133.

Suryawan, A., P. M. J. O'Connor, J. A. Bush, H. V. Nguyen, and T. A. Davis. 2009. Differential regulation of protein synthesis by amino acids and insulin in peripheral and visceral tissues of neonatal pigs. *Amino Acids* 37: 97–104.

Tadera, K., M. Arima, and F. Yagi. 1988. Participation of hydroxyl radical in hydroxylation of pyridoxine by ascorbic acid. *Agric Biol Chem* 52: 2359–2360.

Tan, L. C., W. P. Koh, J. M. Yuan, R. Wang, W. L. Au, J. H. Tan, E. K. Tan, and M. C. Yu. 2008. Differential effects of black versus green tea on risk of Parkinson's disease in the Singapore Chinese health study. *Am J Epidemiol* 167: 553–560.

Thornalley, P. J. 2007. Dietary AGEs and ALEs and risk to human health by their interaction with the receptor for advanced glycation endproducts (RAGE)—an introduction. *Mol Nutr Food Res* 51: 1107–1110.

Thornalley, P., S. Wolff, G. Crabbe, and A. Stern. 1984. The autoxidation of glyceraldehydes and other simple monosaccharides under physiological conditions catalyzed by buffer ions. *Biochim Biophys Acta* 797: 276–287.

Törnwall, U. 2010. Pinpointing oxidative modifications in proteins—Recent advances in analytical methods. *Anal Methods* 2: 1638–1650.

Torres, D. P. M., M. D. F. Goncalves, J. A. Teixeira, and L. R. Rodrigues. 2010. Galacto-oligosaccharides: Production, properties, applications, and significance as prebiotics. *Compr Rev Food Sci Food Saf* 9: 438–454.

Turner, R., C. H. McLean, and K. M. Silvers. 2006. Are the health benefits of fish oils limited by products of oxidation? *Nutr Res Rev* 19: 53–62.

Vlassara, H., W. J. Cai, S. Goodman, R. Pyzik, A. Yong, X. Chen, L. Zhu, T. Neade, M. Beeri, J. M. Silverman, L. Ferrucci, L. Tansman, G. E. Striker, and J. Uribarri. 2009. Protection against loss of innate defenses in adulthood by low advanced glycation en products (AGE) intake: Role of the anti-inflammatory AGE receptor-1. *J Clin Endocrinol Metab* 94: 4483–4491.

Wang, X. D., C. Liu, R. T. Bronson, D. E. Smith, N. I. Krinsky, and R. M. Russell. 1999. Retinoid signaling and activator protein-1 expression in ferrets given β-carotene supplements and exposed to tobacco smoke. *J Natl Cancer Inst* 91: 60–66.

Wang, W. W., S. Y. Qiao, and D. F. Li. 2009. Amino acids and gut function. *Amino Acids* 37: 105–110.

Wang, D., R. Xiao, X. Hu, K. Xu, Y. Hou, Y. Zhong, J. Meng, B. Fan, and L. Liu. 2010. Comparative safety evaluation of Chinese Pu-erh green tea extract and Pu-erh black tea extract in wistar rats. *J Agric Food Chem* 58: 1350–1358.

Wang, S., K. A. Meckling, M. F. Marcone, Y. Kakuda, and R. Tsao. 2011a. Can phytochemical antioxidant rich foods act as anti-cancer agents? *Food Res Int* 44: 2545–2554.

Wang, Z. M., B. Zhou, Y. S. Wang, Q. Y. Gong, Q. M. Wang, J. J. Yan, W. Gao, and L. S. Wang. 2011b. Black and green tea consumption and the risk of coronary artery disease: A meta-analysis. *Am J Clin Nutr* 93: 506–515.

Waterhouse, A. L., and V. F. Laurie. 2006. Oxidation of wine phenolics: A critical evaluation and hypotheses. *Am J Enol Viticult* 57: 306–313.

Weber, F., and W. Grosch. 1976. Co-oxidation of a carotenoid by the enzyme lipoxygenase: Influence on the formation of linoleic acid hydroperoxides. *Z Lebensm-Unters-Forsch* 161: 223–230.

White, J. S. 2009. Misconceptions about high-fructose corn syrup: Is it uniquely responsible for obesity, reactive dicarbonyl compounds, and advanced glycation endproducts? *J Nutr* 139: 1219S–1227S.

Woodall, A. A., G. Britton, and M. J. Jackson. 1997. Carotenoids and protection of phospholipids in solution or in liposomes against oxidation by peroxyl radicals: Relationship between carotenoid structure and protective ability. *Biochim Biophys Acta* 1336: 575–586.

Woodcock, E. A., J. J. Warthesen, and T. P. Labuza. 1982. Riboflavin photochemical degradation in pasta measured by high performance liquid chromatography. *J Food Sci* 47: 545–555.

Wu, G. 2009. Amino acids: Metabolism, functions, and nutrition. *Amino Acids* 37: 1–17.

Xu, G., and M. R. Chance. 2007. Hydroxyl radical-mediated modification of proteins as probes for structural proteomics. *Chem Rev* 107: 3514–3543.

Yuan, J. P., J. A. Peng, K. Yin, and J. H. Wang. 2011. Potential health-promoting effects of astaxanthin: A high-value carotenoid mostly from microalgae. *Mol Nutr Food Res* 55: 150–165.

Zamora, R., and F. J. Hidalgo. 2001. Inhibition of proteolysis in oxidized lipid-damaged proteins. *J Agric Food Chem* 49: 6006–6011.

Zamora, R., and F. J. Hidalgo. 2005. Coordinate contribution of lipid oxidation and Maillard reaction to nonenzymatic food browning. *Crit Rev Food Sci Nutr* 45: 49–59.

Zamora, R., M. Alaiz, and F. J. Hidalgo. 1999. Modification of histidine residues by 4,5-epoxy-2-alkenals. *Chem Res Toxicol* 12: 654–660.

Zeisel, S. H., and K. A. da Costa. 2009. Choline: An essential nutrient for public health. *Nutr Rev* 67: 615–623.

9 Natural Antioxidants in Food Systems

Petras Rimantas Venskutonis

CONTENTS

9.1 INTRODUCTION

The title of this chapter contains two key terms: "natural antioxidants" and "food systems." Fifty years ago, Chipault (1962) defined antioxidants in foods as "substances that in small quantities are able to prevent or greatly retard the oxidation of easily oxidisable materials such as fats." Later, Halliwell and Guteridge (1989) suggested another widely used definition covering all oxidizable substrates, lipids, proteins, DNA, and carbohydrates: "any substance that when present in low concentrations compared to those of an oxidisable substrate significantly delays or prevents oxidation of that substance." In food additive regulations, the antioxidant is a substance prolonging food's shelf life by protecting it from oxidation-induced deterioration, such as fat rancidity and color changes. These generalized definitions do not confine antioxidant activity to any specific group of chemical compounds nor do they refer to any particular mechanism of action. The concept of antioxidants has become very broad for the *in vivo* situation, including antioxidant enzymes, iron binding and transport proteins, and other compounds affecting signal transduction and gene expression (Rice-Evans 2004). The complexity of the question—what kind of molecules should be classified as antioxidants for the *in vivo* situation?—has been intensively discussed in the scientific community (Becker et al. 2004). In the case of foods and beverages, this question is not so complicated in so far as antioxidants may be directly related to the protection of specific oxidation substrates or the formation of specific oxidation products for which threshold values may be defined for different products.

Depending on the origin and the method of production, all food components may be divided into natural and synthetic. For the purpose of medicines, a natural product, as defined almost 100 years ago in *Webster's Revised Unabridged Dictionary*, is "a chemical compound or substance produced by a living organism—found in nature that usually has a pharmacological or biological activity for use in pharmaceutical drug discovery and drug design" (a natural product can be considered as such even if it can be prepared by total synthesis). There are no official internationally accepted definitions for the term "natural antioxidant" in relation to food systems. In food additive regulations, the term "natural" is applied to a large group of flavorings, which are classified as natural, nature identical, and artificial. Thus, natural flavorings are defined as "flavoring substances obtained from plant or animal raw materials, by physical, microbiological or enzymatic processes; they can be either used in their natural state or processed for human consumption, but cannot contain any nature-identical or artificial flavouring substances." By applying the same approach to natural antioxidants, they might be defined as "substances (compounds) possessing various types of antioxidant properties and which are produced in living organisms by biochemical pathways, and also are being formed during handling and processing of such organisms after harvesting (plant origin) or post mortem (animal origin) in the course of food production, or obtained from biological origin raw materials by physical, microbiological or enzymatic processes."

Another term included in the chapter title is "food systems." It has usually been conceived of as a set of activities ranging from production through to consumption (the "from farm to fork" concept). The definitions of food systems may also include nutritional aspects; Sobal et al. (1998) defined food system as "the set of operations and processes involved in transforming raw materials into foods and transforming nutrients into health outcomes, all of which functions as a system within biophysical and sociocultural contexts." A broader definition of food systems includes the interactions between and within biogeophysical and human environments determining a set of activities, the activities themselves (from production through to consumption), outcomes of the activities (contributions to food security, environmental security, and social welfare), and other determinants of food security (Ericksen 2007). Consequently, a food system encompasses many important aspects, such as nutrition, food, health, community economic development, and agriculture, and includes all processes and infrastructure involved in feeding a population: growing, harvesting, processing, packaging, transporting, marketing, consumption, and disposal of food and food-related items (Wilkins and Eames-Sheavly n.d.). Food systems are either conventional, operating on economies of scale, or alternative (including organic agriculture, fair-trade, and food localization movements), according to their model of food lifespan from origin to plate (Scrinis 2007). It is also important to note that the character of a food system and the nature of food policy are both changing, as urbanization, technical change, and the industrialization of the food system transform the way food is produced, marketed, and consumed (Maxwell and Slater 2003). For instance, the traditional use of noncultivated vegetables has decreased with the development of agriculture and global supply chains. Such changes may have an impact on individual nutrients and/or their groups, including natural antioxidants, which are present in agricultural crops and foods. Briefly, the concept of a food system is widely used in agriculture, food science, nutrition, and medicine to describe the complex set of activities involved in providing food for sustenance and nutrients for maintaining human health (Sobal et al. 1998).

Considering the fact that a broader definition of a food system together with technological production aspects also includes societal, environmental, and other elements, there is a challenging question about how to link natural antioxidants with all these aspects. It is evident that natural antioxidants, as biologically active and protective food constituents, are integral components in the production of agricultural crops and the processing of foods as well as in nutrition and human health, while other aspects of a food system may also have some indirect associations with the topic of natural antioxidants. Some links between the elements of a food system and natural antioxidants are presented in Figure 9.1. For instance, the potential for competitive and healthy food chains, which may supply foods enriched with natural

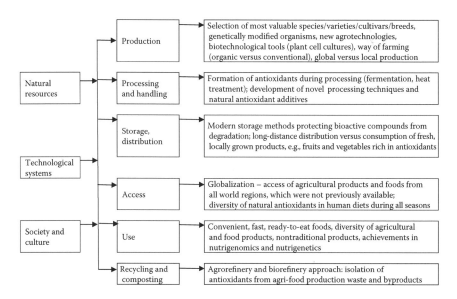

FIGURE 9.1   Elements of food system and their links to natural antioxidants.

dietary antioxidants, of benefit to the countryside was reviewed, emphasizing that agricultural policy liberalization, concern about unhealthy diets, and growing recognition of the importance of sustainable land use have fostered interest in the development of competitive food chains based around products that are beneficial to the rural environment (Traill et al. 2008). Consumers' increasing interest in the relationship between diet and health has become a strong message for food producers to pay more attention to potential health-protecting compounds in new product development and food processing (Van der Sluis et al. 2001). From this point of view, natural antioxidants have become a topical issue for all stakeholders in the agri-food chain, which undergoes remarkable changes resulting from the development and selection of new, more productive agricultural organisms via genetic modifications; modernization of conventional and expansion of organic agricultural practices; development of new technological and handling methods and processes for the food industry; increasing demand for natural, chemical additive-free foods; and rapid development of functional foods and nutraceuticals. All these changes influence agri-food chain elements and compositional characteristics of foods, including the content of such biologically active nutrients as dietary antioxidants. For instance, the number of synthetic antioxidant intervention strategies available for foods is limited and will likely decline as the consumer demand for "all-natural" products increases, causing a clear demand for new antioxidant technologies (Elias et al. 2008). Therefore, the comparison of quality characteristics of produce generated by different food systems, for example, based on conventional or organic agriculture, has become a popular topic for researchers, producers, governmental institutions, health professionals, and consumers.

In terms of nutritional composition, the production of agricultural crops, processing of foods, nutrition, and health are the most important food system components, which are directly linked to various aspects of natural antioxidants, including their diversity, discovery, characterization, application, industrial valorization, impact on human health, etc. Therefore, for the content of this chapter, the term "food system" is restricted to the agri-food production chain, which primarily involves growing and storage of agricultural raw materials and their conversion into concrete food products for human consumption in the course of food processing. The main raw materials for food systems are derived from the biological products, which may be of a plant, animal, marine, or microbial origin. All biological organisms possess their own antioxidant defense systems, consisting of enzymes and various classes' compounds. These natural chemicals comprise a large pool of natural antioxidants, which remain the main sources of antioxidatively active constituents in food systems. The amount of natural antioxidants accumulated in biological systems depends on various factors, such as genetic properties, agrotechnological practices, climate, and others. For instance, because of the demand for more natural and chemical-free food, organic or "ecological" as it is referred to in some countries, agriculture has been rapidly developing in the past few decades. Antioxidatively active compounds are also formed during food processing, which is another important element of a food system; however, antioxidants generated in foods as a result of processing are discussed in another chapter of this book and will not be covered in the present chapter. The content of this chapter is restricted to natural antioxidants present in various agri-food materials and how existing food production systems influence the formation of these compounds in plant- and animal-origin foods. Shortly, a natural antioxidant in a food system shall be understood as an antioxidatively active compound produced in living organisms or in foods during their processing.

The majority of foods are complex systems consisting of organic and inorganic, macro, intermediate, and micro components belonging to various classes of chemicals. Antioxidants are usually minor components in such systems; however, they are naturally present in almost all agri-food materials. During food handling (storage, processing), these components play an important role as protective agents against oxidation of other, major food-system components, particularly unsaturated fats, and in nutrition, they may help to maintain human redox homeostasis as an exogenous compound protecting against the damaging effects of the excessive free radicals, which may occur in living cells under certain conditions. Consequently, natural antioxidants in food systems are playing two key roles: protecting food biomolecules, particularly unsaturated fatty acids containing lipids from oxidation and resulting food deterioration, and supplementing the human body with exogenous substances, which, when necessary, may support its defense system against reactive species. The evaluation of natural antioxidants in foods is a much easier task than the assessment of their possible effects *in vivo*, for example, after consumption by humans. The existing instrumental and analytical methods enable us to assess antioxidant concentrations in foods as well as their effectiveness in preventing oxidation of food components, but measuring the effects of natural dietary antioxidants in a living organism is a much more complex task because of the uncertainties of their fate in the human body, for example, bioavailability, structural changes, optimal effective dosages, and mechanisms of action. Therefore, the question "antioxidants in food: mere myth or magic medicine?"—which was used as a title of a recently published critical review (Berger et al. 2012)—will remain a topical issue in the area of natural antioxidant research, which has been steadily expanding during the last few decades. The scope of antioxidant research may be illustrated by the increasing number of records containing the key terms "natural antioxidant" and "food" in various information databases. For instance, searching the databases SCI-EXPANDED, SSCI, A&HCI, CPCI-S, and CPCI-SSH for the combination of these key words resulted in 2146 records (accessed on August 19, 2012), including 270 review papers. Several reviews on natural food antioxidants of a general nature have been published since 1990, both in the scientific journals (Shahidi 2000; Benzie 2003; Halvorsen et al. 2002; Augustyniak et al. 2010; Brewer 2011) and books (Pratt and Hudson 1990; Schuler 1990; Shahidi 1997; Cuppett et al. 1997; Shi et al. 2001; Wanasundara and Shahidi 2005); however, many more reviews focused on specific groups of agricultural crops, individual species, different types of foods, chemical classes of natural antioxidants, or individual compounds are available in the various literature sources. Some natural antioxidants, their sources, and their formation during food processing are discussed in the other chapters of this book; therefore, this chapter will be restricted to some selected aspects of natural antioxidants in food systems, which have received less coverage in the other parts of this book or other literature sources. The information in this chapter is based mainly on abundant reviews in this scientific area, which have been recently published on various classes of natural antioxidants as well as their sources; therefore, the reader will be redirected to the relevant references to find more comprehensive data on the selected topic in this very broad area, called "natural antioxidants in food systems."

9.2 CLASSIFICATION OF NATURAL ANTIOXIDANTS

The antioxidants in food systems may be classified by using diverse indicators. Depending on the origin and the methods of production, food antioxidants may be synthetic or natural; however, synthetic compounds are beyond the scope of this chapter and will not be discussed. By the mechanisms of performance, the antioxidants are classified into primary and secondary, whereas by their physical properties, they may be water- and lipid-soluble (Wanasundara and Shahidi 2005). From the pharmaceutical perspective, the antioxidants are primarily classified into enzymatic (primary and secondary enzymes) and nonenzymatic (minerals, vitamins, carotenoids, organosulfur compounds, low molecular weight (MW) antioxidants, antioxidant cofactors, and polyphenols) (Venkat Ratnam et al. 2006). Regarding the origin and chemical nature, natural antioxidants most often have been associated with plant secondary metabolites, such as well-known vitamins C and E (ascorbic acid and tocopherols) and numerous plant phytochemicals (phenolic acids, flavonoids, terpenoids, and other chemical classes); however, an increasing number of studies demonstrate that almost all constituents naturally present in agri-food products may possess antioxidant activity. It is not surprising because, fundamentally, the mechanism of antioxidant or radical scavenging actions involves an exchange of electrons/protons, whereas many compounds present in food systems possess functional group(s), which may participate in such molecular processes. Moreover, many biomolecules possess the ability to chelate or reduce the catalysts of oxidation reactions, polyvalent metal ions, and therefore, such biomolecules also may be an important antioxidative factor in a food system. There are many classifications of antioxidants in various literature sources; however, it would be rather difficult to elaborate a comprehensive and exhaustive classifying scheme because of the enormous chemical diversity of natural antioxidants, their properties and mechanisms of action, applications, as well as the sources of origin.

By the mechanism of action, natural antioxidants may be (i) primary chain-breaking compounds; (ii) secondary (or preventive): enzymatic, chelating/sequestering, oxygen adsorbing, and singlet oxygen scavenging; and (iii) multifunctional: depending on the oxidation media, they may act as primary and/or as secondary antioxidants. By the origin and by the way of formation, in some cases, it is convenient to classify natural antioxidants into compounds that are (i) biosynthesized and accumulated in plant-origin agri-food materials, (ii) animal-origin agricultural materials, (iii) marine sources, (iv) produced by microorganisms, and (v) formed during processing of agricultural raw materials (mainly heating and fermentation). By the physical properties, the natural antioxidants may be water- or lipid-soluble and possess both hydrophilic and lipophilic moieties in the molecule. This is a very important characteristic considering lipid-containing food systems, for example, emulsion-type products. Natural antioxidants may be colorless or possess various colors (e.g., anthocyanins); they also may differ in taste or odor, which are important characteristics affecting an overall sensory quality of antioxidant-containing foods.

TABLE 9.1
Examples of Chemical Classes of Natural Antioxidants and Selected Individual Antioxidant Compounds

Antioxidants	Short Characterization
Enzymes: superoxide dismutase, catalase, glutathione peroxidase	SOD catalyzes the transformation of the superoxide radical into hydrogen peroxide; CAT transforms hydrogen peroxide into water and molecular oxygen; GPx reduces lipid peroxides into a stable hydroxyl fatty acid, present in many agri-food materials
Proteins	May act as primary and secondary antioxidants; present in various agri-food sources of animal and plant origin, marine materials, their by-products; an example is potato tuber protein patatin
Protein complexes with other compounds	Binds prooxidative iron ions, demonstrated antioxidant activity in various assay systems; an example is glycoprotein lactoferrin (80 kDa) present in milk (whey) at 20 ± 200 mg/L levels (bovine milk)
Phosphorylated proteins	Metal chelators inhibit metal ions mediated oxidation of phospholipids; an example is that egg yolk phosvitin is the most phosphorylated protein in nature
Peptides	May act as primary and secondary antioxidants; present in various plant and animal origin sources, formed during fermentation, produced by enzymatic hydrolysis with proteinases; examples are carnosine, anserine, common in muscle-type materials
Amino acids	May act as primary and secondary antioxidants; present in various plant and animal origin sources in small amounts, formed during food production by fermentation; an example is histidine, one of the strongest antioxidants among amino acids
PSs	Naturally present in various plant origin sources and obtained by hydrolysis; an example is 120–6300 kDa MW rice bran PSs consisting of Glu:Man:Gal:Rib:Ara at the molar ratio 54.1:10.5:21.7:7.4:6.3
OSs	Naturally present in various plant and marine origin sources and obtained by hydrolysis; an example is 229.21–593.12 Da MW OSs produced from crab chitin by acid hydrolysis
PS complexes with phenolic acids	Present in plant cell walls; examples are feruloyl arabinoxylans (feraxans) in rice and ragi; hydroquinones, substituted by β-$(1 \rightarrow 6)$-linked in wheat germ and bran
Vitamins C, E, A	Perform as radical scavengers, metal chelators, synergists; lipid soluble: tocopherols and tocotrienols and retinol (green leafy vegetables, nuts, seeds, vegetable oils, wheat germ); water soluble: ascorbic and dehydroascorbic acids (present almost in all agri-food sources, high amounts in fruits and vegetables)
Anthocyanins (plant pigments)	Radical scavengers; examples are anthocyanidins: cyanidin, delphinidin, malvinidin, pelarginidin, peonidin, petunidin, their glycosides anthocyanins; present in various plant materials, especially those possessing red-blue colors

(continued)

TABLE 9.1 (Continued)
Examples of Chemical Classes of Natural Antioxidants and Selected
Individual Antioxidant Compounds

Antioxidants	Short Characterization
Lignans	Present in various plant origin sources; examples are pinoresinol, podophyllotoxin, steganacin, syringaresinol, sesamin, lariciresinol, secoisolariciresinol, matairesinol
Lignin	A natural phenolic polymer, mostly synthesized by radical coupling of three hydroxypropanoids: coumaryl, coniferyl, and sinapyl alcohols
Phenolic acids, their esters, oligomeric constituents	Effective radical scavengers, may act as secondary antioxidants; examples are chlorogenic, cinnamic, ferulic, gallic, ellagic, chicoric, rosmarinic, salicylic, caffeic (hydrocinnamic); present in various plant-origin materials
Hydrolyzable tannins	Formed when ellagic acid esterifies and binds with the hydroxyl group of a polyol carbohydrate, such as glucose; examples are ellagitannins, present in raspberries
Rosmarinic acid	An ester of caffeic acid with 3,4-dihydroxyphenyl lactic acid, very strong radical scavenger; present in many Lamiaceae herbs, lemon balm, rosemary, oregano, sage, thyme
Flavonoids, their derivatives, oligomeric constituents	Effective radical scavengers, may act as secondary antioxidants; present in various plant-origin materials; high amounts in berries, fruits, vegetables, herbs, tea
Flavones	Examples are apigenin, luteolin, tangeritin
Flavonols	Examples are qurcetin, myricetin, kaempferol, isorhamnetin
Flavanones	Examples are hesperitin, naringenin, eriodictyol
Flavonols, their polymers	Examples are catechin, gallocatechin, gallate esters; epicatechin, epigallocatechin, and their gallate esters; theaflavin and its galate esters, thearubigins
Isoflavones	Natural phytoestrogens, present in high concentrations in soya, flax seed; examples are daidzein, genistein, glycitein
Condensed tannins	Polymers formed by the condensation of flavans (proanthocyanidins, prodelphinidins); examples are polyflavonoid tannins, catechol-type tannins, nonhydrolyzable tannins or flavolans
Simple volatile phenols	Frequently present in herbs and spices as flavor compounds; examples are vanillin, thymol, eugenol
Various nonflavonoid phenolics	Examples: curcumin possessing several functional groups, the aromatic ring systems, which are phenols, are connected by two α,β-unsaturated carbonyl groups, present in popular Indian spice turmeric; mangostin, a natural xanthonoid, isolated from various parts of the mangosteen tree (*Garcinia mangostana*)
Carotenoids: carotenes (hydrocarbons) and xanthophylls (oxygenated compounds)	Electron donors, radical and singlet oxygen scavengers, may react with other ROS because of conjugated double bonds and hydroxyl groups in xanthophylls; examples are α-, β-carotenes, lycopene; astaxanthin, lutein, canthaxanthin, zeaxanthin; present in many plant sources, eggs

(continued)

TABLE 9.1 (Continued)
Examples of Chemical Classes of Natural Antioxidants and Selected Individual Antioxidant Compounds

Antioxidants	Short Characterization
Coumarines	Benzopyranone chemical class compounds, found in many plants; examples are 5,8-dihydroxycoumarin from sweet grass (*Hierochloe odorata*), a very strong radical scavenger and lipid oxidation inhibitor
Stilbenoids	Strong radical scavengers; examples are resveratrol found in grapes and wine, pterostilbene, a phytoalexin found in blueberries and grapes
Terpenoids	A large and diverse class of naturally occurring compounds similar to terpenes, derived from 5-C isoprene units assembled and modified in thousands of ways; present in most of the plants
Steviol glycosides	Diterpenes, isolated from *Stevia rebaudiana* and identified as stevioside, steviolbioside, rebaudioside A, B, C, D, E, F and dulcoside; used as natural sweeteners
Phosphates (di-, tri-, oligo-)	Component of biological membranes and can be obtained from a variety of readily available sources, such as egg yolk or soy beans; examples are phosphatidylcholine, phosphatidylethanolamine
Biothiols	Glutathione (L-glutamyl-L-cysteinyl glycine), N-acetylcysteine, captopril, cysteine, and γ-glutamyl cysteine; present in asparagus, spinach, green beans, red peppers
Thiosulfinates	Allicin, glutamylcysteinyl glycine, and other sulfur compounds; high amounts in *Allium* species onions, leeks, garlic
Vitamin cofactors and minerals	Coenzyme Q10 (ubiquinone, ubiquinol found in foods from less than 1 to more than 50 mg/kg), manganese (when in its +2 valence state as part of the enzyme MnSOD); iodide, selenium (as selenocysteine in glutathione peroxidase and in thyroxine deiodase)
Betalains	Red and yellow indole-derived pigments; include powerful antioxidant pigments, such as those found in beets (betanin)
Phlorotannins	A type of tannins found in brown algae; eckol, phlorofucofuroeckol A, dieckol, 8,8′-bieckol; inhibited phospholipid peroxidation in a liposome system; effectively scavenge radicals
Squalene	Antioxidant branched hydrocarbon with six double bonds; present in shark-liver oil, amaranth seed, rice bran, wheat germ, and olives
CLAs	Isomers of linoleic acid containing the conjugated double bonds with only one single bond between them; found mainly in the meat and dairy products
Oryzanols (γ-oryzanol)	Phytosteryl ferulate mixture extracted from rice bran oil with a wide spectrum of biological activities in particular, antioxidant effects; in rice bran oil may be present at around 2% of crude oil content
Oleuropein and related compounds	Tyrosol esters of elenolic acid that are further hydroxylated and glycosylated; present in olive leaf together with other closely related compounds, such as 10-hydroxyoleuropein, ligstroside, and 10-hydroxyligstroside

(*continued*)

TABLE 9.1 (Continued)

Examples of Chemical Classes of Natural Antioxidants and Selected Individual Antioxidant Compounds

Antioxidants	Short Characterization
Alkylresorcinols	A class of phenolic lipids exhibiting antioxidant properties; examples are 1,3-dihydroxy-5-n-alkylbenzenes, known as 5-alkylresorcinols; found in cereals, wheat, rye bran, germ
Saponins	Amphipathic glycosides grouped by their composition of one or more hydrophilic glycoside moieties combined with a lipophilic triterpene; found in particular abundance in various plant species, legumes, spinach
Hydroquinones, substituted by β-1,6-linked OSs	4-Hydroxy-3-methoxyphenyl β-D-glucopyranosyl-(1→6)-β-D-glucopyranosyl-(1→6)-β-D-glucopyranoside present in wheat germ (>6 g/kg) and bran
Avenanthramides	Oat phytoalexins; exist predominantly in the groats of oat seeds; inhibited oxygen consumption in a linoleic acid system 3- to 9-fold stronger than caffeic acid
Dehydroferulates and their oligomers	Are mainly found in cereal grains and their abundance is more prominent in the insoluble bound fraction
Phytic acid	Inositol hexaphosphate; present in nuts, seeds, and grains
Maillard reaction products (melanoidins)	Produced in all proteinaceous thermally produced foods; demonstrated *in vitro* antioxidant protective effects on lipids, metal chelating capacity, radical-scavenging activity
Carnosol and carnosic acid	Benzenediol abietane diterpenes; abundant in rosemary and common (dried leaves of rosemary or sage contain 1.5%–2.5% carnosic acid)
Capsaicin	8-Methyl-*N*-vanillyl-6-nonenamide, the active component of chile peppers
Citric acid, oxalic acid	Metal chelators, antioxidant synergists; present in various fruits and vegetables
R-α-Lipoic acid	(*R*)-5-(1,2-dithiolan-3-yl) pentanoic acid; found in almost all foods, but slightly more so in kidney, heart, liver, spinach, broccoli, and yeast extract
Hormone melatonin	N-acetyl-3-(2-aminoethyl)-5-methoxyindole and its major metabolite, *N*1-acetyl-*N*2-formyl-5-methoxykynuramine; many of the organs of higher plants (leaves, fruits and seeds), from several picograms to nanograms per gram to 80 μg/g, or even 10 mg/g tissue

The structures of natural antioxidants fall into many chemical classes. They may be macromolecules (plant and animal biopolymers—proteins, polysaccharides (PSs), complex macromolecules—glycoproteins, phosphorylated proteins, complexes of PSs with phenolic acids); intermediate-size molecules—oligomers (peptides, oligosaccharides [OSs], proanthocyanidines, tanins, lignans); smaller-size, nonpolymeric molecules (amino acids, phenolic acids, flavonoids, terpenoids, thiols, carotenoids, and others); and complex molecules (esters of carbohydrates and phenolic compounds, glycosides, bound to complex biological matrices, cell walls). The examples of natural antioxidants belonging to various chemical classes are given in Table 9.1.

Most of these compound classes, subclasses, and even individual compounds were comprehensively reviewed, some of them several times. Research data are regularly updated, and during the last few years, reviews were published on dietary phenolics (Balasundram et al. 2006; Crozier et al. 2009); anthocyanins (Castaneda-Ovando et al. 2009; Bueno et al. 2012a,b); carotenoids (Kiokias and Gordon 2004; Jaswir et al. 2011) and their antioxidant function (Jauregui et al. 2011); antioxidant vitamins (Nuñez-Cordoba and Martinez-Gonzalez 2011); betalains (Azeredo 2010; Pavokovic and Krsnik-Rasol 2011); coenzyme Q10 contents in foods and fortification strategies (Pravst et al. 2010); ferulic acid (Zhao and Moghadasian 2008); flavonoids (Es-Safi et al. 2007); antioxidant activity of proteins and peptides (Elias et al. 2008); antioxidant peptidic hydrolysates from muscle protein sources and by-products (Di Bernardini et al. 2011); antioxidant peptides from marine processing waste and shellfish (Harnedy and FitzGerald 2012); meat and fish (Ryan et al. 2011); production, assessment, and potential applications of food-derived peptidic antioxidants (Samaranayaka and Li-Chan 2011); antioxidative peptides from food proteins (Sarmadi and Ismail 2010); bioactive peptides in milk and their biological and health implications (Xu 1998); antioxidative peptides from milk proteins (Pihlanto 2006); production, assessment, and applications of fish-derived antioxidants and antimicrobials (Najafian and Babji 2012); bioactives from sea cucumbers (Bihel and Birlouez-Aragon 1998; Bordbar et al. 2011); natural antioxidants and their effects on oxidative status, odor, and quality of fresh beef (Descalzo and Sancho 2008); antioxidant activities of non enzymatic browning reaction products (Lee and Shibamoto 2002); antioxidants from spices and herbs (Nakatani 1997), and *in vitro* activity of vitamins, flavonoids, and natural phenolic antioxidants against the oxidative deterioration of oil-based systems (Kiokias et al. 2008).

9.3 AMINO ACIDS, PEPTIDES, AND PROTEINS

9.3.1 GENERAL ASPECTS

Proteins are the most important biopolymers in food systems supplying human organisms with energy and biologically essential biochemical building materials. The ability of proteins to inhibit lipid oxidation also makes them an important component of the antioxidant defense of biological tissues from which foods are produced. Therefore, it may be possible to increase the oxidative stability of a food by protecting endogenous antioxidant enzymes, by enhancing the activity of proteins found naturally in foods by altering the protein structure, by introducing antioxidant proteins by genetic engineering, or through the use of proteins or peptides with antioxidant activity as food additives (Elias et al. 2008). Smaller amino acid-based polymeric and oligomeric structures, peptides, as well as free amino acids are also present in protein-containing agri-food materials; however, their content in most of them is comparatively low except for in some products, particularly those that are produced by using fermentation and ripening processes. Although proteins, peptides, and amino acids naturally present in food systems until now have not been regarded as natural antioxidants that are as important as plant polyphenolics, tocopherols, or ascorbic acid, their antioxidant activities were discovered a long time ago, for example, amino acids and peptides have been known as typical metal chelators, amino acids were found to exhibit a mild antioxidant effect in nonaqueous media, etc. Proteins are present in the majority of agri-food sources and may serve as a source of antioxidatively active peptides produced by the hydrolysis of animal-, plant-, and marine-origin raw materials and their processing by-products and waste. Exploring the advantage of protein's antioxidant properties, manufacturers could have an added tool to improve the oxidative stability of foods. However, proteins may impact food texture (through gelation and viscosity enhancement), color (through light scattering and formation of Maillard browning products), and flavor (as flavor reactants and bitter compounds); therefore, the use of proteins to inhibit lipid oxidation in some cases might be limited. The production of peptides through hydrolytic reactions seems to be the most promising technique to form protein-derived antioxidants because the peptides, as a rule, exhibit substantially higher antioxidant activity than the intact proteins (Elias et al. 2008). There were many attempts to use antioxidatively active protein sources, specific proteins, protein hydrolysates, and/or peptides in food systems. For instance, porcine blood plasma containing such antioxidant proteins as serum albumin and transferrin retarded the formation of thiobarbituric acid reactive substances (TBARS) in both salted ground pork and cooked ground beef; whey protein concentrate (WPC) exerted antioxidative effects in cooked beef and inhibited lipid oxidation in oil-in-water emulsions; whey and soy (more effective) proteins inhibited lipid oxidation in cooked pork patties; soy protein inhibited the oxidation of ethyl esters of eicosapentaenoic acid dried in a maltodextrin-stabilized, freeze-dried emulsion powder system; whey, casein, soy, and egg yolk hydrolysates inhibited lipid oxidation in beef, pork, and tuna (Elias et al. 2008 and references therein). Proteins and peptides can potentially act as multifunctional antioxidants that can inhibit several different lipid oxidation pathways, by inactivating reactive oxygen species, scavenging free radicals, chelating prooxidative transition metals, reducing hydroperoxides, enzymatically eliminating specific oxidants, and altering the physical properties of food systems in a way that separates reactive species (Elias et al. 2008).

Antioxidant properties of amino acids were reported in the early 1970s when it was determined that 12 amino acids present in the water phase of herring exhibited antioxidant activity in an emulsion of herring oil and linoleic acid model system with histidine and tryptophan being the strongest antioxidants in these assays, whereas proline and lysine were also found to be active in bulk oils (Shahidi 1997 and references therein). A large number of characterized antioxidatively active peptides usually contain 3–20 amino acid residues, whereas their activities are based on the amino acid composition and sequence. These short chains of amino acids are inactive within the sequence of the parent protein but can be released during gastrointestinal digestion, food processing, or fermentation. Amino acids and peptides are found in abundance in protein hydrolysates, and because the antioxidant effect of peptides was first reported more than 50 years ago (Marcuse 1960), numerous studies have investigated protein hydrolysates and peptide antioxidant properties isolated from plant, animal, marine, and other sources, such as rice bran, sunflower protein, alfalfa leaf protein, quinoa seed protein, buckwheat protein, casein, egg-yolk protein, mackerel muscle protein, squid skin gelatine, fish skin gelatine, bovine skin gelatine, porcine myofibrillar proteins, tuna backbone, tuna cooking juice, aquatic by-products, etc. (Sarmadi and Ismail 2010; Gómez-Guillén et al. 2011; Najafian and

Babji 2012). An increasing interest in food-derived antioxidant peptides encouraged rapid expansion of investigations in this area, the results of which were reviewed in a number of articles, most of them published during the last few years. These include the reviews of a general nature, as antioxidative peptides from food proteins (Sarmadi and Ismail 2010), production, assessment, and potential applications of food-derived peptidic antioxidants (Samaranayaka and Li-Chan 2011), and antioxidant activity of proteins and peptides (Elias et al. 2008), as well as the reviews more focused on specified protein sources, such as fish-derived antioxidant peptides (Najafian and Babji 2012), antioxidative peptides derived from milk proteins (Pihlanto 2006), antioxidant and antimicrobial peptidic hydrolysates from muscle protein sources and their by-products (Di Bernardini et al. 2011), and antioxidative factors in milk (Lindmark-Månsson and Åkesson 2000). In addition, general reviews on bioactive peptides, although mainly focused on antihypertensive, immunomodulatory, and other bioactivities, also include information on their antioxidative properties (Xu 1998; Kitts 2005; Hartmann and Meisel 2007; Haque et al. 2008; Shahidi and Zhong 2008; Hernández-Ledesma et al. 2008, 2010; Korhonen 2009; Ryan et al. 2011; Harnedy and FitzGerald 2012; Walther and Sieber 2012).

The presence of histidine in the chain of antioxidatively active peptides was observed a long time ago, and it was acknowledged as an important factor in the antioxidant properties of peptides. For instance, tripeptide GHG produced remarkably stronger complexes with copper than GGG. GGH and β-AH inhibited the antioxidation of egg yolk phosphatidylcholine both in the presence of copper and in the photosensitized oxidation; it was present in the fraction of antioxidative peptides from soy 7S protein, egg white albumin hydrolysates, and many other peptides (Shahidi 1997 and references therein). Histidine-containing hydrophilic dipeptides carnosine (β-alanyl-L-histidine), anserine (β-alanyl-L-1-methylhistidine), and homocarnosine (γ-aminobutyrylhistidine) (Figure 9.2), which are found in relatively high amounts in muscles, were proved to be effective antioxidants a long time ago. They perform both as primary and secondary antioxidants by scavenging free radicals and singlet oxygen and by chelating metals. Antioxidant activity of carnosine, which is commonly present in mammalian tissue and, in particular, in skeletal muscle cells, as well as carnosine-related antioxidants were extensively studied, and the results were reviewed (Decker et al. 1997; Guiotto et al. 2005). It was suggested that aromatic acids (Y, H, W, F) may convert radicals to stable molecules by donating an electron while keeping their own stability via resonance structure. In addition, hydrophobic amino acids may improve the radical-scavenging properties of the amino acid

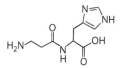

Carnosine: (2S)-2-[(3-Amino-1-oxopropyl)amino]-3-(3H-imidazol-4-yl)propanoic acid

Anserine: (2S)-2-[(3-Amino-1-oxopropyl)amino]-3-(3-methyl-4-imidazolyl)propanoic acid

Homocarnosine: N-(4-Amino-1-oxobutiryl) histidine

FIGURE 9.2 Structures of some antioxidatively active dipeptides.

TABLE 9.2
Characterization of Selected Antioxidant Proteins, Peptides, and Amino Acids from Different Sources (TE = Trolox Equivalents)

Product, Source	Characterization, Antioxidant Properties	References
Amino acids present in protein hydrolysates, muscle foods	Y, C, W, A, F; inhibited photooxidation of ascorbic acid, scavenged radicals; W > H > G ~ M	Jung et al. 1995; Pihlanto 2006; Pazos et al. 2006
Muscle dipeptides carnosine, anserine, and homocarnosine from muscle sources	Hydrophilic dipeptides contained H; primary and secondary antioxidants; scavenged free radicals and singlet oxygen; chelated metals, quenched active oxygen, were antioxidants in linoleic acid system	Decker et al. 1997; Guiotto et al. 2005
Peptides (hydrolysate of porcine myofibrillar proteins, soy peptides)	Contain H; chelated metal ions, quenched active oxygen, scavenged DPPH·, HO· radicals, were antioxidants in linoleic acid system	Pihlanto 2006
WPC and α-lactoglobulin from milk	The antioxidant activities of WPC and α-La were 0.96 and 1.12 mmol TE/mg hydrolyzed protein, respectively	Tavares et al. 2011 and references therein
Buttermilk solids	Sequestered ferrous and ferric ions; scavenged Fenton-induced HO· radicals, protected against lipid peroxidation	Wong and Kitts 2003
Albumin, β-lactoglobulin, lactoferrin	Bovine milk proteins; reduced free radicals; scavenged oxygen radical	Pazos et al. 2006; Elias et al. 2008
Serum albumin from whey	Protein consisting of 582 amino acids; protected lipids against phenolic induced oxidation	Elias et al. 2008
Hydrolysates of α-lactalbumin and β-lactoglobulin A	Bovine whey proteins; possessed antioxidant activity in ORAC assay with the values of 2.315 and 2.151 μmol of TE/mg of protein	Hernández-Ledesma et al. 2005
Peptide from β-lactoglobulin hydrolysate	WYSLAMAASDI amino acids: scavenged radicals (2.62 μmol TE/μmol peptide)	Hernández-Ledesma et al. 2005
Phosphorylated caseins	Milk; chelated transition metals in food emulsions	Pihlanto 2006
Caseins; α-, β-, and κ-caseins	Milk; inhibited lypoxygenase-catalyzed lipid autooxidation, inhibited Fe-induced peroxidation of arachidonic acid	Laakso 1984; Cervato et al. 1999
Hydrolysate of κ-casein	Possessed antioxidant activity in ORAC assay with the value of 7.07 μmol TE/mg protein	Tavares et al. 2011 and references therein
α-La Corolase PP hydrolysate	Possessed antioxidant activity in ORAC assay with the value of 2.95 μmol TE/mg protein	Tavares et al. 2011 and references therein

(continued)

TABLE 9.2 (Continued)

Characterization of Selected Antioxidant Proteins, Peptides, and Amino Acids from Different Sources (TE = Trolox Equivalents)

Product, Source	Characterization, Antioxidant Properties	References
κ-Casein derived peptide	Milk fermented with *Lactobacillus delbrueckii* ssp. *Bulgaricus;* scavenged DPPH	Kudoh et al. 2001
Casein phosphopeptides (CPP) derived from spray-dried whole tryptic digests of bovine casein	Unidentified peptides < 6 KDa; sequestered Fe^{2+}; suppressed Fenton reaction-induced deoxyribose oxidation; reduced AAPH- and Fe^{2+}-induced liposomal peroxidation; scavenged $ABTS^{\cdot+}$ radical	Kitts 2005 and references therein
Glycoprotein lactoferrin	Milk (whey) 80 kDa at 20 ± 200 mg/L levels in bovine milk; bind prooxidative Fe ions, inhibited the oxidation of ascorbic acid and tryptophan, tested in other model systems	Lindmark-Månsson and Åkesson 2000 and references therein
Proteins: transferrin, ovotransferrin (conalbumin), lactoferrin, and ferritin	Blood plasma serum, eggs, milk; control iron reactivity by binding iron in its less active ferric state and by sterically hindering metal-peroxide interactions	Elias et al. 2008 and references therein
Porcine blood plasma containing albumin and transferrin	Possessed iron binding capacity; additive retarded the formation of TBARS in salted ground pork and cooked ground beef	Elias et al. 2008 and references therein
Egg yolk phosvitin	Phosphorylated protein; chelated metals, inhibited Fe^{2+} and Cu^{2+} mediated oxidation of phospholipids	Samaraweera et al. 2011
Peptide of hen egg white lysozyme hydrolyzed with papain, trypsin	NTDGSTDYGILQINSR, 1753.98 ± 0.5 Da; scavenged $DPPH^{\cdot}$, $ABTS^{\cdot+}$, chelated metal ions, inhibited lipid peroxidation; EC_{50} = 1.21 ± 0.051 ($DPPH^{\cdot}$) and 1.35 ± 0.065 mg/mL (ferrous ion chelating); 2.24 µmol TE/mg protein in $ABTS^{\cdot+}$ scavenging assay	Memarpoor-Yazdi et al. 2012
Zein hydrolysate	Up to 6.5% free amino acids, peptides < 500 Da; chelated and scavenged radicals	Adapted from Sarmadi and Ismail 2010
Peptide from frog skin	LEELEEELEGCE; inhibited lipid oxidation, scavenged $DPPH^{\cdot}$, $O_2^{\cdot-}$ and peroxyl radicals	Adapted from Sarmadi and Ismail 2010
WSPs from broad beans, *Vicia faba*	Two fractions (70 kDa and 28 kDa) with small amounts of sulfhydryl groups; scavenged $O_2^{\cdot-}$, other free radicals and H_2O_2; inactivated ROS, chelated prooxidative metals, reduced hydroperoxides, altered the physical properties of food systems	Okada and Okada 1998; Elias et al. 2008; Kitts and Weiler 2003

(continued)

TABLE 9.2 (Continued)

Characterization of Selected Antioxidant Proteins, Peptides, and Amino Acids from Different Sources (TE = Trolox Equivalents)

Product, Source	Characterization, Antioxidant Properties	References
Protein isolates from mature stored, immature, and sprouted potato tubers and by-products	Scavenged ABTS[+]: IC_{50} μg/mL of dm = 12–815 (three for Trolox); active in TRAP assay; the potato liquid alcalase hydrolysate (strongest) = 0.48 g dry matter = 1 mmol TE in TRAP method	Pihlanto et al. 2008
Potato tuber storage protein patatin and its hydrolysates	A glycoprotein 45 kDa; scavenged DPPH[•], inhibited low-density lipoprotein peroxidation, protected against HO[•]-mediated DNA damages and peroxynitrite-mediated dihydrorhodamine 123 oxidations; purified peptides inhibited linoleic acid oxidation in β-carotene decolorization assay, ferric thiocyanate assay system, repressed lipid oxidation in the erythrocyte membrane ghost assay system	Kudoh et al. 2003; Liu et al. 2003
Protein hydrolysates of defatted rapeseed meal and fractionated peptides	Strongly inhibited lipid oxidation in a liposomal model; IC_{50} values from 0.002 to 0.056 mg protein/mL	Mäkinen et al. 2012
Chickpea protein hydrolysate peptide	NRYHQ; quenched DPPH[•], O_2^- and HO[•] radicals; chelated Cu^{2+} and Fe^{2+}	Zhang, T. et al. 2011
Proteolytic digests of a soybean protein β-conglycinin	Six peptides with 5–14 amino acids; the smallest one LLPHH; inhibited linoleic acid peroxidation; antioxidant activity was more dependent on HH segment	Chen et al. 1995
Soy protein fractions	<10 kDa; possessed antioxidant activity in emulsions and reducing power, scavenged radicals	Adapted from Sarmadi and Ismail 2010
Rice endosperm protein	FRDEHKK and KHDRGDEF: inhibited autooxidation, scavenged DPPH[•], O_2^- and HO[•] radicals	Adapted from Sarmadi and Ismail 2010
Peanut kernel protein	3–5 kDa; inhibited LDL oxidation, scavenged DPPH[•], chelated metals, possessed reducing power	Adapted from Sarmadi and Ismail 2010
Peanut protein	Inhibited linoleic acid autoxidation and liver lipid oxidation, scavenged radicals, possessed reducing power	Adapted from Sarmadi and Ismail 2010
Sunflower protein hydrolysate	Enriched with His, Arg; chelated copper	Adapted from Sarmadi and Ismail 2010
Alfalfa leaf protein	<1 kDa; possessed reducing power, chelated and scavenged radicals	Adapted from Sarmadi and Ismail 2010

(continued)

TABLE 9.2 (Continued)
Characterization of Selected Antioxidant Proteins, Peptides, and Amino Acids from Different Sources (TE = Trolox Equivalents)

Product, Source	Characterization, Antioxidant Properties	References
Corn gluten meal	500–1500 Da, 41.12 hydrophobic amino acids; inhibited lipid peroxidation, possessed reducing power, scavenged radicals	Adapted from Sarmadi and Ismail 2010
Algae protein waste	VECYGPNRPQF; scavenged peroxyl, DPPH', O_2^- and HO' radicals, protected DNA and cellular damage	Adapted from Sarmadi and Ismail 2010
Yam ichyoimo tubers	Inhibited linoleic acid autoxidation, scavenged radicals	Adapted from Sarmadi and Ismail 2010

Note: One-letter abbreviations of amino acids: A = alanine; C = cysteine; D = asparagic acid; E = glutamic acid; F = phenylalanine; G = glycine; H = histidine; I = isoleucine; K = lysine; L = leucine; M = methionine; N = asparagine; P = proline; Q = glutamine; R = arginine; S = serine; T = threonine; V = valine; W = tryptophan; Y = tyrosine.

residues by enhancing the solubility of peptide in lipid and facilitating the accessibility to hydrophobic radical species and to hydrophobic polyunsaturated fatty acids. Glycine may act as a hydrogen donor, and carboxyl and amino groups in the side chains of acidic and basic amino acids may perform as metal ion chelators and hydrogen donors, whereas the cysteine SH group may scavenge radicals, thus protecting the tissue from oxidative stress and improving the glutathione activity (Sarmadi and Ismail 2010 and references therein). Antioxidatively active biopeptides obtained from various dietary proteins after enzymatic hydrolysis also were effective against enzymatic and nonenzymatic peroxidation of lipids and essential fatty acids as free radical scavengers and metal ion chelators and in adduct formation (Pihlanto 2006 and references therein). The examples of the selected proteins, peptides, and amino acids and their main characteristics are presented in Table 9.2, whereas different sources of antioxidant peptides are shortly discussed in the next subsections.

9.3.2 Marine Origin Sources

Marine sources, other than traditionally used products, such as fish and crustaceans, have become very promising novel sources for human nutrition, including the production of biologically active ingredients all over the world and, in particular, in Asian countries. Fish processing also generates an enormous volume of waste annually; therefore, waste-derived peptides may be considered as a promising source of natural antioxidants for food and nutraceutical applications. Some such wastes are rich in proteins and are good sources of protein-based antioxidants, which may be produced by enzymatic hydrolysis and other processes, whereas in fermented marine food products, such as blue mussel and oyster sauces, enzymatic hydrolysis has already been done by microorganisms, and bioactive peptides can be purified from such products without further hydrolysis. Marine processing by-products also contain bioactive peptides with valuable functional properties (Ngo et al. 2011 and references therein). A number of antioxidatively active peptides consisting of 5–14 amino acid sequences were isolated from marine products, and these findings were comprehensively reviewed (Zhang et al. 2012). These peptides were present in diverse marine sources, such as yellowfin sole (RPDFPLEPPY), horse mackerel (NHRYDR), sardinelle (GALAAH), croaker (GNRGFACRHA), conger eel (LGLNGDDVN), rotifer (LLGPGLTNHA), oyster (LKEELEDLLEKEE), jumbo squid (FDSGPAGVL), blue mussel (FGHPY), microalgae (VECYGPNRPEF), and tuna (VKAGFAWTANEELS) (Zhang et al. 2012 and references therein).

Effective antioxidant peptides may be produced from alternative sources, such as collagen and gelatin, by using various enzymes. A commercial protease alcalase isolated from a microbial source was recognized as one of the most effective in gelatine or collagen hydrolysis because of its broad specificity as well as the high degree of hydrolysis that can be achieved in a relatively short time under moderate conditions (Gómez-Guillén et al. 2011 and references therein). Strong antioxidant activity exhibited hydrolysates with low average MW obtained from the skin gelatine of Alaska pollack, squid *Todarodes pacificus*, and giant squid. Collagen and gelatine peptides are rich in the residues of G, A, P, Hyp, Glx, and Asx but poor in M, C, H, and Y; they usually have repeated unique GPHyp sequences in their structure, and the observed antioxidative properties have presumably been associated with this unique amino acid composition (Gómez-Guillén et al. 2011 and references therein). These findings demonstrate that His might not be a structural prerequisite for the strong antioxidant activity of peptides. According to some studies, gelatin peptides could inhibit lipid peroxidation more efficiently than antioxidative peptides derived from many other protein sources. In addition, it was reported that collagen and gelatin antioxidative peptides may protect living cells against free radical-mediated oxidative damage.

9.3.3 ANIMAL ORIGIN SOURCES

Proteins are the most important component of animal-origin raw materials, particularly milk and muscle-based products. Milk proteins, consisting of 30–35 g/L of milk, are well documented as versatile food ingredients that have functional and nutritional properties and therefore are recognized as an exceptional biomaterial and a very good source of natural antioxidants and other bioactive compounds. Various native milk protein components possess antioxidant activity in their natural form; however, milk peptides derived from diverse and unique milk proteins during digestion in the gut, fermentation processes in the course of production of various dairy products, as well as their fractions obtained by intentional hydrolysis usually are stronger antioxidant agents. Native milk proteins, such as bovine serum albumin, β-lactoglobulin (β-La), and lactoferrin, were shown to inhibit radical formation from the Fe(II)/CumOOH system, lactoferrin being the most efficient (Pazos et al. 2006).

Bovine WPC, α-lactalbumin (α-La), and caseinomacropeptide (CMP) were used to produce hydrolysates by aqueous extracts of *Cynara cardunculus*. The antioxidant activities of bovine WPC and α-La were 0.96 ± 0.08 and 1.12 ± 0.13 μmol TE/mg hydrolyzed protein, respectively, and although it was higher than that of CMP hydrolysates, none of them possessed any significant antioxidant activity with other milk protein hydrolysates, which were used as a reference in this study, for example, a pepsin-mediated hydrolysate of κ-casein (κ-CN) with an ORAC value of 7.07 μmol TE/mg protein or an α-La Corolase PP hydrolysate with an ORAC value of 2.95 μmol TE/mg protein (Tavares et al. 2011 and references therein). Antioxidant activity has been found specifically in whey proteins; the underlying mechanism of action may be scavenging radicals via Tyr and Cys amino acid residues or chelation of transition metals (Pihlanto 2006).

Milk proteins may act both as primary and secondary antioxidants as it was shown for casein phosphopeptides (CPPs), which may directly scavenge radicals and sequester prooxidants. Phosphoseryl residues in CPP play an important role by catalyzing iron oxidation from the ferrous to the ferric state and thereby forming a highly stable iron-phosphoprotein complex; CPPs that bind up to 4 mM of ferrous iron protected soybean (phosphatidylcholine) liposomes from oxidation initiated by the addition of such ions or peroxyl free radicals, as was demonstrated by the reduced formation of TBARS in peroxyl radical treated phosphatidylcholine liposomes exposed to casein hydrolysates, and a CPP mixture. CPPs are effective at lowering ferrous-induced oxidation in liposomes over a wide range of concentrations; however, prooxidant activity of a CPP mixture in ferric-ascorbate redox cycling assays was observed using lecithin liposomes when the CPP concentration exceeded the concentration of iron (Kitts 2005 and references therein). CPPs exhibited direct ABTS$^{•+}$ scavenging activity in aqueous medium, while an isolated 1 kDa peptide (YFYPEL) from a peptic hydrolysate of casein scavenged $O_2^{•-}$, HO$^•$, and DPPH$^•$ radicals. In the latter case, EL residue was important, and because CPPs do not contain this particular peptide sequence, it was suggested that the functional domain in CPP with the sequence SerP–SerP–SerP–EE also possesses comparable activity not only in metal sequestration but also in hydrogen/electron donation; the combination of both resulted in the reduced presence of reactive oxygen species (Kitts 2005 and references therein). A CPP preparation derived from spray-dried whole tryptic digests of bovine casein contained unidentified peptides with MW less than 6 kDa and an affinity to sequester Fe^{2+}. Associated with this activity, the CPP also effectively suppressed Fenton reaction-induced, site-specific, and non-site-specific deoxyribose oxidation. In addition, CPP was effective at reducing AAPH- and Fe^{2+}-induced liposomal peroxidation and showed direct scavenging affinity for the hydrophilic ABTS$^{•+}$ radical.

Caseins seem to favor the autoxidation of iron as it was shown in the experiments with α-, β-, and κ-caseins, which inhibited Fe-induced peroxidation of arachidonic acid inserted into multilamellar liposomes of dipalmitoylphosphatidylcholine (Cervato et al. 1999). Buttermilk solids possessed greater sequestering activity for ferrous than ferric ion; they scavenged Fenton-induced HO$^•$ radicals and protected against lipid peroxidation (Wong and Kitts 2003). Antioxidant peptides were isolated from various milk proteins, and their amino acid sequences were elucidated (the figures in brackets indicate the amino acid sequence of the related protein): αs1-casein YFYPEL (144–149), β-casein VKEAMAPK (89–105), AVPYPQR (177–183), KVLPVPEK (169–, 170–176), β-lactoglobulin WYSLAMAASDI (19–29), MHIRL (145–149), YVEEL (42–46), and fermented milk ARHPHPHLSFM (κ-casein 96–106) (Walther and Sieber 2012).

An interesting protein, phosvitin, which is the most phosphorylated protein found in nature, is present in egg yolk. Its antioxidant properties have been recently reviewed: Because of high phosphoric acid bound to serine residues, the protein can behave as a polyelectrolyte (polyanion) in the liquid state, and therefore, phosvitin possesses different functionalities, such as metal chelating, antioxidant, and emulsifying capacities. It was observed that phosvitin can efficiently inhibit Fe^{2+}- and Cu^{2+}-mediated oxidation of phospholipids; however, it was sensitive to heat and its efficiency was dependent on pH: At pH 6.1 it was maximum, while it became not effective enough to inhibit the Cu^{2+}-induced oxidation at pH 7.8 in a phospholipid emulsion system. Conjugation of phosvitin with galactomannan significantly increased the antioxidant and radical scavenging activities, which, in contrast to pure protein, were not affected by autoclaving (Samaraweera et al. 2011 and references therein). Phosvitin and its tryptic hydrolysate were found to be more effective than other iron-binding proteins or synthetic metal chelators (ferritin, transferrin, EDTA, diethylenetriamine pentaacetic acid, and citrate) in inhibiting Fe^{2+}-catalyzed $HO^{\bullet}$ radical production in Fenton reaction systems by accelerating the autoxidation of Fe^{2+} to Fe^{3+} and, thus, reducing the availability of Fe^{2+}. Phosvitin and its tryptic hydrolysate also showed a protective effect against $OH^{\bullet}$-mediated damages of DNA *in vivo*, and because of all these antioxidant properties, phosvitin can be exploited in the production of natural antioxidant agents (Ishikawa et al. 2004).

Porcine myofibrillar proteins were hydrolyzed with either actinase E or papain, and it was determined that in the acid system, antioxidant activity of the papain hydrolysates was similar to the activity of α-tocopherol, and in the $DPPH^{\bullet}$ radical scavenging assay, the hydrolysates showed lower antioxidant activities than α-tocopherol. Five peptides were identified in the papain hydrolysate containing H, Y, and M, and their radical scavenging activities could be attributed to these amino acids. Antioxidant peptides were also obtained and isolated from porcine protein actomyosin, collagen, meat meal of cows, scale and bone from yellowfish, keratin of feather meal of chickens, and a mixture of horn and hoof from cows and buffalo, bovine skin (rich in collagen), bovine protein elastin, and hydrolysates of venison (Di Bernardini et al. 2011 and references therein).

9.3.4 Plant Origin Sources

ACE-inhibitory and antioxidant properties of protein isolates obtained from mature stored, immature, and sprouted potato tubers and by-products (pulp fraction, liquid, and peel fraction) were studied by Finnish scientists (Pihlanto et al. 2008). They reported that before hydrolysis, the scavenging activity of the peel fractions was approximately nine times higher than that of the protein isolate of mature tubers, whereas after 5 h of hydrolysis with added proteases, the scavenging activities increased in most cases. For instance, the radical-scavenging value in $ABTS^{\bullet+}$ assay expressed as IC_{50} μg/mL of dry matter was from 12 to 815 (three for Trolox) and was dependent on the protein source, enzyme, and hydrolysis time. The results of the $ABTS^{\bullet+}$ scavenging measurements were confirmed by the TRAP method, and the most active sample was the potato liquid alcalase hydrolysate, which produced an antioxidant capacity of 0.48 g dry matter—equivalent to 1 mmol of Trolox in the TRAP assay. Wang and Xiong (2005) also observed that hydrolysis of potato proteins by alcalase increases their radical-scavenging activity. The main tuber storage protein, patatin-scavenged DPPH$^•$ (IC$_{50}$ was 0.582 mg/mL), inhibited human low-density lipoprotein peroxidations and protected against HO$^•$-mediated DNA damage and peroxynitrite-mediated dihydrorhodamine 123 oxidations (Liu et al. 2003), whereas, after hydrolysis, the purified peptides FGER, FDRR, and FGERR inhibited linoleic acid oxidation in a β-carotene decolorization assay, possessed antioxidant activity in a ferric thiocyanate assay system, and repressed lipid oxidation in the erythrocyte membrane ghost assay system (Kudoh et al. 2003). It was suggested that cysteine and tryptophan residues in patatin might contribute to its antioxidant activities against radicals. During enzymatic treatment, the increased scavenging activity probably resulted in structural changes of proteins and release of peptides. It was reported that the accessibility to the oxidant-antioxidant test system is greater for small peptides and amino acids than for large peptides and proteins (Moosman and Behl 2002). On the other hand, nonprotein compounds, such as phenols and pigments, which might be present in the tested media, should be taken into account when evaluating the antioxidant activities of plant-origin hydrolysates.

The hydrolysate generated by alcalase from industrial defatted rapeseed meal possessed a high inhibitory capacity against lipid oxidation in a liposomal model: There were some differences between the studied samples as two of the controls were less effective with higher IC$_{50}$ values (0.056 and 0.023 mg protein/mL), whereas the others were remarkably stronger with IC$_{50}$ values between 0.002 and 0.004 mg protein/mL. The amino acid composition of peptides had an effect on their antioxidant capacity and hydrophobic amino acids acting as antioxidants by increasing peptide solubility in lipids, and thereby facilitating better interaction with free radicals might be the most important factor (Mäkinen et al. 2012). The differences in antioxidant activity are at least partly a result of the different peptides and amino acids released during hydrolysis. This leads to a difference in their ability to donate protons to radicals or chelate ions, either to stop oxidative chain reactions or prevent their initiation. One factor that also may have an effect is the distribution at the interface in the o/w liposome system (ability to interact with free radicals), which is related to the amino acid composition of the sample.

An antioxidant peptide (717.37 Da) with amino acid sequence NRTHE, which was purified using consecutive chromatographic methods from chickpea protein hydrolysates, efficiently quenched DPPH$^•$, HO$^•$, and O$_2^-$ radicals, chelated Cu^{2+} and Fe^{2+} (77% and 63% at the concentration of 50 μg/mL, respectively), and inhibited lipid peroxidation more efficiently than α-tocopherol (Zhang, T. et al. 2011). Insoluble rapeseed (*Brassica napus*) meal proteins were digested by alcalase and flavorzyme in order to convert them into functionally active ingredients for food application. Rapeseed crude hydrolysates and different MW fractions separated from them exhibited a dose-dependent reducing antioxidant power and HO$^•$ scavenging ability and inhibited malonyldialdehyde (MDA) generation (Xue 2009). Water soluble proteins (WSPs) of 70 and 28 kDa MW, which were isolated from broad beans (*Vicia faba*), exhibited a marked scavenging effect on superoxide and also an effect on hydrogen peroxide, but not so much on DPPH$^•$ (Okada and Okada 1998). As they have only a small amount of sulfhydryl groups, they were considered not to be responsible for the scavenging activity of the WSP.

9.3.5 FACTORS AFFECTING ANTIOXIDANT ACTIVITY OF AMINO ACIDS AND PEPTIDES

The exact mechanism underlying the antioxidant activity of peptides is not fully understood, but many studies showed that they are lipid peroxidation inhibitors, free radical scavengers, and transition metal ion chelators. The following factors are important to the antioxidant capacity of protein hydrolysates containing peptides: (i) the average MW (usually higher in the fractions with lower MW), (ii) amino acid composition, (iii) structure, (iv) hydrophobicity, (v) correct amino acid positioning in the peptide sequence, and (vi) peptide conformation (may show synergistic and antagonistic effects). The results obtained by Pazos et al. (2006) with bovine serum albumin, β-La, and lactoferrin suggested that proteins with higher inhibitory activity on lipid oxidation promoted by the transition metal catalytic decomposition of hydroperoxides should be those with elevated metal chelating and radical-scavenging properties as well as low concentration and accessibility of reducing groups from amino acids capable of activating metals, such as sulfhydryl groups. The radical-scavenging ability of amino acids may be associated mainly with the presence of phenolic, sulfhydryl, and amine-heterocyclic groups where hydrogen atoms can be easily abstracted by radical species. For this reason, W, H, and C have the ability to scavenge DPPH•, whereas the higher inhibitory activity of W and H can be related to their dual behavior as chelating and radical-scavenging agents. G and M, which were reported as less effective in reducing radicals generated by Fe(II) and CumOOH, exhibit only chelating properties (Pazos et al. 2006 and references therein). In addition, Trp showed a higher inhibitory activity than H in agreement with its superior radical-scavenging activity; however, C promoted the generation of radicals despite its high ability to scavenge radicals. It was also reported that dipeptides containing Y and W at their amino terminus and H and M at their carboxyl terminus showed stronger antioxidant activity in an aqueous system than the constituent amino acid mixtures (Suetsuna 2000).

9.4 NATURAL PS AND OS ANTIOXIDANTS

For many years, the antioxidant properties of plants have usually been assigned to the presence of antioxidant vitamins C and E and various classes of phytochemicals, particularly phenolic acids, flavonoids, carotenoids, terpenoids, and others. More recently, other constituents present in agri-food materials or the substances derived thereof have attracted the attention of scientists and food producers as natural antioxidants. In recent years, there has been an increasing interest in utilizing plant-derived PSs and OSs as sources of therapeutic agents in medicine and cosmetics, and as a consequence, some PSs and OSs were commercially developed into important components of therapeutic drugs and skin-care products. They also are of interest for food systems, particularly as promising ingredients for functional foods and nutraceuticals. PSs and OSs as bioactive healthy ingredients, possessing immunomodulatory, hepatoprotective, antitumor, radioprotective, antidiabetic, prebiotic, and other properties, have been in the focus of numerous studies for a long time, whereas the number of articles on isolation, characterization, and application of antioxidatively active PSs and OSs from different sources, such as cereals, legumes, marine-origin materials, herbal plants, mushrooms, agri-food by-products, and others, has been steadily increasing during the last decade. The published data indicate that PSs and OSs isolated from plant-origin materials or derived from them by various treatments have certain antioxidant activity on free radicals and can be explored as novel potential antioxidants (Chen et al. 2012; Capek et al. 2009; Luo et al. 2010; Moure et al. 2006). The selected examples of antioxidatively active PSs and OSs isolated from various plant materials, their main characteristics, and antioxidant properties are given in Table 9.3. It may be observed that many antioxidant PSs and OSs were reported in medicinal plants and mushrooms that were rarely used for foods; however, they are considered as promising components for functional foods and therefore are of interest for food systems in general.

Comprehensive reviews of a general nature, which would be focused exceptionally on antioxidant properties of PSs and OSs, have not been published until now; however, antioxidant activities of PSs and OSs from several specific sources were reviewed as a part of their overall biological properties; most of these reviews were published in the past few years. They include biological activities of chitin (Park et al. 2010), yeast cell wall PSs (Kogan et al. 2008), fucose-rich sulfated PSs and fucoidans isolated from brown seaweed (Wijesinghe and Jeon 2012), edible macromycetes (Stachowiak and Regula 2012), tropical fruits (Sun et al. 2011), sulfated PSs derived from marine algae (Ngo et al. 2011; Jiao et al. 2011), and PSs of *Angelica sinensis* (Jin et al. 2012c).

Compared to small monomeric phytochemical molecules, characterization of natural PS and OS antioxidants is associated with some specific difficulties, such as the rather complicated procedure of isolation, fractionation, and purification; determination of MW; and elucidation of the exact composition and molar ratio of their sugar monomers, the type of glycosidic linkages in the chain, the substitutions in the polymeric chain, and the presence of other molecules, that is, the properties that may have a bigger or smaller influence on the overall antioxidant activity of individual purified PSs or OSs. Therefore, many previously published articles did not present the exact structure of antioxidatively potent PSs and OSs. In some cases, active PS and OS fractions may also contain some amount of proteins and polyphenolic compounds, which are antioxidants themselves, and therefore, the input of pure PSs and OSs in the total antioxidant capacity of the tested fractions is not fully known.

Many methods and procedures were applied to evaluate the antioxidant properties of PSs and OSs, including *in vitro*, *in vivo*, and *in situ* (added to real foods) assays; however, simple *in vitro* assays, such as the scavenging capacity of DPPH$^\bullet$, HO$^\bullet$, O$_2^{\bullet-}$, and ABTS$^{\bullet+}$ radicals, and reduction and chelation of ferrous ions are dominant in the majority of previously performed studies. The antioxidant activity of PSs and OSs was compared with various reference compounds, such as the well-known synthetic antioxidant BHT and ascorbic acid. These studies indicate that the antioxidant power of PSs and OSs may depend on the following factors: (i) degree of polymerization (DP) and MW; (ii) monomer composition and the ratio of monosaccharide

TABLE 9.3

PS and OS Antioxidants (Ratio of Monomers Expressed in Molar %)

PS Origin	Characterization	Reference
Salvia officinalis L. PS (crude and purified fractions)	2–120 kDa: Rha, Fuc, Ara, Xyl, Man, Glc, methyl-Glc, uronic acid; inhibited liposome lipid peroxidation, scavenged DPPH• radicals (crude water-soluble fraction better than purified)	Capek et al. 2009
Fruitshell of *Camellia oleifera* Abel. PS	WEP2: 362 kDa; Rha:Fuc:Ara:Man:Gal:Glc = 4.0 5:11.62:1.78:3.91:8.76:27.06; scavenge HO• and O_2^- radicals	Jin 2012
Rice bran PS (hot-water soluble PW1, PW2, and PW3)	PW1 (120–6300 kDa): Glu:Man:Gal:Rib:Ara = 54.1: 10.5:21.7:7.4:6.3; PW2 (35–74 kDa): Glu:Gal:Rib:Ara = 60.9:26.0:10.7:2.4; PW3 (5.3–23 kDa): Glu:Man:Gal:Rib:Ara = 50.7: 10.1:32.7:2.4:4.1%. Scavenged O_2^-, HO•, DPPH•, ABTS•+ radicals and H_2O_2, inhibited lipid peroxidation chelated ferrous ions, were reducing agents	Zha et al. 2009
Chroogomphis rutilus fruiting bodies PS (edible mushrooms)	Scavenging capacity for HO• radicals (0.25 to 4 mg/ mL) was comparable to ascorbic acid; however, the purity of PS was 57.7% ± 0.77%	Sun et al. 2010
Sarcanda glabra PS (SPP1)	10.6 kDa; Glc:Gal:Man = 8.38:3.13:1.00; inhibit HO•, O_2^-, DPPH• and ABTS•+ radicals	Jin et al. 2012a
Dictyophora indusiata mushroom PS (DIP I and DIP II)	DIP I (2100 kDa); Glc:Man = 5.6:1.0; DIP II (18.16 kDa) Glc:Man:Xyl:Gal(3):Gal(6) = 4.9:15.5:7.8:1.0:5.7; decreased the MDA, lipofuscin levels and increased the SOD, GSH-Px activities in mice	Hua et al. 2012
Scutellaria barbata D. Don PS (SBP)	Contained 0.3 ± 0.1 g/100 g dw of phenolics; scavenge O_2^-, HO• and DPPH•	Ye and Huang 2012
Fibrous pulp of *Mangifera pajang* fruits PS (four fractions)	Neutral F1 (7 kDa):Er:Rh:Ara:Man:Fru:Glc + 5, 7, 21, 42, 4 and 21 mg/100 mg; acidic (13, 24, and 9 kDa): F2: Rha:Xyl:Ara = 33, 7, and 51; F3: Fru:Glc = 14, 72; F4: Ara:Man:Fru:Glc = 32, 36, 2, and 10. Ferric-reducing antioxidant power; scavenging of DPPH•	Al-Sheraji et al. 2012
Ginkgo biloba exocarp PS	Four acidic and one neutral purified to GBEP-NN, and GBEP-AA) GBEP-NN: Rha:Ara:Man: Glc:Gal; GBEP-AA:Man:Rha:GlcA: GalA:GalN:Glc:Gal:Xyl:Ara:Fuc; the crude GBEP scavenged HO• radical better than ascorbic acid	Chen et al. 2012
Dendrobium nobile Lindl PS (DNP1-1, DNP2-1, DNP3-1, DNP4-2)	Av. MW = 136, 27.7, 11.8, and 11.4 kDa; Man, Glc, Gal (major), Rha, Ara, Xyl (smaller). DNP4-2 scavenged ABTS•+, HO• and DPPH• radicals better than the other	Luo et al. 2010

(continued)

TABLE 9.3 (Continued)
PS and OS Antioxidants (Ratio of Monomers Expressed in Molar %)

PS Origin	Characterization	Reference
Ligusticum chuanxiong Hort. PS (crude LC; purified LCA, LCB, and LCC)	LCA (28.3 kDa): Ara:Glc:Man = 0.25:1.00:0.05 (α-glucoside linkaged pyranose); LCB (12.3 kDa): Ara:Glc:Gal:Man = 1.00:0.03:0.13:0.20; LCC (63.1 kDa): Ara:Glc:Gal = 1.00:0.07:0.04 (both β-glucoside linkaged pyranose); antioxidant in DPPH·, HO·, O_2, β-carotene, chelating, reducing, lipid peroxidation inhibiting assays (LCB > LCA > LCC)	Yuan et al. 2008
Root of *Angelica sinensis* PS (APF1, APF2, APF3, and ASP)	APF1: Ara:Glc:Rha:Gal:GalA = 11.0:2.6:1.0:3.5: 2.5; APF2 Ara:Glc:Rha:Gal:Man:GalA = 18.2:7.4:1.0:8.4:0.5:12.3; APF3: Ara:Glc:Rha: Gal:GlcA:GalA = 9.4:8.7:1.0:6.0:0.3:12.1; active against H_2O_2 mediated oxidative stress in mouse peritoneal macrophages; ASP:Man:Rha:GlcA: GalA:Glc:Gal:Ara:Fuc = 1.2:4.5:1.0:10.5:17.8: 37.5:8.7:4.9; reduced lipid peroxidation level	Jin et al. 2012c
Guarana powder PS (purified pectic fraction)	70% uronic acid; Glc (2), Ara (19), Gal (6), Xyl (3), and Rha (2); scavenged DPPH· and HO· radicals (capacity much lower than that of the methanolic extract at low concentrations)	Dalonso and de Oliveira Petkowicz 2012
Native and enzymatically degraded chitosans	30, 90, and 120 kDa; reduced TBARS of salmon during storage; scavenged DPPH· (30 kDa comparable to BHT), HO· radicals, inhibited herring and beef lipid oxidation; chelated metal ions	Kim and Thomas 2007 and references therein
Wolfberry fruit (WFPs) acid heterogeneous PS	GalA:Gal:Ara:Glc = 24.9:21.3:18.5:15.9; scavenged DPPH·, HO· and O_2^- radicals, inhibited the peroxidation of linoleic acid and $FeCl_2$-egg yolk induced lipid peroxidation, reduced Fe^{3+}	He et al. 2012
Eugenia jambolana PS (WE)	116 kDa; arabinogalactan containing *p*-coumaric and ferulic acids in monomeric and dimeric forms; antioxidant in DPPH·, FRAP assays	Bandyopadhyay et al. 2012
Rhizoma of *Ligustici wallichii* PS	Four fractions; FrI: Glc:Man:Gal:Ara = 521:1:4.6:3.3; inhibited MDA production *in vivo*	Fu et al. 2012
Longan (*Dimocarpus longan*) fruit pericarp	PS scavenged DPPH· and O_2^- radicals; methylation of OH groups reduced scavenging capacity	Yang et al. 2010
Water-soluble feraxans from native and malted rice and ragi	High uronic acid, ferulic acid, Gal contents and Ara substitution; in DPPH· and FRAP assays exhibited several folds higher activity than the expected activity because of their bound ferulic acid content	Rao and Muralikrishna 2006

(continued)

TABLE 9.3 (Continued)
PS and OS Antioxidants (Ratio of Monomers Expressed in Molar %)

PS Origin	Characterization	Reference
The green alga, *Ulva pertusa* sulfated heteroPS (ulvan)	Main disaccharide units: β-D-Glcp A-(1→4)-α-L-Rhap 3s] and [α-L-Idop A-(1→4)-α-L-Rhap 3s]; scavenged HO• and O_2^- radicals, chelated ferrous ions, reduced the Fe^{3+}	Qi et al. 2006
Litchi chinensis fruit pericarp tissues PS	Neutral (14 kDa): Man:Gal:Ara = 65.6:33.0:1.4; glycosidic linkages: 8.7% (1→2), 83.3% (1→3), 8.0% (1→6); scavenged DPPH•, HO• and O_2^- radicals	Yang et al. 2006
Okara (by-product from soymilk) cell wall PS	3 Alkali-soluble fractions; strongest: Rha:Fuc:Ara: Xyl:Man:Gal:Glc:UA = 1.3:2.3:18.0:5.5:1.5:26.3: 3.4:41.7; scavenged $ABTS^{+}$, reduced Fe^{3+}	Mateos-Aparicio et al. 2010
Mung bean (*Vigna radiata* L.) hull PS (MSP)	Water-soluble MP1 (83 kDa): uronic acid 9.9%; Ara:Xyl:Man:Gal:Glc = 8.3:2.2:67.2:20.1:2.3; MP2: (45 kDa) uronic acid 36.4%, Rha:Fuc:Ara:Xyl:Man:Gal:GlC = 31.8:3.5:16.7: 4.6:11.7:39.1:2.5. Scavenged DPPH•, HO• and O_2^-, reduced the Fe^{3+}, inhibited self-oxidation of 1,2,3-phentriol	Lai et al. 2010
Chitosan OS (COS)	COS I (>10 kDa); COS II (5–10 kDa); COS III (3–5 kDa); COS IV (1–3 kDa); COS V (<1 kDa); scavenged DPPH•, HO• and O_2^- and alkyl radicals (ESR spectroscopy); COS IV strongest antioxidant	Park et al. 2003
Asparagus officinalis AO-OS-4, 6, 8	AOP4 (57.5 kDa); strongly scavenged HO•; DPPH• and O_2^- scavenging capacity was weaker	Zhao, Q. S. et al. 2012
Chinese truffle *Tuber sinense*	Water-soluble (W-CTCP) and alkali-soluble (A-CTCPI, A-CTCPII); scavenged HO• and O_2^-, reduced the Fe^{3+} (W-CTCP strongest)	Zhao, L. et al. 2012
Corn cobs heteroxylan	130 kDa: Xyl:Ara:Gal:Glc = 5.0:1.5:2.0:1.2; total antioxidant activity = 48.5 mg of ascorbic acid equivalent/g; strong ferric chelating	Melo-Silveira et al. 2012
Chinese truffle *Tuber indicum* (TIP1-1, TIP2-1)	TIP1-1 (17.5 kDa): Man:Glc:Gal:Rha = 3.93:1.24:0.75:1.26; TIP2-1 (5.73 kDa): Man:Glc:Ara = 5.27:1.44:0.43; protective effect on PC12 cells injured by H_2O_2, free radicals scavenging activity	Luo et al. 2011
Boletus edulis, edible mushroom	BEPF30: Fuc:Xyl:Man:Glc:Gal = 1:0.279:8.221: 9.582:0.963 BEPF60: Rha:Fuc:Xyl:Man:Glc:Gal = 0.407:1:0.144:2.709:4.571:2.236; BEPF80: Rha:Fuc:Xyl:Man:Glc:Gal = 0.779:1:0.130: 4.580:6.864:1.333; scavenged HO• and O_2^- radicals, chelated ferrous ions, reduced the Fe^{3+} (BEPF60 strongest antioxidant)	Zhang, A. Q. et al. 2011

(continued)

TABLE 9.3 (Continued)
PS and OS Antioxidants (Ratio of Monomers Expressed in Molar %)

PS Origin	Characterization	Reference
Out-of-date tea leaves (TPS), three types of tea	1–800 kD: Rh, Ara, Gal, Glc, Xyl, Man, GalA; TPS composed of PS, protein and uronic acids; scavenged DPPH⁺ and O_2^-	Xiao et al. 2011
Xylo-OS from xylan-containing lignocellulosic materials	DPPH⁺ radical scavenging; antioxidant activity in erythrocyte hemolysis assay; protective effect against lipid LDL peroxidation	Moure et al. 2006 and references therein
Wheat bran feruloyl OS (FOs)	Protect rat erythrocytes against *in vitro* oxidative damage; in *in vitro* models, more effective antioxidants toward low-density lipoproteins oxidation and DPPH⁺ scavenging than free ferulic acid; enhance antioxidative enzyme activity, reduce oxidized glutathione and malondialdehyde levels in rat plasma *in vivo*	Wang et al. 2010 and references therein
Fructo-OS Raftilose P95 (commercial)	10.12 ± 0.55 µmol TE/g of sample in peroxyl scavenging ORAC assay	Amigo-Benavent et al. 2010
Hydroquinones, substituted by β-(1→6)-linked OS from wheat germ and bran	4-Hydroxy-3-methoxyphenyl β-D-glcp-(1→6)-β-D-glcp-(1→6)-β-D-glcp antioxidant power in 1 L of ethanol water extract was equivalent to approximately 6.8 µmol Trolox equivalents	Zhokhov et al. 2010
Purified longan fruit pericarp OS (OLFP)	Glc:Gal:GalA = 71.5:24.6:3.9; →3)-Gal-(1→,→6)-Gal-(→f, Glc-(→ and →3)-GalA-(1→ ≈ 13:5:6:1; scavenged DPPH⁺ and O_2^- (IC$_{50}$ value =145.09 µg/mL, lower than that of BHT 471.58 µg/mL)	Jiang et al. 2009
Citrus pectin-OS	Inhibited β-carotene–linoleic acid bleaching; possessed electron donating ability; antioxidant power increased by irradiation at 20 kGy and dialysis (<10 kDa)	Kang et al. 2006
OSs (NA-COS) produced from crab chitin by acid hydrolysis	MW = 229.21–593.12 Da; scavenged DPPH, HO⁺, and alkyl radicals with IC$_{50}$ values at 0.8, 1.75, and 1.14 mg/mL, respectively; scavenged free radicals in live cells in dose- and time-dependent manners	Ngo et al. 2010
Agaro-OS from agarose hydrolysate	Degrees of polymerizations (DP) of 2, 4, 6, 8, and 10: scavenged DPPH: agarohexaose IC$_{50}$ = 1.85 mg/mL, agarooctaose IC$_{50}$ of 2.62 mg/mL; acted as an efficient antioxidant in liver cell	Chen and Yan 2005

in the chain; (iii) the presence of functional groups (hydroxyl, methyl, acetyl, sulfur, nitrogen-containing); and (iv) the presence of uronic acids.

Regarding the DP and MW, there is no strict border separating OSs from PSs. The DP tested for antioxidant activity OSs starts from the lowest possible, that is, DP = 2 (Chen and Yan 2005), while the MW of antioxidatively active PSs may be up to

2100 kDa (Hua et al. 2012) and most likely bigger. Chen and Yan (2005) evaluated the antioxidant activity of agaro-OSs with different DPs (2, 4, 6, 8, and 10) and found that agarohexaose displayed the highest ability toward DPPH$^\bullet$ scavenging activity, followed by agarooctaose. Agarobiose and agarotetraose showed relatively low scavenging activity at a concentration lower than 8 mg/mL but exhibited almost the same ability at a high concentration (20 mg/mL), while agarodecaose showed good activity at a low concentration, which did not further increase by increasing the concentration. Consequently, the antioxidant activity did not correlate with their DPs regularly. In addition, it was shown that agarohexaose can permeate across the cell membrane and act as an efficient antioxidant in liver cells by scavenging ROS generated by electron leakage. Antioxidatively active PSs and OSs may be composed of various monomers, from comparatively simple polymers, such as one isolated from *Dictyophora indusiata* mushroom and consisting mainly of Glc and Man (Hua et al. 2012), to a very complex ones, such as a PS purified from the acidic fraction of *Ginkgo biloba* ecocarp and consisting of 10 different types of monomers, namely, Man, Rha, GlcA, GalA, GalN, Glc, Gal, Xyl, Ara, and Fuc (Chen et al. 2012).

The number of PSs and OSs obtained from various sources depends on their isolation procedure, which usually consists of several extraction, fractionation, and purification steps. For instance, the crude PSs (MW = 2–100 kDa) were isolated from the aerial parts of sage by sequential extraction with water, hot ammonium oxalate, dimethyl sulfoxide, and 1 and 4 M potassium hydroxide solutions and further separated into six fractions (MW = 2–120 kDa) by an ion-exchange method (Capek et al. 2009). However, crude PSs were more effective for their ability to inhibit peroxidation of liposome lipids by HO$^\bullet$ radicals and to reduce DPPH$^\bullet$ radical content than the separated fractions. Crude and purified PSs were composed of Rha, Fuc, Ara, Xyl, Man, Glc, methyl-Glc, and uronic acid at various ratios, while crude PSs also contained 7.5–19 wt% of proteins. Sage is widely used for foods; therefore, it is interesting to note that antioxidant activities of PSs isolated from sage were higher than the effects of the previously characterized PSs, which were isolated from various purely medicinal plants (Kardošova and Machová 2006). The selection of the extraction procedure can give PSs, which may exert their antioxidant properties by different mechanisms. For instance, three water-soluble PSs were isolated from rice bran (PW1, PW2, and PW3) by using multiple extraction, fractionation, and purification steps. All of them possessed antioxidant activity in several tested assays; however, their antioxidant power was different: PW1 was the best scavenger of HO$^\bullet$, O$_2^{\bullet-}$ radicals and inhibitor of lipid peroxidation, whereas PW3 was the best DPPH$^\bullet$, ABTS$^{\bullet+}$, and H$_2$O$_2$ scavenger, ferrous ion chelator, and reducing agent. The pure antioxidant reference compounds BHT, ascorbic acid, and EDTA were stronger antioxidants, except for FeCl$_2$–ascorbic acid-induced lipid peroxidation in rat liver, when PW1 was more effective than ascorbic acid (Zha et al. 2009). Generally, the antioxidant capacity of isolated PSs is lower than that of pure synthetic reference antioxidants; however, in some cases, PSs, like the fraction isolated from *Ligusticum chuanxiong*, showed with a high ability to prevent the bleaching of β-carotene, scavenge O$_2^{\bullet-}$ as the synthetic antioxidant BHT, and inhibit lipid peroxidation as the vitamin C (Yuan et al. 2008). The IC$_{50}$ value of PS extracted from *Scutellaria barbata* in the HO$^\bullet$ scavenging assay was lower than that of ascorbic acid, indicating on its slightly higher scavenging activity than that of ascorbic acid;

however, the effectiveness of the same PS in scavenging $O_2^{\cdot-}$ and DPPH$^{\cdot}$ radicals was lower as compared to the ascorbic acid (Ye and Huang 2012).

Plant origin materials contain polyphenolic antioxidants; therefore, in assessing the activity of PSs and OSs, it is important to measure the input of polyphenolic compounds. For this purpose, in one of the studies, antioxidant activity tests were performed with a methanolic extract containing phenolic antioxidants and the pectic fraction, which was isolated by the complex extraction/fractionation/purification procedure. The methanolic extract exhibited a strong DPPH$^{\cdot}$ scavenging capacity (90.9% at 10 mg/mL), which was almost similar to BHA and ascorbic acid, whereas the DPPH$^{\cdot}$ scavenging by PS at the same concentration was lower, 68.4%. At a higher concentration, the methanolic extract and the PS exhibited similar HO$^{\cdot}$ scavenging effects (Dalonso and de Oliveira Petkowicz 2012).

The fraction of PSs and OSs may contain substances other than saccharides, particularly when more simple extraction procedures are applied, for example, using acidified water with subsequent filtration and dialysis. Nonstarch PSs in some foods are bound with phenolic acids, for example, feruloyl arabinoxylans (feraxans) in rice and ragi. In this case, phenolic acids may add to the total antioxidant capacity of a complex; however, it was demonstrated that antioxidant activity of feraxans was several (4.9–1400) times higher than the expected activity because of their bound ferulic acid content (Rao and Muralikrishna 2006). A water-soluble carbohydrate polymer of *Eugenia jambolana* containing inter alia, arabinogalactan, *p*-coumaric, and ferulic acids was isolated and found to possess an antioxidative capacity similar to standard antioxidants. It was suggested that the bioactivity of this carbohydrate polymer is mainly a result of the structural features, although phenolic acids may play a role. A study on feruloyl-OS also confirmed that it had a higher antioxidant capacity than free ferulic acid (Bandyopadhyay et al. 2012 and references therein).

Other agricultural products were used as a source of PS/OS antioxidants as well. After several steps of fractionation and purification, a strong radical-scavenging PS was isolated from *Litchi chinensis* with a MW of 14 kDa, composed of Man:Gal:Ara (65.6:33.0:1.4%), and linked with 8.7% of (1→2), 83.3% of (1→3), and 8.0% of (1→6)-glycosidic linkages in the PS (Yang et al. 2006). Strong antioxidant OSs were isolated and purified from logan fruit pericarp (yield = 32.9 mg glucose equivalents/g dw); its $O_2^{\cdot-}$ scavenging capacity with the IC_{50} value of 145.09 µg/mL was three times lower than that of a synthetic antioxidant BHT (471.58 µg/mL) (Jiang et al. 2009).

It is important that valuable PSs and OSs may be obtained from agri-food and marine by-products. Two water-soluble antioxidatively active acidic PS fractions, MP1 and MP2, were isolated from mung bean (*Vigna radiata* L.) hulls by ultrasonic-assisted extraction. Their antioxidant power was different in the applied assays: MP2 was a stronger HO$^{\cdot}$ scavenger, whereas MP1 exhibited a higher reducing power and stronger $O_2^{\cdot-}$ and DPPH$^{\cdot}$ scavenging capacity as well as higher inhibition on self-oxidation of 1,2,3-phentriol. Possibly, different content of uronic acids in MP1 and MP2 was responsible for these differences (Lai et al. 2010). Three alkali-soluble fractions (12.7% yield) and an insoluble residue (58.7% yield) were obtained from okara, a by-product from soymilk, by the sequential extraction procedure. Soluble PS fractions showed *in vitro* reduction power, which was equivalent to 11–26 µmol

TE/g dw, and free radical-scavenging activity (63–78 μmol TE/g dw). The highest antioxidant activity possessed 0.05 M NaOH-soluble fraction, which was rich in pectins and was characterized by the highest ratio of uronic acids (Mateos-Aparicio et al. 2010). PSs, OSs, and other components, which may present in their fractions can possess a synergistic effect. For instance, glycation mixtures of defatted soy flour (DSF) or soy protein isolate (SPI) with fructo-OS (FOS, Raftilose P95) possessed a synergistic effect in an ORAC assay; moreover, heating of SPI, DSF, FOS, and their glycation mixtures at 150°C for different times led to the formation of Maillard reaction neoantioxidants able to act against peroxyl radicals (Amigo-Benavent et al. 2010). Antioxidant activity of OSs may be enhanced by irradiation as was shown in the case of citrus pectin-OS, which was obtained by dissolving pectin in water and irradiating it at 20 kGy using a Co^{60} γ-ray; dialyzed (<10 kDa) and irradiated OS was an even stronger antioxidant (Kang et al. 2006). Antioxidant compounds that are substituted with OSs were found in wheat-based food products. Seven antioxidant hydroquinones substituted by β-(1→6)-linked OSs were quantified with 4-hydroxy-3-methoxyphenyl β-D-glcp-(1→6)-β-D-glcp-(1→6)-β-D-glcp being the most abundant (6.3 g/kg in germ and 0.7 g/kg in bran); this constituent contributed 38% in total antioxidant power of water-ethanol extracts of germ and bran, which in μmol TE/L of extract was 2.56 and 0.76, respectively (Zhokhov et al. 2010).

Biological activities of xylo-OSs are mainly associated with their modulatory gut effects; however, they were also reported as antioxidant substances that may be produced by various methods from different sources: hydrothermal treatment of rice hulls and enzymatic hydrolysis of wheat flour arabinoxylan (DPPH·-radical scavenging); enzymatic hydrolysis of wheat bran (antioxidant activity in the erythrocyte hemolysis assay); hydrothermal processing of bagasse and enzymatic processing (antioxidant activity); and feruloyl xylo-OSs from enzymatic reactions (protective effect against lipid low-density lipoprotein [LDL] peroxidation). OSs may be obtained from such byproducts as corn cobs, barley hulls, brewery spent grains, almond shells, corn stover, corn fiber, rice hulls, flax shive, and wheat straw by various types of treatments and hydrothermal processing and further purified by enzymatic hydrolysis, thermal treatment, or their combinations. The scheme of a possible process for utilization of xylan-containing lignocellulosic materials to obtain purified OS with prebiotic properties and nonvolatile components with antioxidant activity was proposed (Moure et al. 2006 and references therein).

Regarding the antioxidative mechanism of PS/OS, it has been proposed that they are able to reduce the stable DPPH· radical to yellow diphenylpicrylhydrazine because of the hydroxyl group of the monosaccharide units, which can donate a proton to reduce the DPPH· radical. Methylation experiments performed with PS of longan fruit pericarp indicated the important role of hydroxyl groups of monosaccharide units in the radical-scavenging activity of PS: It was demonstrated that for the same PS, the substitution of the hydroxyl group by methoxyl groups decreased the scavenging effect (Yang et al. 2010). According to Rao and Muralikrishna (2006), the presence of sugars with uronyl/acetyl groups imparts a strong antioxidant activity to PS. The antioxidant activities can be attributed to the mechanism, PS neutralizing the linoleate free radical and other free radicals formed in the applied model system.

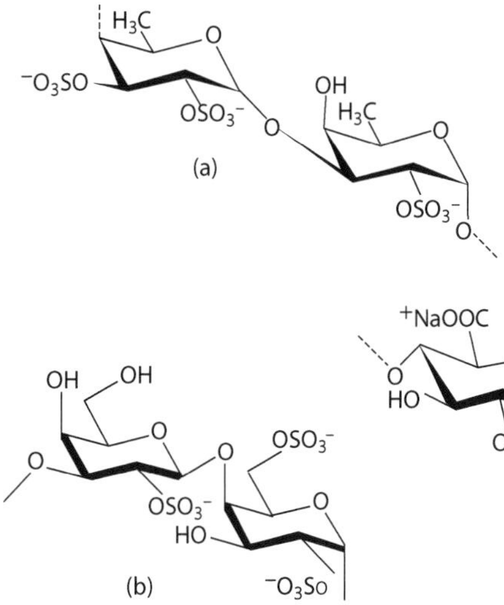

FIGURE 9.3 Antioxidative sulfated PSs derived from marine algae: (a) fucoidan, (b) carrageenan, and (c) ulvan. (From Zhang, C. et al. 2012, *Food Sci Biotechnol* 21: 625–631.)

PSs with special conformations, hydrogen in OH bonds, could be easily liberated and thus could stabilize $O_2^{\cdot-}$. The mechanism of PS on scavenging $O_2^{\cdot-}$ may be associated with the dissociation energy of OH bond (Jin et al. 2012a).

Marine-origin raw materials are attracting and increasing interest as a cheap and abundant source of bioactive compounds. Interesting and promising antioxidatively active PSs were isolated from sea products. The major sulfated compounds found in marine algae (Figure 9.3) include fucoidan and laminarans of brown algae, carrageenan of red algae, and ulvan of green algae (Zhang et al. 2012 and references therein). Sulfated hetero-PS (ulvan) isolated from the green algae *Ulva pertusa* scavenged HO$^{\cdot}$ and $O_2^{\cdot-}$ radicals, chelated ferrous ions, reduced the $Fe^{3+}/K_3Fe(CN)_6$ complex to Fe^{2+}, and was suggested as a promising candidate for functional foods. The antioxidant power of acetylated and benzoylated derivatives of this PS was even higher than that of the native compound (Qi et al. 2006); however, in this case, new derivatives would not fall into the group of natural antioxidants. The acetyl groups, which could substitute at C-2 and/or C-3 of the PS, could activate the hydrogen atom of the anomeric carbon. According to the authors, the higher the activation capacity of the group, the stronger the hydrogen atom-donating capacity. Acetylated PSs function as good hydrogen atom donors and are able to terminate radical chain reactions by converting free radicals to more stable products (Qi et al. 2006). Certain derivatives of the carrageenan OSs, such as oversulfated and acetylated (scavenge $O_2^{\cdot-}$), phosphorylated, and low-DS acetylated (scavenge HO$^{\cdot}$), and the phosphorylated derivatives (scavenge DPPH$^{\cdot}$) exhibited higher antioxidant activity than the PSs and OSs in certain antioxidant systems (Yuan et al. 2005); however, chemically produced compounds—even those synthesized from the natural sources—may not be considered as natural antioxidants in food systems.

Naturally abundant muco-PS chitin, which is distributed in the shell of crusta-ceans, in the cuticle of insects, and also in the cell wall of some fungi and micro-organisms, as well as its derivatives were the focus of numerous studies because of their exceptional biological properties, including the antioxidative activity of chitin-derived PSs and OSs (Park et al. 2010). Antioxidatively active chito-OSs were prepared from chitosan, which is an N-deacetylated derivative of chitin; chito-OSs exhibited strong $HO^{\bullet}$ and $O_2^{\bullet-}$ scavenging activity and weak scavenging activity on alkyl and $DPPH^{\bullet}$ radicals. The radical scavenging activity of chyto-OSs increased with the increment of concentration, and it was also dependent on their MW (Park et al. 2003). Chitin OSs with low MW distribution of 229.21–593.12 Da were produced from crab chitin by acid hydrolysis and possessed a free radical-scavenging effect on $DPPH^{\bullet}$, $HO^{\bullet}$, and alkyl radicals with IC_{50} values of 0.8, 1.75, and 1.14 mg/mL, respec-tively. They also scavenged free radicals in live cells in dose- and time-dependent manners (Ngo et al. 2010). Antioxidant activity of chitosan and its enzymatically degraded derivatives was tested in salmon, herring, and beef, and it was found that chitosans retarded lipid oxidation of these muscle foods, most likely as a result of their metal-chelating capacities (Kim and Thomas 2007 and references therein).

9.5   NATURAL ANTIOXIDANTS FROM AGRI-FOOD WASTE AND BY-PRODUCTS

9.5.1   General Aspects

Dietary antioxidants as ubiquitous nutrients in food systems have become an impor-tant issue in society, and there is a clear tendency toward increasing their supply to the food industry, which has been caused by two main factors: first, the negative attitude of consumers and health professionals toward synthetic food additives and, second, the links between the consumption of antioxidants and health, particularly in preventing cancer and cardiovascular and some other diseases. Although, in some cases, both of these reasons are not sufficiently supported by the existing scientific evidence, the work in the replacement of synthetic antioxidants by natural ones as well as the rapid development of healthy and functional foods enriched with natural antioxidants, which may also possess various other beneficial biological activities in the human body, will continue. These tendencies are challenging, both for the scientists who search for new natural antioxidant sources and develop new technolo-gies and producers who try to implement innovations for the needs of consumers. One of the promising ways to satisfy the increasing demand for natural antioxidants to be used as food additives (preservatives protecting oxidizable substrates in foods) and functional food ingredients (supplementing the human organism with exogenous antioxidants) is their isolation from waste and/or by-products, which, every year, are produced in enormous amounts in the agri-food chain all over the world.

The first comprehensive review on natural antioxidants from residual sources was published more than 10 years ago (Moure et al. 2001). A great number of articles published in the last decades of the previous century show that antioxidant activity, the presence of antioxidants, and the possibilities of their isolation and application were intensively studied, including such residual sources as potato peel waste; rape of olive; olive mill wastewaters; grape seeds; grape pomace and its peels; apple pomace; citrus seeds and peels; carrot pulp waste; old tea leaves; cocoa by-products; hulls from peanuts, mung beans, and buckwheat; wheat and rye bran; the coating of tamarind seeds; nonvolatile residues from essential oil production; soybean molasses; spent ground coffee, etc. A large number of antioxidatively active constituents, mainly polyphenolic compounds, were found in the analyzed plant residues; however, at that time, the literature on studies of antioxidatively potential by-products, other than those of plant origin, was rather scarce. Some studies were performed on shrimp shell waste, dipeptide carnosine, protein hydrolysates, soluble elastin peptides, water-soluble proteins, and pressure-treated β-lactoglobulin.

Usually, the entire body of many vegetables, fruits, cereals, legumes, and other plant-origin crops is rich in bioactive compounds, such as phenolic constituents, carotenoids, vitamins, OSs, and dietary fiber. However, the processing industry of plant-origin agricultural materials deals with the large percentage of by-products, such as peels, seeds, unused flesh, and husks generated in the different steps of the processing chain. Some parts of animal- and marine-origin raw materials, such as skin or bones, which are not directly processed into food products also contain biologically valuable molecules. In many cases, the wasted by-products can present similar or even higher contents of bioactive compounds, including natural antioxidants, than the final product does. Therefore, there is an obvious need to promote the application of so-called agro and biorefinery concepts in the production and processing of agricultural crops, highlighting the possibility of the integral exploitation of by-products rich in bioactive compounds. Rational utilization of agricultural materials is an important issue of a food system; therefore, valorization of agricultural and food-origin by-products increases business opportunities for stakeholders in the industry. The approach also paves the way for structuring an eco-efficient industry that recognizes the importance of sustainable development for continued growth and competitiveness and, consequently, may have a very positive impact on enhancing the efficiency of food systems in general (Tan et al. 2007). However, nowadays, regardless of the increasing number of residual sources studied within the antioxidant literature (mainly as a result of value-adding recycling interest in the agro- and food industries and increasing information on the specific location of active compounds and their modification during processing), only a few by-product-derived antioxidants have been developed successfully from the vast quantities of plant residues produced by the food processing industry in Europe, primarily based on grape seed and olive waste extracts. This might be caused by three limiting factors: the effectiveness of recovery and extraction, the marketability of resulting extracts, and the practical suitability for the food and other products (Peschel et al. 2006 and references therein). Therefore, there is intensive ongoing research in an attempt to enhance the release of bioactive constituents from plant cells. This may be achieved by cell disruption and extraction through the cell using enzyme preparations either alone or in mixtures, processes that have been recently reviewed (Puri et al. 2012). The authors of the review concluded that the enzyme-assisted extraction of natural compounds can save processing time and energy and potentially provide a more reproducible extraction process at the commercial scale; however, the biotechnological application of enzymes is not currently exploited to its maximum

TABLE 9.4

Recovery and Presence of Phenols and Other Natural Antioxidants from 100 g of Waste Dry Matter

Food Waste Source	Natural Antioxidants
Olive oil wastewater[1]	1.0; 4.7 for total phenols; 2.8 for hydroxytyrosol, 1.6 for tyrosol (in g/100 g waste dry matter)
Sea buckthorn berries pomace[1]	1.2 for total phenols; 0.1 for isorhamnetin 3-O-rutinoside (microwave-assisted extraction); 0.7 for total phenols, 0.2 for isorhamnetin 3-O-rutinoside (solid-liquid extraction) (in g/100 g waste dry matter)
Mango peel[1]	0.14, 0.12 for total phenols; 0.12, 0.08 for mangiferin (depending on extraction method) (in g/100 g waste dry matter)
White grape pomace[1]	0.26 (water extraction); 0.44 (water extraction and high-voltage electrical discharge) for total phenols (in g/100 g waste dry matter)
Rice bran[2]	γ-Oryzanol: 0.168 (hexane/isopropanol extraction); 0.539 (supercritical fluid extraction) (in g/100 g waste dry matter)
Palm fatty acid distillate[3]	Extractable tocopherols and tocotrienols (0.4%–0.8%), squalene (0.6%, 2128–13,504 mg/kg)
Wheat germ and bran[4]	4-Hydroxy-3-methoxyphenyl β-D-glcp-(1→6)-β-D-glcp-(1→6)-β-D-glcp, which was present at 6.3 g/kg in germ and 0.7 g/kg in bran
Pearled wheat and roller-milled fractions[5]	Total phenols: 1st and 2nd pearlings (>4000 mg/kg); 3rd and 4th pearlings (>3000 mg/kg); bran and shorts 4000 mg/kg, bran flour ~3000 mg/kg, first middlings flour <1000 mg/kg
Bran samples of seven wheat varieties[6]	Ferulic acid (99–231 μg/g; 46%–67% of total phenolic acids); a-, d-, g-tocopherols (1.28–21.29, 0.23–7.0, 0.92–6.90 μγ/g, respectively); lutein, cryptoxanthin (0.50–1.80, 0.18–0.64 μg/g, respectively); zeaxanthin (up to 2.19 μg/g); β-carotene (0.09–0.40 μg/g)
Wheat bran fractions[7]	Up to 400 mg of insoluble ferulate and 39.9 mg total diferulic acids/100 g (d.m.) 9 and 8 (and 20.1 mg of total diFAs/100 g (d.m.))
Rye bran product[7]	Up to 230 mg of insoluble ferulate and 22.5 mg total diferulic acidase/100 g (d.m.)
Triticale[8]	Total phenols in bran, flakes, straw, leaves 284.9 ± 0.4, 89.6 ± 0.73, 65.3 ± 1.2, 226.6 ± 0.5 mg/100 g (Folin-Ciocalteu)
Tannin fraction from buckwheat groats[9]	Total phenols: 371 mg catechin equiv/g
Apple pomace[10]	Chlorogenic acid, phloridzin, procyanidin B2, epicatechin, quercetin 3-rhamnoside and glucoside, catechin: up to 14.3, 11.4, 9.3, 9.3, 4.7, 3.9, and 2.4 g/kg DM, respectively

Source: [1]Adapted from Galanakis 2012; [2]Patel, M., and S. N. Naik, 2004, *J Sci Ind Res India* 63: 569–578; [3]Tan, Y. A. et al. 2007, *Eur J Lipid Sci Tech* 109: 380–393; [4]Zhokhov, S. S. et al. 2010, *Food Chem* 121: 645–652; [5]Beta, T. et al. 2005, *Cereal Chem* 82: 390–393; [6]Zhou, K. et al. 2004, *J Agric Food Chem* 52: 6108–6114; [7]Gallardo, C. et al. 2006, *Food Chem* 99: 455–463; [8]Hosseinian, F. S., and G. Mazza, 2009, *J Funct Foods* 1: 57–64; [9]Karamać, M., 2010, *J Am Oil Chem Soc* 87: 559–566; [10]Bhushan, S. et al. 2008, *Crit Rev Biotechnol* 28: 285–296.

potential within the food industry. Although a large variety of by-products of plant origin represent an abundant source of bioactive compounds, their concentration in the residues is usually rather low. Therefore, to exploit these resources, commercially relevant strategies for their extraction must be developed. Pressurized liquid extraction and supercritical CO_2 extraction with pretreatment by novel nonthermal processing techniques in order to enhance extraction (Wijngaard et al. 2012) as well as the use of solid-state fermentation, a bioprocess that may convert inexpensive agro-industrial residues in a great variety of valuable compounds including bioactive phenolic compounds (Martins et al. 2011), were shown to be promising alternative techniques for increasing the effectiveness of isolation and fractionation of natural antioxidants from various plant-origin by-products. Some examples of the recovery and the presence of phenols and other natural antioxidants from 100 g of waste dry matter are presented in Table 9.4, and the structures of strong antioxidants present in various by-products are presented in Figure 9.4.

9.5.2 FRUITS AND VEGETABLES

The technologies and commercialized applications for the recovery of high added-value components from food wastes and the agro-industrial potential of exotic fruit by-products as a source of food additives have been recently reviewed (Ayala-Zavala et al. 2011; Galanakis 2012). The results reviewed in the former article estimated that the concentration of natural antioxidants in the peels and seeds of exotic fruits is remarkably higher than in the pulp. For instance, the content of phenolics in banana, avocado, mango, and pomegranate peel was higher than in the pulp by 4, 2.6, 29, and 10 times, respectively. Therefore, by-products from such fruits may serve as a source for antibrowning additives (antioxidants avoiding browning and lipid oxidation and as functional food ingredients), antimicrobial and flavoring agents, colorants, and dietary fiber additives. The group of scientists screened 11 fruit and vegetable by-products and 2 minor crops for industrial polyphenol exploitation potential by determination of their extraction yield, total phenolic content, and antioxidant activity (Peschel et al. 2006). They included the residues from juice production (apple, strawberry, pear, red beet), waste from a canning factory (artichoke, asparagus, tomato), harvest remains (broccoli, cucumber, endive, chicory), and minor crops (goldenrod or *Solidago virdaurea* and woad or *Isatis tinctoria*). The extracts with the highest activity, economic justification, and phenolic content were obtained from apples (48.6), pears (60.7), tomatoes (61.0), goldenrod (251.4), and artichokes (514.2) (in milligram gallic acid equivalents in gram of dry extract). Based on laboratory-scale results, apple, goldenrod, and artichoke by-products were extracted at pilot plant scale, and it was estimated that the antioxidative effect of the three extracts was similar to the established commercial antioxidants Oxynex K at 0.1% (tocopherols, ascorbyl palmitate, and ascorbic and citric acids), Controx KS at 0.15% (70%–100% tocopherols, 10%–20% hydrogenated palm glycerides, and citrate), and BHT at 0.01% (Peschel et al. 2006). A number of strong antioxidants (catechins, procyanidins, caffeic and chlorogenic acids, phloridzin, phloretin, and quercetin glycosides, etc.—in total, 50 phenolic compounds) are present in apple pomace, a by-product obtained during the processing of apple fruits for juice, cider, or wine. The possibilities of

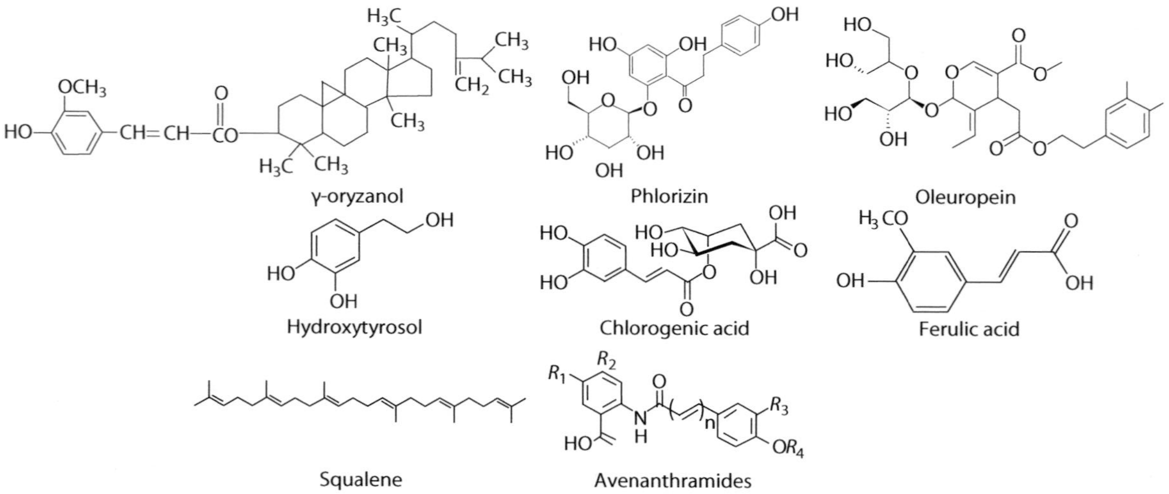

FIGURE 9.4 Structures of some efficient antioxidants obtained from agri-food by-products: phlorizin (apple pomace), γ-oryzanol (rice bran), oleuropein and hydroxytyrosol (olive by-products), chlorogenic acid (coffee by-products, apple pomace), ferulic acid (plant cell walls), squalene (palm fatty acid distillate), and avenanthramides (the groats of oat seeds).

their recovery were reviewed, and it was concluded that the content of some of them may be sufficiently high for efficient commercial extraction; for example, the content of the main apple phenolic compounds chlorogenic acid, phloridzin, procyanidin B2, epicatechin, quercetin 3-rhamnoside and glucoside, and catechin may be as high as 14.3, 11.4, 9.3, 9.3, 4.7, 3.9, and 2.4 g/kg dm, respectively (Bhushan et al. 2008 and references therein). It was estimated that in total, apple pomace lyophylisate may contain 60 g/kg dm of valuable phenolic natural antioxidants (Schieber et al. 2003).

Large amounts of valuable by-products are obtained in the processing of another extremely important fruit: grapes, particularly in the form of wine waste. Grape seeds contain a high amount of total phenols (8.58 g per 100 g dm), total flavonoids (8.36 g catechin equivalents per 100 g dm), and proanthocyanidins (5.95 g cyanidin equivalents per 100 g dm) (Negro et al. 2003); grape seed oil is rich in vitamin E (80–120 mg/100 g). The by-products obtained after winery exploitation, either seeds or pomaces, constitute a very cheap source for the extraction of antioxidant flavonols, which can be used as dietary supplements or in the production of phytochemicals, thus providing an important economic advantage: The number of grape-based by-products of health relevance in the United States already in 2000 were 34 items (Arvanitoyannis et al. 2006 and references therein).

9.5.3 Cereals, Seeds, and Nuts

Processing wastes from cereals and seeds could offer cheap, natural antioxidants for the industry, such as ascorbic and dehydroascorbic and phenolic acids, flavanoids, lignans, stilbenes, carotenes, xanthophylls, tocopherols, and others. For instance, it was estimated that rice bran, a by-product of the rice-milling process, contains most of the phytochemicals, the contents of which, depending on product color, were in the following range (in dry weight): vitamin E antioxidants (tocopherols and toco-trienols), 319.67–443.73 µg/g; γ-oryzanols, 3862–5911 µg/g; anthocyanins, 0.02–40.65 mg kuromarin equivalents/g; proanthocyanidins, 0.10–22.61 mg catechin equivalents/g; total phenols, 9.60–81.85 mg gallic acid equivalents/g; and flavonoids, 3.31–23.98 mg catechin equivalents/g (Min et al. 2011b). The concentration of phytochemicals in rice brans and their antioxidant activities, in many cases, were higher than the same characteristics of antioxidant-rich broccoli and blueberries. Rice bran oil is rich in γ-oryzanol, the compound that was first presumed to be a single component but was later determined to be a fraction containing ferulate esters of triterpene alcohol and plant sterols; they occur in rice bran oil at a level of 1%–2% and present a good source of valuable natural antioxidants, which have already been exploited commercially in foods, cosmetics, and nutraceuticals (Patel and Naik 2004).

An increasing number of studies have reported the high antioxidant activity of wheat fractions and, in particular, of germ and bran fractions (Beta et al. 2005; Martínez-Tomé et al. 2004; Yu et al. 2005; Zhou et al. 2004). Biological activities of xylo-OSs, in addition to those related to their modulatory gut effects, also include antioxidant activities: hydrothermal treatment of rice hulls and enzymatic hydrolysis of wheat flour arabinoxylan (DPPH· scavenging); enzymatic hydrolysis of wheat bran (antioxidant activity in an erythrocyte hemolysis assay); hydrothermal processing of bagasse and enzymatic processing (antioxidant activity); and feruloyl xylo-OSs from enzymatic reactions (protective effect against lipid LDL peroxidation). OSs may be obtained from such by-products as corn cobs, barley hulls, brewery spent grains, almond shells, corn stover, corn fiber, rice hulls, flax shive, and wheat straw by various types of treatments and hydrothermal processing and further purified by enzymatic hydrolysis, thermal treatment, or their combinations. The scheme of a possible process for utilization of xylan-containing lignocellulosic materials to obtain purified OSs with prebiotic properties and nonvolatile components with antioxidant activity was proposed (Moure et al. 2006 and references therein). Some antioxidants in plant-origin residues are strongly bound in cell wall matrices and may be released by using enzymes. For instance, ferulic acid, which is the most abundant hydroxycinnamic acid in the plant world (maize bran contains 3.1% w/w) and therefore may be considered as a very promising natural antioxidant presents in the plant cell wall in dehydrodimeric form and serves to enhance wall rigidity and strength. The applications of ferulic acid and feruloyl esterase enzymes for releasing ferulic acid from various substrates (cereal brans, sugar beet pulp, pectin, and xylan) were reviewed (Mathew and Abraham 2004). 4-Hydroxy-3-methoxyphenyl β-D-glucopyranosyl-(1→6)-β-D-glucopyranosyl-(1→6)-β-D-glucopyranoside, which was present at 6.3 g/kg in germ and 0.7 g/kg in bran, contributed 38% in total antioxidant power of water-ethanol extracts, which in μmol TE/L was 2.56 and 0.76, respectively (Zhokhov et al. 2010).

Total phenols in pearled wheat and roller-milled fractions were from 1000 up to more than 4000 mg/kg (Beta et al. 2005). The antioxidant power that was measured in lipid peroxidation, deoxyribose, and peroxidase assays as well as the rancimat test and expressed in a micromolar concentration of a Trolox solution showing the antioxidant capacity equivalent to the dilution of the substance under investigation at 24 h of various oat and wheat bran products was in the range of 9.90–10.53 and 8.41–18.08, respectively. Among bran antioxidants, avenanthramide showed a higher antioxidant level than each of the following typical cereal components: ferulic, gentisic, p-hydroxybenzoic, protocatechuic, syringic, vanillic, and phytic acids and vanillin (Martínez-Tomé et al. 2004). Triticale bran and straw were assessed as potential new sources of phenolic acids, proanthocyanidins, and lignans. Triticale bran, flakes, straw, and leaves as well as wheat, rye, and oat bran contained 284.9 ± 0.4, 89.6 ± 0.73, 65.3 ± 1.2, 226.6 ± 0.5, 442.7 ± 0.8, 257.3 ± 0.9, and 94.2 ± 0.5 mg/100 g of total phenolics, respectively, measured with a Folin–Ciocalteu reagent. Triticale straw was the richest source of proanthocyanidins, containing 862.5 mg catechin equivalents/100 g of tissue; it also contained 0.27 mg/100 g of lignin secoisolariciresinol diglucoside, whereas the bran had only 0.01 mg/100 g (Hosseinian and Mazza 2009).

Sesame seed coats (testae) contained 9.9 mg polyphenols in gram of seed coat dry matter; however, the content of lignin (a natural phenolic polymer, mostly synthesized by radical coupling of three hydroxypropanoids: coumaryl, coniferyl, and sinapyl alcohols), which is also a strong radical scavenger, was 5.42 g/100 g seed coat dry matter (Elleuch et al. 2012). Using a methodology that combined alkaline extraction and ultrasound, antioxidatively active water-soluble heteroxylan (MW = 130 kDa, yield 40% ± 5% w/w) was isolated from corn cobs (Melo-Silveira et al. 2012). Almond kernels and by-products (skin, shell, and hull) were shown to contain a large variety of polyphenolic compounds, such as hydroxybenzoic acids and aldehydes (skin), hydroxycinnamic acids (skin, hull), anthocyanidins and procyanidins (skin), flavonol glycosides (skin), flavonone glycosides (skin), flavonol aglycones (skin), and dihydroflavonol aglycones (skin). The total content of phenolics may reach 413 µg/g in skin, 2.2 g gallic acid equivalents (GAE)/100 g in shells, and 78.2 mg GAE in 1 g methanolic extract of hulls (Esfahlan et al. 2010 and references therein).

9.5.4 OIL PRODUCTION BY-PRODUCTS

Olive by-products, olive leaves, and olive-mill wastewater (OMWW) contain diverse strong antioxidants: The leaves are rich in apigenin-7-O-glycoside and oleuropein, which, depending on its variety, may reach 2.68 and 2.81 g as o-coumaric acid/kg dry weight, respectively (in chemlali olive-leaf extract, oleuropein reached 4.32 g/100 g dry weight), while hydroxytyrosol and tyrosol were the major compounds in the OMWW extract (up to 3.1 and 0.345 g/L, respectively). Other compounds, p-hydroxyphenyl acetic, caffeic, and p-coumaric acids, were present in lower concentrations. It should be considered that the concentration of natural antioxidants in the by-products may vary in a wide range, depending on plant variety, harvesting time, harvesting year, and storage. For instance, hydroxytyrosol concentration increased during storage, varying over a 5-month period from 0.98 to 3.5 g/L (2004–2005) and from 0.77 to 3.1 g/L (2005–2006) after 4 months of storage (Taamalli et al. 2012 and references therein). Some products and processes of obtaining them from food waste are already patented, for instance, strong antioxidant hydroxytyrosol from olive oil waste (Hidrox and Hytolive), olive phenols and dietary fibers containing powders, lycopene from tomato waste, soybean albumin from SPI wastewater, chitosan from shrimp and crab shells, proanthocyanidin from grape and cranberry seed, and ellagic acid and punicalagin from pomegranate rind and seedcase residues (Galanakis 2012). Commercialization of such natural antioxidant-containing products depends on several factors, first of all the technological and economic feasibility of their production on an industrial scale. Laboratory- or even pilot-scale isolation, fractionation, and purification procedures sometimes are difficult to implement on the industrial scale.

A number of natural antioxidants, both water- and lipid-soluble, may be obtained from oil-seed processing by-products (the distillate from soybean and corn oil contains 10%–14% and 7%–10% of tocopherols, respectively) as was demonstrated in the case of extraction of palm oil, which results in product-specific by-products—empty fruit bunches (EFBs), palm pressed fibers (PPFs), shells—and process-specific by-products, such as aqueous waste or sediment. PPF oil is high in antioxidants, such as carotenoids (up to 7000 mg/kg), tocopherols and tocotrienols (2400–3500 mg/kg), and squalene (1000–1800 mg/kg). The Malaysian Palm Oil Board developed a novel patented process for the recovery of valuable antioxidants, including flavonoids (rutin hydrate), polyphenols and phenolic acids (p-hydroxybenzoic, cinnamic, ferulic, and coumaric), water-soluble vitamins, and organic acids from the water-soluble or bioaqueous fraction of the palm oil industry. Malaysian refineries produced approximately 0.6 million MT of palm fatty acid distillate, containing extractable tocopherols and tocotrienols (0.4%–0.8%), squalene (0.6%, 2128–13,504 mg/kg), and phytosterols (0.6%). The potential availability of squalene from such by-products is estimated at 2205 MT in 2010 (Tan et al. 2007 and references therein).

9.5.5 OTHER BY-PRODUCTS AND WASTE

In vitro experiments have indicated that the residue left from ground soybeans after obtaining the water-extractable fraction used to produce bean curd (tofu) or soymilk, called okara, is a potential source of antioxidant components, such as isoflavones (genistein and daidzein), lignans, phytosterols, coumestans, saponins, and phytates (Mateos-Aparicio et al. 2010). Protease hydrolysate from okara possessed *in vitro* reduction power of 11–26 μmol TE/g dw and free-radical scavenging activity of 63–78 μmol TE/g dw. More than 50% of the coffee fruit is not used for production of commercialized green coffee and, therefore, is discarded during processing. The antioxidants in coffee husks, peel, and pulp, which comprise nearly 45% of the cherry, as well as less-studied processing by-products, mucilage, and the parchment, the possibilities of using the roasted coffee silverskin as a dietary fiber-rich ingredient and for its antioxidative properties, and finally, the constituents of interest in low-grade green coffee and spent coffee have been recently reviewed (Esquivel and Jiménez 2012). Coffee pulp contains such natural antioxidants as chlorogenic (42.2% of the total of identified phenolic compounds), dicaffeoylquinic, protocatechuic, ferulic, and 5-feruloylquinic acids, epicatechin, catechin, rutin, and condensed tannins (proanthocyanidins). Cyanidin-3-rutinoside was the main antioxidant in fresh coffee husks; peels and pulp contain cyanidin-3-rutinoside and glucoside and its aglycone. Silverskin, although containing a low content of free phenol compounds, possessed high antioxidant activity because of melanoidins generated during roasting, and finally, the extracts from low-grade green and spent coffee possessed strong radical-scavenging and antioxidant power because of the presence of caffeine, trigonelline, and chlorogenic acids (Esquivel and Jiménez 2012 and references therein).

Different terms, such as fish waste, by-product, and rest raw materials, have been used for marine-origin by-products. Bioactive peptides possessing antioxidant power may be isolated from marine processing waste and shellfish (Harnedy and FitzGerald 2012), while nutritionally valuable proteins and peptides may be obtained from various fish industry by-products, which can account for up to 75% of the catch, depending on postharvest or industrial-preparation processes (Rustad et al. 2011). The authors suggest that preparation of fish protein hydrolysates (FPHs) with antioxidant properties will enable the production of protein-enriched and oxidatively stable seafood. Recently, FPH was found to be a potential source of antioxidants, such as peptides, with anticancer properties. Even tuna bone was shown to exhibit antioxidant activities: The results demonstrated that an antioxidant peptide from tuna backbone protein significantly inhibited lipid peroxidation in a linoleic acid emulsion system and also quenched DPPH$^{\bullet}$, HO$^{\bullet}$, and O$_2^{\bullet-}$ free radicals in a dose-dependent manner (Herpandi et al. 2011 and references therein). The procedure of isolation, purification, and characterization of the natural antioxidant-containing amine group from shrimp waste was also reported (Li et al. 1997). Antioxidatively active peptides that may be produced from marine- and animal-origin by-products were also discussed in Sections 9.3.2 and 9.3.3.

9.6 NATURAL ANTIOXIDANTS IN CONVENTIONAL ORGANIC FOOD SYSTEMS

9.6.1 GENERAL ASPECTS

A food system includes the inputs needed and outputs generated at each of its steps.

Conventional food systems operate on economies of scale and are geared toward a production model that requires maximizing efficiency in order to lower consumer costs and increase overall production, and they utilize economic models, such as vertical integration, economic specialization, and global trade (Scrinis 2007). The term "conventional," used when describing food systems, is in large part a result of comparisons made to it by proponents of other food systems, collectively known as alternative food systems. Organic food systems, which, in some countries, are also referred to as "ecological," are, first of all, characterized by the reduced dependence on chemical inputs. Demand for organically grown products is increasing, largely as a result of concerns consumers have about health and nutrition. The term "organically grown food" denotes products that have been produced in strict accordance with the principles and practices of organic agriculture. The use of alternatives to synthetic fertilizers is an important issue in organic systems: Organic products are grown without the chemical fertilizers and pesticides of conventional food systems, and livestock is reared without the use of antibiotics or growth hormones. Organic nutrient sources, including compost, manure, compost extract, and authorized fertilizers could be combined and used in order to achieve a balanced nutrient supply and an improved organic product yield and quality. Knowledge of cultivars with naturally higher antioxidant levels could assist producers in growing the species that may provide a competitive advantage and the opportunity to capitalize on the increasing popularity of locally grown, high-quality, fresh produce for the community food systems. The reduced inputs of organic agriculture can also lead to a greater reliance on local knowledge, creating a stronger knowledge community among farmers, which is also important to community food systems (Morgan and Murdoch 2000). Organic agriculture is promoted for the ecological benefits of reduced application of chemicals, the health benefits of lower consumption of hazardous contaminants, the economic benefits that accrue to farmers through a price premium, and the social benefits of increased transparency in the food system. The customers expect organic food to be authentic and healthy and, therefore, the organic market is growing rapidly. The awareness of pesticide residues is one main point in customers' decisions to choose organic food; however, organically produced foods are also expected to contain more secondary plant compounds, such as natural antioxidants.

Do the organic food systems provide foods with higher concentrations of healthy nutrients than the conventional food systems? Is the content of natural antioxidants in organic agri-food products higher than in conventional ones? In general, the public believes that products of organic farming are healthier and safer; however, the increased market for organic food needs to quantify the differences in crops grown under organic and integrated systems. Numerous research data demonstrated that some crops under organic farming practices contained more bioactive substances, such as phenolic acids, flavanoids, vitamin C, and carotenoids; they also contained less toxic residues, such as pesticides, nitrates, and nitrites. Some research studies also confirmed better biological activity of organic products versus conventional because of the higher content of bioactive compounds. However, scientific data on how organic and conventional production practices influence the nutritional quality of food, especially the accumulation of phenols and other important antioxidants are still limited and insufficient for making unquestionable conclusions. The number of studies focused on this important issue has been steadily increasing during recent years. The cost of organic foods is higher compared to conventional foods, and consumers should know that they pay a higher price for scientifically proven higher value. However, until now, data obtained on the effect of organic agriculture on the accumulation of antioxidants are rather controversial. The concentration of antioxidants and other nutrients in agri-food materials depends on many factors and, therefore, it is rather difficult to estimate the effect of mere organic practices on their production and accumulation. The factors beyond the agricultural method, such as plant genotype, plant tissue, product size, development stage, ripening, disease and pests, fertilization, irrigation, pesticide application, season, location, climatic conditions, variety, and environmental stresses, such as UV radiation, drought, soil conditions, and tillage, may have an important influence on the accumulation of phytochemicals (Traill et al. 2008).

Natural antioxidants have become an important issue in recent years, and this tendency commits producers and merchandisers of organic food to claim that there are more antioxidants and other healthy nutrients in organic food than in conventional foods. There are two theories explaining the production of bigger amounts of antioxidants in the plants. First is to ward off insect and fungal attack: Because conventional crops are protected by pesticides, they do not need to synthesize these protective materials (Rosen 2010). However, organic farmers may use "natural" pesticides, such as copper sulfate, and physical methods to suppress insect and fungal activity, and some pesticides may increase secondary metabolite formation while others decrease it. For instance, chitosan, which can be used as a pesticide in organic and conventional farming, has an effect on flavonoid content (Ren et al. 2001). A second theory, which was lent some credence in several published articles, assumes that the higher availability of nitrogen in soils with synthetic fertilizer leads to production of nitrogen-containing metabolites at the expense of carbon-containing metabolites, such as the phenolic antioxidants (Brandt and Molgaard 2001 and references therein). Synthetic fertilizers frequently make nitrogen more available for the plants than do the organic fertilizers and may accelerate plant development, allocating plant resources for growth purposes and causing a decrease in the production of secondary metabolites, such as polyphenolic compounds. For instance, the studies that compared conventionally and organically grown cereals determined higher levels of proteins and amino acids in the conventionally produced grain with a higher N-fertilization rate, which is very likely to explain this difference (Huber et al. 2011 and references therein). It was suggested that limited nutrient accessibility and higher levels of pest and disease occurrence in organic farming systems may increase the biosynthesis of secondary metabolites, including flavonoids (Strissel et al. 2005). The plants manufacture and accumulate an array of defense-related phytochemicals under herbivore and pathogen attack; the accumulation of phenolic compounds may be also accelerated as a result of a deficiency in nitrogen, phosphate, and iron (Zhao et al. 2006 and references therein).

Hundreds of studies aimed at comparing the composition of diverse organic and conventional crops, their antioxidant properties, and their *in vivo* effects have been performed, and the data from these studies were extensively reviewed (Woese et al. 1997; Worthington 2001; Magkos et al. 2003; Brandt et al. 2004; Winter and Davis 2006; Zhao et al. 2006; Dangour et al. 2009; Lairon 2009; Rosen 2010; Huber et al. 2011). The aims of the studies as well as the reviews summarizing their findings were focused on various topics; however, the majority of them also compared the concentration of nutrients in organic products with conventional ones. The conclusions on this matter, both from the individual experimental studies and from the reviews, are rather diverse, controversial, and even contradictory. In the earlier published reviews, it was concluded that there were trends toward higher vitamin C content in organic products (Woese et al. 1997; Worthington 2001). Afterward, more than 200 papers concerning the nutrient content of organic versus conventionally produced foods were summarized in a review by Dutch scientists, who, although focusing on the impact of organic foods on human health, also included data on the comparative studies on the content of nutrients, such as vitamin C, carotenoids, and phenolic compounds (Huber et al. 2011). This review demonstrated rather controversial results on the content of natural antioxidants in organic crops. A higher vitamin C content was found in many organic products, for example, peaches and tomatoes, although other studies reported a similar or lower content of vitamin C in organic tomatoes, broccoli, bell peppers, pears, and peaches. A higher carotenoid content was found in organically grown sweet peppers, yellow plums, tomatoes, and carrots, whereas others found a lower or similar content of carotenoids in organic blanched carrots and tomatoes. A number of studies reported a higher content of phenolics in organic products, whereas other studies found a similar or lower content of phenolic compounds in organic products than in conventional ones. The inconsistency in the findings in the reviewed studies might be explained by the fact that the content of carotenoids may depend on soil type and genotype as well as the fertilizers and pesticides used.

Regarding animal-origin products, some studies found a higher content of conjugated linoleic acids (CLA) in milk from organically raised animals, especially in the summertime when they have their outdoor grazing facilities. However, a study from the United Kingdom showed that milk from low input systems, both organic and nonorganic, has higher contents of CLA, although the highest contents were found in the nonorganic low-input system. Outdoor grazing, a high biodiversity in the pastures, low levels of concentrates, and no silage feeding were found to be predominant factors for beneficial milk fatty acid composition (Huber et al. 2011 and references therein). Several of the systematic and nonsystematic reviews on the nutritional content and quality of organic produce concluded that organic produce has a higher nutrient content (Worthington 2001; Magkos et al. 2003), whereas others concluded that there are no consistent differences between conventionally and organically grown foods (Bourn and Prescott 2002; Woese et al. 1997; Dangour et al. 2009).

Generally, all agricultural crops accumulate antioxidants; however, fruits and vegetables always have been regarded as the main sources of antioxidatively active phytochemicals. The first review discussing the factors that can influence the levels of phytochemicals in crops as well as the results of published studies that compared the effect of organic and conventional production systems on the phytochemical content in fruits and vegetables was published by Zhao et al. (2006). The overall evidence from this review seems to be in favor of enhancement of phytochemical content in organically grown produce, but it is also recognized that there was little systematic study of the factors that may contribute to the increased phytochemical content in organic crops. Therefore, the consistency of the differences and the extent to which biotic and abiotic stresses, soil biology, and other factors contribute to those differences should be carefully investigated. Various problems associated with many completed studies tend to weaken the validity of the comparisons, and therefore data very frequently are rather controversial and even unreliable because of shortcomings in experimental design, incomplete methodology, lack of proper statistical data handling, etc. For instance, the type and the number of compounds that were reported for the same species of organic and conventional origin differ between the performed studies. Some studies on antioxidants are limited to measuring the radical-scavenging and/or antioxidant capacity using *in vitro* assays, whereas such an approach does not provide sufficiently sound scientific data for conclusive statements. For comprehensive assessment of the effects of an organic system, it is advisable that the total content of phenolics, anthocyanins, flavonoids, flavanols, and, even better, the concentrations of individual phytochemicals would be measured at precisely controlled growing conditions (Zhao et al. 2006 and references therein). Some *in vitro* studies comparing the health-related properties of organic versus conventional foods showed higher antioxidative and antimutagenic activity as well as better inhibition of cancer cell proliferation in organically produced food (Huber et al. 2011); higher plasma antioxidant status was reported, followed by the diet, which was based on organic products (fruits and vegetables, wine, milk) possessing higher ORAC values than conventional ones (Di Renzo et al. 2007); however, most of such studies were strongly criticized for their inconsistencies in experimental design and evaluation methodologies (Dangour et al. 2009). It may also be observed that with the small impact of agricultural practice on major plant nutrients, research interest has shifted toward plant secondary metabolites and antioxidants (Bourn and Prescott 2002; Rosen 2010). Many of these plant compounds are still unknown, and only a very narrow range of compounds and their bioavailability have been studied in relation to the healthfulness of organic produce. Further, in this section, some studies on the comparison of organically and conventionally grown crops will be briefly reviewed.

9.6.2 Berry Fruits

Some berry fruit species have been recognized as "antioxidant champions" among all types of plant-origin products. Antioxidatively active berry nutrients as well as the possibility of enhancing their concentrations were the focus of many studies. Comparison of the phytochemical composition of various berry accessions cultivated under specified conditions also was the aim of such studies. It was reported that total anthocyanin (TAnC) and phenolic (TPC) contents in berries as well as the total antioxidant activity were not influenced by the agricultural production system; however, antioxidant activity varied significantly between the studied cultivars (Sablani et al. 2010). However, in another report, statistically higher levels of TPC were consistently found in organically grown marionberries and strawberries as compared to those produced by conventional agricultural practices (Asami et al. 2003). Regardless of the high TPC, TAnC, and ORAC activity in all investigated blueberries, not all the organic berries showed significantly higher TPC, TAnC, and ORAC than the conventional berries, thus demonstrating only subtle differences in bioactive phytochemicals between the organically and conventionally grown fruits. For instance, TPC, TAnC, and ORAC in organically cultivated powder blue cultivar were significantly higher than in conventionally grown, while in the case of some other cultivars, these differences were not significant (You et al. 2011). Organic blueberries (*Vaccinium corymbosum* L.) had significantly higher TPC, TAnC, and ORAC values than the fruits from conventional culture: In organic fruits, the average ORAC, TAnC, and TPC values in fresh weight were 46.14 μmol of TE/g, 131.2 mg/100 g, and 319.3 mg/100 g, respectively, whereas, in conventionally cultured berries, they were 30.8 μmol of TE/g, 82.4 mg/100 g, and 190.3 mg/100 g, respectively. The organic fruits had higher contents of myricetin-3-arabinoside, quercetin-3-glucoside, delphinidin-3-galactoside, glucoside and arabinoside, petunidin 3-galactoside and glucoside, and malvidin 3-arabinoside (Wang et al. 2008). The application of high amounts of N and K fertilizers resulted in high amounts of all nutrients and bioactive compounds in blackberry fruit except ellagic acid (Ali et al. 2012). In general, no consistent differences were observed between the phytochemical concentrations in fresh conventional and organic blueberries (Duke and Reka) and Meeker red raspberries; however, the effect of drying on the retention of phytochemicals depended on the drying technique, cultivar, and production system (Sablani et al. 2011). The organically grown high bush blueberry had the highest flavonol oligomer and chlorogenic acid contents but lower anthocyanidin content than its conventionally grown counterpart (Rodriguez-Mateos et al. 2012). Organic fertilizer also increased the soil biota activity, mycorrhizal colonization, and high bush blueberry leaf antioxidant content relative to a conventional N source (Montalba et al. 2010).

The TAnC during ripening of conventionally grown grapes was significantly higher compared with organic production. In all samples, grapes from the conventional agriculture presented higher proportions of delphinidin, petunidin, malvidin, and acylated malvidin glucosides compared to grapes from organic agriculture (Vian et al. 2006); however, no differences were found in the TPC as well as in the antioxidant activity in two types of organic and conventional red grapes in another study (Mulero et al. 2010). Organic grape juices showed statistically higher values of TPC and resveratrol as compared to conventional grape juices (Dani et al. 2007).

Raspberries are known as a very good source of strong antioxidant ellagic acid and its derivatives. Organic raspberries exhibited higher antioxidant capacities and individual flavonoid content, and also enhanced activities of antioxidant enzymes. In addition, essential oil treatments (natural phytochemicals) promoted the activities of antioxidant enzymes as well as the antioxidant capacities of raspberries. Postharvest essential oil treatments had a positive effect on enhancing antioxidant capacities in raspberries from both organic and conventional cultures (Jin et al. 2012b). In another study, the response of three raspberry cultivars within specific site conditions was often more pronounced than the system of cultivation, and the values of vitamin C, TPC, and DPPH˙ scavenging capacity between organic and conventional methods did not show an unequivocal prevalence (Skupien et al. 2011).

Strawberries grown from organic cultures exhibited generally higher activities in antioxidant enzymes and produced fruits with higher level of antioxidants (Jin et al. 2011). Organic farms had strawberries with a longer shelf life, higher antioxidant activity, and concentration of ascorbic acid and phenolic compounds (Reganold et al. 2010). It was also demonstrated that strawberry fruits from plants grown in compost socks had significantly higher ORAC values and content of flavonoids, anthocyanins, and citric acid than fruit produced in the black plastic mulch or matted row systems; in addition, preplanting a vinegar treatment increased cyanidin-based and pelargonidin-based anthocyanins (Wang and Millner 2009). The ratio of ascorbate to dehydroascorbate was significantly higher in organically cultivated strawberries, and their extracts had a higher antiproliferative activity in the cells at the highest concentration than the conventionally grown, and this might indicate a higher content of secondary metabolites with anticarcinogenic properties in the organically grown berries. When the organically grown strawberry cultivars as a group were compared to the conventionally grown cultivars, the levels of each antioxidant in the group (vitamin C, TPC) grown organically were higher although not always significantly. However, for some cultivars, the findings were diverse: TPCs were higher in the conventionally grown honeoye strawberries; the levels of ellagic acid, hydroxycinnamic acids (HCA, not significantly), TAnC, cyanidin and pelargonidin, and TPC were higher in the organic cavendish cultivar, whereas flavonols were lower in the organically cultivated strawberries; the level of HCA (not significantly) was higher in organic honeoye, while the levels of ellagic acid, TAnC, cyanidin, pelargonidin, and TPC were lower in the organically grown strawberries (Olsson et al. 2006).

Statistically significant differences between blackcurrants grown on different farms were found for almost all compounds, namely, conjugates of hydroxycinnamic acids, flavonols, and anthocyanins; the differences between the highest and the lowest measured values of major phenolic compounds of different phenolic classes ranged from 24% to 77%. Principal component analysis quite effectively separated farms from each other but did not cluster them according to cultivation technique, and therefore it was concluded that the biochemical quality of organically grown blackcurrant fruits did not differ from those grown conventionally (Anttonen and Karjalainen 2006).

9.6.3 Fruits

A great number of studies were carried out with apples as they are one of the most commercially important fruit species. Roussos and Gasparatos (2009) reported that conventionally grown apple trees produced almost twice the yield of the organically managed ones, and the flesh plus peel portion of the conventionally produced fruits exhibited higher total flavonoid and o-diphenol concentrations. Antioxidant activities of fruit extracts isolated from five apple cultivars grown by organic and conventional agricultural methods on neighboring farms were also relatively similar and well correlated to their polyphenolic content. The most important polyphenolics (chlorogenic acid, catechin, epicatechin, procyanidin B1 and B2, cyanidin 3-galactoside, phloridzin, quercetin 3-galactoside, and arabinoside) in the studied fruit cultivars showed that their concentrations do not differentiate significantly between the organic and conventional apples (Valavanidis et al. 2009). The study of four apple cultivars grown in different Italian regions also did not reveal any consistent effect of organic farming on the content of flavanols, anthocyanidins, flavonols, and proanthocyanidins (Lamperi et al. 2008). The average content of identified and quantified polyphenols in the organically and conventionally produced apples was 308 and 321 µg/g fresh weight, respectively, and no significant differences in the sum of phenolic compounds or in either of the polyphenol classes were found between the agricultural methods (Briviba et al. 2007). Maturity and quality of fruit harvested from an orchard of disease-resistant liberty apple (*Malus* x *domestica* Borkh.) trees was investigated during and after the transition from conventional to integrated and organic fruit production systems (a 4-year study), and it was found that the TPC and antioxidant capacity of the fruit were similar between treatments (Peck et al. 2009). Phenolic content in the apple peel of 11 apple cultivars from Austria and Slovenia was not different between organically grown cultivars and apples from integrated production; however, organically grown apples exhibited a higher content of phenolic substances in the apple pulp. This may be a result of either the different genotype source or the growing technology (Veberic et al. 2005). No significant differences in the polyphenol content and the antioxidant capacity from the organic and conventional farming system of apples were observed by Stracke et al. (2010). On the contrary, Petkovsek et al. (2010) determined that the levels of all analyzed groups of phenolics (hydroxycinnamic acids, flavanols, dihydrochalcones, flavonols, and anthocyanins) were higher, although not always significantly, in the organically grown apple leaves and fruits than in the leaves or apples from the integrated production. For instance, the leaves from organic trees had 10%–20% higher TPC than the leaves from trees in the integrated growing system, whereas organic apples had higher TPC, hydroxycinnamic acids, flavanols, dihydrochalcones, and quercetins than the integrated-grown ones. Generally, the studies on apples tend to show that the effects of organic culture might be less important than other factors.

A parallel increase in polyphenol content and polyphenoloxidase activity of organic peaches and pears as compared with the corresponding conventional samples was found (Carbonaro and Mattera 2001). The content of ascorbic and citric acids were higher in organic than conventional peaches, whereas α-tocopherol was increased in organic pears (Carbonaro et al. 2002). Ascorbic acid, α- and γ-tocopherols, and β-carotene were higher in organic plums grown in soil covered with natural meadow, whereas the highest content of phenolic acids was detected in plums grown on soil covered with trifolium. TPC and quercetin content was higher in conventional plums, while myricetin and kaempferol were higher in organic plums. Under the same cultivar and climate conditions, the type of soil management turned out to be of primary importance in influencing the concentration of health-promoting compounds in plums (Lombardi-Boccia et al. 2004). There were no significant differences in the content of TPC, the total *o*-diphenol, the total flavonoid, hesperidin, and narirutin between organically and integrated produced oranges; however, β-carotene concentration (0.43 mg/L) was detected in higher concentrations in organically produced fruit (Roussos 2011). Another study concluded that organic red oranges have a higher phytochemical content (phenolics, anthocyanins, and ascorbic acid), total antioxidant activity, and bioactivity than red oranges of integrated systems (Tarozzi et al. 2006). The mean concentrations of the flavanone glycosides, narirutin, hesperidin, and didymin were several-folds higher in peeled fruit than in tangerine juice and significantly higher in organic tangerines. Narirutin and hesperidin in juice from organic products as well as narirutin in juice from agrochemical-safe products were significantly higher than the respective mean concentrations in juice from agrochemical-based products. Ascorbic acid concentrations were not predicted by the type of cultivation, whereas α-tocopherol was significantly higher in juice from organic products (Stuetz et al. 2010).

The study on polyphenol content and antioxidant capacity in various organically and conventionally grown fruits (bananas, apples, oranges, papayas, mangos, tangerines) and vegetables (potatoes, carrots, tomatoes, broccoli, onions, white cabbage) showed that organic fruits tend to have higher hydrolyzable polyphenol contents than conventional ones with the values ranging from 11.5% (orange peels) to 72.6% (papaya peels) higher for hydrolyzable polyphenols. However, polyphenol content and antioxidant capacity varied among organic and conventional vegetables with no prevalence from either agricultural type. Based on these findings, it was suggested that the effect of organic practices results in different effect patterns, according to the plant species analyzed, with fruits being more susceptible to the induction of polyphenol synthesis and the greatest accumulation of polyphenols in external plant tissues, while, in general, organic agriculture results in products with similar or slightly higher polyphenol content and antioxidant capacity (Faller and Fialho 2010).

9.6.4 Vegetables

Among numerous species of vegetables, the effect of agriculture systems on tomatoes was most frequently studied. Aggregation of farms by type across 2 years resulted in no significant differences between organic and conventional farming systems for all tomato-fruit parameters measured, including the content of bioactive compounds with antioxidant activity (β-carotene, lycopene, ascorbic acid, and TPC) and antioxidant activity. On the other hand, farm-management skills combined with site-specific effects contributed to high lycopene levels, and the choice of variety significantly influenced the content of bioactive compounds, particularly ascorbic acid and TPC (Juroszek et al. 2009). Tomato cultivars (10 tested) and year had an effect in all conducted tests, while growing method influenced yield, soluble solid content, ascorbic acid, and radical-scavenging capacity. The ratio of organic to conventional in TPC was 0.94:1.14, in ascorbic acid was 1.10:1.13, in ABTS$^{•+}$ was 1.14:1.37, and in DPPH$^•$ was 0.97:1.13. Year-to-year variability and the production method affected tomato quality and nutritional characteristics, although the trends were not consistent (Aldrich et al. 2010). Treatments with chicken manure or grass or clover mulch did not significantly affect tomato lycopene and TPC (Toor et al. 2006). No effect was found on lycopene and TPC in all tomato cultivars grown in Tunisia, whereas marketable organic yield when averaged across four field tomato cultivars was only about 63% of conventional yield (Riahi et al. 2009a). TPC and lycopene contents in tomatoes were not affected by different organic fertilizer treatments, such as various combinations of codahumus, mixed compost, olive husk, horse manure, poultry manure, and sheep manure (Riahi et al. 2009b). In another study for all nutrients examined, including antioxidants lycopene, β-carotene, ascorbic and citric acids, and phenolic compounds, tomato cultivar differences were greater than differences because of a cultivation method (Ordóñez-Santos et al. 2011).

The above-mentioned studies agree that the most important variable in the micronutrient content of tomatoes is the cultivar; organically grown tomatoes are no more nutritious than the conventionally grown vegetables when soil fertility is well managed. However, there are some reports claiming a superior quality of organically grown tomatoes in terms of their phytochemical content. Polat et al. (2010) reported that the application of organic fertilizers positively affected the micronutritional element content of tomato fruits compared to the conventional treatment. Comparing organic and integrated agricultures, significantly higher levels of quercetin, kaempferol, and ascorbic acid (by 30%, 17%, and 26%, respectively) were found for Burbank tomatoes, while only the levels of kaempferol (by 20%) were significantly higher in organic Ropreco tomatoes. However, year-to-year variability was significant, and high values from 2003 influenced the 3-year average value of quercetin reported for organic Burbank tomatoes, which generally had higher levels of quercetin, kaempferol, TPC, and ascorbic acid than Ropreco tomatoes. In addition, total carotenoid concentration and antioxidant activity were higher in organic tomatoes (De Pascale et al. 2006). Organic tomatoes had higher vitamin C, carotenoid, and polyphenol contents (except for chlorogenic acid) than conventional tomatoes when the results were expressed in fresh matter; however, no significant difference was found for lycopene and naringenin when the results were expressed in dry matter. Moreover, for the nutritional intervention (3 weeks, 96 g/day of tomato puree), no significant difference was found between the two purees produced from organic and conventional tomatoes with regard to their ability to affect the plasma levels of vitamin C and lycopene (Caris-Veyrat et al. 2004). Organic cultivation was found to provide tomatoes and tomato-derived products with a significantly higher content of TPC and individual antioxidant microconstituents as caffeic acid and its hexosides, neochlorogenic, cryptochlorogenic, chlorogenic, dicaffeoylquinic acids, ferulic acid-O-hexoside, rutin, quercetin, kaempferol-3-O-rutinoside, naringenin, and naringenin-7-O-glucoside (Vallverdú-Queralt et al. 2011). Tomato fruits of three cultivars from conventional greenhouse production observed higher levels of sugars and vitamin C, while those grown organically contained substantial amounts of lycopene and carotenoids; the results also showed differences between cultivar and season of production (Kapoulas et al. 2011). The main polyphenols in tomatoes in conventional and organic extracts were quercetin (33.90 ± 6.31 and 17.92 ± 1.09 mg/kg), chlorogenic (3.52 ± 0.74 and 2.82 ± 0.92 mg/kg), and caffeic (3.61 ± 0.71 and 3.29 ± 0.33 mg/kg) acids. Although statistical differences were found between organic and conventional extracts in several target compounds, no difference in biological effect was observed using cell models (Durazzo et al. 2010). It seems that compared to production practices and environmental effects of years that are generally beyond the control of small-scale producers, the choice of cultivar provides the simplest and most effective means of increasing antioxidant properties of tomatoes (Aldrich et al. 2010).

The influence of a protected environment, organic fertilization, and the growth stage on the ORAC values of spinach, pak choi, red leaf lettuce, and romaine lettuce were also studied, and it was found that pak choi grown in high tunnels had significantly lower ORAC than field-grown plants, while organic fertilizer markedly increased the antioxidant capacity of pak choi compared with conventional treatment. However, in contrast to the first trial, organic fertilization did not cause an increase in the antioxidant capacity of the leafy vegetables. The fertilizer effect may have been confounded by nutrient availability and insect attack, resulting in significant yield reduction under organic treatment. The total antioxidant capacity of pak choi decreased as the fertilizer rate increased, especially under conventional fertilization, whereas a significant decline in ORAC under high tunnel production was observed only in spinach (Zhao et al. 2007). None of the studies performed on pak choi, lettuce, and spinach showed consistent enhancement of phytochemical levels or taste superiority of organic versus conventional produce; however, they did reveal various intriguing differences, including a tendency for phytochemical or antioxidant levels to be higher in organic production plots and for these levels to be higher in field-grown than in high tunnel-grown crops (Carey and Zhao 2007). Antioxidant activity and TPC in pak choi were higher under organic compared with synthetic fertilization; however, vermicompost teas generally decreased phenolics under organic fertilization and increased them under synthetic fertilization compared with the control (Pant et al. 2009).

Experimental results showed that organic farming provided peppers (*Capsicum annuum*) with the highest intensities of red and yellow colors, contents of minerals, antioxidant activity, and total carotenoids, which were found at the levels of 3231, 2493, and 1829 mg/kg for organic, integrated, and conventional sweet peppers, respectively (Pérez-López et al. 2007b). The highest content of total carotenoids was found in the soilless red peppers, which reached a maximum of 148 mg/100 g fw, while slightly lower contents were found in integrated and organic red peppers. TPC in sweet peppers, which ranged from 1.2 to 4.1 mg/100 g fw, was significantly affected by the harvest time but not by the production system assayed. Soilless peppers showed similar or even higher concentrations of bioactive compounds (vitamin C, provitamin A, total carotenoid, hydroxycinnamic acids, and flavonoids) than peppers grown under organic and integrated practices (Marín et al. 2008). The content of ascorbic acid, flavonoids (apigenin, luteolin, and quercetin), and TPC in the organically grown hot pepper was significantly higher than that of conventionally grown peppers regardless of fruit color. In addition, the ABTS[•+] scavenging activity of organic red fruits was significantly higher than that of conventional red fruits. Moreover, regardless of the color of the fruits, higher antioxidative activity was observed in blood plasma from rats that were administered with the organic fruit extracts (Kim et al. 2010). Organic farming increased antioxidant activity but reduced both chlorophylls and β-carotene in sweet peppers (Del Amor 2007), while in another study, the peppers grown under organic culture had higher vitamin C, phenolic, and carotenoid levels (Pérez-López et al. 2007). Bell peppers were influenced less by the environment and did not display cropping system differences (Chassy et al. 2006).

No statistically significant differences were observed in the total carotenoid contents (121 µg/g organic vs. 116 µg/g conventional) and the antioxidant capacities (0.43 and 0.32 µmol TE/g organic vs. conventional, respectively) of carrots. The bioavailability of carotenoids and antioxidant, antigenotoxic, and immunological effects as assessed in a human intervention study also did not depend on the agricultural system (Stracke et al. 2009b). The yield of Batavia lettuce from conventional farming was the highest, while polyphenol content of these plants was lower (1.36 mg/g) than the content in the plants from organic and biodynamic farming (1.74 and 1.85 mg/g, respectively). Biodynamic agriculture falls into the category of general organic agriculture; the main differences are in the use of biodynamic preparations for soil, plants, and compost (Heimler et al. 2012). For most parameters, significant differences between Chinese cabbage and maize foods obtained by conventional and certified organic procedures had not been observed; however, it was noticed that organically grown samples tend to have higher TPC than traditionally grown ones; on the contrary, organic raw Chinese cabbage leaves contained lower amounts of phenolics than conventional (Lima et al. 2009).

There were differences in the antioxidant activity of 14 potato clones grown at four production sites; however, there was no consistent effect of the production system (organic versus conventional) (Rosenthal and Jansky 2008). A Danish study also concluded that organically grown onions, carrots, and potatoes do not contain higher levels of health-promoting secondary metabolites in comparison to conventionally cultivated ones (Søltoft et al. 2010). The two genotypes of cauliflower showed a contrasting response to organic practices: The phytochemical content of Emeraude was generally reduced, while in Magnifico, most of the quality parameters were unaffected or increased. In addition, under organic management, the use of higher fertilization levels significantly increased the phytochemical production of Magnifico, in particular, ascorbic acid and polyphenols. However, the same treatments decreased the phytochemical production of Emeraude, particularly glucosinolates and ascorbic acid. This genotype was identified as a key factor in the determination of cauliflower quality under different management practices (Picchi et al. 2012).

The content of soluble polyphenolics was higher in all raw organic vegetables (potatoes, carrots, onions, broccoli, and white cabbage) except for onions, while the content of hydrolyzable polyphenolics was higher in all raw organic vegetables except for potatoes. In addition, organic vegetables showed a higher sensitivity to heat processing than did conventionally grown vegetables (Faller and Fialho 2009). The mean levels of ascorbic acid and flavonoids in 27 spinach varieties grown in certified organic and conventional cropping systems were significantly higher in the organically grown (40.48 ± 6.16 and 2.83 ± 0.03 mg/kg fw) spinach compared to the conventionally grown spinach (25.75 ± 6.12 and 2.27 ± 0.02 mg/kg fw) (Koh et al. 2012). Organic melons (10 cultivars) had significantly higher ascorbic acid content in a 2-year study, whereas TPC was higher only in the first year (Salandanan et al. 2009). Eggplant is ranked among the top 10 vegetables in terms of antioxidant capacity: The polyphenol content of the conventional Blackbell variety was marginally higher than the organically grown sample, whereas significantly higher yields of TPC were observed in a Millionaire eggplant cultivar grown in an organic environment. However, measurement of the antioxidant activity by two different

LDL-dependent biological assays showed a similar trend for organic and conventional produce (Singh et al. 2008). The antioxidant activity against the DPPH• radical for the studied vegetables was in the following order: organic arugula > organic chicory > organic lettuce > conventional arugula > conventional chicory > conventional lettuce; the TPC was also higher in the organic vegetables (Arbos et al. 2010). The highest value of antioxidant and anticancer activities was obtained for basil plants grown in 50% and 75% compost treatments in the presence of biofertilizer. The authors suggest that the use of bioorganic fertilizers is important for enhancement of the antioxidant activity of phenolics, flavonoids, and essential oils of basil (Taie et al. 2010). The results of a study comparing organic and nonorganic vegetable soups showed significantly higher concentrations of salicylic acid, which acts as an anti-inflammatory compound in organic soups (median 117 ng/g vs. 20 ng/g) (Baxter et al. 2001).

Among sulfur constituents, glutathione (GSH), N-acetylcysteine (NAC), captopril (CAP), cysteine (CYS), and γ-glutamyl cysteine (GGC) in a variety of organic versus conventional (industrially produced) asparagus, spinach, green beans, and red peppers, only the contents of CYS or CYS with NAC were detected as significantly higher in organic green beans or organic asparagus, respectively. However, conventional spinach contained significantly higher amounts of all investigated thiols than the organic spinach. The results also showed that conventional or organic production methods did not significantly affect the contents of CAP, GSH, or CYS in asparagus, green beans, or red peppers (Demirkol and Cagri-Mehmetoglu 2008).

9.6.5 CEREALS

Cereal-based foods are very important in the diet of many countries; therefore, high natural antioxidant content crops are of great interest. The combination of NPK fertilizers did not significantly affect the ferulic acid concentration in wheat varieties; on the other hand, the year (climate conditions) significantly influenced the soluble conjugated ferulic acid content in all fungicide-treated varieties. It was concluded that organic farming did not affect ferulic acid concentration, and climate factors have a greater impact on the phytochemical concentrations in whole wheat than the production method (Gasztonyi et al. 2011). Organically grown wheat (40 spring- and winter-grown genotypes) had similar amounts of tocochromanols as previously found in conventionally grown wheat. However, organic wheat grain could be a good source of tocochromanols because such wheat is more commonly consumed as whole and sprouted grain when compared to conventionally produced wheat (Hussain et al. 2012). There were no statistically significant differences between the two farming systems for wheat varieties grown under comparable organic and conventional conditions over 3 years as part of a long-term field trial; the sum of carotenoids in μg/g for organic versus conventional in 2003 was 0.91 ± 0.55 and 0.96 ± 0.34; in 2005, 1.61 ± 0.22 and 1.33 ± 0.19; and in 2006, 0.87 ± 0.33 and 0.83 ± 0.11; the sum of phenolic acids in 2003 was 448.4 ± 151.1 and 327.3 ± 232.8; in 2005, 502.8 ± 168.3 and 484.4 ± 111.2; and in 2006, 659.1 ± 112.5 and 945.9 ± 353.6. However, statistically significant year-to-year differences by up to 55% were observed. Taken together with these results, it was concluded that climate factors have a greater impact on the phytochemical concentrations in whole wheat than the production method (Stracke et al. 2009a). Organic agriculture did not lead to a significant increase in ferulic, sinapic, *p*-coumaric, vanillic, and *p*-hydroxybenzoic acids in winter wheat. Only a small, statistically irrelevant trend toward higher levels of phenolic acids in organic wheat samples was observed (Žuchowski et al. 2009). The influence of the farming system on the content of xanthophylls, lutein, and zeaxanthin content in hard wheat was very small; the differences were mainly caused by different kernel sizes (thousand-kernel weight), which were found correlating to the lutein content (Roose et al. 2009).

There were significant differences between years, cultivars, and N rate for avenanthramide (AVA) concentration in oat grains, but there were no differences as a consequence of the conventional or organic system. The HCA showed cultivar and year differences but were not influenced by N rates or the cropping system. It seems that factors affecting the yield and/or the specific weight also affect the concentrations of AVAs, HCAs, and TASE in oat grains (Dimberg et al. 2005). The levels of rutin, epicatechin, catechin, and epicatechin gallate were measured in buckwheat groats (hulled achenes), and it was found that only rutin and epicatechin gallate reached a significantly higher level in organic groats. The differences were also influenced by environmental conditions in the given year and variety (Kalinova and Vrchotova 2011).

9.6.6 OTHER CROPS AND PRODUCTS

A three-year study of extra-virgin olive oils showed that organic versus conventional cultivation did not consistently affect the measured parameters, which included the concentrations of phenols, *o*-diphenols, tocopherols, and the antioxidant capacity; it was concluded that genotype and year-to-year changes in climate had more marked effects (Ninfali et al. 2008). No significant trends were found in the oil samples for TAG and FA composition, but organically grown samples had a higher total antioxidant activity compared with the conventional samples (Perretti et al. 2005). The organic coffee contained higher levels of chlorogenic acid, caffeine, and trigonelline than conventional; however, this difference did not significantly affect biomarkers measured in Wistar rats (Do Carmo Carvalho et al. 2011). ABTS$^{•+}$ and DPPH$^{•}$ radical scavenging was found to be systematically higher in Croatian organic wines compared to conventional ones. Higher concentrations of chlorogenic and ferulic acids, catechin, *trans*-resveratrol, all measured hydroxybenzoic acids, and flavonols were found in the organically produced wines (Vrček et al. 2011). The levels of ellagic acid and catechin found in pecan kernels of the organically grown cultivar Desirable were fourfold and twofold higher than in conventional samples, respectively (Malik et al. 2009). Total phenolics, (–)-epigallocatechin gallate, (–)-gallocatechin gallate, and (–)-epicatechin gallate, as well as the antioxidant and antidiarrheal properties of tea leaves were investigated, and it was found that organic fertilization resulted in higher polyphenol content and better antioxidant properties. This study supports the importance of organic agricultural practices in tea for quality improvement and sustainability of the food chain system (Palit et al. 2008). Organic systems based on livestock manure and green manure and conventional systems with mineral fertilizers and pesticides were shown to have an impact on the nutritional quality, for example, affecting γ-tocopherol levels (slightly lower in organically grown crops); however, the differences in dietary treatments composed of ingredients from different cultivation systems did not lead to significant differences in the measured health biomarkers except for a significant difference in plasma IgG levels (Jensen et al. 2012).

ACKNOWLEDGMENTS

Support of Research Council of Lithuania is highly appreciated (grant no. SVE06/2011).

REFERENCES

Aldrich, H. T., K. Salandanan, P. Kendall, M. Bunning, F. Stonaker, O. Kulen, and C. Stushnoff. 2010. Cultivar choice provides options for local production of organic and conventionally produced tomatoes with higher quality and antioxidant content. *J Sci Food Agric* 90: 2548–2555.

Ali, L., B. W. Alsanius, A. K. Rosberg, B. Svensson, T. Nielsen, and M. E. Olsson. 2012. Effects of nutrition strategy on the levels of nutrients and bioactive compounds in blackberries. *Eur Food Res Technol* 234: 33–44.

Amigo-Benavent, M., M. D. del Castillo, and V. Fogliano. 2010. Are the major antioxidants derived from soy protein and fructo-oligosaccharides model systems colored aqueous soluble or insoluble compounds? *Eur Food Res Technol* 231: 545–553.

Amodio, M. L., G. Colelli, J. K. Hasey, and A. A. Kader. 2007. A comparative study of composition and postharvest performance of organically and conventionally grown kiwifruits. *J Sci Food Agric* 87: 1228–1236.

Anttonen, M. J., and R. O. Karjalainen. 2006. High-performance liquid chromatography analysis of black currant (*Ribes nigrum* L.) fruit phenolics grown either conventionally or organically. *J Agric Food Chem* 54: 7530–7538.

Arbos, K. A., R. J. S. de Freitas, S. C. Stertz, and M. F. Dornas. 2010. Antioxidant activity and phenolic content in organic and conventional vegetables. *Ciencia Tecnol Alime* 30: 501–506.

Arvanitoyannis, I. S., D. Ladas, and A. Mavromatis. 2006. Potential uses and applications of treated wine waste: A review. *Int J Food Sci Technol* 41: 475–487.

Asami, D. K., Y. J. Hong, D. M. Barrett, and A. E. Mitchell. 2003. Comparison of the total phenolic and ascorbic acid content of freeze-dried and air-dried marionberry, strawberry, and corn grown using conventional, organic, and sustainable agricultural practices. *J Agric Food Chem* 51: 1237–1241.

Augustyniak, A., G. Bartosz, A. Čipak, G. Duburs, L. Horáková, W. Łuczaj, M. Majekova, A. D. Odysseos, L. Rackova, E. Skrzydlewska, M. Stefek, M. Štrosová, G. Tirzitis, P. R. Venskutonis, J. Viskupicova, P. S. Vraka, and N. Žarković. 2010. Natural and synthetic antioxidants: An updated overview. *Free Radical Res* 44: 1216–1262.

Ayala-Zavala, J. F., V. Vega-Vega, C. Rosas-Domínguez, H. Palafox-Carlos, J. A. Villa-Rodriguez, M. Wasim Siddiqui, J. E. Dávila-Aviña, and G. A. González-Aguilar. 2011. Agro-industrial potential of exotic fruit byproducts as a source of food additives. *Food Res Int* 44: 1866–1874.

Azeredo, H. M. C. 2010. Betalains: Properties, sources, applications, and stability—a review. *Int J Food Sci Technol* 44: 2365–2376.

Balasundram, N., K. Sundram, and S. Samman. 2006. Phenolic compounds in plants and agri-industrial byproducts: Antioxidant activity, occurrence, and potential uses. *Food Chem* 99: 191–203.

Bandyopadhyay, S. S., D. Ghosh, V. Micard, S. Sinha, U. R. Chatterjee, and B. Raya. 2012. Structure, fluorescence quenching and antioxidant activity of a carbohydrate polymer from *Eugenia jambolana*. *Int J Biol Macromol* 51: 158–164.

Baxter, G. J., A. B. Graham, J. R. Lawrence, D. Wiles, and J. R. Paterson. 2001. Salicylic acid in soups prepared from organically and non-organically grown vegetables. *Eur J Nutr* 40: 289–292.

Becker, E. M., L. R. Nissen, and L. H. Skibsted. 2004. Antioxidant evaluation protocols: Food quality or health effects. *Eur Food Res Technol* 219: 561–571.

Benzie, I. F. F. 2003. Evolution of dietary antioxidants. *Comp Biochem Physiol A* 136: 113–126.

Berger, R. G., S. Lunkenbein, A. Ströhle, and A. Hahn. 2012. Antioxidants in food: Mere myth or magic medicine? *Crit Rev Food Sci* 52: 162–171.

Beta, T., S. Nam, J. E. Dexter, and H. D. Sapirstein. 2005. Phenolic content and antioxidant activity of pearled wheat and roller-milled fractions. *Cereal Chem* 82: 390–393.

Bhushan, S., K. Kalia, M. Sharma, B. Singh, and P. S. Ahuja. 2008. Processing of apple pomace for bioactive molecules. *Crit Rev Biotechnol* 28: 285–296.

Bihel, S., and I. Birlouez-Aragon. 1998. Inhibition of tryptophan oxidation in the presence of iron-vitamin C by bovine lactoferrin. *Int Dairy J* 8: 637–641.

Bordbar, S., F. Anwar, and N. Saari. 2011. High-value components and bioactives from sea cucumbers for functional foods: A review. *Mar Drugs* 9: 1761–1805.

Bourn, D., and J. Prescott. 2002. A comparison of the nutritional value, sensory qualities, and food safety of organically and conventionally produced foods. *Crit Rev Food Sci Nutr* 42: 1–34.

Brandt, K. L. Christensen, P. J. Hansen-Moeller, S. L. Hansen, J. Haraldsdottir, L. Jespersen, S. Purup, A. Kharazmi, V. Barkholt, H. Frøkiær, and M. Kobæk-Larsen. 2004. Health promoting compounds in vegetables and fruits: A systematic approach for identifying plant components with impact on human health. *Trends Food Sci Technol* 15: 384–393.

Brandt, K., and J. P. Molgaard. 2001. Organic agriculture: Does it enhance or reduce the nutritional value of plant foods? *J Sci Food Agric* 81: 924–931.

Brewer, M. S. 2011. Natural antioxidants: Their sources, compounds, mechanisms of action, and potential applications. *Compr Rev Food Sci F* 10: 221–247.

Briviba, K., B. A. Stracke, C. E. Rüfer, B. Watzl, F. P. Weibel, and A. Bub. 2007. Effect of consumption of organically and conventionally produced apples on antioxidant activity and DNA damage in humans. *J Agric Food Chem* 55: 7716–7721.

Bueno, J. M., F. Ramos-Escudero, P. Sáez-Plaza, A. M. Muñoz, M. J. Navas, and A. G. Asuero. 2012a. Analysis and antioxidant capacity of anthocyanin pigments. Part I: General considerations concerning polyphenols and flavonoids. *Crit Rev Anal Chem* 42: 102–125.

Bueno, J. M., P. Sáez-Plaza, F. Ramos-Escudero, A. M. Jiménez, R. Fett, and A. G. Asuero. 2012b. Analysis and antioxidant capacity of anthocyanin pigments. Part II: Chemical structure, color, and intake of anthocyanins. *Crit Rev Anal Chem* 42: 126–151.

Capek, P., E. Machová, and J. Turjan. 2009. Scavenging and antioxidant activities of immunomodulating polysaccharides isolated from *Salvia officinalis* L. *Int J Biol Macromol* 44: 75–80.

Carbonaro, M. M., and M. Mattera. 2001. Polyphenoloxidase activity and polyphenol levels in organically and conventionally grown peach (*Prunus persica* L., cv. Regina bianca) and pear (*Pyrus communis* L., cv. Williams). *Food Chem* 72: 419–424.

Carbonaro, M., M. Mattera, S. Nicoli, P. Bergamo, and M. Cappelloni, M. 2002. Modulation of antioxidant compounds in organic vs conventional fruit (peach, *Prunus persica* L., and pear, *Pyrus communis* L.). *J Agric Food Chem* 50: 5458–5462.

Carey, T., and X. Zhao. 2007. Are organic vegetables more nutritious? Fresh and postharvest assessment of nutritional quality of organically- and conventionally-grown lettuce and other salad greens. *Organic Farming Research Foundation Project Report*.

Caris-Veyrat, C., M. J. Amiot, V. Tyssandier, D. Grasselly, M. Buret, M. Mikolajczak, J. C. Guilland, C. Bouteloup-Demange, and P. Borel. 2004. Influence of organic versus conventional agricultural practice on the antioxidant microconstituent content of tomatoes and derived purees: Consequences on antioxidant plasma status in humans. *J Agric Food Chem* 52: 6503–6509.

Castañeda-Ovando, A., M. D. Pacheco-Hernández, M. E. Páez-Hernández, J. A. Rodríguez, and C. A. Galán-Vidal. 2009. Chemical studies of anthocyanins: A review. *Food Chem* 113: 859–871.

Cervato, G., R. Cazzola, and B. Cestaro. 1999. Studies on the antioxidant activity of milk caseins. *Int J Food Sci Nutr* 50: 291–294.

Chassy, A. W., L. Bui, E. N. C. Renaud, M. van Horn, and A. E. Mitchell. 2006. Three-year comparison of the content of antioxidant microconstituents and several quality characteristics in organic and conventionally managed tomatoes and bell peppers. *J Agric Food Chem* 54: 8244–8252.

Chen, H. M., K. Muramoto, and F. Yamauchi. 1995. Structural analysis of antioxidative peptides from soybean β-Conglycinin. *J Agric Food Chem* 43: 574–578.

Chen, H. M., and X. J. Yan. 2005. Anatioxidant activities of agaro-oligosaccharides with different degrees of polymerization in cell-based system. *BBA Gen Subjects* 1722: 103–111.

Chen, J., T. Zhang, B. Jiang, W. Mu, and M. Miao. 2012. Characterization and antioxidant activity of *Ginkgo biloba* exocarp polysaccharides. *Carbohydr Polym* 87: 40–45.

Chipault, J. R. 1962. Antioxidants for food use. In W. O. Lundberg, ed., *Autoxidation and Antioxidants*, 477–542. New York: Wiley.

Crozier, A., I. B. Jaganath, and M. N. Clifford. 2009. Dietary phenolics: Chemistry, bioavailability and effects on health. *Nat Prod Rep* 26: 1001–1043.

Cuppett, S., M. Schnepf, and C. Hall III. 1997. Natural antioxidants: Are they a reality? In F. Shahidi, ed., *Natural Antioxidants: Chemistry, Health Effects, and Applications*, 12–24. Champaign, IL: AOCS Press.

Dalonso, N., and C. L. de Oliveira Petkowicz. 2012. Guarana powder polysaccharides: Characterisation and evaluation of the antioxidant activity of a pectic fraction. *Food Chem* 134: 1804–1812.

Dangour, A., S. K. Dodhia, A. Hayter, E. Allen, K. Lock, and R. Uauy. 2009. Nutritional quality of organic foods: A systematic review. *Am J Clin Nutr* 90: 680–685.

Dani, C., L. S. Oliboni, R. Vanderlinde, D. Bonatto, M. Salvador, and J. A. P. Henriques. 2007. Phenolic content and antioxidant activities of white and purple juices manufactured with organically- or conventionally-produced grapes. *Food Chem Toxicol* 45: 2574–2580.

De Pascale S., R. Tamburrino, A. Maggio, G. Barbieri, V. Fogliano, and R. Pernice. 2006. Effects of nitrogen fertilization on the nutritional value of organically and conventionally grown tomatoes. In F. Tei, P. Benincasa, and M. Guiducci, eds., Proceedings of the International Symposium Towards Ecologically Sound Fertilisation Strategies for Field Vegetable Production. *Acta Horticult* 700: 107–110.

Decker, E. A., W. K. M. Chan, D. Mei, G. L. McNeill-Tompkins, and S. A. Livisay. 1997. Antioxidant activity of carnosine, a skeletal muscle dipeptide. In *Natural Antioxidants: Chemistry, Health Effects, and Applications*, F. Shahidi, ed., 271–282. Champaign, IL: AOCS Press.

Decker, E. A., and Y. Park. 2010. Healthier meat products as functional foods. *Meat Sci* 86: 49–55.

Del Amor, F. M. 2007. Yield and fruit quality response of sweet pepper to organic and mineral fertilization. *Renew Agricult Food Sys* 22: 233–238.

Demirkol, O., and A. Cagri-Mehmetoglu. 2008. Biologically important thiols in various organically and conventionally grown vegetables. *J Food Nutr Res* 47: 77–84.

Descalzo, A. M., and A. M. Sancho. 2008. A review of natural antioxidants and their effects on oxidative status, odor and quality of fresh beef produced in Argentina. *Meat Sci* 79: 423–436.

Di Bernardini, R., P. A. Harnedy, D. Bolton, J. Kerry, E. O'Neill, A. M. Mullen, and M. Hayes. 2011. Antioxidant and antimicrobial peptidic hydrolysates from muscle protein sources and byproducts. *Food Chem* 124: 1296–1307.

Di Renzo, L., D. Di Pierro, M. Bigioni, V. Sodi, F. Galvano, and R. Cianci. 2007. Is antioxidant plasma status in humans a consequence of the antioxidant food content influence? *Eur Rev Med Pharmacol Sci* 11: 185–192.

Dimberg, L. H., C. Gissen, and J. Nilsson. 2005. Phenolic compounds in oat grains (*Avena sativa* L.) grown in conventional and organic systems. *AMBIO* 34: 331–337.

Do Carmo Carvalho, D., M. R. P. L. Brigagão, M. H. dos Santos, F. B. A de Paula, A. Giusti-Paiva, and L. Azevedo. 2011. Organic and conventional *Coffea arabica* L.: A comparative study of the chemical composition and physiological, biochemical and toxicological effects in Wistar rats *Plant Foods Hum Nutr* 66: 114–121.

Durazzo, A., E. Azzini, M. S. Foddai, F. Nobili, I. Garaguso, A. Raguzzini, E. Finotti, V. Tisselli, S. del Vecchio, C. Piazza, M. Perenzin, L. Plizzari, and G. Maiani. 2010. Influence of different crop management practices on the nutritional properties and benefits of tomato—*Lycopersicon esculentum* cv Perfectpeel. *Int J Food Sci Technol* 45: 2637–2644.

Elias, R. J., S. S. Kellerby, and E. A. Decker. 2008. Antioxidant activity of proteins and peptides. *Crit Rev Food Sci* 48: 430–441.

Elleuch, M., D. Bedigian, S. Besbes, C. Blecker, and H. Attia. 2012. Dietary fibre characteristics and antioxidant activity of sesame seed coats (testae). *Int J Food Prop* 15: 25–37.

Ericksen, P. J. 2008. Conceptualizing food systems for global environmental change research. *Global Environ Chang* 18: 234–245.

Esquivel, P., and V. M. Jiménez. 2012. Functional properties of coffee and coffee byproducts. *Food Res Int* 46: 488–495.

Es-Safi, N. E., S. Ghidouche, and P. H. Ducrot. 2007. Flavonoids: Hemisynthesis, reactivity, characterization and free radical scavenging activity. *Molecules* 12: 2228–2258.

Faller, A. L. K., and E. Fialho. 2009. The antioxidant capacity and polyphenol content of organic and conventional retail vegetables after domestic cooking. *Food Res Int* 42: 210–215.

Faller, A. L. K., and E. Fialho. 2010. Polyphenol content and antioxidant capacity in organic and conventional plant foods. *J Food Compos Anal* 23: 561–568.

Fu, Y. R., G. Chen, J. W. Wu, X. H. Wu, C. L. Luo, and Y. F. He. 2012. Compositional features of carbohydrate compound from rhizoma *Ligustici wallichii* and ethanol extract of danshen and its bioactivity. *Carbohydr Polym* 87: 1224–1230.

Galanakis, C. M. 2012. Recovery of high added-value components from food wastes: Conventional, emerging technologies and commercialized applications. *Trends Food Sci Technol* 26: 68–87.

Gallardo, C., L. Jiménez, and M.-T. García-Conesa. 2006. Hydroxycinnamic acid composition and *in vitro* antioxidant activity of selected grain fractions. *Food Chem* 99: 455–463.

Gasztonyi, M. N., R. T. Farkas, M. Berki, I. M. Petróczi, and H. G. Daood. 2011. Content of phenols in wheat as affected by varietal and agricultural factors. *J Food Comp Anal* 24: 785–789.

Gómez-Guillén, M. C., B. Giménez, M. E. López-Caballero, and M. P. Montero. 2011. Functional and bioactive properties of collagen and gelatin from alternative sources: A review. *Food Hydrocolloid* 25: 1813–1827.

Guiotto, A., A. Calderan, P. Ruzza, and G. Borin. 2005. Carnosine and carnosine-related antioxidants: A review. *Curr Med Chem* 12: 2293–2315.

Halliwell, B., and J. M. C. Gutteridge. 1989. *Free Radicals in Biology and Medicine*, 2nd ed., 22–85. Oxford: Clarendon.

Haque, E., R. Chand, and S. Kapila. 2008. Biofunctional properties of bioactive peptides of milk origin. *Food Rev Int* 25: 28–43.

Harnedy, P. A., and R. J. FitzGerald. 2012. Bioactive peptides from marine processing waste and shellfish: A review. *J Funct Foods* S4: 6–24.

Hartmann, R., and H. Meisel. 2007. Food-derived peptides with biological activity: From research to food applications. *Curr Opin Biotech* 18: 63–169.

He, N. W., X. B. Yang, Y. D. Jiao, L. M. Tian, and Y. Zhao. 2012. Characterisation of antioxidant and antiproliferative acidic polysaccharides from Chinese wolfberry fruits. *Food Chem* 133: 978–989.

Heimler, D., P. Vignolini, P. Arfaioli, L. Isolania, and A. Romani. 2012. Conventional, organic and biodynamic farming: Differences in polyphenol content and antioxidant activity of Batavia lettuce. *J Sci Food Agric* 92: 551–556.

Hernández-Ledesma, B., A. Dávalos, B. Bartolomé, and L. Amigo. 2005. Preparation of antioxidant enzymatic hydrolysates from α-lactalbumin and β-lactoglobulin: Identification of active peptides by HPLC-MS/MS. *J Agric Food Chem* 53: 588–593.

Hernández-Ledesma, B., M. Ramos, and J. A. Gómez-Ruiz. 2010. Bioactive components of ovine and caprine cheese whey. *Small Ruminant Res* 101: 196–204.

Hernández-Ledesma, B., I. Recio, and L. Amigo. 2008. β-Lactoglobulin as source of bioactive peptides. *Amino Acids* 35: 257–265.

Herpandi, N. H., A. Rosma, and W. A. W. Nadiah. 2011. The tuna fishing industry: A new outlook on fish protein hydrolysates. *Compr Rev Food Sci F* 10: 195–207.

Hosseinian, F. S., and G. Mazza. 2009. Triticale bran and straw: Potential new sources of phenolic acids, proanthocyanidins, and lignans. *J Funct Foods* 1: 57–64.

Hua, Y. L., B. Yang, J. Tang, Z. H. Ma, Q. Gao, and M. M. Zhao. 2012. Structural analysis of water-soluble polysaccharides in the fruiting body of *Dictyophora indusiata* and their *in vivo* antioxidant activities. *Carbohydr Polym* 87: 343–347.

Huber, M., E. Rembiałkowska, D. Średnicka, S. Bügel, and L. P. L. van de Vijver. 2011. Organic food and impact on human health: Assessing the status quo and prospects of research. *NJAS* 58: 103–109.

Hussain, A., H. Larsson, M. E. Olsson, R. Kuktaite, H. Grausgruber, and E. Johansson. 2012. Is organically produced wheat a source of tocopherols and tocotrienols for health food? *Food Chem* 132: 1789–1795.

Ishikawa, S., Y. Yano, K. Arihara, and M. Itoh. 2004. Egg yolk phosvitin inhibits hydroxyl radical formation from the Fenton reaction. *Biosci Biotechnol Biochem* 68: 1324–1331.

Jaswir, I., D. Noviendri, R. F. Hasrini, and F. Octavianti. 2011. Carotenoids: Sources, medicinal properties and their application in food and nutraceutical industry. *J Med Plants Res* 5: 7119–7131.

Jauregui, M. E. C., M. D. C. Carrillo, and F. P. G. Romo. 2011. Carotenoids and their antioxidant function: A review. *Arch Latinoam Nutr* 61: 233–241.

Jensen, M. M., H. Jørgensen, U. Halekoh, J. E. Olesen, and C. Lauridsen. 2012. Can agricultural cultivation methods influence the healthfulness of crops for foods? *J Agric Food Chem* 60: 6383–6390.

Jiang, G. X., Y. M. Jiang, B. Yang, C. Y. Yu, R. Tsao, H. Y. Zhang, and F. Chen. 2009. Structural characteristics and antioxidant activities of oligosaccharides from longan fruit pericarp. *J Agric Food Chem* 57: 9293–9298.

Jiao, G. L., J. Z. Zhang, and H. S. Ewart. 2011. Chemical structures and bioactivities of sulfated polysaccharides from marine algae. *Marine Drugs* 9: 196–223.

Jin, L., X. Guan, W. Liu, X. Zhang, W. Yan, W. Yao, and X. Gao. 2012a. Characterization and antioxidant activity of a polysaccharide extracted from *Sarcandra glabra*. *Carbohydr Polym* 90: 524–532.

Jin, M., K. Zhao, Q. Huang, C. Xu, and P. Shang. 2012c. Isolation, structure and bioactivities of the polysaccharides from *Angelica sinensis* (Oliv.) Diels: A review. *Carbohydr Polym* 89: 713–722.

Jin, P., S. Y. Wang, H. Gao, H. Chen, Y. Zheng, and C. Y. Wang. 2012b. Effect of cultural system and essential oil treatment on antioxidant capacity in raspberries. *Food Chem* 132: 399–405.

Jin, P., S. Y. Wang, C. Y. Wang, and Y. H. Zheng. 2011. Effect of cultural system and storage temperature on antioxidant capacity and phenolic compounds in strawberries. *Food Chem* 124: 262–270.

Jin, X. C. 2012. Bioactivities of water-soluble polysaccharides from fruit shell of *Camellia oleifera* Abel: Antitumor and antioxidant activities. *Carbohydr Polym* 87: 2198–2201.

Jung, M. Y., S. K. Kim, and S. Y. Kim. 1995. Riboflavin-sensitized photooxidation of ascorbic acid: Kinetics and amino acid effects. *Food Chem* 53: 397–403.

Juroszek, P., H. M. Lumkin, R. Y. Yang, D. R. Ledesma, and C. H. Ma. 2009. Fruit quality and bioactive compounds with antioxidant activity of tomatoes grown on-farm: Comparison of organic and conventional management systems. *J Agric Food Chem* 57: 1188–1194.

Kalinova, J., and N. Vrchotova. 2011. The influence of organic and conventional crop management, variety and year on the yield and flavonoid level in common buckwheat groats. *Food Chem* 127: 602–608.

Kang, H. J., C. Jo, J. H. Kwon, J. H. Son, B. J. An, and M. W. Byun. 2006. Antioxidant and cancer cell proliferation inhibition effect of citrus pectin-oligosaccharide prepared by irradiation. *J Med Food* 9: 313–320.

Kapoulas, N., Z. S. Ilić, M. Durovka, R. Trajković, and L. Milenković. 2011. Effect of organic and conventional production practices on nutritional value and antioxidant activity of tomatoes. *Afr J Biotechnol* 10: 15938–15945.

Karamać, M. 2010. Antioxidant activity of tannin fractions isolated from buckwheat seeds and groats. *J Am Oil Chem Soc* 87: 559–566.

Kardošova, A., and E. Machová. 2006. Antioxidant activity of medicinal plant polysaccharides. *Fitoterapia* 77: 367–373.

Kim, G. D., Y. S. Lee, J. Y. Cho, Y. H. Lee, K. J. Choi, Y. Lee, T. H. Han, S. H. Lee, K. H. Park, and J. H. Moon. 2010. Comparison of the content of bioactive substances and the inhibitory effects against rat plasma oxidation of conventional and organic hot peppers (*Capsicum annuum* L.). *J Agric Food Chem* 58: 12300–12306.

Kim, K. W., and R. L. Thomas. 2007. Antioxidative activity of chitosans with varying molecular weights. *Food Chem* 101: 308–313.

Kiokias, S., and M. H. Gordon. 2004. Antioxidant properties of carotenoids *in vitro* and *in vivo*. *Food Rev Int* 20: 99–121.

Kiokias, S., T. Varzakas, and V. Oreopoulou. 2008. *In vitro* activity of vitamins, flavonoids, and natural phenolic antioxidants against the oxidative deterioration of oil-based systems. *Crit Rev Food Sci* 48: 78–93.

Kitts, D. D. 2005. Antioxidant properties of caseinphosphopeptides. *Trends Food Sci Technol* 16: 549–554.

Kogan, G., M. Pajtinka, M. Babincova, E. Miadokova, P. Rauko, D. Slamenova, and T. A. Korolenko. 2008. Yeast cell wall polysaccharides as antioxidants and antimutagens: Can they fight cancer? Minireview. *Neoplasma* 55: 387–393.

Koh, E., S. Charoenprasert, and A. E. Mitchell. 2012. Effect of organic and conventional cropping systems on ascorbic acid, vitamin C, flavonoids, nitrate, and oxalate in 27 varieties of spinach (*Spinacia oleracea* L.). *J Agric Food Chem* 60: 3144–3150.

Korhonen, H. 2009. Milk-derived bioactive peptides: From science to applications. *J Funct Foods* 1: 177–187.

Kudoh, Y., S. Matsuda, K. Igoshi, and T. Oki. 2001. Antioxidative peptide from milk fermented with *Lactobacillus delbrueckii* subsp. *bulgaricus* IFO13953. *J Jpn Soc Food Sci* 48: 44–55.

Kudoh, K., M. Matsumoto, S. Onodera, Y. Takeda, K. Ando, and N. Shiomi. 2003. Antioxidative activity and protective effect against ethanol-induced gastric mucosal damage of a potato protein hydrolysate. *J Nutr Sci Vitaminol* 49: 451–455.

Laakso, S. 1984. Inhibition of lipid peroxidation by casein: Evidence of molecular encapsulation of 4,4-pentadiene fatty acids. *Biochim Biophys Acta* 792: 11–15.

Lai, F., Q. Wen, L. Li, H. Wu, and X. Li. 2010. Antioxidant activities of water-soluble polysaccharide extracted from mung bean (*Vigna radiata* L.) hull with ultrasonic assisted treatment. *Carbohydr Polym* 81: 323–329.

Lairon, D. 2010. Nutritional quality and safety of organic food: A review. *Agron Sustain Dev* 30: 33–41.

Lamperi, L., U. Chiuminatto, A. Cincinelli, P. Galvan, E. Giordani, L. Lepri, and A. del Bubba. 2008. Polyphenol levels and free radical scavenging activities of four apple cultivars from integrated and organic farming in different Italian areas. *J Agric Food Chem* 56: 6536–6546.

Lee, K. G., and T. Shibamoto. 2002. Toxicology and antioxidant activities of non-enzymatic browning reaction products: Review. *Food Rev Int* 18: 151–175.

Li, S. J., T. A. Seymour, and M. T. Morrissey. 1997. Isolation of a natural antioxidant from shrimp waste. In *Natural Antioxidants: Chemistry, Health Effects, and Applications*, F. Shahidi, ed., 283–295. Champaign, IL: AOCS Press.

Lima, G. P. P., T. do Vale Cardoso Lopes, T. M. R. M. Rossetto, and F. Vianello. 2009. Nutritional composition, phenolic compounds, nitrate content in eatable vegetables obtained by conventional and certified organic grown culture subject to thermal treatment. *Int J Food Sci Technol* 44: 1118–1124.

Lindmark-Månsson, H., and B. Åkesson. 2000. Antioxidative factors in milk. *Br J Nutr* 84: S103–S110.

Liu, Y., C. Han, M. Lee, F. Hsu, and W. Hou. 2003. Patatin, the tuber storage protein of potato (*Solanum tuberosum* L.), exhibits antioxidant activity *in vitro*. *J Agric Food Chem* 51: 4389–4393.

Lombardi-Boccia, G., M. Lucarini, S. Lanzi, A. Aguzzi, and M. Cappelloni. 2004. Nutrients and Antioxidant molecules in yellow plums (*Prunus domestica* L.) from conventional and organic productions: A comparative study. *J Agric Food Chem* 52: 90–94.

Luo, A. X., X. J. He, S. D. Zhou, Y. J. Fan, A. S. Luo, and Z. Chun. 2010. Purification, composition analysis and antioxidant activity of the polysaccharides from *Dendrobium nobile* Lindl. *Carbohydr Polym* 79: 1014–1019.

Luo, Q., J. Zhang, L. Yan, Y. L. Tang, X. Ding, Z. R. Yang, and Q. Sun. 2011. Composition and antioxidant activity of water-soluble polysaccharides from *Tuber indicum*. *J Med Food* 14: 1609–1616.

Magkos, F., F. Arvaniti, and A. Zampelas. 2003. Organic food: Nutritious food or food for thought? A review of the evidence. *Int J Food Sci Nutr* 54: 357–371.

Mäkinen, S., T. Johannson, E. Vegarud Gerd, J. Matti Pihlava, and A. Pihlanto. 2012. Angiotensin I-converting enzyme inhibitory and antioxidant properties of rapeseed hydrolysates. *J Funct Foods* 4: 575–583.

Malik, N. S. A., J. L. Perez, L. Lombardini, R. Cornacchia, L. Cisneros-Zevallos, and J. Braforda. 2009. Phenolic compounds and fatty acid composition of organic and conventional grown pecan kernels. *J Sci Food Agric* 89: 2207–2213.

Marcuse, R. 1960. Antioxidative effect of amino acids. *Nature* 186: 886–887.

Marín, A., M. I. Gil, P. Flores, P. Hellín, and M. V. Selma. 2008. Microbial quality and bioactive constituents of sweet peppers from sustainable production systems. *J Agric Food Chem* 56: 11334–11341.

Martínez-Tomé, M., M. A. Murcia, N. Frega, S. Ruggieri, A. M. Jiménez, F. Roses, and P. Parras. 2004. Evaluation of antioxidant capacity of cereal brans. *J Agric Food Chem* 52: 4690–4699.

Martins, S., S. I. Mussatto, G. Martínez-Avila, J. Montañez-Saenz, C. N. Aguilar, and J. A. Teixeira. 2011. Bioactive phenolic compounds: Production and extraction by solid-state fermentation. A review. *Biotechnol Adv* 29: 365–373.

Mateos-Aparicio, I., C. Mateos-Peinado, A. Jiménez-Escrig, and P. Rupérez. 2010. Multifunctional antioxidant activity of polysaccharide fractions from the soybean byproduct okara. *Carbohydr Polym* 82: 245–250.

Mathew, S., and T. E. Abraham. 2004. Ferulic acid: An antioxidant found naturally in plant cell walls and feruloyl esterases involved in its release and their applications. *Crit Rev Biotechnol* 2–3: 59–83.

Maxwell, S., and R. Slater. 2003. Food policy old and new. *Dev Policy Rev* 21: 531–553.

Melo-Silveira, R. F., G. P. Fidelis, M. S. S. P. Costa, C. B. S. Telles, N. Dantas-Santos, S. D. Elias, V. B. Ribeiro, A. L. Barth, A. J. Macedo, E. L. Leite, and H. A. O. Rocha. 2012. *In vitro* antioxidant, anticoagulant and antimicrobial activity and in inhibition of cancer cell proliferation by xylan extracted from corn cobs. *Int J Mol Sci* 13: 409–426.

Memarpoor-Yazdi, M., A. Asoodeh, and J. K. Chamani. 2012. A novel antioxidant and antimicrobial peptide from hen egg white lysozyme hydrolysates. *J Funct Foods* 4: 278–286.

Min, B., J. C. Cordray, and D. U. Ahn. 2011a. Antioxidant effect of fractions from chicken breast and beef loin homogenates in phospholipid liposome systems. *Food Chem* 128: 299–307.

Min, B., A. M. McClung, and M. H. Chen. 2011b. Phytochemicals and antioxidant capacities in rice brans of different color. *J Food Sci* 76: C117–C126.

Montalba, R., C. Arriagada, M. Alvear, and G. E. Zuniga. 2010. Effects of conventional and organic nitrogen fertilizers on soil microbial activity, mycorrhizal colonization, leaf antioxidant content, and *Fusarium* wilt in highbush blueberry (*Vaccinium corymbosum* L.). *Sci Hortic* 125: 775–778.

Moosman, B., and C. Behl. 2002. Secretory peptides hormones are biochemical antioxidants. *Mol Pharmacol* 61: 260–268.

Moure, A., J. M. Cruz, D. Franco, J. M. Domínguez, J. Sineiro, H. Domínguez, M. J. Núñez, and J. C. Parajó. 2001. Natural antioxidants from residual sources. *Food Chem* 72: 145–171.

Moure, A., P. Gullón, H. Domínguez, and J. C. Parajó. 2006. Advances in the manufacture, purification and applications of xylo-oligosaccharides as food additives and nutraceuticals. *Process Biochem* 41: 1913–1923.

Morgan, K., and J. Murdoch. 2000. Organic vs. conventional agriculture: Knowledge, power and innovation in the food chain. *Geoforum* 31: 159–173.

Mulero, J., F. Pardo, and P. Zafrilla. 2010. Antioxidant activity and phenolic compounds in conventional and organic red grapes (var. Monastrell). *Cyta-J Food* 8: 185–191.

Najafian, L., and A. S. Babji. 2012. A review of fish-derived antioxidant and antimicrobial peptides: Their production, assessment, and applications. *Peptides* 33: 178–185.

Nakatani, N. 1997. Antioxidants from spices and herbs. In *Natural Antioxidants: Chemistry, Health Effects, and Applications*, F. Shahidi, ed., 64–75. Champaign, IL: AOCS Press.

Negro, C., L. Tommasi, and A. Miceli. 2003. Phenolic compounds and antioxidant activity from red grape marc extracts. *Bioresource Technol* 87: 41–44.

Ngo, D. N., M. M. Kim, Z. J. Qian, W. K. Jung, S. H. Lee, and S. K. Kim. 2010. Free radical-scavenging activities of low molecular weight chitin oligosaccharides lead to antioxidant effect in live cells. *J Food Biochem* 34: 161–177.

Ngo, D. H., I. Wijesekara, T. S. Vo, Q. V. Ta, and S. K. Kim. 2011. Marine food-derived functional ingredients as potential antioxidants in the food industry: An overview. *Food Res Int* 44: 523–529.

Ninfali, P., M. Bacchiocca, S. Biagiotti, S. Esposto, M. Servili, A. Rosati, and G. Montedoro. 2008. A 3-year study on quality, nutritional and organoleptic evaluation of organic and conventional extra-virgin olive oils. *J Am Oil Chem Soc* 85: 151–158.

Nuñez-Cordoba, J. M., and M. A. Martinez-Gonzalez. 2011. Antioxidant vitamins and cardio-vascular disease. *Curr Top Med Chem* 11: 1861–1869.

Okada, Y., and M. Okada. 1998. Scavenging effect of water soluble proteins in broad beans on free radicals and active oxygen species. *J Agric Food Chem* 46: 401–406.

Olsson, M., C. S. Andersson, S. Oredsson, R. H. Berglund, and K. E. Gustavsson. 2006. Antioxidant levels and inhibition of cancer cell proliferation *in vitro* by extracts from organically and conventionally cultivated strawberries. *J Agric Food Chem* 54: 1248–1255.

Ordóñez-Santos, L., M. Vázquez-Odériz, and M. Romero-Rodríguez. 2011. Micronutrient contents in organic and conventional tomatoes (*Solanum lycopersicum* L.). *Int J Food Sci Technol* 46: 1561–1568.

Palit, S., B. C. Ghosh, S. D. Gupta, and D. K. Swain. 2008. Studies on tea quality grown through conventional and organic management practices: Its impact on antioxidant and antidiarrhoeal activity. *T ASABE* 51: 2227–2238.

Pant, A. P., T. J. K. Radovich, N. V. Hue, S. T. Talcott, and K. A. Krenek. 2009. Vermicompost extracts influence growth, mineral nutrients, phytonutrients and antioxidant activity in pak choi (*Brassica rapa* cv. Bonsai, *Chinensis* group) grown under vermicompost and chemical fertilizer. *J Sci Food Agric* 89: 2383–2392.

Park, P. J., J. Y. Je, and S. K. Kim. 2003. Free radical scavenging activity of chitooligo-saccharides by electron spin resonance spectrometry. *J Agric Food Chem* 51: 4624–4627.

Park, P.-J., S. Koppula, and S.-K. Kim. 2010. Antioxidative activity of chitosan, chitooligo-saccharides and their derivatives. In *Chitin, Chitosan, Oligosaccharides and Their Derivatives. Biological Activities and Applications*, S.-K. Kim, ed., 241–250. Boca Raton, FL: CRC Press.

Patel, M., and S. N. Naik. 2004. Gamma-oryzanol from rice bran oil: A review. *J Sci Ind Res India* 63: 569–578.

Pavoković, D., and M. Krsnik-Rasol. 2011. Complex biochemistry and biotechnological pro-duction of betalains. *Food Technol Biotech* 49: 145–155.

Pazos, M., M. L. Andersen, and L. H. Skibsted. 2006. Amino acid and protein scavenging of radicals generated by iron/hydroperoxide system: An electron spin resonance spin trap-ping study. *J Agric Food Chem* 54: 10215–10221.

Peck, G. M., I. A. Merwin, C. B. Watkins, K. W. Chapman, and O. I. Padilla-Zakour. 2009. Maturity and quality of 'Liberty' apple fruit under integrated and organic fruit produc-tion systems are similar. *Hortscience* 44: 1382–1389.

Pérez-López, A. J., F. M. del Amor, A. Serrano-Martínez, M. I. Fortea, and E. Núñez-Delicado. 2007a. Influence of agricultural practices on the quality of sweet pepper fruits as affected by the maturity stage. *J Sci Food Agric* 87: 2075–2080.

Pérez-López, A. J., J. M. López-Nicolas, E. Núñez-Delicado, F. M. Del Amor, and Á. A. Carbonell-Barrachina. 2007b. Effects of agricultural practices on color, carotenoids composition, and minerals contents of sweet peppers, cv. Almuden. *J Agric Food Chem* 55: 8158–8164.

Perretti, G., E. Finotti, S. Adamuccio, R. della Sera, and L. Montanari. 2005. Composition of organic and conventionally produced sunflower seed oil. *J Am Oil Chem Soc* 81: 1119–1123.

Peschel, W., F. Sánchez-Rabaneda, W. Diekmann, A. Plescher, I. Gartzía, D. Jiménez, R. Lamuela-Raventós, S. Buxaderas, and C. Codina. 2006. An industrial approach in the search of natural antioxidants from vegetable and fruit wastes. *Food Chem* 97: 137–150.

Petkovsek, M. M., A. Slatnar, F. Stampar, and R. Veberic. 2010. The influence of organic/integrated production on the content of phenolic compounds in apple leaves and fruits in four different varieties over a 2-year period. *J Sci Food Agric* 90: 2366–2378.

Picchi, V., C. Migliori, R. Lo Scalzo, G. Campanelli, V. Ferrari, and L. F. Di Cesare. 2012. Phytochemical content in organic and conventionally grown Italian cauliflower. *Food Chem* 130: 501–509.

Pihlanto, A. 2006. Antioxidative peptides derived from milk proteins. *Int Dairy J* 16: 1306–1314.

Pihlanto, A., S. Akkanen, and H. J. Korhonen. 2008. ACE-inhibitory and antioxidant properties of potato (*Solanum tuberosum*). *Food Chem* 109: 104–112.

Polat, E., H. Demir, and F. Erler. 2010. Yield and quality criteria in organically and conventionally grown tomatoes in Turkey. *Sci Agric* 67: 424–429.

Pratt, D. E., and B. J. F. Hudson. 1990. Natural antioxidants not exploited commercially. In *Food Antioxidants*, B. J. F. Hudson, ed., 171–192. London: Elsevier Applied Science.

Pravst, I., K. Zmitek, and J. Zmitek. 2010. Coenzyme Q10 contents in foods and fortification strategies. *Crit Rev Food Sci* 50: 269–280.

Puri, M., D. Sharma, and C. J. Barrow. 2012. Enzyme-assisted extraction of bioactives from plants. *Trends Biotechnol* 30: 37–44.

Qi, H. M., Q. B. Zhang, T. T. Zhao, R. G. Hu, K. Zhang, and Z. Li. 2006. *In vitro* antioxidant activity of acetylated and benzoylated derivatives of polysaccharide extracted from *Ulva pertusa* (Chlorophyta). *Bioorg Med Chem Lett* 16: 2441–2445.

Rao, R. S. P., and G. Muralikrishna. 2006. Water soluble feruloyl arabinoxylans from rice and ragi: Changes upon malting and their consequence on antioxidant activity. *Phytochemistry* 67: 91–99.

Reganold, J. P., P. K. Andrews, J. R. Reeve, L. Carpenter-Boggs, C. W. Schadt, J. R. Alldredge, C. F. Ross, N. M. Davies, and J. Zhou. 2010. Fruit and soil quality of organic and conventional strawberry agroecosystems. *PLoS ONE* 5: e12346.

Ren, H., H. Endo, and T. Hayashi. 2001. Antioxidative and antimutagenic activities and polyphenol content of pesticide-free and organically cultivated green vegetables using water-soluble chitosan as a soil modifier and leaf surface spray. *J Sci Food Agric* 81: 1426–1432.

Riahi, A., C. Hdider, M. Sanaa, N. Tarchoun, M. Ben Khedere, and I. Guezal. 2009a. Effect of conventional and organic production systems on the yield and quality of field tomato cultivars grown in Tunisia. *J Sci Food Agric* 89: 2275–2282.

Riahi, A., C. Hdider, M. Sanaa, N. Tarchoun, M. Ben Kheder, and I. Guezal. 2009b. The Influence of different organic fertilizers on yield and physico-chemical properties of organically grown tomato. *J Sustain Agric* 33: 658–673.

Rice-Evans, C. 2004. Flavonoids and isoflavones: Absorption, metabolism, and bioactivity. *Free Radical Biol Med* 36: 827–828.

Rodriguez-Mateos, A., T. Cifuentes-Gomez, S. Tabatabaee, C. Lecras, and J. P. E. Spencer. 2012. Procyanidin, anthocyanin, and chlorogenic acid contents of highbush and lowbush blueberries. *J Agric Food Chem* 60: 5772–5778.

Roose, M., J. Kahl, and A. Ploeger. 2009. Influence of the farming system on the xanthophyll content of soft and hard wheat. *J Agric Food Chem* 57: 182–188.

Rosen, J. D. 2010. A review of the nutrition claims made by proponents of organic food. *Compr Rev Food Sci F* 9: 270–277.

Rosenthal, S., and S. Jansky. 2008. Effect of production site and storage on antioxidant levels in specialty potato (*Solanum tuberosum* L.) tubers. *J Sci Food Agric* 88: 2087–2092.

Roussos, P. A. 2011. Phytochemicals and antioxidant capacity of orange (*Citrus sinensis* (l.) Osbeck cv. *Salustiana*) juice produced under organic and integrated farming system in Greece. *Sci Hortic—Amsterdam* 129: 253–258.

Roussos, P. A., and D. Gasparatos. 2009. Apple tree growth and overall fruit quality under organic and conventional orchard management. *Sci Hortic—Amsterdam* 123: 247–252.

Rustad, T., I. Storrø, and R. Slizyte. 2011. Possibilities for the utilisation of marine by-products *Int J Food Sci Technol* 46: 2001–2014.

Ryan, J. T., R. P. Ross, D. Bolton, G. F. Fitzgerald, and C. Stanton. 2011. Bioactive peptides from muscle sources: Meat and fish. *Nutrients* 3: 765–791.

Sablani, S. S., P. K. Andrews, N. M. Davies, T. Walters, H. Saez, R. M. Syamaladevi, and P. R. Mohekar. 2010. Effect of thermal treatments on phytochemicals in conventionally and organically grown berries. *J Sci Food Agric* 90: 769–778.

Sablani, S. S., P. K. Andrews, N. M. Davies, T. Walters, H. Saez, and L. Bastarrachea. 2011. Effects of air and freeze-drying on phytochemical content of conventional and organic berries. *Dry Technol* 29: 205–216.

Salandanan, K., M. Bunning, F. Stonaker, O. Kulen, P. Kendall, and C. Stushnoff. 2009. Comparative analysis of antioxidant properties and fruit quality attributes of organically and conventionally grown melons (*Cucumis melo* L.). *Hortscience* 44: 1825–1832.

Samaranayaka, A. G. P., and E. C. Y. Li-Chan. 2011. Food-derived peptidic antioxidants: A review of their production, assessment, and potential applications. *J Funct Foods* 3: 229–254.

Samaraweera, H., W.-G. Zhang, E. J. Lee, and D. U. Ahn. 2011. Egg yolk phosvitin and functional phosphopeptides—Review. *J Food Sci* 76: R143–R150.

Sarmadi, B. H., and A. Ismail. 2010. Antioxidative peptides from food proteins: A review. *Peptides* 31: 1949–1956.

Schieber, A., P. Hilt, P. Streker, H. U. Endre, C. Rentschler, and R. Carle. 2003. A new process for the combined recovery of pectin and phenolic compounds from apple pomace. *Innov Food Sci Emerg* 4: 99–107.

Schuler, P. 1990. Natural antioxidants exploited commercially. In *Food Antioxidants*, B. J. F. Hudson, ed., 99–170. London: Elsevier Applied Science.

Scrinis, G. 2007. From techno-corporate food to alternative agri-food movements. *Local Global* 4: 112–140.

Shahidi, F. 1997. Natural antioxidants: An overview. In *Natural Antioxidants: Chemistry, Health Effects, and Applications*, F. Shahidi, ed., 1–11. Champaign, IL: AOCS Press.

Shahidi, F. 2000. Antioxidants in food and food antioxidants. *Nahrung* 44: S158–S163.

Shahidi, F., and J. Zhong. 2008. Bioactive peptides. *J AOAC Int* 91: 914–931.

Shi, H., N. Noguchi, and E. Niki. 2001. Natural antioxidants. In *Antioxidants in Food: Practical Applications*, J. Pokorny, N. Yanishlieva, and M. Gordon, eds., 147–266. Boca Raton, FL: CRC Press.

Singh, A. P., T. Wilson, D. L. Luthria, V. Singh, G. S. Banuelos, S. P. Pasakdee, and N. Vorsa. 2008. ANYL 153-HPLC and LC-MS detection and LDL-antioxidant activity of polyphenols from the pulp of eggplants grown under organic and conventional growing conditions. *Abstr Papers Am Chem Soc* 236: Meeting Abstract: 153-ANYL.

Skupien, K., I. Ochmian, J. Grajkowski, and E. Krzywy-Gawrońska. 2011. Nutrients, antioxidants, and antioxidant activity of organically and conventionally grown raspberries. *J Appl Bot Food Qual* 84: 85–89.

Sobal, J., L. K. Khan, and C. Bisogni. 1998. A conceptual model of the food and nutrition system. *Soc Sci Med* 47: 853–863.

Søltoft, M., J. Neilsen, K. Holst Laursen, S. Husted, U. Halekoh, and P. Knuthsen. 2010. Effects of organic and conventional growth systems on the content of flavonoids in onions and phenolic acids in carrots and potatoes. *J Agric Food Chem* 58: 10323–10329.

Stachowiak, B., and J. Regula. 2012. Health-promoting potential of edible macromycetes under special consideration of polysaccharides: A review. *Eur Food Res Technol* 234: 369–380.

Stracke, B., A. J. Eitel, B. Watzl, P. Mäder, and C. E. Rüfer. 2009a. Influence of the production method on phytochemical concentrations in whole wheat (*Triticum aestivum* L.): A comparative study. *J Agric Food Chem* 57: 10116–10121.

Stracke, B. A., C. E. Rüfer, A. Bub, K. Briviba, S. Seifert, C. Kunz, and B. Watzl. 2009b. Bioavailability and nutritional effects of carotenoids from organically and conventionally produced carrots in healthy men. *Br J Nutr* 101: 1664–1672.

Stracke, B. A., C. E. Rüfer, A. Bub, S. Seifert, F. P. Weibel, C. Kunz, and B. Watzl. 2010. No effect of the farming system (organic/conventional) on the bioavailability of apple (*Malus domestica* Bork., cultivar Golden Delicious) polyphenols in healthy men: A comparative study. *Eur J Nutr* 49: 301–310.

Strissel, T., H. Halbwirth, U. Hoyer, C. Zistler, K. Stich, and D. Treutter. 2005. Growth-promoting nitrogen nutrition affects flavonoid biosynthesis in young apple (*Malus domestica* Borkh.) leaves. *Plant Biol* 7: 677–685.

Stuetz, W., T. Prapamontol, S. Hongsibsong, and H. K. Biesalski. 2010. Polymethoxylated flavones, flavanone glycosides, carotenoids, and antioxidants in different cultivation types of tangerines (*Citrus reticulata Blanco* cv. Sainampueng) from Northern Thailand. *J Agric Food Chem* 58: 6069–6074.

Suetsuna, K. 2000. Antioxidant peptides from the protease digest of prawn (*Penaeus japonicus*) muscle. *Mar Biotechnol* 2: 5–10.

Sun, J., L. Li, X. R. You, C. B. Li, E. Z. Zhang, Z. C. Li, G. L. Chen, and H. X. Peng. 2011. Phenolics and polysaccharides in major tropical fruits: Chemical compositions, analytical methods and bioactivities. *Anal Met* 3: 2212–2220.

Sun, Y.-X., J.-C. Liu, and J. F. Kennedy. 2010. Extraction optimization of antioxidant polysaccharides from the fruiting bodies of *Chroogomphis rutilus* (Schaeff.: Fr.) O.K. Miller by Box-Behnken statistical design. *Carbohydr Polym* 82: 209–214.

Taamalli, A., D. Arráez-Román, M. Zarrouk, J. Valverde, A. Segura-Carretero, and A. Fernández-Gutiérrez. 2012. The occurrence and bioactivity of polyphenols in Tunisian olive products and byproducts: A review. *J Food Sci* 77: R83–R92.

Taie, H. A. A., Z. A. Salama, and S. Radwan. 2010. Potential activity of basil plants as a source of antioxidants and anticancer agents as affected by organic and bio-organic fertilization. *Not Bot Hort Agrobot Cluj* 38: 119–127.

Tan, Y. A., R. Sambanthamurthi, K. Sundram, and M. B. Wahid. 2007. Valorisation of palm byproducts as functional components. *Eur J Lipid Sci Tech* 109: 380–393.

Tarozzi, A., S. Hrelia, C. Angeloni, F. Morroni, P. Biagi, M. Guardigli, G. Cantelli-Forti, and P. Hrelia. 2006. Antioxidant effectiveness of organically and non-organically grown red oranges in cell culture systems. *Eur J Nutr* 45: 152–158.

Tavares, T. G., M. M. Contreras, M. Amorim, P. J. Martín-Álvarez, M. E. Pintado, I. Recio, and F. X. Malcata. 2011. Optimisation, by response surface methodology, of degree of hydrolysis and antioxidant and ACE-inhibitory activities of whey protein hydrolysates obtained with cardoon extract. *Int Dairy J* 21: 926–933.

Toor, R. K., G. P. Savage, and A. Heeb. 2006. Influence of different types of fertilizers on the major antioxidant components of tomatoes. *J Food Compos Anal* 19: 20–27.

Traill, W. B., M. H. P. Arnoult, S. A. Chambers, E. R. Deaville, M. H. Gordon, P. John, P. J. Jonese, K. E. Kliem, S. R. Mortimer, and J. R. Tiffin. 2008. The potential for competitive and healthy food chains of benefit to the countryside. *Trends Food Sci Technol* 19: 248–254.

Valavanidis, A., T. Vlachogianni, A. Psomas, A. Zovoili, and V. Siatis. 2009. Polyphenolic profile and antioxidant activity of five apple cultivars grown under organic and conventional agricultural practices. *Int J Food Sci Technol* 44: 1167–1175.

Vallverdú-Queralt, A., A. Medina-Remón, I. Casals-Ribes, M. Amat, and R. M. Lamuela-Raventós. 2011. A metabolomic approach differentiates between conventional and organic ketchups. *J Agric Food Chem* 59: 11703–11710.

Van der Sluis, A. A., M. Dekker, A. de Jager, and W. M. F. Jongen. 2001. Activity and concentration of polyphenolic antioxidants in apple: Effect of cultivar, harvest year, and storage conditions. *J Agric Food Chem* 49: 3606–3613.

Veberic, R., M. Trobec, K. Herbinger, M. Hofer, D. Grill, and F. Stampar. 2005. Phenolic compounds in some apple (*Malus domestica* Borkh) cultivars of organic and integrated production. *J Sci Food Agric* 85: 1687–1694.

Venkat Ratnam, D., D. D. Ankola, V. Bhardwaj, D. K. Sahana, and M. N. V. Ravi Kumar. 2006. Role of antioxidants in prophylaxis and therapy: A pharmaceutical perspective. *J Controll Release* 113: 189–207.

Vian, M. A., V. Tomao, P. O. Coulomb, J. M. Lacombe, and O. Dangles. 2006. Comparison of the anthocyanin composition during ripening of Syrah grapes grown using organic or conventional agricultural practices. *J Agric Food Chem* 54: 5230–5235.

Vrček, I. V., M. Bojić, I. Žuntar, G. Mendaš, and M. Medić-Šarić. 2011. Phenol content, antioxidant activity and metal composition of Croatian wines deriving from organically and conventionally grown grapes. *Food Chem* 124: 354–361.

Walther, B., and R. Sieber. 2012. Available at http://www.agroscope.admin.ch/data/publikationen/1313057378_Walther_Bioaktive_Proteine_Peptide_15_11.pdf.

Wanasundara, P. K. J. P. D., and F. Shahidi. 2005. Antioxidants: Science, technology, and applications. In *Bailey's Industrial Oil and Fat Products*, 6th ed., F. Shahidi, ed., 431–489. New York: John Wiley & Sons.

Wang, J., B. G. Sun, Y. P. Cao, and C. T. Wang. 2010. Wheat bran feruloyl oligosaccharides enhance the antioxidant activity of rat plasma. *Food Chem* 123: 472–476.

Wang, L. L., and Y. L. L. Xiong. 2005. Inhibition of lipid oxidation in cooked beef patties by hydrolyzed potato protein is related to its reducing and radical scavenging ability. *J Agric Food Chem* 53: 9186–9192.

Wang, S. Y., C.-T. Chen, W. Sciarappa, C. Y. Wang, and M. J. Camp. 2008. Fruit quality, antioxidant capacity, and flavonoid content of organically and conventionally grown blueberries *J Agric Food Chem* 56: 5788–5794.

Wang, S. Y., and P. Millner. 2009. Effect of different cultural systems on antioxidant capacity, phenolic content, and fruit quality of strawberries (*Fragaria x aranassa* Duch.). *J Agric Food Chem* 57: 9651–9657.

Wijesinghe, W. A. J. P., and Y.-J. Jeon. 2012. Biological activities and potential industrial applications of fucose rich sulfated polysaccharides and fucoidans isolated from brown seaweeds: A review. *Carbohydr Polym* 88: 13–20.

Wijngaard, H., M. B. Hossain, D. K. Rai, and N. Brunton. 2012. Techniques to extract bioactive compounds from food byproducts of plant origin. *Food Res Int* 46: 505–513.

Wilkins, J., and M. Eames-Sheavy. n.d. Discovering the food system: A primer on community food systems: Linking food, nutrition and agriculture. Available at http://discoverfoodsys.cornell.edu/primer.html. Accessed August 2012.

Winter, C. K., and S. F. Davis. 2006. Organic foods. *J Food Sci* 71: R117–R124.

Woese, K., D. Lange, C. Boess, and K. W. Bogl. 1997. A comparison of organically and conventionally grown foods—Results of a review of the relevant literature. *J Sci Food Agric* 74: 281–293.

Wong, P. Y. Y., and D. D. Kitts. 2003. Chemistry of buttermilk solid antioxidant activity. *J Dairy Sci* 86: 1541–1547.

Worthington, V. 2001. Nutritional quality of organic versus conventional fruits, vegetables, and grains. *J Altern Complement Med* 7: 161–173.

Xiao, J. B., J. L. Huo, H. X. Jiang, and F. Yang. 2011. Chemical compositions and bioactivities of crude polysaccharides from tea leaves beyond their useful date. *Int J Biol Macromol* 49: 1143–1151.

Xu, R. J. 1998. Bioactive peptides in milk and their biological and health implications. *Food Rev Int* 14: 1–16.

Xue, Z., W. Yu, Z. Liu, M. Wu, X. Kou, and J. Wang. 2009. Preparation and antioxidative properties of a rapeseed (*Brassica napus*) protein hydrolysate and three peptide fractions. *J Agric Food Chem* 57: 5287–5293.

Yang, B., J. Wang, M. Zhao, Y. Liu, W. Wang, and Y. Jiang. 2006. Identification of polysaccharides from pericarp tissues of litchi (*Litchi chinensis* Sonn.) fruit in relation to their antioxidant activities. *Carbohyd Res* 341: 634–638.

Yang, B., M. Zhao, N. Prasad, G. Jiang, and Y. Jiang. 2010. Effect of methylation on the structure and radical scavenging activity of polysaccharides from Longan (*Dimocarpus longan* Lour.) fruit pericarp. *Food Chem* 118: 364–368.

Ye, C. L., and Q. Huang. 2012. Extraction of polysaccharides from herbal *Scutellaria barbata* D. Don (Ban-Zhi-Lian) and their antioxidant activity. *Carbohydr Polym* 89: 1131–1137.

You, Q., B. Wang, F. Chen, Z. Huang, X. Wang, and P. G. Luo. 2011. Comparison of anthocyanins and phenolics in organically and conventionally grown blueberries in selected cultivars. *Food Chem* 125: 201–208.

Yu, L. L., K. Q. Zhou, and J. W. Parry. 2005. Inhibitory effects of wheat bran extracts on human LDL oxidation and free radicals. *LWT Food Sci Technol* 38: 463–470.

Yuan, H. M., W. W. Zhang, X. G. Li, X. X. Lu, N. Li, X. L. Gao, and J. M. Song. 2005. Preparation and *in vitro* antioxidant activity of κ-carrageenan oligosaccharides and their oversulfated, acetylated, and phosphorylated derivatives. *Carbohydr Res* 340: 685–692.

Yuan, J. F., Z. Q. Zhang, Z. C. Fan, and J. X. Yang. 2008. Antioxidant effects and cytotoxicity of three purified polysaccharides from *Ligusticum chuanxiong* Hort. *Carbohydr Polym* 74: 822–827.

Zha, X. Q., J. H. Wang, X. F. Yang, H. Liang, L. L. Zhao, S. H. Bao, J.-P. Luo, Y.-Y. Xu, and B.-B. Zhou. 2009. Antioxidant properties of polysaccharide fractions with different molecular mass extracted with hot water from rice bran. *Carbohydr Polym* 78: 570–575.

Zhang, A. Q., N. N. Xiao, P. F. He, and P. L. Sun. 2011. Chemical analysis and antioxidant activity *in vitro* of polysaccharides extracted from *Boletus edulis*. *Int J Biol Macromol* 49: 1092–1095.

Zhang, C., X. Li, and S.-K. Kim. 2012. Application of marine biomaterials for nutraceuticals and functional foods. *Food Sci Biotechnol* 21: 625–631.

Zhang, T., Y. Li, M. Miao, and B. Jiang. 2011. Purification and characterisation of a new antioxidant peptide from chickpea (*Cicer arietium* L.) protein hydrolysates. *Food Chem* 128: 28–33.

Zhao, L., K. Y. Wang, R. Q. Yang, X. Wang, D. F. Chen, and F. Shi. 2012. Antioxidant activity of the water-soluble and alkali-soluble polysaccharides from Chinese Truffle *Tuber sinense*. *J Anim Vet Adv* 11: 1753–1756.

Zhao, Q. S., B. X. Xie, J. Yan, F. C. Zhao, J. Xiao, L. Y. Yao, B. Zhao, and Y. X. Huang. 2012. *In vitro* antioxidant and antitumor activities of polysaccharides extracted from *Asparagus officinalis*. *Carbohydr Polym* 87: 392–396.

Zhao, X., E. E. Carey, W. Q. Wang, and C. B. Rajashekar. 2006. Does organic production enhance phytochemical content of fruit and vegetables? Current knowledge and prospects for research. *Horttechnology* 16: 449–456.

Zhao, X., T. Iwamoto, and E. E. Carey. 2007. Antioxidant capacity of leafy vegetables as affected by high tunnel environment fertilisation and growth stage. *J Sci Food Agric* 87: 2692–2699.

Zhao, Z. H., and M. H. Moghadasian. 2008. Chemistry, natural sources, dietary intake and pharmacokinetic properties of ferulic acid: A review. *Food Chem* 109: 691–702.

Zhou, K., L. Su, and L. L. Yu. 2004. Phytochemicals and antioxidant properties in wheat bran. *J Agric Food Chem* 52: 6108–6114.

Zhokhov, S. S., A. Broberg, L. Kenne, and J. Jastrebova. 2010. Content of antioxidant hydroquinones substituted by β-1,6-linked oligosaccharides in wheat milled fractions, flours and breads. *Food Chem* 121: 645–652.

Żuchowski, J., I. Kapusta, B. Szajwaj, K. Jończyk, and W. Oleszek. 2009. Phenolic acid content of organic and conventionally grown winter wheat. *Cereal Res Commun* 37: 189–197.

10 Antioxidants Generated in Foods as a Result of Processing

María Dolores del Castillo,
Elena Ibáñez, and Miguel Herrero

CONTENTS

10.1 INTRODUCTION

In a recent review published by a group of experts from the International Life Sciences Institute, ILSI Europe, Process-Related Compounds and Natural Toxins Task Force (van Boekel et al. 2010), the beneficial aspects of food processing were identified and widely discussed—mainly to ensure safety and food quality while guaranteeing consumer acceptability.

Some of the beneficial aspects to consider include (1) food safety and food quality improvement (by destruction or inactivation of unwanted compounds and microorganisms, such as pathogens, enzymes, etc.); (2) enhancement of nutritional value (by improvement of digestibility and bioavailability); (3) improvement of sensory quality (by releasing of flavor compounds or improving texture and taste); and (4) formation of bioactives with associated health benefits: These compounds might be either released or generated during food processing, mainly heat processing, and can provide benefits for human health. Among the different compounds released or generated during food processing, those with antioxidant capacity will be reviewed and discussed in the present chapter.

Food processes that can lead to the release or generation of health-promoting compounds can be based on either thermal or nonthermal processing. In both cases, processes should be optimized in order to promote beneficial effects while avoiding undesired side effects (losses of nutrients; formation of toxic compounds and formation of off-flavors). Even considering that thermal processes are better known, including their positive and negative effects, nonthermal processes are receiving a lot of attention as alternative processes to minimize the negative effects of heat processing. Nonthermal processes, such as those based on fermentation, enzymatic treatment, high pressure, electric field, etc., may provide fewer risks and equal or better benefits than thermal processes and can also generate or release antioxidants with health-related benefits. Those with some potential to be used on an industrial scale are discussed in the present chapter, mainly referring to how they contribute to the generation of unique antioxidants with new structures and health benefits.

10.2   PROCESSING BY APPLICATION OF HEAT

Traditionally, thermal processes have been used extensively in food technology with two main goals: (1) to preserve foods and (2) to transform raw foods. The intensity of the thermal processing conditions for either food preservation or transformation is very different. Pasteurization and sterilization are two food-preservation processes used to ensure microbiological safety and to eliminate some enzymatic activity that might reduce food shelf life, while baking and roasting serve mainly to transform food by obtaining particular sensory or textural features. The most popular thermal food preservation processes can be classified according to the intensity of the heat treatment as follows: pasteurization (70°C–80°C), sterilization (110°C–120°C), and UHT (140°C–160°C). Transformation processes, such as roasting and baking, are much more intense heat treatments. On the other hand, microwave treatment also is considered a thermal food process that can be used to achieve both goals: food preservation or transformation. As mentioned, in the present chapter, we attempt to review the effects of all these processes on the antioxidant profile of food.

It is well known that some reactions occur during food processing, causing the formation of both beneficial and harmful compounds. Although a lot of work has been performed on the risks derived from thermal food processing, recently, there has been a lot of interest in the enhancement of functional properties as key benefits derived from thermal processing (Henle 2005; Silván et al. 2006; van Boekel et al. 2010). Some of the beneficial properties of heated foods included increased antioxidants or antibacterial effectiveness. The antioxidant power of the heated foods may be ascribed to both natural antioxidants existing in the food and newly formed compounds generated during food processing. Natural bioactives might be released to some extent during processing by disruption of cell walls, breakdown of complex molecular structures, and dissociation of molecular linkages between food components; these compounds can be secondary plant metabolites, such as carotenoids, glucosinolates, and polyphenols. The new bioactive compounds can derive from several chemical reactions undergone during food processing, for instance, the Maillard reaction, which is the key chemical event taking place during thermal food processing (Henle 2005; Silván et al. 2006). In Figure 10.1, the chemical structure of some

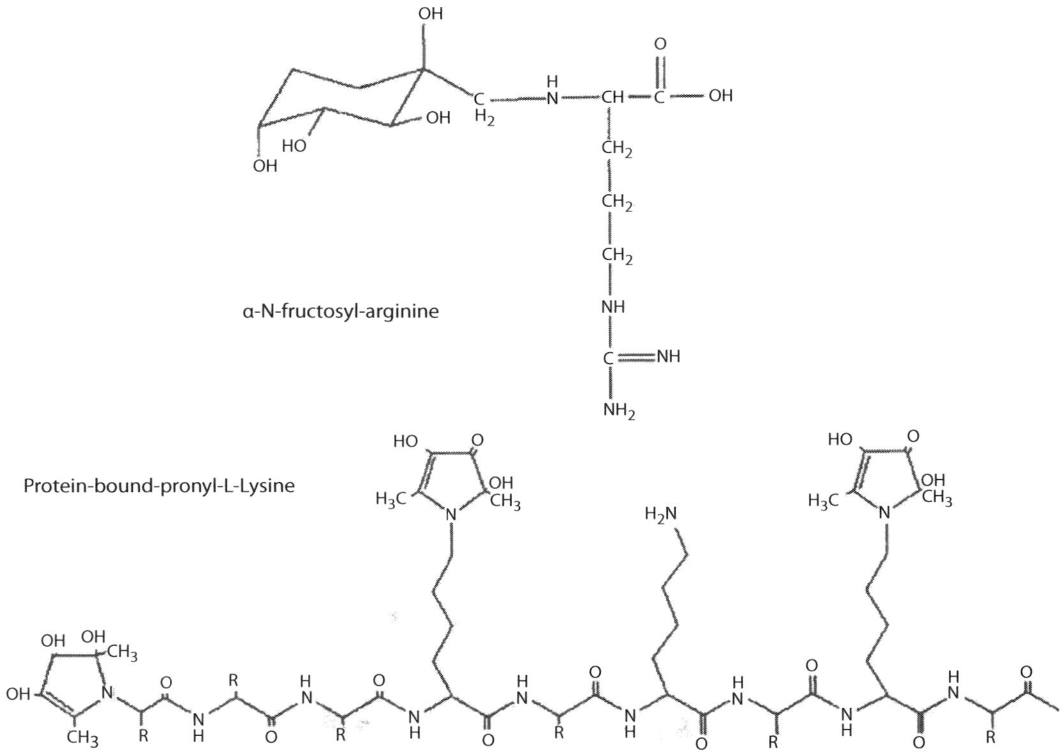

FIGURE 10.1 Maillard reaction products with known structure and antioxidant properties. (Reprinted from *J Pharm Biomed Anal*, 41, Silván, J. M., van Lagemaat, J., Olano, A., del Castillo, M. D., Analysis and biological properties of amino acids derivatives formed by Maillard reaction in foods, 1543–1551, Copyright 2006, with permission from Elsevier.)

of the antioxidant compounds that might be formed through Maillard reactions is shown.

The rate of release and/or formation of antioxidants along with their type depend on food composition and on the intensity of thermal food processing and, therefore, will be different for preservation or transformation events. In agreement, in this section, we will provide some examples of the effect of both types of thermal food processing on the antioxidant profile (natural and newly formed antioxidants) of processed foods. We will focus our discussion on frequently consumed foods, such as coffee, bread, fruit, and vegetables, with natural (polyphenols) and also newly formed antioxidants, exposed to thermal conditions able to favor the simultaneous occurrence of several chemical reactions, including Maillard reactions, and with epidemiological evidence of health effects. The overall antioxidant activity (total antioxidant capacity (TAC) of some foods will be also discussed as they are affected by thermal processes because the TAC increase cannot be merely attributed to the release of antioxidants from plant matrix but also to other reactions favored at higher temperature, such as *trans–cis* isomerization of carotenoids, intramolecular *trans*-esterification of polyphenols, etc., that may lead to the formation of nonidentified compounds with very high antioxidant power.

10.2.1 THERMAL PROCESSES FOR FOOD PRESERVATION

At present, there is a clear correlation between a diet high in fruits and vegetables and a healthy life and prevention of chronic diseases. It is believed that there is a link between antioxidant content and the health benefits of fruits and vegetables; antioxidants, mainly phenols, are ubiquitously present in plant-based foods, and therefore, humans consume them daily. These bioactive compounds have received a lot of attention (Robbins 2003). However, few studies are available on the effects of thermal treatment on dietary antioxidants, such as phenolic compounds, as well as on their availability in heat-processed foods. Dietary antioxidants undergo several enzymatic and chemical reactions during processing. Moreover, the consequences of food processing on natural antioxidant behavior may dramatically differ depending on several variables, such as concentration, chemical structure, oxidation state, localization in the cell, possible interaction with other components, and type and intensity of the thermal processing applied. Therefore, food processing may cause a decrease, increase, or minor changes in content and functionality of these natural dietary antioxidants (Patras et al. 2009; van Boekel et al. 2010). On the other hand, there is some evidence about the generation or improvement of antioxidant levels and total antioxidant capacity in processed foods.

Regular consumption of tomatoes and tomato-based products has been associated with reduced incidence of some types of cancer and heart disease. These beneficial properties have been partially attributed to their content of various bioactive compounds, such as carotenoids and, among them, lycopene, which exhibits high oxygen-radical scavenging and quenching capacities, and β-carotene, which is the main carotenoid with provitamin A activity. Studies on the changes in antioxidant profiles during cold storage of tomato juice stabilized by thermal or high-intensity pulsed electric field treatments performed by Odriozola-Serrano et al. (2008)

indicated higher lycopene and lower vitamin C levels in pasteurized tomato juices (90°C for 1 min or 30 s), while no significant changes in the total phenolic content and antioxidant capacity were detected between treated and fresh juices just after processing. The influence of food processing on the chemical and physical properties of lycopene in tomatoes has been reviewed by Shi and Le Maguer (2000). The main chemical reactions causing lycopene degradation during processing are isomerization and oxidation. For instance, during heat processing, all-*trans*-lycopene isomers are converted into *cis*-isomer with higher bioavailability than *all-trans* isomers. In Figure 10.2, the most important occurring lycopene *cis*-isomers are shown. The analysis of lycopene isomerization has been proposed as a measure of the health benefits of tomato-based foods. According to Shi and Le Maguer (2000), lycopene availability in processed tomato products is higher than in unprocessed fresh tomatoes.

The consumption of citrus juices, especially orange juice, has been reported to be beneficial for the prevention of several diseases. Citrus juices are very popular, consumed daily, and considered a dietary source of provitamin A. The health benefits of citrus could be attributed to the richness in various antioxidants: vitamin C, polyphenols, carotenoids, etc. (Dhuique-Mayer et al. 2007). Thermal treatments could cause undesirable reactions, such as nonenzymatic browning and nutrient losses. Vitamin C (L-ascorbic acid) is a typical heat-sensitive micronutrient, and its degradation plays a major role in nonenzymatic browning reactions (Villamiel et al. 2012). The thermal degradation kinetics of vitamin C, carotenoids (β-carotene and β-cryptoxanthin), and hesperidin, as a function of temperature, has been determined for citrus juice (*Citrus sinensis* L.). The authors found that thermal treatments corresponding to classical pasteurization conditions do not damage provitamin A carotenoids, polyphenols as hesperidin, and vitamin C in citrus juice. Moreover, the model developed by them may predict the optimal processing conditions to minimize degradation of vitamin C and carotenoids in citrus juice. The authors also reported that xanthophyll carotenoids were more heat-sensitive than carotene and more likely to generate degradation products, such as furanoids and *cis* isomers. Violaxanthin was the most heat-sensitive, and its complete conversion to auroxanthin results in a visually colorless

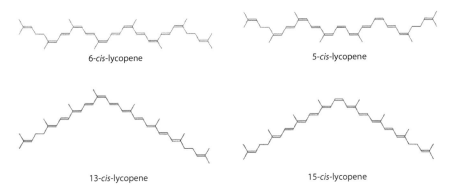

6-*cis*-lycopene

5-*cis*-lycopene

13-*cis*-lycopene

15-*cis*-lycopene

FIGURE 10.2   Chemical structures of *cis*-isomers of lycopene.

juice. Further information regarding the antioxidants' modification pathways during juice processing has been described by Grajek and Olejnik (2010).

Fiore et al. (2005) assessed the antioxidant capacity of pasteurized and sterilized commercial red orange juice with the aim of finding any relationship between the antioxidant properties and the anthocyanin's composition in juices subjected to different thermal treatments. They concluded that the healthy antioxidant properties of red orange juice associated with anthocyanins can be attributed only to short shelf life products containing 100% pure juice and subjected to mild thermal processing conditions (pasteurization). Huge differences in the antioxidant profile of short shelf life (mild pasteurized ~80°C) and long shelf life sterilized juices were found and were attributed to the intensity of the heat treatment. This is a common conclusion in most of the works done comparing low- and high-intensity thermal treatment processes; evidence supports that low-intensity thermal treatment of food and vegetables provides healthier foods because of the preservation of antioxidant bioactives and total antioxidant capacity.

Food by-products, such as grape-seed extracts, can be used as functional food ingredients, mainly for their content of phenolic acids, flavan-3-ols (catechins and their isomers), and proanthocyanidins. An important aspect to consider is the stability of the functional food ingredient during food processing in terms of composition and bioavailability. Little work has been done so far regarding the effects of heat treatment on potential functional food ingredients. Recently, new information has been provided on the kinetics of thermal modifications in grape-seed extracts. Mathematical models have been proposed as the appropriate way to predict thermal stability and quantify changes in individual antioxidant compounds, antioxidant capacity, and browning (Davidov-Pardo et al. 2011). In this work, grape-seed extracts were submitted to thermal treatments of 60°C, 90°C, and 120°C for 5, 10, 15, 30, 45, and 60 min; these heating conditions simulated those commonly used in the food industry for food preservation. Results showed that the individual antioxidants behave differently during heating: Both proanthocyanidins and gallic acid increased, while catechin and epicatechin decreased. In addition, no statistically significant changes in total antioxidant capacity were observed after thermal treatment. The authors concluded that during the heating of grape-seed extract, the release of gallic acid units, epimerization and polymerization of catechins, and darkening of the samples occurred.

Several extraction methods have been suggested to obtain natural antioxidant extracts from different natural sources, such as food by-products and algae. Obviously, the stability of natural antioxidants to extraction conditions is a critical issue because it will determine the extract composition and the bioavailability of the extract's bioactive components. Among the different methods available for natural antioxidant extraction, green and safe processes, such as those based on the use of subcritical and supercritical fluids, are preferred by the consumers and producers. Although these processes provide important advantages compared to traditional ones, they commonly imply the use of thermal treatments of different intensities to improve extraction yields and selectivity. A promising procedure for obtaining natural extracts with important antioxidant activity in a sustainable way is subcritical water extraction (SWE), which is based on the use of water at high temperatures and enough pressure to be kept in a liquid state. Very recently, our research team probed the feasibility of this approach to obtain extracts with potent antioxidant activity and provided novel information related to the chemical reactions occurring during SWE, such as thermoxidation, caramelization, and Maillard reactions, that overall contribute to the antioxidant character of the extracts (Plaza et al. 2010a,b). Results showed that pressurized water extraction at mild thermal conditions (50°C for 20 min) seems to be adequate to achieve good antioxidant extracts while avoiding further degradation of natural antioxidants and generation of other undesirable substances. Heating to higher temperatures may generate new antioxidants with a different mechanism of action than those naturally existing in the raw matrix. Extraction conditions should be carefully optimized for any particular application, considering the different matrix composition and the stability of their components.

10.2.2   Thermal Processes for Food Transformation

Most of the food products that have been identified as health promoting are, for instance, heat-processed foods, such as coffee, cocoa, bread, and barley, in which the Maillard reaction played a very important role.

Recent epidemiological studies on coffee effects provide evidence of its beneficial effects on human health (van Boekel et al. 2010). The health-promoting properties of coffee brews are associated with their composition of antioxidant phenolic compounds. The most prevalent phenolic compounds in foods are hydroxycinnamic acids, being the major component of the class caffeic acid, which occurs in food mainly as an ester, known as chlorogenic acid. Coffee is the major source of chlorogenic acid in the human diet; the daily intake in coffee drinkers is approximately 0.5–1 g.

During roasting, which is a typical food-transformation thermal process, coffee beans are heated to 200°C–250°C during a given time (from 0.75 to 25 min), depending on the degree of roasting required. Many complex physical and chemical changes take place during this process, including the obvious change in color from green to brown. The major compositional changes occurring are decreases in protein, amino acids, arabinogalactan, reducing sugars, trigonelline, chlorogenic acid, sucrose, and water as well as the formation of melanoidins. Many of these changes are related to the Maillard reaction. Although compounds with antioxidant properties (mainly chlorogenic acid) are lost during roasting, the overall antioxidant properties of coffee brews can be maintained or even enhanced by the development of compounds possessing antioxidant activity, including Maillard reaction products (MRPs). MRPs formed in foods under heating have been reported to possess antioxidant activity and even prooxidant properties (Silván et al. 2006). Although a huge number of studies have been carried out to achieve a better degree of understanding of the effects of food transformation processes on the antioxidant profile and total antioxidant capacity of coffee brews (Farah and Doanangelo 2006; Alves et al. 2010; Renouf et al. 2011), this information is still not complete. This fact might be a result of the complex network of reactions that may take place simultaneously during the roasting process. Figure 10.3 summarizes most of the reactions taking place during coffee roasting that affect antioxidant properties of coffee brews and antioxidant intake as a result of coffee drinking.

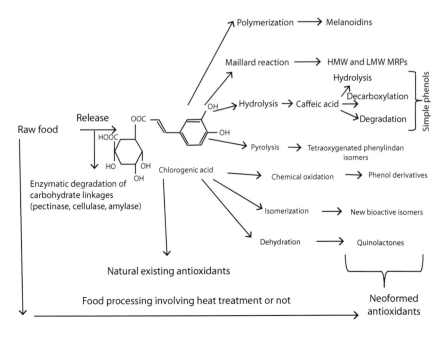

FIGURE 10.3 Chemical and enzymatic reactions affecting chlorogenic acid during processing. LMW: low molecular weight compounds, HMW: high molecular weight compounds.

This complexity has been illustrated by analyzing Colombian Arabica coffee beans roasted at three different levels. A progressive decrease in antioxidant activity (associated mainly with a decrease in chlorogenic acids) was observed with the increasing degree of roasting together with the simultaneous generation of high (HMW) and low molecular weight (LMW) compounds possessing antioxidant activity. The highest antioxidant activity was observed in the medium-roasted coffee, with the contribution to the overall antioxidant activity of the LMW fraction being greater than that of the HMW fraction (Del Castillo et al. 2002).

Besides Maillard reactions, other chemical events could also take place during roasting, such as pyrolysis. In fact, an increase in the antioxidant activity of pyrolysated chlorogenic and caffeic acids (11-fold and 460-fold, respectively) after a heat treatment equivalent to roasting has been observed (Guillot et al. 1996). Tetraoxygenated 1,3-*cis* and 1,3-*trans*-phenyllindan isomers were identified as the main active components in caffeic acid pyrolysates.

Similar observations have been obtained from the roasting of small black soybeans. Roasted soybeans (at 250°C for 30 min) showed significantly higher antioxidant activity than unroasted small black soybeans *in vitro*. This enhancement of antioxidant properties of the roasted samples was ascribed to an increase in phenolic acid and MRPs resulting from roast processing (Kim et al. 2011). Thus, the roasting process under controlled conditions might be a feasible and helpful way to obtain food with optimal antioxidant properties. However, further research to confirm this hypothesis has to be undertaken considering also that the identity of some of the newly formed antioxidants is still unknown.

Baking is another very common food transformation process. Baked products, such as bread, are part of the human daily diet worldwide. It has been observed that the baking process can positively influence the overall antioxidant capacity of the obtained products, mainly through Maillard reactions, of rye bread (Michalska et al. 2008). Baking favored the formation of antioxidant compounds during the manufacture of rye bread made of whole grains. The bread crust, where the heating is more intense, was the portion of the bread where the main changes resulting from Maillard reactions were observed. However, not all the MRPs provide the same antioxidant activity; for instance, it was demonstrated that advanced MRPs showed good scavenging of peroxyl and ABTS radicals, whereas early MRPs did not seem to be linked to overall antioxidant capacity (Michalska et al. 2008).

10.2.3 Microwave Heating

Microwave heating has been employed either to assist an extraction process or as an alternative to traditional heating processes. Depending on the particular application, the intensity of the treatment differs, and as a result, the concentrations of antioxidants and the total antioxidant capacity of the treated foods also change. Microwaves have been used in food processing to inactivate enzymes from vegetable products that otherwise might induce sensory and chemical changes. It has been shown that, although the treatment with microwaves was enough to inactivate enzymes from red peppers, the amount of phenolic compounds was reduced by approximately 20%. Nevertheless, interestingly, the total antioxidant capacity of the samples was significantly enhanced after the treatment. These results were associated with the emergence of new phenol derivatives that increased the overall antioxidant capacity of the treated samples (Dorantes-Alvarez et al. 2011).

Other investigations have revealed that a microwave treatment can also promote changes in the chemical composition of the food toward the release of free phenolic acids, reducing the amount of bound phenolics and producing an increase in the overall antioxidant capacity. This fact has been observed in mandarin pomace (Hayat et al. 2010) where a correlation between the intensity of the microwave treatment and the stability of flavonol compounds was detected; whereas the amount of total flavonol compounds increased with the treatment power, long irradiation times caused a degradation of these components (Hayat et al. 2010). Therefore, it was concluded that an efficient control of microwave treatment might improve the composition and antioxidant properties of mandarin pomace by increasing both the content and bioavailability of the bioactive components present.

From the information provided in this section, it can be deduced that moderate heat treatments might be considered as a useful tool to improve the health properties of some vegetables, considering that increases in the amounts of phenolic compounds and total antioxidant activities may be observed. Nevertheless, processing conditions should be carefully optimized, and the composition of the food has to be closely studied in order to assure its safety and health-promoting effects. In this sense, it is important to consider the safety and health-promoting properties of neo-antioxidants generated during processing, such as some MRPs like hydroxymethylfurfural (HMF). For instance, some controversy exists in the literature about the positive effects and the safety issues related to HMF consumption (Zhao and Hall 2008; Li et al. 2009; Herrero et al. 2012).

10.3 NONTHERMAL PROCESSING OF FOODS

Although, as mentioned in previous sections, some of the most-used processes in the food industry for increasing shelf life deal with the use of heat, it is also true that with the increasing interest of the consumer in high-quality food, including preservation of both sensory and nutritional parameters, new nonthermal processes are being further developed. For instance, processes such as irradiation or application of high pressure are gaining importance in inactivating microorganisms while preserving food quality parameters. In this section, the main nonthermal processes used, or that have the potential to be used, in the food industry are briefly described, focusing on the formation of antioxidants during their application. In this regard, some basic food treatments that do not imply the use of heat, including wet cleaning, sorting, knife peeling, size reduction, mixing, or separations, will not be described considering their little, if not null, effect on the generation of antioxidants.

10.3.1 Enzymatic Treatments

Enzymes are widely used in the food industry because of their broad applicability (Fellows 2000); the use of enzymes presents a series of advantages, such as the reaction's specificity at mild conditions of temperature and pH. In addition, enzymes are active at quite low concentrations. Besides the technology-related applications of these compounds, such as texture improvement, viscosity reduction, or flavor production, enzymes used in different processes allow the formation of new antioxidant compounds that were not present before the treatment. Among the most-employed enzymes in the food industry, α-amylases, invertases, cellulases and hemicellulases, lipases, and some proteases, including rennet, are pointed out.

One of the main fields of generation of antioxidant compounds derived from enzyme application is the production of antioxidant peptides, mainly in dairy products (Pihlanto 2006). In fact, during cheese elaboration, different enzymes produce the proteolysis of casein and other milk proteins, and as a result, different peptides might be formed, depending on the type of milk and the enzymes added as well as on the particular manufacturing process followed. It is also well known that new peptides also can be formed during cheese ripening and that these bioactive peptides might differ depending on the type of cheese (Sousa et al. 2011).

The formation of antioxidant peptides after treatment with other enzymes also has been assessed. For instance, a peptide composed of 11 amino acid residues was isolated after the treatment of algae protein waste with pepsin, showing potent antiradical activity measured by using TEAC, ORAC, DPPH, as well as other antiradical assays (Sheih et al. 2009). The use of this enzyme also has been widely explored for the generation of active peptides from different protein sources, including chickpea proteins, milk casein, and fish proteins, among others.

The effect of the use of enzymes during processing on the formation of other antioxidant compounds has been also studied. For instance, it has been shown that the enzymatic treatment of the highly viscous puree resulting from the mechanical crushing of carrots allows a better recovery of the carrot juice directly by pressing. In fact, it has been observed that the treatment with cell wall-degrading pectinases before pressing enhanced the recovery of antioxidants in the juice, significantly improving the bioactivity of the resulting product (Khandare et al. 2011). This strategy, based on the treatment of vegetable products with pectinases, is potentially applicable to other vegetable-derived products in which the recovery of antioxidants can be effectively enhanced (Oszmianski et al. 2011).

10.3.2 FERMENTATION

Fermentation can be classified as a nonthermal process usually employed in the food industry to produce beneficial effects in food. During fermentation, different microorganisms are utilized to induce a series of chemical changes that, in the end, provide a food conservation method. After fermentation, the food products treated have significantly changed not only from an organoleptic point of view but also from a chemical perspective. In fact, the digestion of food components by microorganisms (bacteria and yeast, most frequently) is responsible for the modification and formation of new components derived from the action of the microorganisms' enzymes. Beyond shelf life extension, fermentation produces other beneficial effects in foods, such as the enrichment of nutritional value, the elimination of anti-nutrients, and the improvement of the sensory properties of food. Besides, new compounds not formerly present in the original food can be also formed, and among them, the formation of antioxidants is a possibility.

Indeed, among the antioxidants formed from fermentation processes, antioxidant peptides derived from food proteins are pointed out. Several antioxidative peptides have been described in fermented foods, although their mechanism of action is still not fully understood. Generally, these peptides possess 2 to 10 amino acid residues and can act through three different actions: as metal chelators, scavenging radicals, or proton donors.

The generation of antioxidant peptides in different fermented foods has been assessed. For instance, it was found that peptides derived from milk fermented by *Lactobacillus delbruekii* spp. *bulgaricus* had a potential antioxidant activity among other interesting bioactivities (Qian et al. 2011). Similarly, other antioxidant peptides have been described from commercial fermented milk-based products (Hernandez-Ledesma et al. 2005). Although dairy products are one of the most studied food products regarding the occurrence of bioactive peptides generated after fermentation processes, other examples can also be found, such as, for instance, fermented mussel (*Mytilus edulis*) sauce. An interesting study performed using this product allowed the identification of a heptapeptide, the amino acid sequence of which was HFGBPFH (MW 962 kDa) and which possessed a good radical-scavenging activity (Rajapakse et al. 2005). After the purification of this peptide from the mussel sauce, its radical-scavenging properties against superoxide and hydroxyl radicals were assessed, showing an activity approximately two times higher than that of α-tocopherol. Likewise, this peptide also showed metal ion chelation activities as well as lipid peroxidation inhibition properties. In fact, as can be observed in Figure 10.4, the isolated peptide

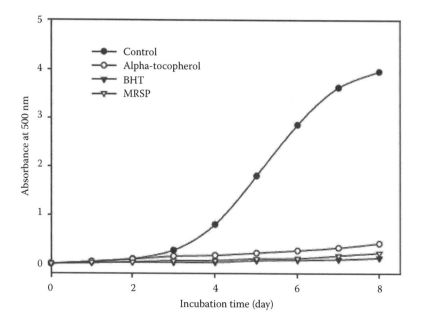

FIGURE 10.4 Lipid peroxidation inhibitory activity of the peptide (54 μM) isolated from fermented mussel sauce (MRSP). The activity was measured in linoleic acid oxidation system for 8 days using butylated hydroxytoluene (BHT) and α-tocopherol as positive controls at same concentrations. (From Rajapakse, N. et al. 2005, *Food Res Int* 38: 175–182. With permission.)

derived from the fermentation process showed an inhibition of the lipid peroxidation higher than α-tocopherol, which is a well-known lipid-soluble antioxidant. The activity was attributed to the ability of the peptide to interfere in the propagating cycle of lipid peroxidation, slowing radical-mediated linoleic oxidation; the presence of several hydrophobic amino acids in its sequence would help to enhance the solubility of the peptide in the lipid fraction facilitating its interaction with the radicals (Rajapakse et al. 2005).

Other fermented food-derived peptides have been also described as possessing antioxidant properties against a wide range of radicals. An example is the isolation of antioxidant peptides from a fermented mushroom, *Ganoderma lucidum* (Sun et al. 2004).

10.3.3 IRRADIATION

Irradiation is a nonthermal food processing technique, involving the exposure of food products to ionizing or nonionizing radiation and enabling processing at nearly ambient temperatures. The use of ionizing radiation, mainly through the application of gamma-irradiation, improves the hygienic quality of food products without having a critical impact on the sensory characteristics of the treated products. Besides considering that packaged food can be also treated, recontamination during food production and consumption chains is low. On the other hand, the nonionizing radiation employed is electromagnetic radiation that does not possess energy enough to ionize atoms or molecules as they are ultraviolet rays (UV-A, UV-B, UV-C), the most frequently used. During the irradiation process, reactive ions are produced, which destroy or damage microorganisms in quite a fast way by changing the cell membrane structure and affecting the metabolic enzyme activity. The safety of food irradiation at 10 kGy and above has been assured (Alothman et al. 2009).

It has been observed that the irradiation of several foods and food products can have a different effect on the antioxidants naturally present in the treated matrix. In this sense, it has been commonly assessed that the antioxidant capacities of the irradiated products and/or their antioxidant contents were raised compared to non-irradiated counterparts. The effect of radiation on the antioxidants has been shown to be dependent on the dose and exposure time as well as on the matrix being irradiated itself. Table 10.1 presents a summary of some of the most recently published reports in which positive effects have been observed. In general, the increase in antioxidants after irradiation has been related to an enhancement of the enzyme activity or to an improvement of extractability from the tissues in which they are contained. For instance, the increasing synthesis of phenolic compounds observed during storage of different vegetables after irradiation was suggested as being responsible for the enhancement of the antioxidant capacity and total phenolic contents observed in those vegetables after ionizing radiation treatments, even at doses below 1 kGy (Fan 2005).

These observations allow us to conclude that irradiation treatments can be a useful tool not only in assuring the microbiological safety of food products but also in increasing their quality. This fact also can be applicable to nonionizing radiation. In this sense, UV-C has been proposed as a useful tool to improve the postharvest quality of fruits. In a recent work, authors demonstrated that a UV-C irradiation treatment of mango fruit, at levels between 2.46 and 4.93 kJ m^{-2}, produced a significant increase on the total phenol and total flavonoid content of the fruits during the storage following the irradiation treatment, whereas fungi infections were reduced (Gonzalez-Aguilar et al. 2007a). Results suggested a response to the stress generated by UV radiation in plants that may act by inducing enzymes related to scavenging radical oxygen species as well as to the synthesis of flavonoids and phenolic compounds. Thus, UV-C was proposed as a useful alternative to maintain the postharvest quality of the mango fruit (Gonzalez-Aguilar et al. 2007b).

It is also important to remark that the enhancement or decrease in antioxidants present in the samples might happen as a result not only of the type of treatment (type of radiation, intensity, and time, among others) but also of the solvents used for the extraction. For instance, it was observed that the scavenging activity after irradiation treatments at dose levels from 2 to 16 kGy of *Nigella sativa* seeds (black cumin), a spice employed in a wide variety of food products, significantly varied among three different tested extraction solvents (i.e., water, methanol, and acetone) (Khattak and Simpson 2008). The free radical-scavenging activity of the methanol and acetone extracts was enhanced after the treatment with gamma radiation, as well as the total phenolic contents.

Other antioxidants can also be formed after treatment with gamma radiation, for instance, neoantioxidants derived from the Maillard reaction after irradiation. The

TABLE 10.1

Positive Effects on Antioxidants Observed after Irradiation Treatment of Food Products

Product	Antioxidants	Irradiation Type	Observations	Reference
Romaine lettuce, iceberg lettuce, endive	Phenolic compounds	γ-Radiation (up to 2 kGy)	Increased antioxidant capacity and total phenolic content after irradiation	Fan 2005
Mushrooms (*Agaricus blazei*)	Phenolic compounds	γ-Radiation (from 2.5 to 20 kGy)	Antioxidant capacity of extracts increased	Huang and Mau 2006
Mango (fresh cut)	Phenolics, flavonoids	UV-C	Total phenolic and flavonoid accumulation during storage	Gonzalez-Aguilar et al. 2007a
Carrot juice	Phenolic compounds	γ-Radiation (10 kGy)	Total phenolics and antioxidant capacity increased	Song et al. 2006
Almond skin	Phenolic compounds	γ-Radiation (0–16 kGy)	Increased antioxidant capacity and total phenolic content after irradiation	Harrison and Were 2007
Apple	Anthocyanins, flavonols, quercetin glycosides, phenolic compounds	UV-B	Antioxidant activity increased	Hagen et al. 2007
Rosemary	Phenolic compounds	γ-Radiation (30 kGy)	Antioxidant capacity and total phenolic contents increased in extracts	Perez et al. 2007
Broccoli	Phenolic compounds, ascorbic acid	UV-C (8 kJ m^{-2})	Increased phenolics and ascorbic acid contents as well as antioxidant capacity	Lemoine et al. 2007
Nigella sativa seeds	Phenolic compounds	γ-Radiation (2–16 kGy)	Antioxidant capacity and total phenol content increased depending on solvent	Khattak et al. 2008
Strawberries	Anthocyanins	UV-C	Increased antioxidant capacity and anthocyanin content	Erkan et al. 2008
Soybean	Phenolic compounds	UV-C	Increased flavonoid content	Winter and Rostas 2008
Hizikia fusiformis alga	Polyphenolic compounds	γ-Radiation (1 kGy)	Antioxidant activity increased	Choi et al. 2010
Beet (fresh cut)		γ-Radiation (1–2 kGy)	Antioxidant activity increased	Latorre et al. 2010

formation of this kind of compound from cheese whey has been confirmed (Chawla et al. 2009). The presence of reducing sugars and proteins in this important food by-product allows the occurrence of Maillard reactions under certain conditions. Different irradiation intensities, using gamma radiation, were tested, and a dose-dependent increase in browning and fluorescence as well as a decrease in free amino groups were observed. Based on these results, the occurrence of Maillard reactions could be confirmed after irradiation. Besides, it was clearly observed that the anti-oxidant capacity of the products after irradiation, using different *in vitro* assays, was significantly higher. Thus, it could be concluded that an irradiation treatment, under certain conditions, of cheese whey can have a positive effect not only on the microbiological safety of the product but also on the final antioxidant profile because it was able to produce new antioxidants related to Maillard reactions, which could potentially increase the interest in the final product (Chawla et al. 2009).

10.3.4 HIGH PRESSURES

At present, the use of high pressures in food processing is an interesting alternative for the nonthermal inactivation of microorganisms and pathogens in general. Nevertheless, its use is not widely distributed, mainly because of the expensive equipment required to apply this treatment to food products. When high pressures, typically up to 1000 MPa, are applied to packaged food immersed in a liquid, this pressure is uniformly and instantly distributed throughout the food, causing the destruction of the microorganisms present. Considering that pressure transmission is not time-dependent—times required to apply these treatments are very short—under these conditions, the break of covalent bonds does not occur, helping to maintain the sensory properties and nutritional value of the foods. Instead, high hydrostatic pressure (HHP) produces changes in membrane structures, resulting in bacterial inactivation as well as in the structure of macromolecules, such as enzymes, fostering their inactivation.

Because of these intrinsic characteristics, HHP will not generally produce significant changes in the nutritional composition of the treated foods. Nevertheless, some changes have been reported in several applications. For instance, it has been shown how the content of naringenin and hesperitin present in orange juice could be increased after treatment at 400 MPa (Sanchez-Moreno et al. 2005). A similar effect was detected in cashew apple juice when it was pressurized between 250 and 400 MPa. Under these conditions, the juice presented a higher content of soluble poly-phenols, demonstrating that HHP treatments could be potentially employed in the food industry to obtain products with higher nutritional quality (Queiroz et al. 2010). The treatment of onions with high pressures improved the extractability of glycoside flavonoids and aglycones when compared to untreated samples.

On the other hand, even if high-pressure treatments could not increase the anti-oxidant content in the treated foods, the changes promoted by high pressures in the food structures might derive a better accessibility and availability of important food components, such as antioxidants and minerals. This has been demonstrated with apples treated with 500 MPa for 10 min, which showed, in comparison with untreated samples, higher antioxidant capacities, minerals, and starch contents.

Consequently, the consumption of this kind of fruit could provide further potential health-promoting effects than their corresponding untreated counterparts (Briones-Labarca et al. 2011). The same has been observed for other kinds of food components, such as carotenoids; HHP treatments have been shown to have a positive effect on the availability of carotenoids present in some vegetables (McInerney et al. 2007).

10.3.5 OTHERS (SEPARATION, PULSED ELECTRIC FIELDS)

Other nonthermal processes that may affect the antioxidant profile of food products are, for example, pulsed electric fields and pulsed light.

The application of pulsed electric fields has raised some attention for the possibility of obtaining microbial inactivation in extremely short times. This technique is based on the application of a pulsed high voltage field (usually between 20 and 80 kV cm^{-1}) to food products during times generally shorter than 1 s and by applying short-duration pulses (less than 5 μs each). The effects on the microorganisms include electrical breakdown as well as electroporation, inducing the rupture of the cells by changing the structure of the membrane. Figure 10.5 illustrates the effects of pulsed electric fields on the membrane of *Saccharomyces cerevisiae* cells.

(a)
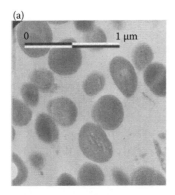

(b)
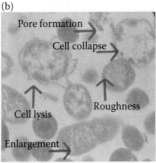

FIGURE 10.5 Transmission electron microscopy of (a) untreated cells of *Saccharomyces cerevisiae* and (b) cells of *S. cerevisiae* suspended in peach juice by PEF for 600 μs at 35 kV cm^{-1}. (With kind permission from Springer Science+Business Media: *Food Bioprocess Technol*, Combination of pulsed electric fields with other preservation techniques, 4, 2011, 954–968, Martín-Belloso, O., Sobrino-Lopez, A.)

Although, obviously, heat is produced as a result of the application of high voltage, this heat is controlled, and the sample is never heated. Besides, the effects observed on the microorganisms are a result of the electric field and not of any thermal effect. During these extremely short treatment times, the food properties are mainly unchanged, minimizing the chance of finding undesirable side effects in the nutritional or sensory properties. Even if these changes are minimal, some effects on the antioxidant composition of foods treated with pulsed electric fields have been reported. This is the case when this technique is applied as a pretreatment during juice production; the application of pulsed electric fields before pressing allows the attainment of apple juices with increased content on polyphenols and a higher antioxidant capacity (Grimi et al. 2011) (see Figure 10.3 for examples). Other researchers have found that carrot juices stabilized by using pulsed electric fields (35 kV cm^{-1} for 1500 µs using 6-µs pulses at 200 Hz) had a higher β-carotene content than untreated juices (Quitao-Teizeira et al. 2009). Besides, the treatment using this technique allowed better retention of the quality parameters than using heat treatments. The same observations were obtained for other juices as well (Odriozola-Serrano et al. 2008). The effect of this treatment on the vegetable matrix also could be useful for the subsequent extraction of bioactively interesting compounds, such as anthocyanins. A fast-pulsed electric field treatment (2.5 kV cm^{-1}, 15-µs pulse width, and 50 pulses) allowed the improvement of more than twofold the extraction of anthocyanins from red cabbage (Gachovska et al. 2010).

Pulsed-light processing is being explored as a nonthermal technique and is based on the ability of pulsed light to treat food surfaces, eliminating the microorganisms present. The light employed in this technique is broad-spectrum white light, basically similar to that of sunlight but also including some UV wavelengths. The light is applied in single or a short series of short pulses (ms) with an intensity between 20,000 and 90,000 times higher than that of the sunlight. The mechanisms employed would include photochemical effects and DNA damage as well as short-term thin-layer photothermal effects. The influence on the natural antioxidants present in foods as well as on the generation of new components is still scarcely studied. Nevertheless, it has been observed that these treatments would not imply a destruction of the nutritional quality of different products (Caminiti et al. 2011; Muñoz et al. 2012).

10.4 CONCLUSIONS

Food processing seems to generate some controversy in terms of the risks and benefits associated with its use. Although some risks have been stressed during recent years and a lot of research has been concentrated in order to minimize them (e.g., production of acrylamide or heterocyclic amines, losses of essential nutrients, formation of artifacts), it is clear that food processing is a need in terms of food safety requirements. Moreover, the new trends are focused on the possibility of using controlled food processes to improve the health benefits of certain foods, that is, food processing understood beyond its own basic function. Food processes susceptible to being fine-tuned to generate beneficial compounds are based on thermal and nonthermal treatments and are discussed in the present chapter based on their ability to produce antioxidant compounds or to improve the overall antioxidant activity of the food commodity. Although it is true that evidence has been presented widely that demonstrated the *in vitro* effects of antioxidants either released or generated in foods during processing, a lot of research is still needed to provide scientific evidence of the real effect of such compounds in human health. Therefore, in the future, more research will be needed in order to decipher the molecular mechanisms of such products in the human body, and new approaches, such as those based on -omics technologies, will be required. In this sense, the development of Foodomics, together with metabolomics, proteomics, and transcriptomics, can be the key for a holistic approach to the real effect of antioxidants generated during food processing as functional food ingredients. More research will be also needed in terms of systematic studies on food processing conditions (thermal and nonthermal), on their effects on different types of foods, and also on the development of industrial applications of new technologies (e.g., nonthermal) able to minimize the risks and maximize the benefits of the food processing. By building all this new knowledge, the possibility of "producing" new compounds with antioxidant activity able to provide a health benefit might be a reality.

To conclude, only research carried out considering multidisciplinary teams (chemists, biochemists, food technologists, nutritionists, medical doctors, etc.) can guarantee the real effects of such antioxidant compounds, generated during food processing, as relevant for human health.

REFERENCES

Alothman, M., Bhat, R., Karim, A. A. 2009. Effects of radiation processing on phytochemicals and antioxidants in plant produce. *Trends Food Sci Technol* 20: 201–212.

Alves, R. C., Costa, A. S. G., Jerez, M., Casal, S., Sineiro, J., Nuñez, M. J., Oliveira, B. 2010. Antiradical activity, phenolic profile and hydroxymethylfurfural in espresso coffee: Influence of technological factors. *J Agric Food Chem* 58: 1221–1229.

Briones-Labarca, V., Vargas-Cubillos, G., Ortiz-Portilla, S., Chacana-Ojeda, M., Maureira, H. 2011. Effects of high hydrostatic pressure (HHP) on bioaccessibility, as well as antioxidant activity, mineral and starch contents in Granny Smith apple. *Food Chem* 128: 520–529.

Caminiti, I. M., Noci, F., Muñoz, A., Whyte, P., Morgan, D. J., Cronin, D. A., Lyng, J. G. 2011. Impact of selected combinations of non-thermal processing technologies on the quality of an apple and cranberry juice blend. *Food Chem* 124: 1387–1392.

Chawla, S. P., Chander, R., Sharma, A. 2009. Antioxidant properties of Maillard reaction products obtained by gamma-irradiation of whey proteins. *Food Chem* 116: 122–128.

Choi, J., Kim, H. J., Kim, J. H., Chun, B. S., Ahn, D. H., Kim, G. H., Lee, J. W. 2010. Changes in colour and antioxidant activities of *Hizikia fusiformis* cooking drips by gamma irradiation. *LWT-Food Sci Technol* 43: 1074–1078.

Davidov-Pardo, G., Arozamena, I., Martin-Arroyo, M. R. 2011. Kinetics of thermal modifications in grape seed extract. *J Agric Food Chem* 59: 7211–7217.

Del Castillo, M. D., Ames, J. M., Gordon, M. H. 2002. Effect of roasting on the antioxidant activity of coffee brews. *J Agric Food Chem* 50: 3698–3703.

Dhuique-Mayer, C., Tbatou, M., Carail, M., Caris-Veyrat, C., Dornier, M., Amiot, M. J. 2007. Thermal degradation of antioxidant micronutrients in citrus juice: Kinetics and newly formed compounds. *J Agric Food Chem* 55: 4209–4216.

Dorantes-Alvarez, L., Jaramillo-Flores, E., González, K., Martínez, R., Parada, L. 2011. Blanching peppers using microwaves. *Procedia Food Sci* 1: 178–183.

Erkan, M., Wang, S. Y., Wang, C. Y. 2008. Effect of UV treatment on antioxidant capacity, antioxidant enzyme activity and decay in strawberry fruit. *Postharvest Biol Technol* 48: 163–171.

Fan, X. 2005. Antioxidant capacity of fresh-cut vegetables exposed to ionizing radiation. *J Sci Food Agric* 85: 995–1000.

Farah, A., Doanangelo, C. M. 2006. Phenolic compounds in coffee. *Braz J Plant Physiol* 18: 23–26.

Fellows, P. J. 2000. *Food Processing Technology: Principles and Practice*. Boca Raton, FL: CRC Press.

Fiore, A., La Fauci, L., Cervellati, R., Guerra, M. C., Speroni, E., Costa, S., Galvano, G., De Lorenzo, A., Bacchelli, V., Fogliano, V., Galvano, F. 2005. Antioxidant activity of pasteurized and sterilized commercial red orange juices. *Mol Nutr Food Res* 49: 1129–1135.

Gachovska, T., Cassada, D., Subbiah, J., Hanna, M., Thippareddi, H., Snow, D. 2010. Enhanced anthocyanin extraction from red cabbage using pulsed electric field processing. *J Food Sci* 75: E323–E329.

Gonzalez-Aguilar, G. A., Villegas-Ochoa, M. A., Martinez-Tellez, M. A., Gardea, A. A., Ayala-Zavala, J. F. 2007a. Improving antioxidant capacity of fresh-cut mangoes treated with UV-C. *J Food Sci* 72: S197–S202.

Gonzalez-Aguilar, G. A., Zavaleta-Gatica, R., Tiznado-Hernandez, M. E. 2007b. Improving postharvest quality of mango "Haden" by UV-C treatment. *Postharvest Biol Technol* 45: 108–116.

Grajek, W., Olejnik, A. 2010. The influence of food processing and home cooking on the antioxidant stability in foods. In *Functional Food Product Development*, J. Smith, E. Charter (eds.), Oxford: Wiley-Blackwell.

Grimi, N., Mamouni, F., Labovka, N., Vorobiev, E., Vaxelaire, J. 2011. Impact of apple pressing modes on extracted juice quality: Pressing assisted by pulsed electric fields. *J Food Eng* 103: 52–61.

Guillot, F. L., Malnoe, A., Stadler, R. H. 1996. Antioxidant properties of novel tetraoxygenated phenylindan isomers formed during thermal decomposition of caffeic acid. *J Agric Food Chem* 44: 2503–2510.

Hagen, S. F., Borge, G. I. A., Bengtsson, C. B., Bilger, W., Berge, A., Haffner, K. 2007. Phenolic contents and other health and sensory related properties of apple fruit (*Malus domestica Borkh* cv. Aroma): Effect of post-harvest UV-B irradiation. *Postharvest Biol Technol* 45: 1–10.

Harrison, K., Were, L. M. 2007. Effect of gamma irradiation on total phenolic content yield and antioxidant capacity of almond skin extracts. *Food Chem* 102: 932–937.

Hayat, K., Zhang, X., Faroog, U., Abbas, S., Xia, S., Jia, C., Zhong, F., Zhang, J. 2010. Effect of microwave treatment on phenolic content and antioxidant activity of citrus mandarin pomace. *Food Chem* 123: 423–429.

Henle, T. 2005. Protein-bound advanced glycation end products (AGEs) as bioactive amino acid derivatives in foods. *Amino Acids* 29: 313–322.

Hernandez-Ledesma, B., Miralles, B., Amigo, L., Ramos, M., Recio, I. 2005. Identification of antioxidant and ACE-inhibitory peptides in fermented milk. *J Food Sci Agric* 85: 1041–1048.

Herrero, M., Castro-Puyana, M., Rocamora-Reverte, L., Ferragut, J. A., Cifuentes, A., Ibáñez, E. 2012. Formation and relevance of 5-hydroxymethylfurfural in bioactive subcritical water extracts from olive leaves. *Food Res Int* 47: 31–37.

Huang, S. J., Mau, J. L. 2006. Antioxidant properties of methanolic extracts of *Agaricus blazei* with various doses of γ-irradiation. *LWT-Food Sci Technol* 39: 707–716.

Khandare, V., Walia, S., Singh, M., Kaur, C. 2011. Black carrot (*Daucus carota* ssp. *sativus*) juice: Processing effects on antioxidant composition and color. *Food Bioprod Process* 89: 482–486.

Khattak, K. F., Simpson, T. J. 2008. Effect of gamma radiation on the extraction yield, total phenolic content and free radical scavenging activity of *Nigella sativa* seed. *Food Chem* 110: 967–972.

Kim, H. G., Kim, G. W., Oh, H., Yoo, S. Y., Kim, Y. O., Oh, M. S. 2011. Influence of roasting on the antioxidant activity of small black soybean (*Glycine max* L. Merrill). *LWT-Food Sci Technol* 44: 992–998.

Latorre, M. E., Narvaiz, P., Rojas, A. M., Gerschenson, L. N. 2010. Effects of gamma irradiation on bio-chemical and physico-chemical parameters of fresh-cut red beet (*Beta vulgaris* L. var. *conditiva*) root. *J Food Eng* 98: 178–191.

Lemoine, M. L., Civello, P. M., Martinez, G. A., Chaves, A. R. 2007. Influence of post-harvest UV-C treatment on refrigerated storage of minimally processed broccoli (*Brassica oleracea* var. *italica*). *J Sci Food Agric* 87: 1132–1139.

Li, Y. X., Li, Y., Quian, Z. J., Kim, M. M., Kim, S. K. 2009. In vitro antioxidant activity of 5-HMF isolated from marine red alga *Laurencia undulata* in free radical mediated oxidative systems. *J Microbiol Biotechnol* 19: 1319–1327.

Martín-Belloso, O., Sobrino-Lopez, A. 2011. Combination of pulsed electric fields with other preservation techniques. *Food Bioprocess Technol* 4: 954–968.

McInerney, J. K., Seccafien, C. A., Stewart, C. M., Bird, A. R. 2007. Effects of high pressure processing on antioxidant activity, total carotenoid content and availability, in vegetables. *Innovat Food Sci Emerg Technol* 8: 543–548.

Michalska, A., Amigo-Benavent, M., Zielinski, H., del Castillo, M. D. 2008. Effect of bread making on formation of Maillard reaction products contributing to the overall antioxidant activity of rye bread. *J Cereal Sci* 48: 123–132.

Muñoz, A., Caminiti, I. M., Palgan, I., Pataro, G., Noci, F., Morgan, D. J., Cronin, D. A., Whyte, P., Ferrari, G., Lyng, J. G. 2012. Effects on *Escherichia coli* inactivation and quality attributes in apple juice treated by combinations of pulsed light and thermosonication. *Food Res Int* 45: 299–305.

Odriozola-Serrano, I., Soliva-Fortuny, R., Martín-Belloso, O. 2008. Changes of health-related compounds throughout cold storage of tomato juice stabilized by thermal or high intensity pulsed electric field treatments. *Innovat Food Sci Emerg Technol* 9: 272–279.

Oszmianski, J., Wojdylo, A. Kolniak, J. 2011. Effect of pectinase treatment on extraction of antioxidant phenols from pomace for the production of puree-enriched cloudy apple juices. *Food Chem* 127: 623–631.

Patras, A., Brunton, N. P., Da Pieve, S., Butler, F. 2010. Impact of high pressure processing on total antioxidant activity, phenolic, ascorbic acid, anthocyanin content and colour of strawberry and blackberry purées. *Innovat Food Sci Emerg Technol* 10: 308–331.

Perez, M. B., Calderon, N. L., Croci, C. A. 2007. Radiation-induced enhancement of antioxidant activity in extracts of rosemary (*Rosmarinus officinalis* L). *Food Chem* 104: 585–592.

Pihlanto, A. 2006. Antioxidative peptides derived from milk proteins. *Int Dairy J* 16: 1306–1314.

Plaza, M., Amigo-Benavent, M., del Castillo, M. D., Ibáñez, E., Herrero, M. 2010a. Neoformation of antioxidants in glycation model systems treated under subcritical water extraction conditions. *Food Res Int* 43: 1123–1129.

Plaza, M., Amigo-Benavent, M., del Castillo, M. D., Ibáñez, E., Herrero, M. 2010b. Facts about the formation of new antioxidants in natural samples after subcritical water extraction. *Food Res Int* 43: 2341–2348.

Qian, B., Xing, M., Cui, L., Deng, Y., Xu, Y., Huang, M., Zhang, S. 2011. Antioxidant, antihypertensive, and immunomodulatory activities of peptide fractions from fermented skim milk with *Lactobacillus delbruekii* spp. *bulgaricus* LB340. *J Dairy Res* 78: 72–79.

Queiroz, C., Moreira, C. C. F., Lavinas, F. C., Lopes, M. L. M., Fialho, E., Valente-Mesquita, V. L. 2010. Effect of high hydrostatic pressure on phenolic compounds, ascorbic acid and antioxidant activity in cashew apple juice. *High Pres Res* 30: 507–513.

Quitao-Teizeira, L. J., Odriozola-Serrano, I., Soliva-Fortuny, R., Mota-Ramos, A., Martin-Belloso, O. 2009. Comparative study on antioxidant properties of carrot juice stabilized by high intensity pulsed electric fields or heat treatments. *J Sci Food Agric* 89: 2636–2642.

Rajapakse, N., Mendis, E., Jung, W. K., Je, J. Y., Kim, S. K. 2005. Purification of a radical scavenging peptide from fermented mussel sauce and its antioxidant properties. *Food Res Int* 38: 175–182.

Renouf, M., Guy, P. A., Colette, C., Marmet, O., Steilling, H., Cavin, C., Williamson, G. 2011. Method for promoting and selling coffee. United States Patent Application Publication. Pub. Date July 7, 2011, US 2011/0166946 A1.

Robbins, R. J. 2003. Phenolic acids in foods: An overview of analytical methodology. *J Agric Food Chem* 51: 2866–2887.

Sanchez-Moreno, C., Plaza, L., Elez-Martinez, P., de Ancos, B., Martin-Belloso, O., Cano, M. P. 2005. Impact of high pressure and pulsed electric fields on bioactive compounds and antioxidant activity of orange juice in comparison with traditional thermal processing. *J Agric Food Chem* 53: 4403–4409.

Sheih, I. C., Wu, T. K., Fang, T. J. 2009. Antioxidant properties of new antioxidative peptide from algae protein waste hydrolysate in different oxidation systems. *Biores Technol* 100: 3419–3425.

Shi, J., Le Maguer, M. 2000. Lycopene in tomatoes: Chemical and physical properties affected by food processing. *Crit Rev Food Sci Nutr* 40: 1–42.

Silván, J. M., van Lagemaat, J., Olano, A., del Castillo, M. D. 2006. Analysis and biological properties of amino acids derivatives formed by Maillard reaction in foods. *J Pharm Biomed Anal* 41: 1543–1551.

Song, H. P., Kim, D. H., Jo, C., Lee, C. H., Kim, K. S., Byum, M. W. 2006. Effect of gamma irradiation on the microbiological quality and antioxidant activity of fresh vegetable juice. *Food Microbiol* 23: 372–378.

Sousa, M. J., Ardo, Y., McSweeney, P. L. H. 2011. Advances in the study of proteolysis during cheese ripening. *Int Dairy J* 11: 327–345.

Sun, J., He, H., Xie, J. 2004. Novel antioxidant peptides from fermented mushroom *Ganoderma lucidum*. *J Agric Food Chem* 52: 6646–6652.

van Boekel, M., Fogliano, V., Pellegrini, N., Stanton, C., Scholz, G., Lalljie, S., Somoza, V., Knorr, D., Jasti, P. R., Eisenbrand, G. 2010. A review on the beneficial aspects of food processing. *Mol Nutr Food Res* 54: 1215–1247.

Villamiel, M., del Castillo, M. D., Corzo, N. 2012. Browning reactions. In *Food Biochemistry and Food Processing*, 2nd ed. Y. H. Hui (ed.), Blackwell Publishing, Ames, Iowa.

Winter, T. R., Rostas, M. 2008. Ambient ultraviolet radiation induces protective responses in soybean but does not attenuate indirect defense. *Environ Pollut* 155: 290–297.

Zhao, B., Hall, C. A. 2008. Composition and antioxidant activity of raisin extracts obtained from various solvents. *Food Chem* 108: 511–518.

11 Mechanisms of Antioxidant Activity

Klaudia Jomova, Michael Lawson, and Marian Valko

CONTENTS

11.1 INTRODUCTION

Numerous biochemical reactions occurring in living systems in which electron transfer takes place are called redox reactions (Schafer and Buettner 2001). A chemical reaction in which a loss of electrons occurs is called an oxidation reaction; conversely, the gain of electrons by a chemical substance is called a reduction process or a reduction reaction. In recent years, significant progress in the understanding of oxidation/reduction reactions occurring in living systems has been achieved (Chaiswing and Oberley 2010). The theory describing such reactions is termed the redox theory of cellular function.

Each biological compartment contains a particular number of electrons stored in various cellular substances, characterizing thus the overall redox state of cells (Jomova and Valko 2011). Under normal physiological conditions, similarly to regulation of intracellular pH, the redox state of a biological system is tightly controlled and is kept within a narrow range. Fluctuations in cellular redox state levels are typical for various cellular processes, such as the cell cycle control system. A more reducing cellular environment of the cell maintains proliferation, and a slight shift toward an oxidizing environment initiates cell differentiation (Matsuzawa and Ichijo 2005). A highly oxidizing environment in the cell is typical for apoptosis and necrosis.

Under pathological conditions, the redox state can be shifted to lower or higher values. An approximately a 30-mV change in the redox state triggers a tenfold change in the ratio between reductant and oxidant species (Schafer and Buettner 2001). Redox buffering is the tendency of a biological compartment to maintain redox stability, conceptually similar to pH buffering (Buettner et al. 2012). The intracellular "redox buffer" mechanism is substantiated by the antioxidant network of which a primary role is played by glutathione (GSH) and thioredoxin (TRX) (Circu and Aw 2010). Other important antioxidants involved in redox regulation are vitamin C, vitamin E, carotenoids, flavonoids, lipoic acid, and other species. In addition, antioxidant enzymes represent a key group of biomolecules acting in the antioxidant network within the cells. This chapter reports on the roles of both small molecular weight antioxidants and antioxidant enzymes in maintaining the cellular redox balance.

11.2 SOURCES OF FREE RADICALS

11.2.1 REACTIVE OXYGEN SPECIES

Molecular oxygen (O_2, dioxygen) is itself a biradical. The addition of one electron to dioxygen forms the superoxide anion radical $\left(O_2^{\cdot-}\right)$. The superoxide radical is considered the "primary" reactive oxygen species (ROS) and can further interact with other molecules to generate "secondary" ROS, either directly or prevalently through enzyme- or metal-catalyzed processes (Halliwell and Gutteridge 2007).

The production of a superoxide occurs mostly within the mitochondria of a cell. Superoxide is produced from both complexes I and III of the electron transport chain (Brand et al. 2004). Recently, it has been demonstrated that a complex I-dependent superoxide is exclusively released into the matrix and that no detectable levels escape from intact mitochondria (Muller et al. 2004). This finding fits well with the proposed site of an electron leak at complex I, namely, the iron–sulfur clusters of the (matrix-protruding) hydrophilic arm. In addition, experiments on complex III show a direct extramitochondrial release of superoxide, but measurements of hydrogen peroxide production revealed that this could only account for ~50% of the total electron leak, even in mitochondria lacking Cu,Zn-SOD. It has been proposed that the remaining ~50% of the electron leak must be a result of the superoxide released to the matrix.

Nicotine adenine dinucleotide phosphate (NAD(P)H) oxidase is best characterized in neutrophils, where its production of $O_2^{\cdot-}$ generates the respiratory burst necessary for bacterial destruction (Bedard and Krause 2007). The enzyme complex consists of two membrane-bound components, gp91[phox] and p22[phox], which comprise cytochrome b558, the enzymatic center of the complex. After activation, cytosolic components, involving p47phox, p67phox, p40phox, and the small G coupled proteins, Rac and Rap1A, translocate to the membrane to form the active enzyme complex. The nonphagocytic NAD(P)H oxidases produce superoxides at a fraction (1–10%) of the levels produced in neutrophils and are thought to function in intracellular signaling pathways (see also below).

The hydroxyl radical, ·OH, possesses a high reactivity, making it a very dangerous radical with a very short *in vivo* half-life of approximately 10^{-9} s (Chu and Anastasio 1995). When produced *in vivo*, ·OH reacts close to its site of formation with all biomolecules. The *in vivo* formation of hydroxyl radicals is supposed to occur via Fenton reactions. Under stress conditions, the released Fe^{2+} by superoxide, demonstrated for the [4Fe–4S] cluster-containing enzymes of the dehydratase–lyase family (Liochev and Fridovich 1994), can, in turn, participate in the Fenton reaction, generating highly reactive hydroxyl radicals ($Fe^{2+} + H_2O_2 \rightarrow Fe^{3+} + \cdot OH + OH^-$). *In vivo* production of hydroxyl radicals according to the Fenton reaction occurs when M^{n+} is iron, copper, chromium, or cobalt. However, recently reported results have shown that the upper limit of free copper was less than a single atom per cell (Rae et al. 1999). This finding raises serious concerns about the *in vivo* role of copper in Fenton-like generation of hydroxyl radicals. Although Fenton chemistry is known to occur *in vitro*, its significance under physiological conditions is not clear. The main reason for this is the negligible amounts of free catalytically active iron because of its effective sequestration by the various metal-binding proteins (Kakhlon and Cabantchik 2002). However, organisms overloaded by iron (as in the conditions of hemochromatosis, β-thalassemia, hemodialysis) contain higher amounts of free available iron, and this can have deleterious effects. Free iron is transported into an intermediate, labile iron pool (LIP), which represents a steady-state exchangeable and readily chelatable iron compartment (Kakhlon and Cabantchik 2002).

Additional reactive radicals derived from oxygen that can be formed in living systems are peroxyl radicals (ROO·). It has been demonstrated that the hydroperoxyl radical initiates fatty acid peroxidation by two parallel pathways: fatty acid hydroperoxide (LOOH)-independent and LOOH-dependent (Aikens and Dix 1991). The LOOH-dependent pathway of $HO_2^{\cdot}$-initiated fatty acid peroxidation may be relevant to mechanisms of lipid peroxidation initiation *in vivo*.

11.2.2 Reactive Nitrogen Species

Nitric oxide (NO·) is a reactive radical containing one unpaired electron. It acts as an important oxidative biological signaling molecule in a variety of physiological processes, including neurotransmission, regulation of blood pressure, smooth muscle relaxation, and immune and defense regulation (Bergendi et al. 1999). Nitric oxide is generated in biological tissues by nitric oxide synthases (NOSs), which metabolize arginine to citrulline with the formation of nitric oxide via a five-electron oxidative reaction (Ghafourifar and Cadenas 2005). NO· has a short half-life of only a few seconds in an aqueous environment. It has a greater stability in a deoxygenated environment (half-life >15 s). Because of its good solubility in both aqueous and lipid media, it effectively diffuses through the biological membranes (Chiueh 1999). NO· has effects on neuronal transmission as well as on synaptic plasticity in the central nervous system. In the extracellular space, nitric oxide reacts with oxygen and water to form nitrate and nitrite anions. Nitric oxide reacts with transition metal ions; iron reacts in the active site of the enzyme soluble guanylyl cyclase (sGC),

$$Fe^{2+}\{sGC\} + NO^{\bullet} \rightarrow Fe^{2+}\{sGC\} - NO \qquad (11.1)$$

stimulating it to produce the intracellular cyclic Guanosine Mono Phosphate (cGMP), which, in turn, enhances the release of neurotransmitters resulting in smooth muscle relaxation and vasodilation. The resulting complex formed is $\{Fe^{2+} - NO^{\bullet}\}$. However, the ferric complex with nitric oxide $\{Fe^{3+} - NO^{\bullet}\}$ is also commonly seen.

Overproduction of reactive nitrogen species is termed nitrosative stress (Klatt and Lamas 2000). This may occur when the generation of ROS in a system exceeds the system's ability to neutralize and eliminate them. Nitrosative stress may lead to nitrosylation reactions that can alter the structure of proteins and so inhibit their normal function.

$NO^{\bullet}$ toxicity is most commonly linked with its ability to combine with the superoxide radical to form peroxynitrite ($ONOO^-$), an oxidizing agent that can cause DNA damage and oxidation of lipids (Valko et al. 2006):

$$NO^{\bullet} + O_2^{\bullet-} \rightarrow ONOO^- \qquad k = 7.0 \times 10^9 M^{-1} s^{-1} \qquad (11.2)$$

In the mitochondria, $ONOO^-$ acts on the respiratory chain (I–IV) complex and manganese superoxide dismutase (Mn-SOD) to generate superoxide anions and hydrogen peroxide (H_2O_2), respectively.

11.3 ANTIOXIDANT ENZYMES

11.3.1 SUPEROXIDE DISMUTASE

Superoxide dismutase (SOD, EC 1.15.1.1) was isolated in 1939; however, its antioxidant activity was proved 30 years later in 1969 by McCord and Fridovich (1969). SOD is one of the most effective intracellular enzymatic antioxidants that catalyze the dismutation of $O_2^{\bullet-}$ to O_2 and to the less-reactive species H_2O_2 according to the following reaction:

$$2O_2^{\bullet-} + 2H^+ \xrightarrow{\text{SOD}} H_2O_2 + O_2 \qquad (11.3)$$

SOD converts a superoxide anion radical with high reaction rates at the metal active site via a ping-pong-type mechanism (Mates et al. 1999). Under physiological pH, the rate constant for uncatalyzed dismutation is $1.5 \times 10^5 M^{-1} s^{-1}$ (Bielski et al. 1985). The catalyzed reaction depletes the superoxide anion with a much more effective reaction rate of $2.5 \times 10^9 M^{-1} s^{-1}$ (Liochev and Fridovich 2003).

There are several isoforms of SOD, for example, cytosolic Cu,Zn-SOD, mitochondrial Mn-SOD, and extracellular SOD (EC-SOD) (Landis and Tower 2005). In humans, there are only three isoforms of SOD, namely, Cu,Zn-SOD, Mn-SOD, and

EC-SOD. Recently, in streptomyces and cyanobacteria, a distinct class of SOD that contains nickel at the active site (Ni-SOD) was discovered (Barondeau et al. 2004).

Cu,Zn-SOD (molecular weight of about 32 kDa) is composed of two identical subunits (Mates et al. 1999). Each subunit contains a binuclear metal cluster formed by copper and zinc ions. While the copper ion plays an important role in catalytic function, the zinc is required only for the structural stability of this SOD isoform. The activity of this SOD isoform is relatively independent of pH in the range of 5–9.5.

Mitochondrial Mn-SOD is a homotetramer (96 kDa) containing one manganese atom per subunit (Mates et al. 1999). This enzyme oscillates between Mn(III) and Mn(II) during the two-step dismutation of superoxide. Mn-SOD has been documented to be one of the most effective antioxidant enzymes possessing antitumor activity. Overexpressed Mn-SOD exhibited retardation of tumor growth in several cell lines (Valko et al. 2006). However, further work is necessary to clarify Mn-SOD as a tumor-suppressor protein.

In some tumors, decreased levels of various transition metal ions have been noted. In agreement with this is the observation that some tumors exhibited suppressed activity of Mn-SOD. For certain tumors, total SOD activity (Cu,Zn-SOD and Mn-SOD) has been found to be reduced. However, there exist examples of studies that confirmed significantly increased expression of Mn-SOD in some tumors (Behrend et al. 2003). This was observed in gastrointestinal cancers in advanced stages of progression with a metastatic potential. Thus, an excessively increased level of Mn-SOD, on the one hand, suppresses cell growth; however, on the other hand, it enhances the metastatic potential of cancer cells.

An interesting correlation exists between Mn-SOD and the enzymes of the zinc-dependent matrix metalloproteinase (MMP) family (Jiang 2002). MMPs are known to play a key role in tumor invasion. Increased activity of Mn-SOD results in elevated levels of hydrogen peroxide, which, in turn, leads to activation redox sensitive transcription factors, such as AP-1 and nuclear factor-kappa B (NF-κB). The activation of MMPs occurs via activation of both AP-1 and NF-κB. Thus, the imbalance between the formation of superoxide radicals and removal of hydrogen peroxide activates overexpression of Mn-SOD, which triggers the metastatic potential of cancer cells. The exact role of Mn-SOD as an inducer of MMPs in the process of metastasis has yet to be proved.

Extracellular SOD is a tetrameric protein containing copper and zinc. This enzyme has been shown to be involved in the modulation of inflammatory response. Inflammatory cytokines, such as IFN-gamma and IL-4, are known to upregulate expression of EC-SOD. Conversely, EC-SOD is downregulated by TNF-alpha (Stralin and Marklund 2000).

11.3.2 CATALASE

Catalase (EC 1.11.1.6) is a heme-containing redox-active enzyme present in nearly all living systems requiring oxygen. It is a tetramer containing four porphyrin heme groups (Nicholls 2012). The exact mechanism of decomposition of hydrogen peroxide by catalase is not currently known; however, the reaction is believed to proceed in two steps during which the cycling of iron between oxidation states +4 and +3 occur. The enzyme very effectively accelerates the decomposition of hydrogen peroxide to water and molecular oxygen:

$$2H_2O_2 \xrightarrow{\text{catalase}} 2H_2O + O_2 \qquad (11.4)$$

Perturbed levels of catalase are tightly linked with the various disease states of an organism. Decreased activity of catalase has been found in a variety of tumors.

11.3.3 GLUTATHIONE PEROXIDASES

The main role of glutathione peroxidases (GPxs, EC 1.11.1.9) as antioxidant enzymes is to protect cells against oxidative damage. GPxs are a family of enzymes that catalyze the reduction of hydrogen peroxide to water and organic hydroperoxides to alcohols (Lubos et al. 2011). In humans, we find four selenocysteine-containing GPxs that differ in their subcellular localization, tissue distribution, and peroxide substrate preference.

Glutathione peroxidase 1 (GPx1) is found in many tissues and cells of various organs. It is a cytosolic enzyme with a preference for hydrogen peroxide but can also reduce organic hydroperoxides and free lipid hydroperoxides. GPx2 is highly abundant in the cells of the gastrointestinal tract but also in lung cells (Singh et al. 2006). It has been proposed that GPx2 at least partially compensates for the loss of GPx1 (Florian et al. 2010), which may indicate a similar substrate range for both GPx1 and GPx2. GPx3 is a secreted form, present in plasma. Similarly to GPx1, GPx3 reduces hydrogen peroxide very efficiently. GPx4 is capable of efficiently reducing hydrogen peroxide and small organic hydroperoxides in cell membranes and intact liposomes.

The antioxidant activity of GPxs is based on the elimination of peroxides as potential substrates for the Fenton reaction. GPxs act in conjunction with the tripeptide GSH, which is present in cells in high concentrations. The catalytic activity of GPx, which accelerates decomposition of peroxides to water (or alcohol) while simultaneously oxidizing GSH, can be described according to the following reactions:

$$2GSH + H_2O_2 \xrightarrow{\text{GPx}} GSSG + 2H_2O \qquad (11.5)$$

$$2GSH + ROOH \xrightarrow{\text{GPx}} GSSG + ROH + H_2O \qquad (11.6)$$

GPx competes with catalase for H_2O_2 as a substrate and is the major source of protection against low levels of oxidative stress.

11.4 NONENZYMATIC ANTIOXIDANTS

11.4.1 ASCORBIC ACID

Ascorbic acid (vitamin C), also known as L-ascorbic acid, is one of the most important naturally occurring, low molecular weight antioxidants that work in aqueous environments of living systems (Buettner and Schafer 2000). Vitamin C is found in high abundance in many fresh fruits, such as lemons, limes, oranges, grapefruit, tomatoes, potatoes, cabbages, and green peppers.

The body's pool of vitamin C can be exhausted within 1 to 3 months. Severe deficiency in vitamin C in humans results in scurvy, which is characterized by hemorrhages and abnormal bone and dentine formation.

The structure of ascorbic acid contains two hydroxyl groups and, therefore, is a diacid (AscH$_2$). In the course of redox reactions, ascorbate can donate either one or two electrons. At physiological pH, typically around 7, more than 99% of ascorbate is in the monoanion form, AscH$^-$ (carbon-3 hydroxyl pKa = 4.2) (May 1999). Loss of the first electron results in the formation of the resonance stabilized tricarbonyl ascorbate free radical (AscH$^•$), which has a pK = –0.86, and therefore, it is not protonated and is present in the form of the ascorbyl radical anion, Asc$^{•-}$. Thus, the product of the reaction of ascorbate monoanion (AscH$^-$) with ROS is the ascorbyl radical (Asc$^{•-}$) (Figure 11.1). Asc$^{•-}$ has low reactivity and is considered to be a terminal antioxidant. The level of this poorly reactive radical in biological systems is a good measure of the degree of oxidative stress in biological systems (Kasparova et al. 2005). Mild oxidants, such as ethylenediaminetetraacetic acid (EDTA), can remove a second electron and convert the Asc$^{•-}$ to dehydroascorbic acid (DHA) (Gropper et al. 2009).

Vitamin C acts predominantly as an antioxidant and protects biological systems against oxidation (Retsky et al. 1999). While a reasonable protective effect of vitamin C has been reported in lung and colorectal cancers (Knekt et al. 1991), the general benefit of a high intake of vitamin C has never been unambiguously proved. A positive effect of increased intake of vitamin C in high-risk populations may contribute to the suppressed risk of gastric metaplasia or chronic gastritis, both precancerous lesions (You et al. 2000). The protective effect of vitamin C intake in

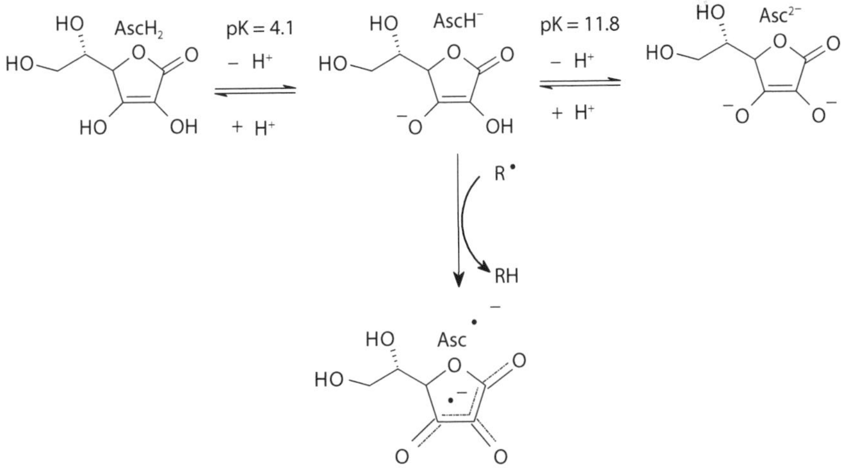

FIGURE 11.1 Various forms of ascorbic acid (vitamin C) and its reaction with radicals (R$^•$).

lowering the incidence of stomach cancer is most probably related to the suppressed formation of N-nitroso compounds by interrupting the reaction between nitrites and amine groups.

Interestingly, vitamin C may act as a prooxidant by reducing certain transition metal ions such as cupric ions (Cu^{2+}) to cuprous ions (Cu^+) and ferric ions (Fe^{3+}) to ferrous (Fe^{2+}) ions, while itself becoming oxidized to an ascorbate radical:

$$AscH^- + Fe^{3+}/Cu^{2+} \rightarrow Asc^{\bullet-} + Fe^{2+}/Cu^+ \tag{11.7}$$

The reduced forms of transition metal ions, such as Fe^{2+} and Cu^+, may catalyze the decomposition of hydrogen peroxide according to the Fenton reaction

$$Fe^{2+}/Cu^+ + H_2O_2 \rightarrow Fe^{3+}/Cu^{2+} + OH^{\bullet} + OH^- \tag{11.8}$$

leading to the formation of damaging hydroxyl radicals.

In several *in vitro* studies, the prooxidant properties of ascorbate were attributed to the release of metal ions from damaged cells (Kang et al. 1998). It has also been reported that vitamin C induces lipid hydroperoxide decomposition to the various reactive electrophiles involving, for example, 4,5-epoxy-2(E)-decenal, a precursor of a highly mutagenic etheno-2'-deoxyadenosine lesion found in human DNA (Lee et al. 2001).

With respect to the potential prooxidant effect of vitamin C, it was concluded that ascorbate may be able to promote metal ion-dependent hydroxyl radical formation in biological fluids but only under unphysiological/*in vitro* conditions (Smith et al. 1997). In addition, it should be noted that clinical trials should be taken with caution as to their choice of biomarkers and methodology to rule out any oxidation effects (Podmore et al. 1998).

Vitamin C has been shown to activate various signaling pathways, including the AP-1 complex. In several studies, vitamin C has been documented to protect against cell death triggered by various stimuli. Antiapoptotic activity of vitamin C has been linked with the modulation of the immune system.

The primary small molecular weight antioxidant partners of vitamin C are vitamin E and the carotenoids. Vitamin C cooperates with vitamin E to regenerate α-tocopherol from α-tocopherol radicals in membranes and lipoproteins (Kojo 2004).

11.4.2   VITAMIN E

Vitamin E is a lipid-soluble membrane-bound antioxidant employed by the cell. Vitamin E is abundant in vegetable oils and derivative foods, such as margarine. Leafy green vegetables are also rich in vitamin E. Generally, the protective effect of vitamin E is a result of the inhibition of free radical formation and activation of endonucleases (Burton and Ingold 1989). Vitamin E deficiency is a relatively rare condition. In humans, it is most frequently linked with lipid malabsorption syndromes, which can occur with genetic or acquired diseases affecting the intestine, pancreas, or liver.

Vitamin E represents a family of eight different forms, α-tocopherol being the most active form. The main antioxidant function of vitamin E is protection against lipid peroxidation (Pryor 2000). Investigations suggest that α-tocopherol and ascorbic acid function together in a cyclic type of process. In the course of the chemical reaction, α-tocopherol is converted to an α-tocopheryl radical by the donation of a labile hydrogen to a lipid or lipid peroxyl radical. The original α-tocopherol can be regenerated from the α-tocopheryl radical by vitamin C (Kojo 2004).

Vitamin E deficiency promotes peroxidation of membrane lipids, resulting in altered membrane transport and decreased mitochondrial energy production. Deficiency in vitamin E in humans (a relatively rare condition, see above) leads to degeneration of the central nervous system and peripheral nerves and impaired fertility in both sexes. In addition, enhanced destruction of red blood cells has been seen as a result of vitamin E deficiency.

Several clinical trials reported the positive effects of the intake of vitamin E supplements. The intake of 200 IU/day of vitamin E suppressed the incidence of colorectal cancer by triggered apoptosis of cancer cells (White et al. 1997). Conversely, another study reported negative results for vitamin E in combination with vitamin C and beta-carotene to prevent colorectal cancer adenoma (Greenberg et al. 1994). Because vitamin C is known to regenerate vitamin E, it has been proposed that the addition of vitamin E hampers the antioxidant effect of vitamin C against the deleterious effects of ROS (Dreher and Junod 1996).

Interestingly, a recent study conducted in the United States reported that daily intake of vitamin E (400 IU or more) can increase the risk of death and should be avoided (Miller et al. 2005). However, half of that dose, corresponding to 200 mg a day appears to be safe.

11.4.3 GLUTATHIONE

GSH is found in mammalian cells in concentrations up to 12–13 mM and represents one of the most important intracellular antioxidant systems (Schafer and Buettner 2001). From a chemical point of view, GSH is the tripeptide consisting of glutamic acid, cysteine, and glycine. GSH has important functions as a cellular antioxidant in detoxifying various xenobiotics. In particular, it is very effective in cellular defense against ROS. GSH directly reacts with a variety of free radicals, and it also acts as an electron donor in the reduction of peroxides catalyzed by the GPx (see above) (Dringen 2000).

The radical reactions of GSH with the radical $R^{\bullet}$ can be described as

$$GSH + R^{\bullet} \rightarrow GS^{\bullet} + RH \tag{11.9}$$

Thiyl radicals ($GS^{\bullet}$) formed may dimerize to form the nonradical product, oxidized glutathione (GSSG):

$$GS^{\bullet} + GS^{\bullet} \rightarrow GSSG \tag{11.10}$$

Oxidized glutathione GSSG is accumulated inside the cells, and the ratio of GSH/GSSG is a good measure of the oxidative stress of an organism (Hwang et al. 1992).

In the course of the detoxification reactions of free radicals, GSH participates in two types of reactions:

(1) Nonenzymatic reactions of GSH with ROS, such as superoxide anion radicals and hydroxyl radicals as well as RNS involving nitric oxide.
(2) In addition, GSH acts as an electron donor for the reduction of peroxides in the GPx reaction.

The final product of the oxidation of GSH is glutathione disulfide (GSSG). GSH is regenerated from GSSG by the reaction catalyzed by glutathione reductase (GR).

The main protective roles of GSH against oxidative stress can be summarized as follows:

(1) GSH is a cofactor of several detoxifying enzymes against oxidative stress, for example, glutathione peroxidase (GPx) (Figure 11.2).
(2) GSH is involved in amino acid transport through the plasma membrane.
(3) Direct ROS-scavenging properties of GSH.
(4) GSH regenerates the most important antioxidants, vitamins C and E, back to their active forms. Glutathione can reduce the tocopherol radical of vitamin E directly or indirectly via reduction of semidehydroascorbate to ascorbate.

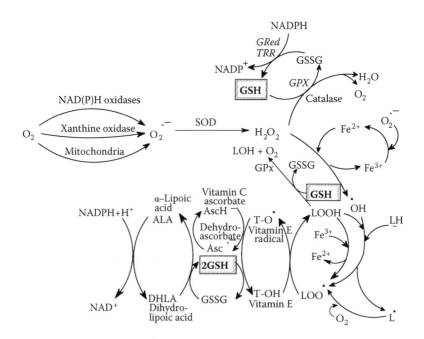

FIGURE 11.2   Role of GSH and other antioxidants in management of oxidative stress.

The presence of cellular oxidants results in rapid modification of protein sulfhydryls (Protein-SH): Two-electron oxidation yields sulfenic acids (Protein-SOH), and one-electron oxidation yields thiyl radicals (Protein-S$^\bullet$) (Ji et al. 1999). The main role of GSH in the nucleus is to protect critical protein sulfhydryls—mainly those necessary for DNA repair and expression. The oxidized products can be restored back with GSH to form glutathiolated protein (Protein-SSG). Protein-SSG is then reduced in the next step by the glutathione reductase cycle to restore protein sulfhydryls (Protein-SH). In the absence of GSH, the process of protein oxidation may proceed further, leading to the formation of irreversibly oxidized products, such as sulfinic (Protein-SO$_2$H) and sulfonic (Protein-SO$_3$H) acids.

Interesting is the behavior of GSH in the brain. The brain cells are able to release glutathione, and the level of extracellular GSH in the brain has been monitored by microdialysis. The release of GSH into extracellular space occurs predominantly during ischemia (Orwar et al. 1994); however, the origin and the detailed mechanism are under investigation. Release of GSH can be triggered by depolarization, and it was concluded that neurons are the glutathione-releasing cell type in the brain.

11.4.4 Lipoic Acid

α-Lipoic acid (ALA) is a disulfide derivative of octanoic acid. It is a natural compound also referred to as thiothic acid found in almost all foods but more abundantly in the kidneys, heart, liver, spinach, broccoli, and yeast extract. ALA is both water- and fat-soluble and is readily absorbed from the diet. In many tissues, ALA rapidly converts to its reduced dithiol form, dihydrolipoic acid (DHLA) (Smith et al. 2004). The antioxidant properties of ALA and DHLA involve (1) quenching of ROS, (2) regeneration of antioxidants (vitamins C and E and GSH), (3) redox metal chelation, and (4) repair of oxidized proteins. The redox potential of the DHLA/ALA couple is very low, approximately –320 mV, making this couple a very effective antioxidant system.

The positive effect of lipoic acid has been associated with cardiovascular disease, ischemia-reperfusion injury, and neurodegenerative disorders (Bustamante et al. 1998). Lipoic acid is a very effective metal chelator and has been used in the treatment of heavy metal poisoning.

11.4.5 Carotenoids

Carotenoids (Car) are found in microorganisms and many plant foods, such as carrots, tomatoes, sweet potatoes, spinach, kale, collard greens, and others. Several epidemiological studies have shown that carotenoids may prevent or inhibit various disease states of an organism, including cancer, cardiovascular disease, age-related muscular degeneration, and other diseases. The most common carotenoids occurring in the diet are alpha-carotene, beta-carotene, beta-cryptoxanthin, lutein, zeaxanthin, and lycopene.

The anticancer and health-protective properties of carotenoids may be related to their antioxidant activity substantiated by the ability of the conjugated double-bonded structure to delocalize unpaired electrons (Mortensen et al. 2001). Carotenoids effectively react with a variety of free radicals, including peroxyl radicals and hydroxyl radicals as well as superoxide anion radicals. In addition, carotenoids are effective quenchers of singlet oxygen, providing humans with protection against skin damage from sunlight. Carotenoids, when present at sufficient concentrations, have been shown to be effective in protecting lipids from peroxidative damage.

There are three major mechanisms proposed for the reaction of free radicals (ROO•, R•) with carotenoids: (1) radical addition, (2) hydrogen abstraction from the carotenoid, and (3) electron transfer reaction (El-Agamey et al. 2004). It has been proposed that beta-carotene may scavenge peroxyl radicals by two different mechanisms, namely, by adduct formation or by hydrogen atom abstraction. An electron transfer reaction between beta-carotene and peroxyl radicals has been proposed to be less probable.

The first communication reporting that beta-carotene may participate in peroxidation of lipids as a prooxidant was published by Burton and Ingold (1984). This proposal was later supported by an epidemiological trial Alpha-Tocopherol/Beta-Carotene (ATBC) carried out in Finland by the US National Cancer Institute. This trial has very surprisingly shown that supplementation of smokers with β-carotene for 5 to 8 years led to an 18% increase in the incidence of lung cancer, which, in turn, contributed to an 8% excess in total mortality. The observed findings were attributed to the prooxidant behavior of β-carotene. The switch of β-carotene from antioxidant to prooxidant has been explained by the high partial pressure of oxygen in lungs. Another important factor is the carotenoid concentration.

At a higher pressure of oxygen, a carotenoid radical, Car•, can react with molecular oxygen to generate a carotenoid-peroxyl radical, Car-OO• (Jomova et al. 2009):

$$Car• + O_2 \rightarrow Car\text{-}OO• \qquad (11.11)$$

The Car-OO• can act as a prooxidant by promoting oxidation of unsaturated lipid (RH):

$$Car\text{-}OO• + RH \rightarrow Car\text{-}OOH + R• \qquad (11.12)$$

Some carotenoids (in particular, β-carotene) exhibit antioxidant properties at low oxygen partial pressures (below 150 torr). Conversely, under increased pressure of oxygen, they may become prooxidants. The carotenoid concentration also influences their antioxidant or prooxidant properties in a similar manner.

Carotenoids are known to regulate transcription factors (Niles 2004). Cells treated with β-carotene and exposed to oxidative stress stimuli exhibited suppressed activation of NF-κB and production of interleukin-6 (IL-6) and TNF-alpha inflammatory cytokines. This suggests a protective effect of β-carotene.

Beta-carotene supplementation has been documented to affect the process of apoptosis in healthy cells. Oxidative stress-induced stimuli followed by supplementation of β-carotene triggered downregulation of proapoptotic BAX protein, while the antiapoptotic protein Bcl-2 was upregulated (McEligot 2005). Lycopene has also been shown to regulate transcription factors and has been documented to inhibit cell cycle progression in breast, lung, and prostate cell lines.

11.4.6 FLAVONOIDS

Flavonoids represent a wide range of secondary plant phenolics containing the flavan nucleus. These compounds are commonly found in the leaves, seeds, bark, and flowers and offer plants protection against radiation, herbivores, and pathogens. The anthocyanin copigments in flowers are responsible for the red and blue colors of wines, berries, and vegetables. The molecular structure of flavonoids consists of two aromatic carbon rings and benzopyran (A and C rings) and benzene (B ring) (Rice-Evans et al. 1996) (Figure 11.3). Flavonoids can be classified into several subgroups on the basis of degree of the oxidation of the C ring, the hydroxylation pattern of the ring structure, and the substitution of the three-position. Flavonoids can be classified into (1) flavonols (quercetin), (2) flavones (luteolin), (3) isoflavones (genistein), (4) flavanones (naringenin), (5) flavanols (epigallocatechin), and (6) anthocyanidins (cyaniding) (Heim et al. 2002).

Flavonoids are benzo-γ-pyrone derivatives, and their chemical structure consists of phenolic and pyrane rings. They are classified according to differences in substitutions and conjugations between the A and B rings. The main differences are in the attachment of hydroxyl groups, methoxy groups, and glycosidic groups.

The protective effects of flavonoids in biological systems are substantiated by their antioxidant capacity to terminate free radicals, chelate redox-active metal, activate various antioxidant enzymes, and inhibit oxidases (Cos et al. 1998). The most important structural feature affecting antioxidant properties of flavonoids is the arrangement of substituents (Rice-Evans 2001). The configuration and total number of hydroxyl groups influence the total antioxidant activity of flavonoids. Generally, free radical-scavenging activity is primarily attributed to the reactivities of hydroxyl groups participating in the reactions of hydrogen abstraction:

$$\text{flavonoid–OH} + \text{R}^\bullet \rightarrow \text{flavonoid–O}^\bullet + \text{RH} \qquad (11.13)$$

The arrangement of hydroxyl groups located on the B ring most significantly affects the ROS scavenging properties of flavonoids. Hydroxyl groups on the B ring donate hydrogen atoms (electrons) to various free radicals, such as hydroxyl radicals, peroxyl

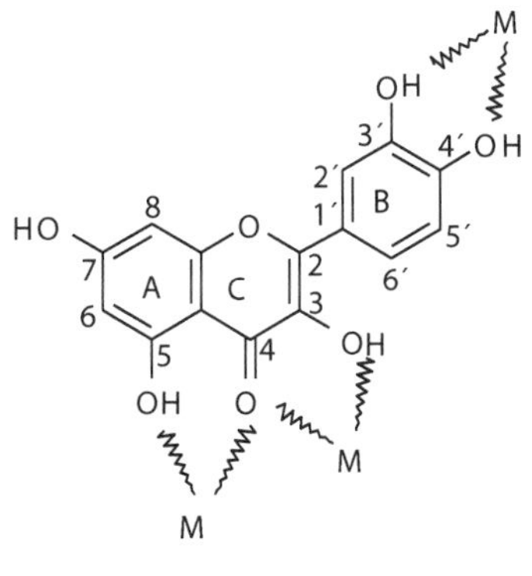

FIGURE 11.3 Structure of flavonoid quercetin (M = coordinated metal ion).

radicals, and peroxynitrite, thus stabilizing them and leaving behind a relatively stable flavonoid radical. A 3'4'-catechol structure in the B ring promotes inhibition of peroxidation of lipids (Cao et al. 1997). It has been documented that the A-ring substitution does not correlate with the antioxidant activity of flavonoids. Other important structural features of flavonoids include 2,3 unsaturation in conjugation with a 4-oxo function in the C ring. Functional groups may participate in the binding of redox-active transition metal ions, such as iron and copper (Rice-Evans et al. 1996).

As previously described, flavonoids are chemically able to prevent oxidation, and their intake has been linked with suppressed oxidative stress markers in animals and humans. However, when assessing the antioxidant activity of flavonoids, one should bear in mind metabolic modifications of flavonoids, mainly structural modifications in the B ring, which plays a key role in the antioxidant nature of flavonoids. Other crucial structural features important for the antioxidant behavior of flavonoids is the presence of 2,3 unsaturation in conjugation with a 4-oxo function in the C ring. Metabolized flavonoids circulating in human plasma, for example, flavonoid adducts with GSH, have a much-reduced ability to donate hydrogen (electrons), and their overall antioxidant efficiency is reduced with respect to the parent forms.

Another important aspect when discussing antioxidant properties of flavonoids is their *in vivo* concentration. It has been determined that the concentrations of flavonoids in plasma, or in various organs, including the brain (nanomolar concentrations), are lower than those observed for small antioxidants, such as vitamins C and E (present in micromolar concentrations). Thus, such low concentrations of flavonoids cannot be attributed to highly beneficial action under *in vivo* conditions through competing antioxidants, such as vitamin C present at higher concentrations (Macready et al. 2009).

A vast majority of papers dealing with flavonoids have focused on their *in vivo* antioxidant properties. However, recent studies confirmed their important role as molecules modulating cell-signaling pathways, such as the mitogen-activated, protein-kinase pathway (MAPK) and the phosphoinositide 3-kinase (PI3 kinase/ Akt) signaling cascade (Williams et al. 2004). Flavonoids have also been shown to interfere with transcription factors, such as NF-κB. NF-κB is important in signal transduction through protein-kinase inhibition (Goyarzu et al. 2004). Isoflavones are a group of flavonoids probably capable of mimicking estrogen and affecting brain function by mediating estrogen receptor processes and inhibiting tyrosine kinase (Lee et al. 2005). Flavonoids are known to affect endothelial function by increasing the formation of nitric oxide, which is a signaling molecule leading to arterial vessel relaxation and the control of blood pressure. Enhanced formation of nitric oxide has been found to inhibit nitric oxide synthase (iNOS) and cyclooxygenase (COX-2), reactive C protein, and the atheromatous plaque adhesion molecules known to be involved in inflammation (Gonzáles-Gallego 2007; see also Chapter 8).

11.5   CONCLUSIONS

ROS are known to participate in the physiology of aerobic organisms and the normal regulation of cell signaling, including the signals triggering antioxidant mechanisms. Conversely, uncontrolled ROS formation leads to oxidation of various cell components involving DNA, proteins, and membrane lipids. The cellular and tissue damage determines the acute pathology of many diseases and various pathological states. The defense against oxidative damage is substantiated by the action of antioxidant enzymes and small molecular weight antioxidants.

Many researchers are trying to understand the role of Mn-SOD for prospective antioxidant therapy in the treatment of various cancers both *in vitro* and *in vivo*. Enhanced expression of Mn-SOD and Cu,Zn-SOD, both superoxide anion radical-scavenging enzymes, has been tested in therapeutic strategies of radioprotection. Investigations suggest that the increase in SOD expression reduced the level of apoptosis, providing the foundation for radioprotective gene therapies in the treatment of cancer.

Small molecular weight antioxidants provide protection against the deleterious action of free radicals. Antioxidants can protect against the redox-metal-catalyzed formation of free radicals by chelating redox-active metal ions and preventing the reaction with molecular oxygen or peroxides. Another aspect of antioxidant functioning is chelating redox-active metal ions and thus maintaining a redox state that makes them unable to reduce molecular oxygen. In addition, antioxidants are capable of direct trapping or terminating of any radicals formed. One of the most effective antioxidants is thiol compounds, especially GSH. GSH provide significant protection by maintaining the redox state of the cell within strict physiological limits. Uncontrolled formation of ROS and RNS results in oxidative or nitrosative stress, which, in turn, is linked with a number of diseases and results at least partly from declined antioxidant mechanisms. Thus, design of dual-functioning antioxidants possessing both metal-chelating and ROS/RNS-scavenging properties is awaited.

ACKNOWLEDGMENTS

This work was supported by Scientific Grant Agency (VEGA Projects #1/0856/11 and #1/0289/12) and Research and Development Agency of the Slovak Republic (Contract No. APVV-0202-10 and APVV-0339-10).

REFERENCES

Aikens, J. and T.A. Dix. 1991. Perhydroxyl radical (HOO•.) initiated lipid peroxidation: The role of fatty acid hydroperoxides. *J Biol Chem* 266: 15091–15098.

Barondeau, D.P., C.J. Kassmann, C.K. Bruns, J.A. Tainer and E.D. Getzoff. 2004. Nickel superoxide dismutase structure and mechanism. *Biochemistry* 43: 8038–8047.

Bedard, K. and K.H. Krause. 2007. The NOX family of ROS-generating NADPH oxidases: Physiology and pathophysiology. *Physiol Rev* 87: 245–313.

Behrend, L., G. Henderson and R.M. Zwacka. 2003. Reactive oxygen species in oncogenic transformation. *Biochem Soc Trans* 31: 1441–1444.

Bergendi, L., L. Benes, Z. Duracková and M. Ferencik. 1999. Chemistry, physiology and pathology of free radicals. *Life Sci* 65: 1865–1874.

Bielski, B.H.J., D.E. Cabelli, R.L. Arudi and A.B. Ross. 1985. Reactivity of HO_2/O_2^{-} radicals in aqueous solution. *J Phys Chem Ref Data* 14: 1041–1100.

Brand, M.D., C. Affourtit, T.C. Esteves, K. Green, A.J. Lambert, S. Miwa, J.L. Pakay and N. Parker. 2004. Mitochondrial superoxide: Production, biological effects, and activation of uncoupling proteins. *Free Radic Biol Med* 37: 755–767.

Buettner, G.R. and F.Q. Schafer. 2000. Free radicals, oxidants, and antioxidants. *Teratology* 62: 234.

Buettner, G.R., B.A. Wagner and V.G. Rodgers. 2012. Quantitative redox biology: An approach to understand the role of reactive species in defining the cellular redox environment. *Cell Biochem Biophys* DOI: 10.1007/s12013-011-9320-3.

Burton, G.W. and K.U. Ingold. 1984. Beta-carotene—An unusual type of lipid antioxidant. *Science* 224: 569–573.

Burton, G.W. and K.U. Ingold. 1989. Vitamin E as an *in vitro* and *in vivo* antioxidant. *Ann NY Acad Sci* 570: 7–22.

Bustamante, J., J.K. Lodge, L. Marcocci, H.J. Tritschler, L. Packer and B.H. Rihn. 1998. Alpha-lipoic acid in liver metabolism and disease. *Free Radic Biol Med* 24: 1023–1039.

Cao, G., E. Sofic and R.L. Prior. 1997. Antioxidant and prooxidant behavior of flavonoids structure-activity relationships. *Free Radic Biol Med* 22: 749–760.

Chaiswing, L. and T.D. Oberley. 2010. Extracellular/microenvironmental redox state. *Antiox Redox Signal* 13: 449–465.

Chiueh, C.C. 1999. Neuroprotective properties of nitric oxide. *Ann NY Acad Sci* 890: 301–311.

Chu, L. and C. Anastasio. 2005. Formation of hydroxyl radical from the photolysis of frozen hydrogen peroxide. *J Phys Chem A* 109: 6264–6271.

Circu, M.L. and T.Y. Aw. 2010. Reactive oxygen species, cellular redox systems, and apoptosis. *Free Radic Biol Med* 48: 749–762.

Cos, P., L. Ying, M. Calomme, J.P. Hu, K. Cimanga, B. Van Poel, L. Pieters, A.J. Vlietnck and D. Vanden Berghe. 1998. Structure-activity relationship and classification of flavonoids as inhibitors of xanthine oxidase and superoxide scavengers. *J Nat Prod* 61: 71–76.

Dreher, D. and A.F. Junod. 1996. Role of oxygen free radicals in cancer development. *Eur J Cancer* 32A: 30–38.

Dringen, R. 2000. Metabolism and functions of glutathione in brain. *Progr Neurobiol* 62: 649–671.

El-Agamey, A., G.M. Lowe, D.J. McGarvey, A. Mortensen, D.M. Phillip and T.G. Truscott. 2004. Carotenoid radical chemistry and antioxidant/pro-oxidant properties. *Arch Biochem Biophys* 430: 37–48.

Florian, S., S. Krehl, M. Loewinger, A. Kipp, A. Banning, S. Esworthy, F.F. Chu and R. Brigelius-Flohé. 2010. Loss of GPx2 increases apoptosis, mitosis, and GPx1 expression in the intestine of mice. *Free Radic Biol Med* 49: 1694–1702.

Ghafourifar, P. and E. Cadenas. 2005. Mitochondrial nitric oxide synthase. *Trends Pharmacol Sci* 26: 190–195.

González-Gallego, J., S. Sánchez-Campos and M.J. Tuñón. 2007. Anti-inflammatory properties of dietary flavonoids. *Nutr Hosp* 22: 287–293.

Goyarzu, P., D.H. Malin, F.C. Lau, G. Taglialatela, W.D. Moon, R. Jennings, E. Moy, D. Moy, S. Lippold, B. Shukitt-Hale and J.A. Joseph. 2004. Blueberry supplemented diet: Effects on object recognition memory and nuclear factor-kappa B levels in aged rats. *Nutr Neurosci* 7: 75–83.

Greenberg, E.R., J.A. Baron, T.D. Tosteson, D.H. Freeman, G.J. Beck and J.H. Bond. 1994. Clinical-trial of antioxidant vitamins to prevent colorectal adenoma. *N Engl J Med* 331: 141–147.

Gropper, S.S., J.L. Smith and J.L. Groff. 2009. *Advanced Nutrition and Human Metabolism*. 5th ed. Stamford, CT: Wadsworth/Cengage Learning.

Halliwell, B. and J.M.C. Gutteridge. 2007. *Free Radicals in Biology and Medicine*. Oxford: Oxford University Press.

Heim, K.E., A.R. Tagliaferro and D.J. Bobilya. 2002. Flavonoid antioxidants: Chemistry, metabolism and structure-activity relationships. *J Nutr Biochem* 13: 572–584.

Hwang, C., A.J. Sinskey and H.F. Lodish. 1992. Oxidized redox state of glutathione in the endoplasmic-reticulum. *Science* 257: 1496–1502.

Ji, Y.B., T.P.M. Akerboom, H. Sies and J.A. Thomas. 1999. S-nitrosylation and S-glutathiolation of protein sulfhydryls by S-nitroso glutathione. *Arch Biochem Biophys* 362: 67–78.

Jiang, Y.F. 2002. Complex roles of tissue inhibitors of metalloproteinases in cancer. *Oncogene* 21: 2245–2252.

Jomova, K., O. Kysel, J.C. Madden, H. Morris, S.J. Enoch, S. Budzak, A.J. Young, M.T.D. Cronin, M. Mazur and M. Valko. 2009. Electron transfer from all-trans beta-carotene to the t-butyl peroxyl radical at low oxygen pressure (an EPR spectroscopy and computational study). *Chem Phys Lett* 478: 266–270.

Jomova, K. and M. Valko. 2011. Thermodynamics of free radical reactions and the redox environment of a cell. In *Oxidative Stress: Diagnostics, Prevention, and Therapy,* eds. Andreescu, S. and M. Hepel, 71–82. ACS Symposium Series, American Chemical Society, Washington DC.

Kakhlon, O. and Z.I. Cabantchik. 2002. The labile iron pool: Characterization, measurement, and participation in cellular processes. *Free Radic Biol Med* 33: 1037–1046.

Kang, S.A., Y.J. Jang and H. Park. 1998. *In vivo* dual effects of vitamin C on paraquat-induced lung damage: Dependence on released metals from the damaged tissue. *Free Radic Res* 28: 93–107.

Kasparova, S., V. Brezova, M. Valko, J. Horecky, V. Mlynarik, T. Liptaj, O. Vancova, O. Ulicna and D. Dobrota. 2005. Study of the oxidative stress in a rat model of chronic brain hypoperfusion. *Neurochem Int* 46: 601–611.

Klatt, P. and S. Lamas. 2000. Regulation of protein function by S-glutathiolation in response to oxidative and nitrosative stress. *Eur J Biochem* 267: 4928–4944.

Knekt, P., R. Jarvinen, R. Seppanen, A. Rissanen, A. Aromaa, O.P. Heinonen, D. Albanes, M. Heinonen, E. Pukkala and L. Teppo. 1991. Dietary antioxidants and the risk of lung-cancer. *Am J Epidemiol* 134: 471–479.

Kojo, S. 2004. Vitamin C: Basic metabolism and its function as an index of oxidative stress. *Curr Med Chem* 11: 1041–1064.

Landis, G.N. and J. Tower. 2005. Superoxide dismutase evolution and life span regulation. *Mech Ageing Dev* 126: 365–379.

Lee, S.H., T. Oe and I.A. Blair. 2001. Vitamin C-induced decomposition of lipid hydroperoxides to endogenous genotoxins. *Science* 292: 2083–2086.

Lee, Y.B., H.J. Lee and H.S. Sohn. 2005. Soy isoflavones and cognitive function. *J Nutr Biochem* 16: 641–649.

Liochev, S.I. and I. Fridovich. 1994. The role of $O_2^{\cdot-}$ in the production of HO.: *In vitro* and *in vivo*. *Free Radic Biol Med* 16: 29–33.

Liochev, S.I. and Fridovich, I. 2003. Reversal of the superoxide dismutase reaction revisited. *Free Radic Biol Med* 34: 908–910.

Lubos, E., J. Loscalzo and D.E. Handy. 2011. Glutathione peroxidase-1 in health and disease: From molecular mechanisms to therapeutic opportunities. *Antioxid Redox Signal* 15: 1957–1997.

Macready, A.L., O.B. Kennedy, J.A. Ellis, C.M. Williams, J.P. Spencer and L.T. Butler. 2009. Flavonoids and cognitive function: A review of human randomized controlled trial studies and recommendations for future studies. *Genes Nutr* 4: 227–242.

Mates, J.M., C. Perez-Gomez and I.N. De Castro. 1999. Antioxidant enzymes and human diseases. *Clin Biochem* 32: 595–603.

Matsuzawa, A. and H. Ichijo. 2005. Stress-responsive protein kinases in redox-regulated apoptosis signaling. *Antiox Redox Signal* 7: 472–481.

May, J.M. 1999. Is ascorbic acid an antioxidant for the plasma membrane? *FASEB J* 13: 995–1006.

McCord, J.M. and I. Fridovich. 1969. Superoxide dismutase: An enzymic function for erythrocuprein (hemocuprein). *J Biol Chem* 244: 6049–6055.

McEligot, A.J., S. Yang and F.L. Meyskens, Jr. 2005. Redox regulation by intrinsic species and extrinsic nutrients in normal and cancer cells. *Ann Rev Nutr* 25: 261–295.

Miller, E.R., R. Pastor-Barriuso, D. Dalal, R.A. Riemersma, L.J. Appel and E. Guallar. 2005. Meta-analysis: High-dosage vitamin E supplementation may increase all-cause mortality. *Ann Intern Med* 142: 37–46.

Mortensen, L.H., T.G. Skibsted and G. Truscott. 2001. The interaction of dietary carotenoids with radical species. *Arch Biochem Biophys* 385: 13–19.

Muller, F.L., Y. Liu and H. Van Remmen. 2004. Complex III releases superoxide to both sides of the inner mitochondrial membrane. *J Biol Chem* 279: 49064–49073.

Nicholls, P. 2012. Classical catalase: Ancient and modern. *Arch Biochem Biophys* 525: 95–101.

Niles, R.N. 2004. Signaling pathways in retinoid chemoprevention and treatment of cancer. *Mutat Res Fund-Mol Mech Mutagen* 555: 81–96.

Orwar, O., X. Li, P. Andiné, C.M. Bergström, H. Hagberg, S. Folestad and M. Sandberg. 1994. Increased intra- and extracellular concentrations of gamma-glutamylglutamate and related dipeptides in the ischemic rat striatum: Involvement of glutamyl transpeptidase. *J Neurochem* 63: 1371–1376.

Podmore, I.D., H.R. Griffiths, K.E. Herbert, N. Mistry, P. Mistry and J. Lunec. 1998. Vitamin C exhibits pro-oxidant properties. *Nature* 392: 559.

Pryor, W.A. 2000. Vitamin E and heart disease: Basic science to clinical intervention trials. *Free Radic Biol Med* 28: 141–164.

Rae, T.D., P.J. Schmidt, R.A. Pufahl, V.C. Culotta and T.V. O'Halloran. 1999. Undetectable intracellular free copper: The requirement of a copper chaperone for superoxide dismutase. *Science* 284: 805–808.

Retsky, J.M., K. Chen, J. Zeind and B. Frei. 1999. Inhibition of copper induced LDL oxidation by Vitamin C is associated with decreased copper-binding to LDL and 2-oxo-histidine formation. *Free Radic Biol Med* 26: 90–98.

Rice-Evans, C.A. 2001. Flavonoid antioxidants. *Curr Med Chem* 8: 797–807.

Rice-Evans, C.A., N.J. Miller and G. Paganga. 1996. Structure-antioxidant activity relationships of flavonoids and phenolic acids. *Free Radic Biol Med* 20: 933–956.

Schafer, F.Q. and G.R. Buettner. 2001. Redox environment of the cell as viewed through the redox state of the glutathione disulfide/glutathione couple. *Free Radic Biol Med* 30: 1191–1212.

Singh, A., T. Rangasamy, R.K. Thimmulappa, H. Lee, W.O. Osburn, R. Brigelius-Flohé, T.W. Kensler, M. Yamamoto and S. Biswal. 2006. Glutathione peroxidase 2, the major cigarette smoke-inducible isoform of GPX in lungs, is regulated by Nrf2. *Am J Respir Cell Mol Biol* 35: 639–650.

Smith, A.R., S.V. Shenvi, M. Widlansky, J.H. Suh and T.M. Hagen. 2004. Lipoic acid as a potential therapy for chronic diseases associated with oxidative stress. *Curr Med Chem* 11: 1135–1146.

Smith, M.A., P.L.R. Harris, L.M. Sayre, J.S. Beckman and G. Perry. 1997. Widespread peroxynitrite-mediated damage in Alzheimer's disease. *J Neurosci* 17: 2653–2657.

Stralin, P. and S.L. Marklund. 2000. Multiple cytokines regulate the expression of extracellular superoxide dismutase in human vascular smooth muscle cells. *Atherosclerosis* 151: 433–441.

Valko, M., C.J. Rhodes, J. Moncol, M. Izakovic and M. Mazur. 2006. Free radicals, metals and antioxidants in oxidative stress-induced cancer. *Chem Biol Interact* 160: 1–40.

White, E., J.S. Shannon and R.E. Patterson. 1997. Relationship between vitamin and calcium supplement use and colon cancer. *Cancer Epidemiol Biomark Prev* 6: 769–774.

Williams, R.J., J.P. Spencer and C. Rice-Evans. 2004. Flavonoids: Antioxidants or signalling molecules? *Free Radic Biol Med* 36: 838–849.

You, W.C., L. Zhang, M.H. Gail, Y.S. Chang, W.D. Liu, J.L. Ma, J.Y. Li, M.L. Jin, Y.R. Hu, C.S. Yang, M.J. Blaser, P. Correa, W.J. Blot, J.F. Fraumeni, G.W. Xu. 2000. Gastric cancer: *Helicobacter pylori*, serum Vitamin C, and other risk factors. *J Natl Cancer Inst* 92: 1607–1612.

12 Measuring the Antioxidant Activity of Food Components

Takayuki Shibamoto

CONTENTS

12.1 INTRODUCTION

Every day, we are subjected to the health risks associated with oxidative damage caused by reactive oxygen species. These reactive oxygen species are derived from all aspects of human endeavors, from automobile exhaust fumes, industrial plants, waste incinerations, and cigarette smoking, to indirect environment consequences, such as UV-light exposure through a depleted ozone layer. Oxidation of various biological substances contributes to many diseases, including AIDS (Sepulveda and Watson 2002), Alzheimer's disease (Moreira et al. 2005), atherosclerosis (Heinecke 1997), cancer (Paz-Elizur et al. 2008), cataracts (Selvi et al. 2011), diabetes (Albright et al. 2004; Itoh et al. 2009), inflammation (Halliwell and Gutteridge 1995), liver disease (Preedy et al. 1998), and Parkinson's disease (Beal 2003; Chaturvedi and Beal 2008), as well as aging (Liu and Mori 2006). Therefore, use of antioxidant supplements has begun to receive much attention as they are substances that might help to prevent these diseases.

Antioxidants found in natural plants, such as vitamin E (α-tocopherol), vitamin C, and polyphenols/flavonoids, have been investigated for their possible role in the prevention of the diseases mentioned above (Nunez-Selles 2005). For example, vitamin E is reported to be effective in preventing diabetes (Levy and Blum 2007). Clinical and research evidence on the effects of vitamin C on cancer and cardiovascular disease were also well discussed in a recent review (Li and Schellhorn 2007). Polyphenols/ flavonoids found in natural plants and plant products, such as red wine, also exhibit potent antioxidant activity and can prevent some cardiovascular diseases (Renaud and de Lorgeril 1992; Kanner et al. 1994; Kinsella et al. 1993; see also Chapter 11).

In addition to natural compounds of plant origin, some antioxidants have been found in heat-treated foods. The antioxidant components in these foods are proposed to be formed by the Maillard reaction during heat treatment. High molecular weight substances, such as melanoidins, produced from a sugar/amino acid model system by the Maillard reaction have been known to have antioxidant activity (Yamaguchi 1986; Daglia et al. 2000; Steinhart et al. 2001). Also, the antioxidant activity of low molecular weight volatile compounds—particularly heterocyclic compounds— obtained from Maillard reaction model systems has also been reported (Shaker et al. 1995; Eiserich and Shibamoto 1994; see also Chapter 10).

The search for new antioxidants, which can be used as food supplements, would therefore be one avenue to pursue in order to find ways to protect people from oxidative damage.

12.2 METHODS FOR MEASURING ANTIOXIDANT ACTIVITY

There are many assays that can be used to measure the antioxidant activity of food components. Two types of assays are widely used for antioxidant studies on foods and their components. The first are assays associated with lipid peroxidations, including the thiobarbituric acid (TBA) assay, the malonaldehyde/high-performance liquid chromatography (MDA/HPLC) assay, the malonaldehyde/gas chromatography (MDA/GC) assay, the β-carotene bleaching assay, and the conjugated diene assay. The second type are assays associated with electron or radical scavenging, including the 2,2-diphenyl-1-picrylhydrazyl (DPPH) assay, the 2,2′-azino-bis (3-ethylbenzothiazoline-6 sulfonic acid) (ABTS) assay, the ferric reducing/antioxidant power (FRAP) assay, the ferrous oxidation-xylenol orange (FOX) assay, the ferric thiocyanate (FTC) assay, and the aldehyde/carboxylic acid (ACA) assay (Moon and Shibamoto 2009). However, it is extremely important to use the appropriate assay for a given target sample. It is generally recommended to use at least three different assays to determine the antioxidant activity of samples. There are enzymatic assays and nonenzymatic assays for antioxidant determination (Moon and Shibamoto 2009). The antioxidant activity of foods and their components is commonly measured by nonenzymatic assays, which are discussed in this chapter.

12.2.1 SPECTROPHOTOMETRIC METHODS

Table 12.1 shows commonly used antioxidant assays using a spectrophotometer. Measuring a product formed by oxidation using a spectrophotometer is a simple and fast method for determining the antioxidant activity of the chemical(s) of interest.

A 2,2-diphenyl-1-picrylhydrazyl (DPPH) assay may be the most commonly and widely used method for determination of the antioxidant activity of food components. DPPH readily forms a stable radical (DPPH•), which accepts hydrogen from an antioxidant (MacDonald-Wicks et al. 2006). The disappearance of DPPH•, which is

TABLE 12.1
Commonly Used Antioxidant Assays Using a Spectrophotometer

Antioxidant Assay	Monitoring Product	Absorbed	Typical Application	Reference
DPPH	DPPH·	517 nm	Medicinal plants	Sone et al. 2011
β-Carotene bleaching	β-Carotene radical	470 nm	Juniper berry	El-Ghorab et al. 2008
Conjugated diene	Conjugated diene	234 nm	Essential oils	Wei and Shibamoto 2010
ABTS	ABTS·	734 nm	Rooibos tea	Bramati et al. 2003
FRAP	Fe^{2+}-TPTZ[a]	593 nm	MRPs[b]	Yilmaz and Akgun 2008
FOX	Fe^{3+}-XOC[c]	550 nm	Plant extract	Pinto et al. 2007
FTC	$Fe(SCN)_3$	500 nm	Cauliflower	Llorach et al. 2003
TBA	TBA/MA adduct	535 nm	Green tea	Lee et al. 2003

[a] Ferrous tripyridyltriazine.
[b] Maillard reaction products.
[c] Fe^{3+}–xylenol orange complex.

proportional to the antioxidant effect, is monitored by a spectrophotometer at 517 nm to determine antioxidant activity. Almost 90% of antioxidant studies on food components have been conducted using the DPPH assay (Moon and Shibamoto 2009).

The theory behind the β-carotene bleaching assay is based on the fact that β-carotene readily absorbs a proxy radical yielded from a lipid upon oxidation to form β-carotene epoxides (Kennedy and Liebler 1991). In this assay, the amount of β-carotene is monitored in a system consisting of a lipid and a chemical of interest to determine antioxidant activity. The antioxidant activity of various phenolic compounds was determined using this assay (Chaillou and Nazareno 2006).

The theoretical basis for the conjugated diene assay is similar to that of the β-carotene bleaching assay. A moiety with two double bonds separated by a single methylene group in a fatty acid changes to a moiety with a conjugated diene moiety in the presence of reactive oxygen species. The diene moiety formed can be monitored by a spectrophotometer at 234 nm. One drawback of this assay is that many substrates absorb 234 nm UV-light and consequently interfere with the diene absorbance. Therefore, it is essential to use a simple fatty acid, such as linoleic acid, in this assay (Moon and Shibamoto 2009).

The 2,2′-azinobis (3-ethylbenzothiazoline-6-sulfonic acid) ABTS assay is based on the theory that decolorization of the ABTS radical cation is caused by the action of an antioxidant. The absorbance of the reaction mixture of ABTS and an antioxidant is compared to that of the Trolox antioxidant standard, and the results are expressed in terms of Trolox equivalent antioxidant capacity (TEAC) (Re et al. 1999). This assay has been used widely for fruits and vegetables because it can be applied in either an aqueous or an organic matrix.

There are also assays involving oxidation of ferrous to ferric ions in an organometallic complex. The basic theory underlying these assays is that color changes of a solution will occur when ferrous ions are oxidized. The organometallic complex is ferrous tripyridyltriazine for the ferric reducing/antioxidant power (FRAP) assay (Liu et al. 1982), Fe^{3+}–Xylenol orange complex for the ferrous oxidation-xylenol orange (FOX) assay (Pinto et al. 2007), and Fe^{3+}–thiocyanate complex for the ferric thiocyanate (FTC) assay (Kikuzaki and Nakatani 1993).

The TBA assay is one of the most conventional methods to measure the anti-oxidant activity of chemical(s). The theory is based on the notion that the forma-tion of a secondary oxidation product, malondialdehyde (MDA), can be prevented by an antioxidant. MDA is known as a secondary product formed from a lipid at the final stage of lipid peroxidation (Frankel and Neff 1983). However, analysis of MDA is extremely difficult because it is highly water-soluble and reactive to nucleophiles (Dennis and Shibamoto 1989). Among the many methods to prepare a stable derivative to determine the amount of MDA formed from a lipid upon oxidation, use of a TBA derivative has been the most popular (Shibamoto 2006). The TBA–MDA adduct is monitored by its absorption at 535 nm. The method is simple, and it is easy to observe the presence of antioxidants. However, TBA reacts not only with MDA but also with many other carbonyl compounds produced from lipid peroxidation. Therefore, the amount of MDA analyzed by this method is susceptible to being overestimated. For this reason, the term "thiobarbituric acid reactive substances" (TBARS) is generally used in reports using this method. Consequently, various chromatographic methods for specific analysis of MDA have been developed.

12.2.2　Chromatographic Methods

As mentioned above, the TBA/spectrometric method is not specific for MDA. More specific measurement of MDA has been performed by GC and HPLC after MDA was derivatized into more stable derivatives. Table 12.2 shows typical chromato-graphic methods used to analyze MDA formed in oxidized lipids for antioxidant studies.

Because the MDA–TBA adduct has a high boiling point, GC is not applicable. Therefore, HPLC has been applied to analyze MDA–TBA to determine specific amounts of MDA in various samples, such as serum (Carbonneau et al. 1991; Esben et al. 2006), plasma (Qian and Liu 1997), and liver (Soares et al. 2004). The spectro-photometric detectors used in these HPLC analyses are somewhat lower than those of GC detectors. However, the recent development of LC/MS has resolved this prob-lem (Alghazeer et al. 2008). For example, MDA formed in oxidized linoleic acid was analyzed by LC/MS, the sensitivity of which was comparable to that of GC detectors (Jardine et al. 2002).

The most widely used derivatives for carbonyl analysis, including MDA, are dinitrophenyl hydrazine (DNPH) derivatives. DNPH derivatives are analyzed by various methods including spectrophotometry, GC/NPD, GC/MS, HPLC/UV, and HPLC/MS (Shibamoto 2006). The DNPH derivatives of low molecular weight car-bonyls, such as formaldehyde, acrolein, acetone, and acetaldehyde, can be analyzed by GC (Deyl and Miksik 1996), whereas those of relatively high molecular weight carbonyl compounds, including MDA, must be analyzed by HPLC. In particular,

TABLE 12.2
Typical Chromatographic Methods Used to Analyze Malonaldehyde (MA) Formed in Oxidized Lipids for Antioxidant Studies

Derivatizing Agent	Derivative	Method	Sample	Reference
TBA	MA-TBA	HPLC/FL[a]	Plasma	Lykkesfeldt 2007
DNPH[b]	MA-DNPH	HPLC/UV	Phospholipid	Moore and Roberts 1998
		HPLC/MS	Beer	Gonçalves et al. 2010
PFPH[c]	MA-PFPH	GC/ECD[d]	Vegetable oils	Stashenko et al. 1997
		GC/MS	Biological fluids	Yeo et al. 1994
NMH[e]	1-Methypyrazole	GC/NPD[f]	Essential oils	Wei and Shibamoto 2007

[a] Fluorescence.
[b] 2,4-Dinitrophenylhydrazine.
[c] Penta-fluorophenylhydrazine.
[d] Electron capture detector.
[e] N-methylhydrazine.
[f] Nitrogen phosphorous detector.

since the development of LC/MS, it has become the mainstream method for DNPH derivatives, even for low molecular weight carbonyl derivatives (Sakuragawa et al. 1999). One recent report demonstrated that the analysis of DNPH derivatives using negative ion MS resulted in highly selective and sensitive detectability to carbonyl compounds (Yasuhara et al. 2011). It is expected that antioxidant studies will be performed primarily using the LC/MS method in the near future.

Nevertheless, although LC/MS will be a mainstream chromatographic method for antioxidant studies, the LC/MS instrument is still expensive and not easy for individual labs to obtain. Therefore, the GC method, instrumentation for which is relatively less expensive compared to that of LC/MS, is still useful. It should also be noted that the relatively simple and effective GC/NPD method was developed and applied to various foods and plant samples, including barley leaves (Nishiyama et al. 1993, 1994), plant essences (Miyake and Shibamoto 1997), beans (Lee et al. 2000), herbs and spices (Lee and Shibamoto 2002a), basil and thyme leaves (Lee et al. 2005), essential oils (Wei and Shibamoto 2007), licorice (Tanaka et al. 2008), and onion sprouts (Takahashi and Shibamoto 2008). This method involves the derivatization of MDA to stable 1-methylpyrazole with N-methylhydrazine. 1-Methylpyrazole contains two nitrogen atoms, which are highly specific and sensitive toward NPD. For example, 3.8–190.2 nmol/mg of MDA was satisfactorily determined in UV-irradiated cod liver oil using this method (Niyati-Shirkhodace and Shibamoto 1992). Also, highly selective and sensitive analysis of MDA using pentafluorophenyl hydrazine (PFPH) has been reported. The volatility of this derivative, N-pentafluorophenyl pyrazole, is suited to GC analysis, and it contains five fluorine atoms, which are highly selective and sensitive to electron-capture detector (ECD) and MS with negative chemical ionization MS (Yeo et al. 1998).

12.2.3 ALDEHYDE/CARBOXYLIC ACID ASSAY

The theory involved in this assay is that aldehyde is oxidized into carboxylic acid by reactive oxygen species. The assay uses a relatively low molecular weight alkyl aldehyde, such as pentanal and hexanal. The assay matrix is very simple. It requires only a 3%–4% dichloromethane solution of pentanal or hexanal. Because dichloromethane contains a trace level of a hydroxyl radical, the oxidation of aldehyde occurs slowly according to the proposed mechanisms shown in Figure 12.1.

Any chemical(s)—in particular, a hydroxyl radical scavenger—that blocks this oxidation process is defined as an antioxidant (Moon and Shibamoto 2009). This assay is useful for monitoring a prolonged oxidation process, such as the shelf life of food. If an aldehyde solution is allowed to stand for aldehyde oxidation, it takes more than 160 days for conversion of the aldehyde to carboxylic acid completely in a 3%–4% dichloromethane solution. However, if the solution is agitated by the addition of H_2O_2, air, or heat, the oxidation could be accelerated. Figure 12.2 shows the results of experiments on agitation with the above three methods.

The assay solution was a 3% dichloromethane solution of hexanal. After 40 days, 24.3% hexanal oxidized to hexanoic without any agitation. On the other hand, when the solution was purged by air for 10 s every day, hexanal oxidized completely after 40 days. Either the addition of 1 mol of H_2O_2 or heating at 60°C also accelerated the oxidation. According to the results from this study, most studies using this assay have been conducted by air purging. This assay is also convenient to test organic compounds because the matrix consists of an organic solvent. A typical result of an antioxidant study on a barley essence using this assay is shown in Figure 12.3.

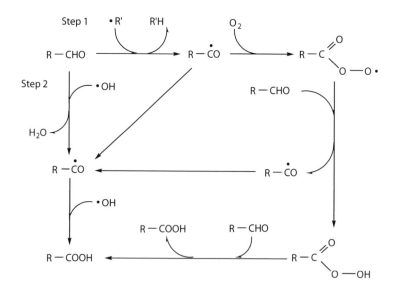

FIGURE 12.1 Proposed oxidation mechanisms from aldehyde to carboxylic acid.

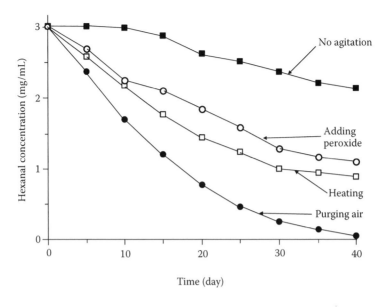

FIGURE 12.2   Oxidation of hexanal to hexanoic acid with or without agitation.

The barley essence extract inhibited hexanal oxidation by 95% at the level of 500 µg/mL over 45 days. It also inhibited hexanal oxidation by 80% and by 20% at the level of 250 and 100 µg/mL, respectively, for 45 days. The blank is a solution with no testing sample.

Most antioxidant study results reported in the following sections were ones obtained using this assay.

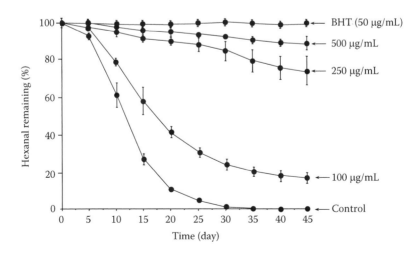

FIGURE 12.3   Antioxidant activity of barley essence tested by aldehyde/carboxylic acid assay.

12.3 ANTIOXIDANT ACTIVITY OF BEVERAGES AND THEIR COMPONENTS

12.3.1 ANTIOXIDANT ACTIVITY OF BEVERAGES: COFFEE, TEA, AND BEER

Most studies on coffee associated with human health have focused on the negative aspects, such as the toxicity of caffeine. Because coffee has been consumed for many years, however, one can argue that there must be some positive benefit, such as antioxidant activity, toward human health. Therefore, investigation of the antioxidant activities of coffee and its components is one avenue to assessing the health benefits of coffee drinking.

The first report on antioxidant activity in brewed coffee demonstrated that one of the fractionated samples of a coffee extract inhibited pentanal oxidation over 14 days (Singhara et al. 1998). The antioxidant activity of this fraction was comparable to those of known antioxidant α-tocopherol and BHT. Later, the antioxidant activity of column chromatographic fractions prepared from brewed coffee was further investigated to assess the benefit of coffee drinking (Yanagimoto et al. 2004). In this study, the dichloromethane extract of brewed coffee inhibited hexanal oxidation by 100% and 50% for 15 and 30 days, respectively, at the level of 5 μg/mL. A GC/MS analysis of the fraction with potent antioxidant activity revealed the presence of various volatile heterocyclic compounds, the antioxidant activity of which is discussed in the next section.

The antioxidant activities of dichloromethane extracts of commercial brewed coffees were investigated by MDA-GC assay and TBA assay (Fujioka and Shibamoto 2006). The highest antioxidant activity obtained by the MDA-GC assay was from regular whole brewed coffee (97.8%) at a level of 20% and by the TBA assay from decaffeinated whole brewed coffee (96.6%) at a level of 5%.

Among 31 chemicals identified in a dichloromethane extract of brewed coffee, chlorogenic acids, caffeic acid, ferulic acid, guaiacol, ethylguaiacol, and vinylguaiacol all exhibited antioxidant activities. Figure 12.4 shows the antioxidant activity of these compounds tested by TBA and MDA/GC assays at the level of 10 μg/mL.

Among nine chlorogenic acids (3-caffeoylquinic acid, 3-feruloylquinic acid, 3-dicaffeoylquinic acid) identified, 5-caffeoylquinic acid contained the greatest amount both in regular (883.5 μg/mL) and in decaffeinated (1032.6 μg/mL) coffees. It exhibited 24.5% and 45.3% antioxidant activity by the MDA-GC and the TBA, respectively. Ethylguaiacol and vinylguaiacol showed a more than 80% antioxidant effect in both assays. Caffeic acid, ferulic acids, and guaiacol showed moderate antioxidant activities in both assays, which were comparable to those of α-tocopherol.

The antioxidant activities of volatile extracts from six teas (one green tea, one oolong tea, one roasted green tea, and three black teas) were determined using an aldehyde/carboxylic acid assay and a conjugated diene assay (Yanagimoto et al. 2003). The results obtained from the two assays were consistent. All extracts except roasted green tea exhibited dose-dependent inhibitory activity in the aldehyde/carboxylic acid assay. A volatile extract from green tea exhibited the most potent activity among the six tea extracts in both assays. It inhibited hexanal oxidation by almost 100% over 40 days at the level of 200 μg/mL. The extract from oolong tea

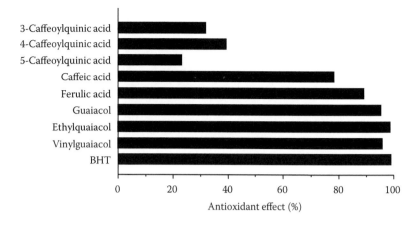

FIGURE 12.4   Antioxidant activity of chemicals identified in brewed coffee.

inhibited hexanal oxidation by 50% in 15 days. In the case of the extract from roasted green tea, the lowest antioxidant activity was obtained at the level of 200 µg/mL, suggesting that the extract from roasted green tea contained some prooxidants. The extracts from the three black teas showed slight anti-activities or pro-activities in both assays. The major volatile constituents of green tea and roasted green tea extracts, which exhibited significant antioxidant activities, were analyzed using gas chromatography/mass spectrometry. The major volatile chemicals with possible antioxidant activity identified were alkyl compounds with double bond(s), such as 3,7-dimethyl-1,6-octadien-3-ol (8.04 mg/kg), in the extract from green tea, and heterocyclic compounds, such as furfural (7.67 mg/kg), in the extract from roasted green tea. Benzyl alcohol, which has been known to exhibit an antioxidant activity, was identified both in a green tea extract (4.67 mg/kg) and a roasted tea extract (1.35 mg/kg).

The antioxidant activity of a dichloromethane extract from commercial beer has also been reported (Wei et al. 2001). The extract inhibited hexanal oxidation by more than 99% at the level of 50 µg/mL over 35 days, comparable to that of the natural antioxidant α-tocopherol.

12.3.2   ANTIOXIDANT ACTIVITY OF MAILLARD REACTION PRODUCTS

Over the last three decades, nutritional, physiological, and biological activities of Maillard reaction products (MRPs) have been intensively investigated (Fujimaki et al. 1986). Some research involving the Maillard reaction has focused on the toxicity of MRPs (Ikan 1996). However, MRPs have also received much attention as products contributing preferable factors to foods, such as giving a pleasant flavor and stabilizing with antioxidants. Higher molecular weight MRPs, such as melanoidins, exhibited antioxidant activity and stabilized some food products (Yamaguchi 1986). Later, some volatile flavor heterocyclic compounds, including pyrroles, furans, thiophenes, thiazoles, oxazoles, pyridines, and pyrazines, were found to possess appreciable antioxidative activity (Lee and Shibamoto 2002b).

Figure 12.5 shows the antioxidant activity of the dichloromethane extract from glucose/amino acids in a Maillard browning model system tested by aldehyde/carboxylic acid assay and DPPH assay at the level of 200 μL/mL. All extracts exhibited antioxidant activity in the two assays.

In the aldehyde/carboxylic acid assay, extracts from glucose/tyrosine, methionine, or asparagine showed strong antioxidant activity, comparable to that of the known antioxidant BHT. The extracts from glucose/glycine, tryptophan, histidine, and phenyl alanine exhibited more than 90% activity. Extracts from glucose/cysteine or threonine exhibited moderate antioxidant activity. In the DPPH assay, the extract from glucose/phenyl alanine showed the highest antioxidant activity (100%), followed by the extracts from glucose/asparagine (85%), glucose/phenyl alanine (83%), and glucose/cysteine (82%). The results indicate that the Maillard browning model systems produce potent antioxidants.

It has been known for some time that many heterocyclic compounds form in various sugar/amino acid Maillard browning model systems (Shibamoto 1983). More than 300 heterocyclic compounds formed by Maillard reactions—including pyrroles, oxazoles, furans, thiazoles, thiophenes, imidazoles, and pyrazines—were reported in brewed coffee (Flament and Bessiere-Thomas 2002). Recent studies have demonstrated the antioxidant activity of these volatile heterocyclic compounds (Fuster et al. 2000; Yanagimoto et al. 2002). In these studies, various heterocyclic compounds found in MRPs were examined for antioxidant activity. Pyrroles exhibited the greatest antioxidant activity among all heterocyclic compounds tested. All pyrroles inhibited hexanal oxidation by almost 100% at the level of 50 μg/mL over

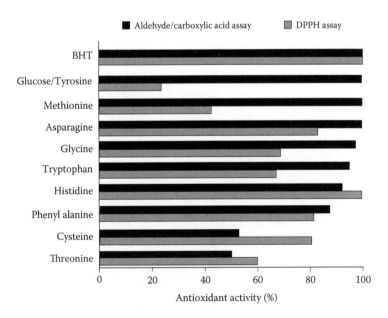

FIGURE 12.5 Antioxidant activity of the dichloromethane extract from glucose/amino acids in Maillard browning model system tested by aldehyde/carboxylic acid assay and DPPH assay at the level of 200 μL/mL.

40 days. Addition of formyl and acetyl groups to a pyrrole ring enhanced antioxidative activity remarkably. Pyrrole-2-carboxaldehyde, 2-acetylpyrrole, 1-methyl-2-pyrrolecarboxaldehyde, and 2-acetyl-1-methylpyrrole inhibited hexanal oxidation by more than 80% at 10 µg/mL. Unsubstituted furan exhibited the greatest antioxidant activity among furans tested. Antioxidant activity of thiophene was increased by the addition of methyl and ethyl groups, but addition of formyl or acetyl groups to thiophene decreased antioxidant activity. Thiazoles and pyrazines exhibited slight antioxidant activity, whereas imidazoles and pyridines did not show appreciable activity.

Figure 12.6 shows the antioxidant activity of typical heterocyclic compounds along with their methyl and acetyl derivatives tested by the aldehyde/carboxylic acid assay (Yanagimoto et al. 2002). Pyrroles and BHT were tested at the level of 50 µg/mL, and all others were tested at 500 µg/mL for 35 days.

It is proposed that a carbon atom with high electron density in a heterocyclic ring scavenges a hydroxyl radical and subsequently reveals antioxidant activity (Shaker et al. 1995). In fact, when *N*-methylpyrrole was reacted with hydrogen peroxide, hydroxyl radical adducts, 1,5-dihydro-1-methyl-2H-pyrrole-2-one, and 1-methyl 2,5 pyrrolidine dione were produced (Yanagimoto et al. 2002), suggesting that pyrroles scavenge hydroxyl radicals. Because the hydroxyl radical-scavenging activity is dependent on the electron density of ring carbons, the nature of the substituent changes the degree of scavenging activity. When a substituent was added at the number 2 ring carbon, the antioxidant activities of furan, thiophene, thiazole, pyrazine, and

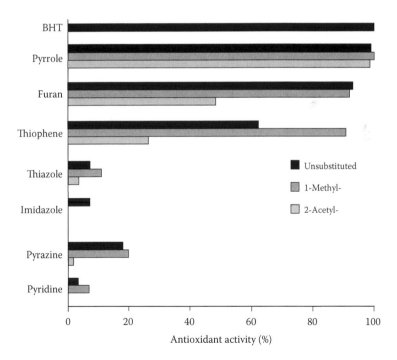

FIGURE 12.6 Antioxidant activity of typical heterocyclic compounds along with their methyl and acetyl derivatives tested by aldehyde/carboxylic acid assay.

pyridine were increased by an electron-donating methyl group, whereas their activity was reduced by an electron withdrawing acetyl group. It is difficult to explain, but the hydroxyl radical-scavenging activity of furan by these substituents did not show significant difference. Both substituents deleted the antioxidant activity of unsubstituted imidazole completely. However, it is obvious that the nature of substituents plays an important role in the antioxidant activity of heterocyclic compounds.

12.4   CONCLUSION

The cells of the human body are subjected to oxidative damage, which is associated with certain biological complications, such as cancer, arteriosclerosis, aging, diabetes, and immune deficiency. Although living systems are protected from active oxidants by enzymatic systems, ingesting additional antioxidants, like ascorbic acid and α-tocopherol, has been recommended to protect living cells from oxidation. We are consuming these natural antioxidants from fruits and vegetables. Moreover, it is obvious that humans consume some quantity of antioxidants formed in heat-treated foods. In particular, ingestion of heterocyclic compounds formed in heat-treated foods and beverages may help to prevent *in vivo* oxidative damage as mentioned above. Therefore, studies focused on the measurement of antioxidants in foods and beverages are critical to the search for ways to protect us from oxidative damage.

REFERENCES

Albright, C.D., Salganik, R.I., and Van Dyke, T. 2004. Dietary depletion of vitamin E and vitamin A inhibits mammary tumor growth and metastasis in transgenic mice. *J Nutr* 134: 1139–1144.

Alghazeer, R., Saeed, S., and Howell, N.K. 2008. Aldehyde formation in frozen mackerel (*Scomber scombrus*) in the presence and absence of instant green tea. *Food Chem* 108: 801–810.

Beal, M.F. 2003. Mitochondria, oxidative damage, and inflammation in Parkinson's disease. *Ann New York Acad Sci* 991: 120–131.

Bramati, L., Aquilano, F., and Pietta, P. 2003. Unfermented rooibos tea: Quantitative characterization of flavonoids by HPLC-UV and determination of the total antioxidant activity. *J Agric Food Chem* 51: 7472–7474.

Carbonneau, M.A., Peuchant, E., Sess, D., Canioni, P., and Clerc, M. 1991. Free and bound malondialdehyde measured as thiobarbituric acid adduct by HPLC in serum and plasma. *Clin Chem* 37: 1423–1429.

Chaillou, L.L., and Nazareno, M.A. 2006. New method to determine antioxidant activity of polyphenols. *J Agric Food Chem* 54: 8397–8402.

Chaturvedi, R.K., and Beal, M.F. 2008. PPAR: A therapeutic target in Parkinson's disease. *J Neurochem* 106: 506–518.

Daglia, M., Papetti, A., Gregotti, C., Bert, F., and Gazzani, G. 2000. *In vitro* antioxidant and *ex vivo* protective activities of green and roasted coffee. *J Agric Food Chem* 48: 1449–1454.

Dennis, K.J., and Shibamoto, T. 1989. Gas chromatographic determination of malonaldehyde formed by lipid peroxidation. *Free Radic Biol Med* 7: 187–189.

Deyl, Z., and Miksik, I. 1996. The effect of high fat diet upon the production of reactive carbonyls in hypoxi heart: The effect upon connective tissue. *Nutr Res* 16: 79–90.

Eiserich, J.P., and Shibamoto, T. 1994. Antioxidative activity of volatile heterocyclic compounds. *J Agric Food Chem* 42: 1060–1063.

El-Ghorab, A., Shaaban, H.A., El-Massry, K.F., and Shibamoto, T. 2008. Chemical composition of volatile extract and biological activities of volatile and less-volatile extracts of juniper berry (*Juniperus drupacea* L.) fruit. *J Agric Food Chem* 56: 5021–5025.

Esben, S., Tor, H., and Azam, M.M. 2006. A novel HPLC method for the measurement of thiobarbituric acid reactive substances (TBARS): A comparison with a commercially available kit. *Clin Biochem* 39: 947–954.

Flament, I., and Bessiere-Thomas, Y. 2002. *Coffee Flavor Chemistry.* John Wiley & Sons, New York.

Frankel, E.N., and Neff, W.E. 1983. Formation of malonaldehyde from lipid oxidation products. *Biochim Biopys Acta* 754: 264–270.

Fujimaki, M., Namiki, M., and Kato, H. 1986. *Amino–Carbonyl Reactions in Food and Biological Systems.* Elsevier, New York.

Fujioka, K., and Shibamoto, T. 2006. Quantitation of volatiles and nonvolatile acids in an extract from coffee beverages: Correlation with antioxidant activity. *J Agric Food Chem* 54: 6054–6058.

Fuster, M.D., Mitchell, A.E., Ochi, H., and Shibamoto, T. 2000. Antioxidative activities of heterocyclic compounds formed in brewed coffee. *J Agric Food Chem* 48: 5600–5603.

Gonçalves, L.M., Magalhäes, P.J., Valente, I.M., Pacheco, J.G., Dostálek, P., Sykora, D., Rodrigues, J.A., and Barros, A.A. 2010. Analysis of aldehydes in beer by gas-diffusion microextraction: characterization by high-performance liquid chromatography-diode-array detection-atmospheric pressure chemical ionization-mass spectrometry. *J Chromatogr A* 1217: 3717–3722.

Halliwell, B., and Gutteridge, J.M. 1995. The definition and measurement of antioxidants in biological systems. *Free Radic Biol Med* 18: 125–126.

Heinecke, J.W. 1997. Mechanisms of oxidative damage of low density lipoprotein in human atherosclerosis. *Curr Opin Lipidol* 8: 268–274.

Ikan, R. 1996. *The Maillard Reaction: Consequences for the Chemical and Life Sciences.* John Wiley & Sons, New York.

Itoh, K., Hirata, N., Masuda, M., Naruto, S., Murata, K., Wakabayashi, K., and Matsuda, H. 2009. Inhibitory effects of citrus hassaku extract and its flavanone glycosides on melanogenesis. *Biol Pharm Bull* 32: 410–415.

Jardine, D., Antolvich, M., Prezzler, P.D., and Robards, K. 2002. Liquid chromatography-mass spectrometry (LC-MS) investigation of the thiobarbituric acid reactive substances (TBARS) reaction. *J Agric Food Chem* 50: 1720–1724.

Kanner, J., Frankel, E., Granit, R., German, B., and Kinsella, J.E. 1994. Natural antioxidants in grapes and wines. *J Agric Food Chem* 42: 64–69.

Kennedy, T.A., and Liebler, D.C. 1991. Peroxy radical oxidation of β-carotene: Formation of β-carotene epoxides. *Chem Res Toxicol* 4: 290–295.

Kikuzaki, H., and Nakatani, N. 1993. Antioxidant effects of some ginger constituents. *J Food Sci* 58: 1407–1410.

Kinsella, J.E., Frankel, E., German, B., and Kanner, J. 1993. Possible mechanisms for the protective role of antioxidants in wine and plant foods. *Food Technol* 47: 85–89.

Lee, K.-G., Mitchell, A.E., and Shibamoto, T. 2000. Determination of antioxidant properties of aroma extracts from various beans. *J Agric Food Chem* 48: 4817–4820.

Lee, K.-G., and Shibamoto, T. 2002a. Determination of antioxidant potential of volatile extracts isolated from various herbs and spices. *J Agric Food Chem* 50: 4947–4952.

Lee, K.-G., and Shibamoto, T. 2002b. Toxicology and antioxidant activities of non-enzymatic browning reaction products: review. *Food Rev Int* 18: 151–175.

Lee, K.-G., Shibamoto, T., Takeoka, G.R., See, S.-E., Kim, J.-H., and Park, B.-S. 2003. Inhibitory effects of plant-derived flavonoids and phenolic acids on malonaldehyde formation from ethyl arachidonate. *J Agric Food Chem* 51: 7203–7207.

Lee, S.-J., Umano, K., Shibamoto, T., and Lee, K.-G. 2005. Identification of volatile components in basil (*Ocimum basilicum* L.) and thyme leaves (*Thumus vulgaris* L.) and their antioxidant properties. *Food Chem* 91: 131–137.

Levy, A.P., and Blum, S. 2007. Pharmacogenomics in prevention of diabetic cardiovascular disease: Utilization of the haptoglobin genotype in determining benefit from vitamin E. *Expert Rev Cardiovasc Ther* 5: 1105–1111.

Li, Y., and Schellhorn, H.E. 2007. New developments and novel therapeutic perspectives for vitamin C. *J Nutr* 137: 2171–2184.

Liu, J., and Mori, A. 2006. Oxidative damage hypothesis of stress-associated aging acceleration: Neuroprotective effects of natural and nutritional antioxidants. *Res Comm Biol Psych Psychiatr Neurosci* 30–31: 103–119.

Liu, T.Z., Chin, N., Kiser, M.D., and Bigler, W.N. 1982. Specific spectrophotometry of ascorbic acid in serum or plasma by use of ascorbate oxidase. *Clin Chem* 28: 2225–2228.

Llorach, R., Espin, J.C., Tomas-Barberan, F.A., and Ferreres, F. 2003. Valorization of cauliflower (*Brassica oleracea L. var botrytis*) by-products as a source of antioxidant phenolics. *J Agric Food Chem* 51: 2181–2187.

Lykkesfeldt, J. 2007. Malonaldehyde as biomarker of oxidative damage to lipids caused by smoking. *Clin Chim Acta* 380: 50–58.

MacDonald-Wicks, L.K., Wood, L.G., and Garg, M.L. 2006. Methodology for the determination of biological antioxidant capacity *in vitro*: A review. *J Sci Food Agric* 86: 2046–2056.

Miyake, T., and Shibamoto, T. 1997: Antioxidative activities of natural compounds found in plants. *J Agric Food Chem* 45: 1918–1822.

Moon, J.-K., and Shibamoto, T. 2009: Antioxidant assays for plant and food components. *J Agric Food Chem* 57: 1655–1666.

Moore, K., and Roberts II, J. 1998. Measurement of lipid peroxidation. *Free Radic Res* 28: 659–671.

Moreira, P., Smith, M.A., Zhu, X., Honda, K., Lee, H.-G., Aliev, G., and Perry, G. 2005. Since oxidative damage is a key phenomenon in Alzheimer's disease, treatment with antioxidants seems to be a promising approach for slowing disease progression. Oxidative damage and Alzheimer's disease: Are antioxidant therapies useful? *Drug News Perspect* 18: 13.

Nishiyama, T., Hagiwara, Y., Hagiwara, H., and Shibamoto, T. 1993. Inhibition of malonaldehyde formation from lipids by an isoflavonoid isolated from young green barley leaves. *J Am Oil Chem Soc* 70: 811–813.

Nishiyama, T., Hagiwara, Y., Hagiwara, H., and Shibamoto, T. 1994. Formation and inhibition of genotoxic glyoxal and malonaldehyde from phospholipids and fish liver oil upon lipid peroxidation. *J Agric Food Chem* 42: 1728–1731.

Niyati-Shirkhodaee, F., and Shibamoto, T. 1992. Formation of toxic aldehydes in cod liver oil after ultraviolet irradiation. *J Am Oil Chem Soc* 69: 1254–1256.

Nunez-Selles, A.J. 2005. Antioxidant therapy: Myth or reality? *J Brazil Chem Soc* 16: 699–710.

Paz-Elizur, T., Sevilya, Z., Leitner-Dagan, Y., Elinger, D., Roisman, L.C., and Livneh, Z. 2008. DNA repair of oxidative DNA damage in human carcinogenesis: Potential application for cancer risk assessment and prevention. *Cancer Lett* 266: 60–72.

Pinto, M. del C., Tejeda, A., Duque, A.L., and Macias, P. 2007. Determination of lipoxygenase activity in plant extracts using a modified ferrous oxidation-xylenol orange assay. *J Agric Food Chem* 55: 5956–5959.

Preedy, V.R., Reilly, M.E., Mantle, D., and Peters, T.J. 1998. Oxidative damage in liver disease. *J Intern Fed Clin Chem* 10: 16–20.

Qian, H., and Liu, D. 1997. The time course of malondialdehyde production following impact injury to rat spinal cord as measured by microdialysis and high pressure liquid chromatography. *Neurochem Res* 22: 1231–1236.

Re, R., Pellegrini, N., Proteggente, A., Pannala, A., Yang, M., and Rice-Evans, C.A. 1999. Antioxidant activity applying an improved ABTS radical cation decolorization assay. *Free Radic Biol Med* 26: 1231–1237.

Renaud, S., and de Lorgeril, M. 1992. Wine, alcohol, platelets, and the French paradox for coronary heart disease. *Lancet* 340: 313–315.

Sakuragawa, A., Yoneno, T., Inoue, K., and Okutani, T.A. 1999. Trace analysis of carbonyl compounds by liquid chromatography–mass spectrometry after collection as 2,4-dinitrophenylhydrazine derivatives. *J Chromatogr* 844: 403–408.

Selvi, R., Angayarkanni, N., Biswass, J., and Ramakrishnan, S. 2011. Total antioxidant capacity in Eales' disease, uveitis and cataract. *Indian J Med Res* 134: 83–90.

Sepulveda, R.T., and Watson, R.R. 2002. Treatment of antioxidant deficiencies in AIDS patients. *Nutr Res* 22: 27–37.

Shaker, E.S., Ghazy, M.A., and Shibamoto, T. 1995. Antioxidative activity of volatile browning reaction products and related compounds in a hexanal/hexanoic acid system. *J Agric Food Chem* 43: 1017–1022.

Shibamoto, T. 1983. Heterocyclic compounds in browning and browning/nitrite model systems: Occurrence, formation mechanisms, flavor characteristics and mutagenic activity, in *Instrumental Analysis of Foods,* G. Charalambous and G. Inglett (Eds.), pp. 229–278, Academic Press, New York, Vol. I.

Shibamoto, T. 2006. Analytical methods for trace levels of reactive carbonyl compounds formed in lipid peroxidation systems. *J Pharm Biomed Anal* 41: 12–25.

Singhara, A., Macku, C., and Shibamoto, T. 1998, Antioxidative activity of brewed coffee extracts, in *Functional Foods for Disease Prevention II: Medicinal Plants and Other Foods.* ACS Symposium Series 701, American Chemical Society, Washington, DC, pp. 101–109.

Soares, M.E., Carvalho, M., Remião, F., Carvalho, F., and de Lourdes, M. 2004. Implementation of HPLC methodology for the quantification of malondialdehyde in cell suspensions and liver. *J Liq Chromatogr Rel Technol* 27: 2357–2369.

Sone, Y., Moon, J.-K, Mai, T.T., Thu, N.N., Asano, E., Yamaguchi, K., Otsuka, Y., and Shibamoto, T. 2011. Antioxidant/anti-inflammatory activities and total phenolic content of extracts obtained from plants grown in Vietnam. *J Sci Food Agric* 91: 2259–2264.

Stashenko, E.E., Ferreira, M.C., Sequeda, L.G., Martinez, J.R., and Wong, J.W. 1997. Comparison of extraction methods and detection systems in the gas chromatographic analysis of volatile carbonyl compounds. *J Chromatogr A* 779: 360–369.

Steinhart, H., Luger, A., and Piost, J. 2001. Antioxidative effect of coffee melanoidins, in *19th Colloque Scientifique International sur le Café,* pp. 67–74.

Takahashi, M., and Shibamoto, T. 2008. Chemical composition and antioxidant/anti-inflammatory activities of steam distillate from freeze-dried onion (*Allium cepa* L.) sprout. *J Agric Food Chem* 56: 10462–10467.

Tanaka, A., Horiuchi, M., Umano, K., and Shibamoto, T. 2008. Antioxidant and anti-inflammatory activities of water distillate and its dichloromethane extract from licorice root (*Glycyrrhiza uralensis*) and chemical composition of dichloromethane extract. *J Sci Food Agric* 88: 1158–1165.

Wei, A., Mura, K., and Shibamoto, T. 2001. Antioxidative activity of volatile chemicals extracted from beer. *J Agric Food Chem* 49: 4097–4101.

Wei, A., and Shibamoto, T. 2007. Antioxidant activities and volatile constituents of various essential oils. *J Agric Food Chem* 55: 1737–1742.

Wei, A., and Shibamoto, T. 2007. Antioxidant activities of essential oil mixture toward skin lipid squalene oxidized by UV irradiation. *Cutaneous Ocular Toxicol* 26: 227–233.

Wei, A., and Shibamoto, T. 2010. Antioxidant/lipoxygenase inhibitory activities and chemical compositions of selected essential oils. *J Agric Food Chem* 58: 7218–7225.

Yamaguchi, N. 1986. Antioxidative activity of the oxidation products prepared from elanoidins, in *Proceedings of the 3rd International Symposium on the Maillard Reaction*, M. Fujimaki, M. Namiki, and H. Kato (Eds.), pp. 291–299. Elsevier, Amsterdam.

Yanagimoto, K., Lee, K.-G., Ochi, H., and Shibamoto, T. 2002. Antioxidative activity of heterocyclic compounds found in coffee volatiles produced by Maillard reaction. *J Agric Food Chem* 50: 5480–5484.

Yanagimoto, K., Ochi, H., Lee, K.-G., and Shibamoto, T. 2003. Antioxidative activities of volatile extracts from green tea, oolong tea, and black tea. *J Agric Food Chem* 51: 7396–7401.

Yanagimoto, K., Ochi, H., Lee, K.-G., and Shibamoto, T. 2004. Antioxidative activities of fractions obtained from brewed coffee. *J Agric Food Chem* 52: 592–596.

Yasuhara, A., Tanaka, Y., Makishima, M., Suzuki, S., and Shibamoto, T. 2011. LC-MS analysis of low molecular weight carbonyl compounds as 2,4-dinitrophenylhydrazones using negative ion mode electron spray ionization mass spectrometry. *J Chromatogr Separ Technol online*. http://dx.doi.org/10.4172/215-7064.1000108.

Yeo, H.C., Helbock, H.J., and Ames, B.N. 1998. Chromatographic analysis of insecticidal carbamates, in *Chromatographic Analysis of Environmental and Food Toxicants*, T. Shibamoto (Ed.), pp. 289–322, Marcel Dekker, New York.

Yeo, H.C., Helbock, H.J., Chyu, D.W., and Ames, B.N. 1994. Assay of malondialdehyde in biological fluids by gas chromatography-mass spectrometry. *Anal Biochem* 220: 391–396.

Yilmaz, Y., and Akgun, F.B. 2008. Ferric reducing/antioxidant power of Maillard reaction products in model bread crusts. *J Food Agric Environ* 6: 56–60.

13 Measuring the Antioxidant Activity of Apple Products

Iwona Wawer

CONTENTS

13.1 INTRODUCTION

In most industrialized countries, cardiovascular disease and cancer are ranked as the top two leading causes of death. The causes of both diseases have been linked to lifestyle and dietary choices. A diet high in fruits and vegetables may provide some protection. People who eat the highest amount of fruits and vegetables have a 20% lower risk for coronary heart disease, and the lowest risks were seen in people who ate more fruits rich in polyphenolic compounds and vitamins. Heart infarct, cancer, and neurodegenerative diseases have been shown to have free radical involvement in their etiology. In order to prevent oxidative reactions in biological tissues, food rich in antioxidants should be consumed.

The aim of numerous studies was to identify and evaluate antioxidants of fruits, vegetables, beverages, and spices. Unfortunately, the methods used in most of these studies were different. The widely employed assays used to assess the antioxidant content of foods include Trolox equivalent antioxidant capacity (TEAC), the ferric-reducing ability of plasma (FRAP), the oxygen radical absorbance capacity (ORAC), and the DPPH˙ radical-scavenging assay.

The analysis of 1113 food samples from the United States (National Food and Nutrient Analysis Program) using a modified version of the FRAP assay showed (Halvorsen et al. 2006) that the products richest in antioxidants were ground spices (cloves, ginger, cinnamon, turmeric powder), which contained more than 10 mmol antioxidants/100 g. Based on typical serving sizes, the berries (blackberries, strawberries, cranberries, raspberries) appeared at the top of the ranked list. The top 50 foods containing the most antioxidants include apple juice with added vitamin C. Systematic measurement of the antioxidant content of more than 3100 foods was performed (Carlsen et al. 2010), and the results are published as the Antioxidant Food Database.

Because plant foods contain many different classes and types of antioxidants, knowledge of their total antioxidant capacity (TAC), which is the cumulative capacity of food components to scavenge free radicals, would be useful for epidemiologic purposes. To accomplish this, a variety of foods commonly consumed in Italy were analyzed (Pellegrini et al. 2006) using different assays (e.g., TEAC, FRAP). Both lipophilic and hydrophilic antioxidant capacities were determined (Wu et al. 2004) using the ORAC (ORAC$_{FL}$) assay on more than 100 different kinds of foods, including fruits, vegetables, nuts, and spices. The results were compiled for the database "Oxygen Radical Absorbance Capacity (ORAC) of Selected Foods—2007" published in the United States (http://www.ars.usda.gov/nutrientdata).

These data may be utilized in identifying potentially good sources of antioxidants, enabling the calculation of total antioxidant content of diets, and also in planning dietary antioxidant interventions.

The activity and mechanism of complex natural antioxidants are affected by many factors, including the composition of the system, the kinetics, and the conditions of oxidation. Therefore, more rigorous guidelines and measurement protocols are required. It seemed interesting to show advantages and disadvantages of a popular antioxidant assay, based on the measurement of the reducing ability of antioxidants toward the DPPH· radical. The data on antioxidant capacity are useful for the food industry in the development of high-quality products; examples are apple juice and apple purée.

13.2 ANTIOXIDANTS OF APPLES

Apples have commonly been considered to be a healthy food. The old adage "an apple a day keeps the doctor away" is still popular in the United States. Recently, apples have been subjected to a number of investigations, which confirmed their health-beneficial effects. Does an apple a day keep the oncologist away? One investigation (Gallus et al. 2005) found a consistent inverse association between apples and the risk of various cancers. Apples, and especially apple peels, can inhibit the growth of liver cancer and colon cancer cells. Apples are a good source of antioxidants in people's diets and had one of the highest levels of antioxidant activity and total concentration of phenolic compounds, when compared to other fruits.

Apples and apple juice showed antioxidant activities when tested both *in vitro* and *in vivo*; the effects have been attributed to the polyphenolic constituents, such as flavan-3-ols, including monomeric (catechins) and polymeric (procyanidins), hydroxycinnamic acids, dihydrochalcones, flavonols, and anthocyanins (in red apple peel). The composition of apple phenolics is known relatively well and has been studied mainly by the HPLC method. Cinnamic acid derivatives and flavanols represent approximately 90% of the phenolic content of the cortex of an apple with wide variations among cultivars. The main compound is chlorogenic acid with significant amounts of

4-coumaroylquinic acid. The flavanols epicatechin and procyanidin B2 are present in high concentrations. Flavonols and dihydrochalcones (phloridzin) are present only in minor quantities but distinguish apples from a number of other fruits. The characteristic flavonol glycosides of apples include quercetin-3-O-galactopyranoside (hyperin), quercitrin, and rutin. The major anthocyanin is cyanidin-3-galactoside. The concentrations of polyphenolic compounds in apple products depend on processing technology.

Of course, the healthiest choice is a fresh apple a day. Nevertheless, sales of fresh-cut product continue to grow because consumers like prepared, ready-to-eat fruit. How to avoid browning in cut apples and loss of phenolic antioxidants during storage? Apple slices dipped in calcium ascorbate and stored at a low temperature in packages with reduced O_2 had a shelf life of 21–28 days. Total antioxidant activity in these treatments was provided by both exogenous ascorbic acid and endogenous phenolic compounds (Aguayo et al. 2010). Changes in antioxidant activity were measured using DPPH· and FRAP assays.

Apples and apple products are of special interest for Polish research teams because Poland processes more than 1.5 million tons of apples yearly, and the production of clear apple juice concentrate reaches 200,000 tons. Apple juice and apple flavoring do appear to be rising in popularity with a noticeable increase in apple drinks appearing on the EU markets. Apple juice is a widely consumed product, although the juice typically contains fewer phenolics than whole apples. The process of clear juice production has greater influence on the content of polyphenolic compounds than the variation of apple cultivars. Commercial technologies of processing are very effective, but most of the valuable bioactive compounds remained in the apple pomace, a waste product after juicing. After apple pulp enzyming, the juice contained 44% less chlorogenic acid and 58% less catechins. However, in the case of cloudy apple juice, the suppressing enzymatic browning conditions and the lack of clarification prevent loss of the polyphenols.

So, cloudy or clear apple juice? At present, clear apple juice is preferred because of the sense of purity it exudes. However, the marketing suggestion that clarity means purity is not rational in the case of apple juice and should be replaced by "cloudy means healthy." Health-conscious consumers looking to increase their overall well-being should drink the cloudy one. The complex process involved in developing a totally clear juice, which has taken years of scientific research to perfect, may no longer be needed if the latest research has enough power to change consumer choice. Reasoning behind cloudy juices apparently bringing far greater health benefits is a result of their higher polyphenol content. These antioxidants have been linked with protecting people from cancer, cardiovascular disease, and even Alzheimer's. According to the studies (Oszmiański et al. 2007), developing a clear solution causes a considerable reduction in the polyphenol content of the resulting juice, thereby lowering its antioxidant and free radical-scavenging activity. The information on high antioxidant activity of cloudy apple juice can help in marketing and promotion of this healthy product.

The apple purée is a valuable product, which can be used as intermediate material for production of nectars, juices with solid particles, apple sauce, baby foods, and many others. In industrial processes of apple purée production raw materials are cooked at 93°C–98°C for 4 to 5 min; it softens the fruit tissue and inactivates the enzyme responsible for enzymatic browning. The stability may be improved by the addition of vitamin C.

Apple pomace is a by-product of the apple processing industry and represents approximately 20%–35% of the original fruit. Disposal of apple pomace added costs to the beverage industry; its use as compost without any pretreatment may not be acceptable, and it is a poor animal feed because of its low protein content. For these reasons, exploration of potential alternative uses for this apple waste is needed. The high phenolic content and antioxidant activity qualify apple pomace as a valuable source of natural antioxidants and bioactive compounds (with antiviral activity). Apple pomace extracts were able to inhibit both HSV-1 and HSV-2 replication (Suárez et al. 2010). Methanolic and acetonic extracts from apple pomace were evaluated to compare their total phenolic content, phenolic profiles, and antioxidant capacity. In the industrial pomace, a total of 12 phenolic compounds (three phenolic acids and nine flavonoids) were identified. The predominant phenolic compounds were quercetin glycosides followed by dihydrochalcones. Minor compounds were phenolic acids, epicatechin, and procyanidin B2. The free radical-scavenging activity of apple pomace extracts was evaluated using the DPPH$^•$ and FRAP assays.

The apple skins as a waste product of the food industry are valuable sources of antioxidants (condensed tannins, anthocyanins, and other phenolics) and dietary fibers (cellulose, hemicellulose, lignin, and pectins). Solid-state NMR was used for characterization of micronized fiber powders from apples and anthocyanin-rich berries (Wawer et al. 2006). The ESR assay with DPPH$^•$ radical confirmed that the extracts of fibers have strong radical-scavenging properties. The scavenging capacity increased in the order apple < bilberry < blackcurrant < aronia in agreement with the increasing intensity of the phenolic signals in the ^{13}C CPMAS NMR spectra of the respective fibers. In conclusion, the dietary fibers with antioxidant properties may be interesting for functional food development.

13.3 DPPH$^•$ RADICAL SCAVENGING: SPECTROPHOTOMETRIC ASSAY

To assess the radical-scavenging activity of foods or food components, radical species, such as ABTS$^{•+}$ and DPPH$^•$, are usually used. They do not reproduce *in vivo*; however, they are useful in evaluating the antioxidant activity in a rapid and inexpensive way. Especially, the DPPH$^•$ radical-scavenging test became popular because it is technically simple and needs only a UV-Vis spectrophotometer to perform. In the presence of free radical-scavenging antioxidants (hydrogen or electron donors, although the assay is considered to be mainly based on an electron-transfer reaction), the absorption intensity is decreased, and the deep purple radical solution is discolored (yellow). However, in the case of color antioxidant compounds, such as carotenoids or anthocyanins having spectra that overlap the absorbance of DPPH$^•$, the use of electron spin resonance (ESR) spectroscopy is preferred.

The DPPH$^•$ assay can be performed in two versions: dynamic and static. In the dynamic version, the rate of DPPH$^•$ decay is measured after the addition of a sample containing phenolics. It characterizes the reactivity, and rate constants can be determined (Gaupy et al. 2003). In the static version, one determines the amount of DPPH$^•$ radical scavenged by a sample tested related to the stoichiometry for the reaction of the individual substance or the quantity of active OH-groups in a complex mixture. The percentage of scavenged DPPH$^\bullet$ is proportional to the antioxidant concentration, and the concentration that causes a decrease in the initial DPPH$^\bullet$ concentration by 50% is defined as EC_{50}. This parameter is independent of the sample concentration, but the time needed to reach the steady state should be determined. Besides reaction time, several factors may influence the method and the interpretation of the results, such as solvent, pH, and reagent concentrations. DPPH$^\bullet$ radicals can only be dissolved in organic solvents, and this fact could be an important limitation in the interpretation of hydrophilic antioxidant properties. All these problems are not discussed in sufficient depth in numerous papers. A standard procedure taking into account the sensitivity range of spectrophotometry was recommended (Sharma and Bhat 2009). Three common standard antioxidants (ascorbic acid, propyl gallate, BHT) have been tested, and their radical-scavenging EC_{50} values were influenced by the reaction medium (methanol, buffered methanol, ethanol).

It seemed worthwhile to show some characteristic features of the DPPH$^\bullet$ assays performed for apple products.

Polyphenols responsible for the antioxidant activity in apples are still present in the pomace. A range of polyphenolic compounds isolated from apple pomace, comprising phloridzin; 3-hydroxyphloridzin; chlorogenic acid; epicatechin; epicatechin dimer (procyanidin B2), trimer, tetramer, and oligomer; and quercetin glycosides, were evaluated (Lu and Foo 2000) for their antioxidant and DPPH$^\bullet$ radical-scavenging properties. The decrease in absorbance at 517 nm was measured every 15 min until the reaction reached a plateau, and the percentage of DPPH$^\bullet$ remaining at the steady state was calculated. The EC_{50} values showed that the DPPH$^\bullet$-scavenging activity decreased in the order quercetin glycosides > procyanidins $\gg$ chlorogenic acid, 3-hydroxyphloridzin $\gg$ phloridzin. All the quercetin glycosides had EC_{50} values of 0.10 ± 0.11, while the procyanidins had comparable or slightly higher EC_{50} values, indicating that these two classes of compounds were the most potent DPPH$^\bullet$ scavengers. Their radical-scavenging activity was significantly better than that of chlorogenic acid ($EC_{50} = 0.24$), the dihydrochalcones, and phloridzin. Procyanidin B2 (dimer) had an EC_{50} value of 0.06, but when calculated on a per epicatechin unit, $EC_{50} = 0.12$. In a similar manner, both the epicatechin trimer and tetramer had an EC_{50} of 0.115 on a per epicatechin unit basis and were slightly more effective scavengers than the dimer procyanidin B2, which, in turn, was superior to its monomer epicatechin ($EC_{50} = 0.135$). However, the higher epicatechin oligomers ($EC_{50} = 0.15$) showed the least activity in the epicatechin series, possibly as a result of increased crowding. In conclusion, all the polyphenols examined were found to possess good DPPH$^\bullet$-scavenging activity, and apple pomace, still underutilized, is a potential source of natural polyphenols for use as dietary or food antioxidants.

The DPPH$^\bullet$ radical-scavenging activity of apple juices was determined (Oszmiański et al. 2007) by measuring the absorbance at 517 nm. The juices are colored; thus, for reliable spectrophotometric measurements, background corrections for absorbance are necessary. The apple juices obtained from two apple cultivars differ in the content of total polyphenols, from 250 mg/L in clear juice of Idared to 1044 mg/L found in the cloudy one of Champion. The concentration of polymeric procyanidins was two to five times lower in clear juices. For example, the cloudy juice of Champion contained 523.8 mg/L of polymeric procyanidins, whereas their content in clear juice was only 197.5 mg/L. However, the higher content of procyanidins and other phenolic compounds in cloudy Champion juice was not reflected by the amount of scavenged DPPH˙ measured by spectrophotometry because the results differ only by 10%–25%. The corrections for background absorbances resulted in higher errors in the determination of concentration, but the most important obstacle is that the sample is not transparent as required.

The problem became more evident in the case of apple purées (Oszmiański et al. 2008). TAC assessed spectrophotometrically as measured by DPPH˙ free radical scavenging ranged from 0.16 to 0.81 mg/g purées of Trolox equivalent. The amount of scavenged DPPH˙ radicals should be proportional to the content of polyphenols in the sample unless antioxidant synergism or other reactions take place. The amount of scavenged DPPH˙ measured by spectrophotometry remained almost unchanged up to approximately 100 mg of polyphenols, whereas at a higher concentration, the data became scarce (Figure 13.1a).

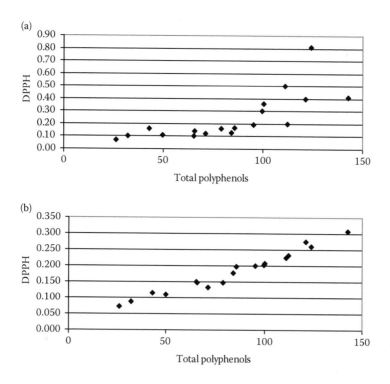

FIGURE 13.1   DPPH˙ radical-scavenging capacity (mg of Trolox equivalent) measured by UV-Vis (a) and ESR spectroscopy (b) versus total polyphenol content (mg/100 g) in apple purées. (From Oszmiański J., Wolniak M., Wojdyło A., and Wawer I.: Influence of apple puree preparation and storage on polyphenol contents and antioxidant activity. *Food Chem.* 2008. 107. 1473–1484. Copyright Wiley-VCH Verlag GmbH & Co. KGaA. Reproduced with permission.)

It is obvious that the spectrophotometric method is not reliable for cloudy juices or purées.

13.4 DPPH' RADICAL SCAVENGING: ESR ASSAY

13.4.1 ESR STUDIES OF APPLE JUICE

Estimating the percentage of scavenged DPPH' radicals using ESR, it became evident that this method is better for assessment of antiradical properties of cloudy and color materials. ESR spectroscopy directly measures the free radical concentration, and the relationship between the signal height and the amount of polyphenols is linear (Figure 13.1b).

Therefore, the radical-scavenging capacity of apple juices was estimated by ESR. Usually, the reaction of DPPH' with an efficient flavonoid antioxidant proceeds very quickly (within seconds). The kinetics of this reaction was investigated using stopped-flow absorption spectroscopy (Madsen et al. 2000), and the majority of the rate data were in seconds; only the reactions with hesperetin, naringenin, and chrysin were slow ($t_{1/2} > 1000$ s). The slow reaction might be expected in the presence of weak antioxidants (with a small number of OH groups, such as chrysin) or polymerized ones.

The reactions of apple polyphenolics with DPPH' were not completed after 2 to 5 min, and the decay of ESR spectrum of DPPH' radicals upon the addition of apple juice had to be followed for 30 min or longer (Figure 13.2).

At the beginning, the reaction DPPH' + Ar-OH → DPPH-H + Ar-O' is very fast and proceeds according to the second-order kinetics. After approximately 7 min, the radical reactions slow down and follow the first-order kinetics. Other, less active scavengers as well as secondary reaction products slowly decrease the amount of DPPH'. The first-order kinetic equation was fitted using nonlinear regression analysis, and the pseudo first-order rate constants (k_{obs}) were obtained. The calculated rate constants are in the range of 0.47–1.45 s^{-1} for clear juices and 1.61–4.11 s^{-1} for cloudy ones and are larger for juices with a higher content of procyanidins. The linear relationship holds: $k_{obs} = 0.08X + 0.06$, where X is the concentration of polymeric procyanidins (mmol/L).

Procyanidins and larger condensed polymeric compounds present in apple juice seemed to be responsible for the long reaction time with DPPH'. Additionally, these compounds may exhibit a variety of radical-scavenging mechanisms.

The ESR spectrum illustrated in Figure 13.3 shows the overlapping lines of two radicals: the decaying DPPH' and remaining a long-living one. This radical, probably a product of the reaction of DPPH' with polymers, is more stable because of the steric obstacles. The spectrum of an oxygen-centered radical, such as a phenoxy radical, is expected at $g = 2.0036$. The intensity of the signal registered after 20 min was proportional to the content of procyanidins, suggesting that these compounds are responsible for the formation of long-living radical species.

It supports the assumption that procyanidins are a major group of compounds responsible for the antioxidant and radical-scavenging activities of apple juices.

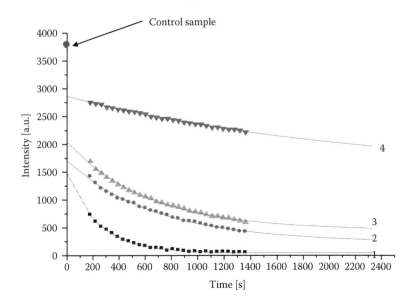

FIGURE 13.2 Decay of DPPH˙ signal (measured in Bruker ELEXSYS E 500 spectrometer) in time after addition of apple juices (1: Champion cloudy, 2: Champion clear, 3: Idared cloudy, 4: Idared clear). The fitted curves were obtained by nonlinear regression, using the equation for a first-order reaction. (From Oszmiański J., Wolniak M., Wojdyło A., and Wawer I.: Comparative study of polyphenolic content and antiradical activity of cloudy and clear apple juices. *J Sci Food Agric.* 2007. 87. 573–579. Copyright Wiley-VCH Verlag GmbH & Co. KGaA. Reproduced with permission.)

Among apple-based beverages, natural cloudy apple juices contain the highest polyphenol amounts. A growing market for natural cloudy apple juice over the last few years (2008–2010) has been observed. For that reason, cloudy juices are the focus of nutrition research. The technological problem of these juices is to stabilize the cloudiness during storage. Because juice particles are negatively charged, the addition of negatively charged colloids, such as carboxymethyl cellulose (CMC) or Arabic gum, in concentrations as low as 0.05% may completely inhibit apple juice clarification.

Studies of the stability and antiradical activity of cloudy apple juice after the treatment with various additives were performed (Ibrahim et al. 2011). The content of total phenolics in fresh and treated cloudy apple juices was determined by the Folin-Ciocalteu assay. The antioxidant activity was evaluated using DPPH˙ free radical-scavenging spectrophotometric and ESR assays. The DPPH˙ radical-scavenging capacity of apple juices was calculated using the height of the second peak in the ESR spectrum of the DPPH˙ radical of the blank and the probe, respectively. Such an approach enables researchers to avoid the problem of long-living radicals overlapping the central peak (see above), although the authors did not report its appearance. The sample treated with a phenol concentrate of apple pomace demonstrated the strongest activity of radical scavenging (95.7%)

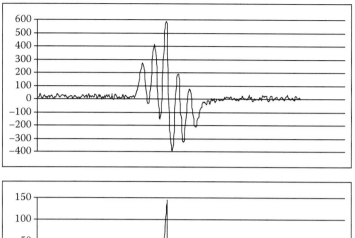

FIGURE 13.3 ESR spectra of DPPH⁺ radical after addition of cloudy apple juice registered after 180 s (upper spectrum) and radical recorded after 1361 s (lower spectrum). (From Oszmiański J., Wolniak M., Wojdyło A., and Wawer I.: Comparative study of polyphenolic content and antiradical activity of cloudy and clear apple juices. *J Sci Food Agric*. 2007. 87. 573–579. Copyright Wiley-VCH Verlag GmbH & Co. KGaA. Reproduced with permission.)

followed by pectin (87.4%), xanthan (70.2%), and CMC. The scavenging activities decrease with prolonged storage time. The addition of phenolic compounds from apple pomace efficiently prevents phenolic degradation during storage of the juice. Therefore, the extract of apple pomace has potential as a value-added ingredient for functional foods.

13.4.2   ESR Studies of Apple Purée

The beneficial effects of apples on health may be better achieved by consuming products that contain not only liquid but also the solid part of the raw material. This kind of product is, for example, the apple purée. The concentrations of phenolic compounds in the purées are related to their content in raw apples but also resulted from the oxidation reactions they undergo during processing. The control of purée oxidation and browning has always been a challenge for the processing industry, and the use of a chemical antioxidant (e.g., ascorbic acid) and high temperature are the most common solutions. The objective of the study (Oszmiański et al. 2008) was to monitor the composition of polyphenols and the antioxidant activity of apple purée during its production and storage.

The amounts of phenolics were determined by HPLC. Microwave heating gave a significant increase in the concentration of chlorogenic acid, polymeric procyanidins, phloretin-2'-glucoside, and quercetin glycosides. During storage (for 3 and 6 months), significant changes were observed in the concentration of procyanidins and cyanidin-3-galactoside.

The intensity of the ESR signal of DPPH$^{\bullet}$ after the addition of methanolic extract of the apple purée was measured after 3 and 30 min. The first-order kinetic equation was fitted using nonlinear regression analysis, and the calculated pseudo first-order rate constants k_{obs} are within 1.5–11.5 s^{-1}.

It seemed interesting to examine the apple purée in detail and to identify the most active radical scavengers among the components. The HPLC method enabled the identification of 18 individual phenolic constituents. An attempt has been made to estimate the influence of particular compounds on the TAC and radical-scavenging activity. Different preparation methods and storage times yielded a sufficient number of variables for multiple regression analysis. The linear model relating compositional data to antioxidant capacity can be written as

$$A = b_0 + b_1 X_1 + b_2 X_2 + \cdots + b_{16} X_{16}$$

where A is the ESR signal intensity measured after 3 or 30 min, and X_n denotes the concentration of particular compounds. Multiple regression analyses performed with A as a dependent variable and up to 15 phenolic constituents of apple purée as the independent variables showed that only few components have significant influence on the ESR signal intensity (Table 13.1). Among the most active are chlorogenic acid, epicatechin, and procyanidins. Although polymerized procyanidins occur in the highest concentration, their impact on A was not the highest ($b_5 = 0.252$) after 3 min, suggesting different radical-scavenging properties. When the measurement is performed after 3 min, radical-scavenging activity depends upon the concentration of six phenolic constituents, namely, chlorogenic acid, (–)-epicatechin, procyanidin B2 and C1, polymeric procyanidins, and quercetin galactoside:

$$A = -0.013 + 0.271 \, X_1 + 0.186 \, X_2 + 0.322 \, X_3 + 0.105 \, X_4 + 0.252 \, X_5 + 0.062 \, X_6$$

Considering the progress of the reaction after a prolonged time, the contributions of these compounds appear to be different, and the radical-scavenging activity can be better reproduced as

$$A = -0.007 + 0.052 \, X_1 + 0.036 \, X_2 + 0.062 \, X_3 + 0.020 \, X_4 + 0.870 \, X_5 + 0.012 \, X_6$$

This clearly shows that the influence of nonpolymeric compounds decreases, and the polymerized procyanidins are mainly responsible for the antioxidant activity of apple purées when the measurements are done after 10 min or later as indicated by the value of $b_5 = 0.870$.

TABLE 13.1

Multiple Regression Analysis Relating Selected Phenolics to Antioxidant Activity of Apple Purée

	Variable	Coefficient b	SE	t	P
	Intensity of DPPH· Signal Measured after 3 min				
1	Chlorogenic acid	**0.271**	0.063	12.90	**0.006**
2	(–)-epicatechin	**0.186**	0.103	5.43	**0.032**
3	Procyanidins B2	**0.322**	0.041	23.83	**0.002**
4	Procyanidins C1	**0.105**	0.065	4.82	**0.040**
5	Polymeric procyanidins	**0.252**	0.045	16.90	**0.003**
6	Quercetin-3-O-galactose	0.062	0.013	14.16	0.005
	Intensity of DPPH· Signal Measured after 30 min				
1	Chlorogenic acid	0.052	0.012	12.90	0.006
2	(–)-epicatechin	0.036	0.020	5.43	0.032
3	Procyanidins B2	0.062	0.008	23.83	0.002
4	Procyanidins C1	0.020	0.012	4.82	0.040
5	Polymeric procyanidins	**0.870**	0.009	304.46	**< 0.001**
6	Quercetin-3-O-galactose	0.012	0.003	14.16	0.005

Source: Oszmiański J. et al., *Food Chem* 107, 1473–1484, 2008.

13.5 CUPRAC ASSAY FOR APPLE JUICE

The variant of the FRAP assay using Cu instead of Fe has been introduced as the cupric ion reducing antioxidant capacity (CUPRAC) method. The assay is based on the reduction of Cu(II) to Cu(I) by the combined action of all antioxidants in a sample. The CUPRAC assay using neocuproine copper complex as the chromogenic reagent is simple, applicable to both hydrophilic and lipophilic antioxidants.

The CUPRAC assay has been recently applied to the study of apple juices of selected apples grown in Turkey (Karaman et al. 2010). The TAC of apple juices was comparatively assayed with the CUPRAC and the ABTS methods. For rapid identification and quantification of individual antioxidants in the juices, HPLC analysis was optimized using synthetic mixtures of antioxidants. The CUPRAC method was first applied to antioxidant standards that possibly exist in apple juice, namely, ascorbic acid, gallic acid, procyanidin B2, catechin, epicatechin, chlorogenic acid, caffeic acid, phloridzin, rutin, isoquercitrin, and quercetin using Trolox as the reference. The essential phenolics that could be quantified in apple juices were catechin, epicatechin, chlorogenic acid, caffeic acid, and phloridzin.

Theoretical TAC was assessed as

$$(TAC) = \sum_i C_i TEAC_i$$

where C_i is the concentration of constituent (i) measured by HPLC; $TEAC_i$ is the TEAC coefficient of constituent (i) measured by the spectrophotometric method.

The theoretically calculated TAC values using the combined HPLC/CUPRAC or HPLC/ABTS methods were lower than the corresponding experimental TAC values because only the HPLC-identifiable constituents were taken into account. There were a few peaks in the chromatograms, which could not be identified because of the lack of appropriate standards. The TAC of HPLC-quantified compounds accounted for between 40% and 70% of the observed CUPRAC capacities of apple juices with respect to apple varieties. Excluding two apple cultivars, Lutz Golden and Granny Smith, which have more unidentified constituents, the approach was capable of estimating 70% of the observed capacity.

The CUPRAC assay is complete in minutes for ascorbic acid, gallic acid, or quercetin, but requires 30 to 60 min for more complex molecules. Thus, the copper reduction assays have similar problems as DPPH$^\bullet$ assays with a complex mixture of antioxidants in terms of selecting an appropriate reaction time.

13.6 PARAMETERS CHARACTERIZING THE ANTIOXIDANT AND FREE RADICAL-SCAVENGING ACTIVITY

By definition, the antioxidant activity is the capability of a compound (mixture) to inhibit oxidative degradation. Although antioxidant activity of polyphenols is associated with various mechanisms, the elevated reactivity of phenolics toward active free radicals is considered as the fundamental mechanism. We should distinguish between the antioxidant capacity (gives the information about the duration of antioxidative action) and the reactivity (characterizes the starting dynamics).

As widely discussed, methods applied to the evaluation of natural antioxidants lack standardization and produce confusing results when working with complex substrates (Frankel and Finley 2008). For example, a nonlinear relationship between the antioxidant concentration and the radical-scavenging activity makes the measurement of the EC_{50} problematic. A method of calculation of the EC_{50} of antioxidants in the DPPH$^\bullet$ radical-scavenging assay has been proposed (Locatelli et al. 2009) together with mathematical software to process the data. The method was employed to compare the antiradical activity of different natural food extracts: phenolic-reach cocoa beans, cocoa hulls, hazelnut skins, and sweet peppers. Even if the extracts show similar EC_{50} values, their antiradical activity curves are totally different. The antioxidant activity appears to be related to the concentration: For the lower concentrations, cocoa hulls were more effective than red peppers, but after the EC_{50}, this trend was inverted. So the EC_{50} parameter is useful but cannot adequately discriminate the antioxidant activity. The differences can be expressed by the parameters describing the corresponding straight lines, namely, the slope a and the intercept with the y-axis b or both the intercepts.

A crucial parameter that could be given together with the EC_{50} value is b (intercept on y-axis).

The rate of reaction is an important parameter for the evaluation of the antioxidant activity, particularly in the case of complex food extracts in which synergistic effects can occur. Another method (Sanchez-Moreno et al. 1998) introduced to express antioxidant activity in the DPPH$^{\bullet}$ assay is the calculation of the antiradical efficiency, AE, defined as $AE = 1/(EC_{50} T_{EC50})$, where T_{EC50} is the reaction time needed to reach the steady state.

The empirical model based on the cumulative function of Weibull's equation was proposed (Murado and Vazquez 2010); it allows the inclusion of the effects of any number of antioxidant concentrations and evaluation of the whole system. The dose of antioxidants, the exposure times, and the size of the experimental unit should be standardized. The parameter τ providing the substrate half-life at a given concentration of the antioxidant is the most important parameter and the most robust. The model enables researchers to estimate the antioxidant concentration necessary for duplicating substrate half-life, the maximum substrate oxidation rate at a given antioxidant concentration, the lag time of the substrate oxidation resulting from the presence of antioxidants, and the action interval (the time that elapses to a given concentration of antioxidants until the conversion of 99% of the substrate). An efficient way to formulate the model is to consider jointly the kinetic series in the presence of all the antioxidant concentrations assayed. By means of this approach, the simultaneous solution of all the kinetics is achieved.

The verification of the multidimensional model with experimental data requires knowledge of the concentrations of all active compounds present in a sample. Plant materials contain thousands of low molecular weight metabolites, which are characteristic for the properties, including antioxidant ones. Proton nuclear magnetic resonance (^{1}H NMR) spectroscopy has become a powerful technique in metabolic profiling and fingerprinting. The advantages of ^{1}H NMR are as follows (1) sample preparation is minimal when compared to HPLC, and (2) the principal component analysis (PCA) can be applied to the spectral NMR data to explore any clustering behavior of the samples. A recent study (Bertram et al. 2010) demonstrated the feasibility of ^{1}H NMR spectroscopy to characterize the metabolite profile of legumes and to perform a high-throughput analysis.

Assessment of the antioxidant capacity of food matrices requires the parallel use of several methods, based on different mechanisms, because no single method is adequate. To standardize reports on antioxidant capacity, four assays have been proposed (Tabart et al. 2009) based on different principles: DPPH$^{\bullet}$ or TEAC (reducing capacity), ORAC (peroxyl radical-scavenging capacity), hemolysis (protection of cells), and ESR (free radical evaluation). A simple mathematical mean is not adequate because two methods (ORAC and ESR) gave much higher values because of the poor performance of Trolox in these assays. A global antioxidant capacity should be calculated as a weighted mean of the results obtained by the four assays. This strategy was used to test the antioxidant capacity of several beverages. The highest antioxidant capacity was observed for red wine, followed by green tea, orange juice, grape juice, vegetable juice, and apple juice. Although the DPPH$^{\bullet}$ results were almost always lower than the others, the results of the TEAC, ORAC, and hemolysis assays were quite similar in the case of apple juice. Red wine showed the best antioxidant capacity regardless of the method used. It would be interesting to know the type of compounds responsible for the antioxidant capacity.

In conclusion, methods for evaluating antioxidant activity suffer the lack of standardization. Under these conditions, many of the experimental data are incomplete, which prevents suitable characterization of the relevant properties of the tested compounds. Bioactive phytochemicals found in plant-based foods exhibit many biological properties that are not necessarily correlated with their antioxidant capacity, including acting as signaling molecules or as gene-expression modulators. Thus, a food low in antioxidant content may have beneficial health effects resulting from other food components or other mechanisms. However, the ultimate goal of the studies still remains: to understand the role of dietary antioxidants in the prevention of cancer, cardiovascular diseases, diabetes, and other chronic diseases related to oxidative stress.

REFERENCES

Aguayo E., Requejo-Jackman C., Stanley R., and Woolf A. 2010. Effects of calcium ascorbate treatments and storage atmosphere on antioxidant activity and quality of fresh-cut apple slices. *Postharvest Biol Technol* 57: 52–60.

Bertram H. Ch., Weisbjerg M. R., Jensen Ch. S., Pedersen M. G., Didion T., Pedersen B. O., Duus J. O., Larsen M. K., and Nielsen J. H. 2010. Seasonal changes in the metabolic fingerprint of 21 grass and legume cultivars studied by nuclear magnetic resonance-based metabolomics. *J Agric Food Chem* 58: 4336–4341.

Carlsen M. H., Halvorsen B. L., Holte K., Bøhn S. K., Dragland S., Sampson L., Willey C., Senoo Y., Umezono H., Sanada C., Barikmo I., Berhe N., Willett W. C., Phillips K. M., Jacobs D. R. Jr., and Blomhoff R. 2010. The total antioxidant content of more than 3100 foods, beverages, spices, herbs and supplements used worldwide. *Nutr J* 9: 3.

Frankel E. N., and Finley J. W. 2008. How to standardize the multiplicity of methods to evaluate natural antioxidants. *J Agric Food Chem* 56: 4901–4908.

Gallus S., Talamini R., Giacosa A., Montella M., Ramazzotti V., Franceschi S., Negri E., and La Vecchia C. 2005. Does an apple a day keep the oncologist away? *Ann Oncol* 16: 1841–1844.

Gaupy P., Dufcur C., Loonis H., and Dangles O. 2003. Quantitative kinetic analysis of hydrogen atom transfer reactions from dietary polyphenols to the DPPH⋅ radical. *J Agric Food Chem* 51: 615–622.

Halvorsen B. L., Carlsen M. H., Phillips K. M., Bøhn S. K., Holte K., Jacobs D. R. Jr., and Blomhoff R. 2006. Content of redox-active compounds (i.e., antioxidants) in foods consumed in the United States. *Am J Clin Nutr* 84: 95–135.

Ibrahim G. E., Hassan I. M., Abd-Elrashid A. M., El-Massry K. F., Eh-Ghorab A. H., Manal M. R., and Osman F. 2011. Effect of clouding agents on the quality of apple juice during storage. *Food Hydrocoll* 25: 91–97.

Karaman S., Tütem E., Baskan K. S., and Apak R. 2010. Comparison of total antioxidant capacity and phenolic composition of some apple juices with combined HPLC–CUPRAC assay. *Food Chem* 120: 1201–1209.

Locatelli M., Gindro R., Travaglia F., Cod'sson J.-D., Rinaldi M., and Arlorio M. 2009. Study of the DPPH-scavenging activity: Development of a free software for the correct interpretation of data. *Food Chem* 114: 889–897.

Lu Y., and Foo L. Y. 2000. Antioxidant and radical scavenging activities of polyphenols from apple pomace. *Food Chem* 68: 81–85.

Madsen H. L., Andersen C. M., Jørgensen L. V., and Skibsted L. H. 2000. Radical scavenging by dietary flavonoids: A kinetic study of antioxidant efficiencies. *Eur Food Res Technol* 211: 240–246.

Murado M. A., and Vazquez J. A. 2010. Mathematical model for the characterization and objective comparison of antioxidant activities. *J Agric Food Chem* 58: 1622–1629.

Oszmiański J., Wolniak M., Wojdyło A., and Wawer I. 2007. Comparative study of polyphenolic content and antiradical activity of cloudy and clear apple juices. *J Sci Food Agric* 87: 573–579.

Oszmiański J., Wolniak M., Wojdyło A., and Wawer I. 2008. Influence of apple puree preparation and storage on polyphenol contents and antioxidant activity. *Food Chem* 107: 1473–1484.

Pellegrini N., Serafini M., Salvatore S., Del Rio D., Bianchi M., and Brighenti F. 2006. Total antioxidant capacity of spices, dried fruits, nuts, pulses, cereals and sweets consumed in Italy assessed by three different *in vitro* assays. *Mol Nutr Food Res* 50: 1030–1038.

Sanchez-Moreno C., Larrauri J. A., and Saura-Calixto F. 1998. A procedure to measure the antiradical efficiency of polyphenols. *J Sci Food Agric* 76: 270–276.

Sharma O. P., and Bhat T. K. 2009. DPPH• antioxidant assay revisited. *Food Chem* 113: 1202–1205.

Suárez B., Álvarez Á. L., García Y. D., del Barrio G., Lobo A. P., and Parra F. 2010. Phenolic profiles, antioxidant activity and *in vitro* antiviral properties of apple pomace. *Food Chem* 120: 339–342.

Tabart J., Kevers C., Pincemail J., Defraigne J.-O., and Dommesa J. 2009. Comparative antioxidant capacities of phenolic compounds measured by various tests. *Food Chem* 113: 1226–1233.

Wawer I., Wolniak M., and Paradowska K. 2006. Solid state NMR of dietary fiber powders from aronia, bilberry, black currant and apple. *Solid State NMR* 30: 106–113.

Wu X., Beecher G. R., Holden J. M., Haytowitz D. B., Gebhardt S. E., and Prior R. L. 2004. Lipophilic and hydrophilic antioxidant capacities of common foods in the United States. *J Agric Food Chem* 52: 4026–4037.

14 Antioxidant and Prooxidant Activity of Food Components

Anna Gliszczyńska-Świgło and Jan Oszmiański

CONTENTS

14.1 INTRODUCTION

Food, especially of plant origin, contains a variety of antioxidant components that can prevent or delay oxidative processes occurring in food. There is also evidence that excessive free radicals in cells and tissues are the causative agents behind some chronic diseases, such as cardiovascular disease and some forms of cancer, and aging. Free radicals are normal species produced during the body's metabolic processes, but if they get out of balance, highly reactive forms of the free radicals can cause oxidative damage to biological systems. Conditions of oxidative stress may be prevented or delayed by the consumption of dietary antioxidants—"substances in foods that significantly decrease the adverse effects of reactive species, such as reactive oxygen and nitrogen species, on normal physiological function in humans," as defined by the Institute of Medicine (Huang et al. 2005). These natural food antioxidants include, for example, antioxidant vitamins (tocopherols and ascorbic acid), plant phenolics, and thiol antioxidants (e.g., glutathione, lipoic acid). Other micronutrients that are involved include some carotenoids, selenium, zinc, and folates (vitamin B9) (Godfrey and Richardson 2002). Some literature data suggest also the antioxidant activity of other water-soluble vitamins (Senapati et al. 2000; Joshi et al. 2001; Nakano et al. 2001; Jung and Kim 2003; Rezk et al. 2003; Stocker et al. 2003; Gliszczyńska-Świgło 2006, 2007; Gliszczyńska-Świgło and Muzolf 2007).

Food antioxidants impair oxidation via different mechanisms, such as free radical scavenging, metal chelating, metal reduction, and antioxidant interactions, within the antioxidant network. They may also function indirectly as antioxidants through their effect on transcription factors and enzyme activities. The effectiveness of natural antioxidants in food and in the human body is dependent on many factors, including water or lipid solubility, stability, matrix interactions, and bioavailability. For antioxidant-type food ingredients at higher doses prooxidant actions may become of importance.

14.2 ANTIOXIDANT AND PROOXIDANT ACTIVITY OF PLANT PHENOLICS

The term "phenolics" covers a very large and diverse group of compounds having one or more hydroxyl groups attached directly to an aromatic ring. There are more than 8000 various phenolic structures, from simple molecules, for example, phenolic acids with C6 ring structure, to highly polymerized compounds, for example, tannins (Kris-Etherton et al. 2002). According to Harborne and Simmonds (1964), they are classified into groups based on the number of carbons in the molecule. The main classes of phenolic compounds present in food are shown in Table 14.1 (Vermerris and Nicholson 2006).

Phenolics are widely distributed in the flowers, leaves, bark, and seeds of edible plants; thus, they are an integral part of the human diet. The content of polyphenols in food may range from 2 to 7500 mg/kg or mg/L (Manach et al. 2004). They exhibit a wide range of chemical and biological effects, including (1) antioxidant (radical-scavenging) activity; (2) the ability to chelate metal ions, such as iron or copper; and (3) the ability to induce or modulate the activity of different enzyme systems. These properties are often claimed to be responsible for antibacterial, antiviral, anti-inflammatory, antiallergic, and vasodilatory actions; inhibition of lipid peroxidation; platelet aggregation; and capillary permeability and fragility (Cook and Samman 1996). They have been reported to protect against cardiovascular and photosensitivity-related diseases, aging, and various forms of cancer (Middleton and Kandaswami 1993; Crespy and Williamson 2004; Galvano et al. 2004; Prior and Gu 2005; Arts and Hollman 2005; Stevenson and Hurst 2007; Tripoli et al. 2007).

TABLE 14.1

Main Classes of Phenolic Compounds, Their Dietary Sources, and Main Representatives

Basic Skeleton/ Chemical Structure	Class	Dietary Sources	Main Representatives
C6–C1	Benzoic acids and aldehydes	Berries, cereals, herbs, and spices	4-Hydroxybenzoic, gallic, protocatechuic, salicylic, vanillic, gentisic, and ellagic acids; vanillin
C6–C3	Cinnamic acids	Apple, cherry, plum, berries, tomato, asparagus, white grape, and herbs	p-Coumaric, caffeic, ferulic, sinapic, and chlorogenic acids
C15 (C6–C3–C6)	Flavonoids	See Table 14.3	See Table 14.3
C6–C2–C6	Stilbenes	Grapes and wine	Resveratrol
C18	Betacyanins	Red beet and opuntia	Betanin and isobetanin
Dimers or oligomers	Lignans	Flaxseed, sesame seed, cereals, legumes, berries, and vegetables	Secoisolariciresinol, secoisolariciresinol diglucoside, isolariciresinol, pinoresinol, and matairesinol
Oligomers or polymers	Tannins	Apples, berries, grapes, and red wine	Procyanidins B1, B2, B3, B4, C, gallotannins, and ellagitannins

14.2.1 Metabolism and Bioavailability of Polyphenols

The estimation of average daily intake of polyphenols by humans is rather difficult because of the lack of comprehensive and uniform nutrient databases related to polyphenol content in food, taking into account species and variety differences, as well as the influence of cultivation and technological conditions during plant growth and processing. It was estimated that depending on region and nutrition habits, the average daily intake of flavonoids is 50–800 mg (Miranda et al. 2000), for example, estimated mean daily total flavonoid intake in US adults is 189.7 mg/day and is mainly from flavan-3-ols (83.5%), followed by flavanones (7.6%), flavonols (6.8%), anthocyanidins (1.6%), flavones (0.8%), and isoflavones (0.6%). The total polyphenol intake probably commonly reaches up to 1 g/day in people who eat several servings of fruit and vegetables per day (Manach et al. 2004). Major sources of polyphenols are beverages (coffee, tea, wine, fruit and vegetable juices) as well as legumes (Chun et al. 2007).

Biological properties of polyphenols depend on their absorption, metabolism, and distribution. The rate and extent of absorption and the nature of metabolites occurring in the plasma or urine are dependent mainly on the chemical structure of the polyphenols (e.g., glycosylation, esterification, and polymerization) and the food matrix. Polyphenols that are the most common in the human diet are not necessarily the most active in the body. This is because of low intrinsic activity or poor absorption, high metabolism, or rapid elimination. Moreover, the biological activity of polyphenol metabolites found in the blood or target organs or their degradation products may significantly differ from the activity of the native compound (Manach et al. 2004).

Polyphenols are mainly absorbed in the small intestine, although, for some flavonoids, absorption from the stomach was also observed (Crespy et al. 2002). Absorption of polyphenols is mainly limited by their solubility. The partition coefficient (log octanol/water), which measures the relative affinity of a compound for organic and aqueous phases (hydrophobicity/hydrophilicity of the compound) for flavonoid aglycones, is not higher than 4 (Yang et al. 2001; Rothwell et al. 2005). Food flavonoids, except flavan-3-ols, are usually glycosylated, and their hydrophilicity is higher than their aglycones. This limits the transport of glucosylated flavonoids across the stomach or small intestine brush border by passive diffusion. Two mechanisms are postulated for glycosylated flavonoid absorption. The first step in the metabolism of glycosylated flavonoids is enzyme deglycosylation by β-glycosidases and then diffusion of aglycones across the cell membrane into the enterocyte. According to the second mechanism, glycosides may enter the enterocytes as intact glycosides via the sodium-dependent glucose transporters (SGLT1) (Gee et al. 1998; Walgren et al. 2000; Walle et al. 2000; Walle and Walle 2003). The intracellular cytosolic β-glycosidases and lactase phloridzin hydrolase release aglycone from its glycosylated form; the aglycone may be subsequently conjugated with glucuronic acid by uridine-5′-diphosphate-glucuronyltransferases (UGT, UDPGT) or with sulfuric acid by phenol sulfotransferases (PST) (Day et al. 1998; Scalbert and Williamson 2000). Moreover, catechol-O-methyltransferase (COMT) may methylate polyphenols. It has been estimated that 90%–95% of absorbed polyphenols are converted to conjugates (Clifford 2004). The aglycone and/or its metabolites enter the bloodstream or can be transported back to the intestinal lumen by specific transporter proteins, such as BCRP1/ABCG2 (breast cancer resistance protein) or multidrug resistance-associated protein 2 (MRP2) (Walle et al. 1999; Imai et al. 2004; Sesink et al. 2005). Anthocyanins are absorbed in glycosylated forms from both the stomach (Passamonti et al. 2003; Talavera et al. 2003) and small intestine (Miyazawa et al. 1999; Talavera et al. 2004), and bilitranslocase was identified as the carrier protein involved (Passamonti et al. 2003, 2005). They circulate in the blood and urine mainly as intact glycosides, methylated, glucurono-, and/or sulfoconjugated forms (Cao et al. 2001; Matsumoto et al. 2001; Wu et al. 2002; Felgines et al. 2003; Kay et al. 2004, 2005).

Flavan-3-ols (catechins), such as (–)-epicatechin, are often acylated, especially by gallic acid, but galloyl substitution changes the partition coefficient only slightly and does not influence their bioavailability as dramatically as glycosylation (Scalbert and Williamson 2000). Hydroxycinnamates, such as ferulic and caffeic acids, are also commonly esterified to sugars, organic acids, and lipids. Esterases with the ability to hydrolyze hydroxycinnamate esters at appreciable rates have been described in humans and rats (Andreason et al. 2001), but the significant site for, for example, chlorogenic acid (ester of caffeic acid and quinic acid) metabolism is the colonic microflora (Plumb et al. 1999; Scalbert and Williamson 2000).

Little is known about the structural features that affect the bioavailability and metabolism of proanthocyanidins. According to Holt et al. (2002) and Sano et al. (2003), the absorption of procyanidins B2 and B1 from a cocoa beverage and grape-seed extract is fast but minor. However, these compounds may have a direct effect on the intestinal mucosa and protect it against oxidative stress and the action of car-cinogens (Manach et al. 2005). It has been shown that plasma antioxidant capacity is increased after the consumption of proanthocyanidin-rich foods, such as cocoa, red wine, or grapeseed extracts (Williamson and Manach 2005).

As mentioned above, polyphenols are extensively metabolized by intestinal and hepatic enzymes and by intestinal microflora. They circulate in the blood and are excreted in urine mainly as methylated, glucurono-, and/or sulfoconjugated forms or as intact glycosides (e.g., anthocyanins) (Wu et al. 2002; Felgines et al. 2003; Kay et al. 2004, 2005; Tripoli et al. 2007). Many polyphenols are broken down into sim-pler phenolic compounds common to various polyphenols (Scalbert and Williamson 2000). The levels of individual flavonoids in fecal water was found to be very low (0.05 to 1.2 µM or even less), whereas monophenol breakdown products of flavonoids are present at much higher concentrations (from 19 to 479 µM) (Jenner et al. 2005; Halliwell 2007).

Animal studies revealed that flavonoids might be present in different organs. Quercetin and quercetin metabolites were widely distributed in rat and pig tissues, mainly in the lungs, liver, and kidneys (de Boer et al. 2005). Anthocyanins were found in digestive system organs (stomach, jejunum, and liver), in excretory tissue (kid-neys), and in the brain of rats fed with a blackberry extract-enriched diet (Talavera et al. 2005). The parent anthocyanins were detected in the stomach, whereas the jejunum, liver, and kidneys contained native, methylated, and glucuronidated antho-cyanins. The jejunum and plasma of rats also contained aglycone forms (Talavera et al. 2005). The presence of intact anthocyanins in the brain of anesthetized rats was reported by Passamonti et al. (2005). Mohsen et al. (2006) demonstrated that metabolites of anthocyanins, such as aglycons, could reach different tissues, includ-ing the brain. The aglycone form (cyanidin) was also present in the jejunum accord-ing to Tsuda et al. (1999). Other flavonoids were also found in various mouse and rat tissues (Suganuma et al. 1998; Chang et al. 2000; Coldham and Sauer 2000; Kim et al. 2000; Datla et al. 2001; Abd et al. 2002; Mullen et al. 2002; Vitrac et al. 2003).

The concentration of polyphenols or their metabolites in serum may range from 0 to approximately 10 µmol/L, and their secretion with urine ranges from 0.02% to 63% depending on the nature of polyphenol and the food source. Time to reach maximal circulatory concentration varies from several minutes to up to 20 h. The half-life for disappearance from circulation ranges from 1.3 h for naringenin and gallic acid up to 28 h for flavonoids from onions (Manach et al. 2005; Stevenson and Hurst 2007). Isoflavones are the best-absorbed flavonoids, whereas the bioavailabil-ity of anthocyanins was reported to be very poor (Lapidot et al. 1998; Manach et al.

2004). Only 0.02%–1.8% of the ingested anthocyanin doses are excreted unchanged or as metabolites. According to Fleschhut et al. (2006), the gut microflora seems to play an important role in the biotransformation of anthocyanins. The bacterial biotransformation leads to the cleavage of the sugar moiety, leading to the formation of the anthocyanin aglycone. The aglycone could be further metabolized by the bacteria or degraded chemically to the phenolic acids. Seeram et al. (2001) confirmed that protocatechuic acid was the predominant degradation product of cyanidin in a cell culture study. The instability of anthocyanidins at physiological pH could explain their absence or low presence in plasma (Miyazawa et al. 1999; Tsuda et al. 1999; Talavera et al. 2005). This instability may also limit the detection of these compounds. Another conceivable pathway is the reaction of anthocyanins with reactive macromolecules, such as free thiols and/or amino groups of proteins (Fleschhut et al. 2006). These two pathways may partially explain the results of many studies indicating the poor bioavailability of anthocyanins.

14.2.2 Antioxidant Properties of Plant Phenolics

14.2.2.1 Hydroxybenzoic and Cinnamic Acids

The most important hydroxybenzoic acids that are present in various fruits and occur mostly as esters are 4-hydroxybenzoic acid, 2-hydroxybenzoic acid (salicylic acid), 2,4-dihydroxybenzoic acid (gentisic acid), 3,4-dihydroxybenzoic acid (protocatechuic acid), 3,4,5-trihydroxybenzoic acid (gallic acid), 3-methoxy-4-hydroxybenzoic acid (vanillic acid), and ellagic acid. The hydroxybenzoic acid content in edible plants is generally rather low with the exception of certain fruits, onions, and black radish. The most important sources of these acids are blackberries, raspberries, black currant, and strawberries, which may contain from 20 to 270 mg/kg fresh weight (Belitz et al. 2009). Gallic acid and ellagic acid are components of complex structures, such as gallotannins and ellagitannins.

The antioxidant activity of phenolic acids depends on the number and substitution pattern of hydroxyl groups in the molecule that would be strengthened by steric hindrance. The electron-withdrawing properties of the carboxyl group present in benzoic acids have a negative influence on the H-donating abilities of the hydroxybenzoic acids. 4-Hydroxybenzoic acid and 2-hydroxybenzoic acid with only one hydroxyl group show low antioxidant activity (Table 14.2) (Rice-Evans et al. 1996; Ma et al. 2011).

The hydroxycinnamic acids are more common than hydoxybenzoic acids. In food sources, they are mainly present as glycosylated derivatives or esters of caffeic, coumaric, ferulic, and sinapic acids with D-quinic, shikimic, or tartaric acids. Chlorogenic acid (5-caffeoylquinic acid), which is an ester of caffeic acid with quinic acid, coumaroylquinic acid, and feruloylquinic acid are present in high concentrations in stone fruits (apple, cherry, plum) and berries (blueberry, blackberry, black currant) (Belitz et al. 2009). The important source of chlorogenic acid is coffee: one cup may contain 70–350 mg (Clifford 1999). Free forms of cinnamic acids can be found in processed foods, for example, fermented, frozen, or heated products, such as fruit juices (Gliszczyńska-Świgło and Tyrakowska 2003; Oszmiański and Wojdyło 2009) or alcoholic beverages (Nardini and Ghiselli 2004; Shahidi and Naczk 2004).

TABLE 14.2

Antioxidant Activity of Selected Hydroxybenzoic and Cinnamic Acids

Hydroxybenzoic and Cinnamic Acids	TEAC (pH 7.4)[a] Trolox eqv. (mM)	H_2O_2– Scavenging Activity[b] ($\times 10^{-3} \mu M^{-1}$)	ORAC[c] Trolox eqv. (μM)	Reducing Capacity[d] (mol of electrons/ mol of phenolic)
p-Hydroxybenzoic acid (4-hydroxybenzoic acid)	0.08	0.89	–	–
Gallic acid (3,4,5-trihydroxybenzoic acid)	3.01	–	–	–
Protocatechuic acid (3,4-dihydroxybenzoic acid)	1.19	17.6	–	–
Salicylic acid (2-hydroxybenzoic acid)	0.04	–	–	–
Vanillic acid (4-hydroxy-3-methoxybenzoic acid)	1.43	2.22	–	–
Syringic acid (4-hydroxy-3,5-dimethoxybenzoic acid)	1.36	–	–	–
Cinnamic acid	–	0.72	–	–
p-Coumaric (4-hydroxycinnamic acid)	2.22	–	–	0.1
Caffeic (3,4-dihydroxycinnamic acid)	1.26	125	1.26	2.2
Ferulic (4-hydroxy-3-methoxycinnamic acid)	1.90	–	2.85	1.9
Sinapic (4-hydroxy-3,5-dimethoxycinnamic acid)	–	–	3.35	–
Chlorogenic acid 3-caffeoylquinic acid	1.30	–	2.28	1.6

[a] Rice-Evans et al. 1995, 1996.
[b] Ma et al. 2011 (H_2O_2–scavenging activity is $1/IC_{50}$).
[c] Zhang et al. 2008.
[d] Medina et al. 2007.

Hydroxycinnamic acids are more effective antioxidants than benzoate counterparts (Table 14.2). *trans*-cinnamic acid with no hydroxyl group on its ring exhibits the lowest H_2O_2-scavenging activity because the phenoxyl radical becomes less nucleophilic as a result of the absence of an OH electron-donating group and the presence of an allyl carboxylic group (Ma et al. 2011). The peroxyl radical-scavenging activities of cinnamic acids are in the order sinapic > ferulic > chlorogenic > caffeic acid (Zhang et al. 2008).

Evaluating the antioxidant activity of caffeic, chlorogenic, o-coumaric, and ferulic acids in a fish muscle system, Medina et al. (2007) found that the capacity of these compounds for donating electrons seems to play the most significant role in delaying rancidity in fish muscle, whereas the ability to chelate metals and the distribution between the oily and aqueous phases are not correlated with the inhibitory activities. The most effective hydroxycinnamic acid was caffeic acid with antioxidant efficiency similar to that of propyl gallate (Table 14.2).

14.2.2.2 Flavonoids

Dietary flavonoids have the basic $C_6C_3C_6$ carbon skeleton (15-carbon flavan structure) differing in the level of C-ring saturation. The major flavonoid classes include flavonols, flavones, isoflavones, flavan-3-ols (catechins), flavanones, anthocyanidins, and chalcones, for which the C-ring is open (Table 14.3). Individual flavonoids within the class differ in the number and substitution of hydroxyl, methoxy, and glycosidic side groups. They occur in food mostly as O-glycosides with glucose being the most common sugar residue. Other glycosidic units include glucorhamnose, galactose, arabinose, and rhamnose (Cook and Samman 1996). Flavan-3-ols, unlike most flavonoids, are not glycosylated; that is, they occur in nature as free aglycones or as polymers (condensed tannins or proanthocyanidins). The differences in the structure and substitution of flavonoids will influence the stability of a phenoxyl radical formed upon the antioxidant action of flavonoids and, thereby, the antioxidant properties of these compounds.

In a large number of *in vitro* studies, flavonoids have been found to be good antioxidants. Mechanisms of their antioxidant action can include (1) the scavenging of highly reactive oxygen species (ROS) and reactive nitrogen species (RNS) and (2) the suppression of the formation of ROS either by inhibition of oxidizing enzymes or chelation of transition metal ions. The low redox potentials of flavonoids thermodynamically allow them to reduce such free radicals as $O_2^{\cdot-}$, $RO^{\cdot}$, and $^{\cdot}OH$ (Buettner 1993). Furthermore, they may act as antioxidants indirectly through (1) regeneration of α-tocopherol, (2) stimulation of phase II and "antioxidant" enzymes, and/or (3) inhibition of oxidases and redox-sensitive transcription factors, such as nuclear factor κB and activator protein AP-1 (Khan et al. 1992; Rice-Evans et al. 1996; Williamson et al. 1997; Yu et al. 1997; Chen et al. 2000; Heim et al. 2002; Cooper et al. 2005a; Zhou et al. 2005). Structure–activity relationships determined for flavonoids have indicated some structural elements in the flavonoid structure that contribute to their antioxidant activity. These include an *ortho* 3′,4′-dihydroxy (catechol) moiety in the B ring and a C2=C3 double bond in combination with both a C4-keto group and a C3-hydroxyl group in the C ring (Bors et al. 1990; Cook and Samman 1996; Rice-Evans et al. 1996). The presence of the same structural elements contributes the prooxidant activity of flavonoids. Moreover, the antioxidant efficiency of flavonoids has been related to the number of hydroxyl groups in the molecule and also to their hydrogen and/or electron-donating abilities (Tyrakowska et al. 1999; Pietta 2000; Lemańska et al. 2001, 2004; Frei and Higdon 2003; Borkowski et al. 2005; Muzolf et al. 2008). Chelating complexes of flavonoids with divalent cations may form between the 5-OH and 4-oxo group or between the 3′- and 4′-OH (catechol group in the B ring) (Heim et al. 2002).

TABLE 14.3

Chemical Structure, Dietary Sources, and Antioxidant Activity of Selected Flavonoids in TEAC, ORAC, and LPO Assays

Flavonoid Class		Dietary Source	Main Representatives	Substitution Pattern	TEAC (pH 7.4) Trolox Equiv. (mM)	ORAC$_{ROO}$-Trolox Equiv./comp. (µM/µM)	LPO IC$_{50}$ (µM)
Flavonols 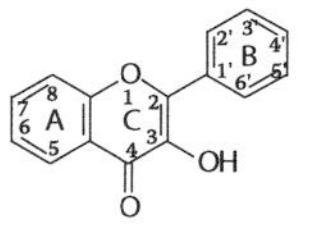		Onion, tomato, apple, broccoli, red wine	Kaempferol	3,5,7,4'-OH	1.34[a]	2.67[d]	19.0[f]
			Quercetin	3,5,7,3',4'-OH	4.72[a]	3.29[d]	8.5[f]
			Myricetin	3,5,7,3',4',5'-OH	3.12[a]	4.32[d]	10.5[f]
			Rutin	3,5,7,3',4'-OH; 3-rutinose	2.40[a]	–	93.5[f]
Flavones 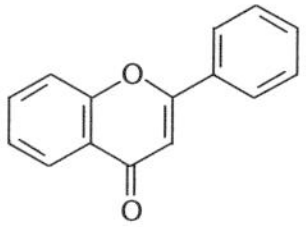		Herbs, celery, parsley, fruit skins	Luteolin	5,7,3',4'-OH	2.09[a]	3.57[d]	26.2[f]
			Apigenin	5,7,4'-OH	1.45[a]	–	>100[f]
			Chrysin	5,7-OH	1.43[a]	–	–
Flavan-3-ols 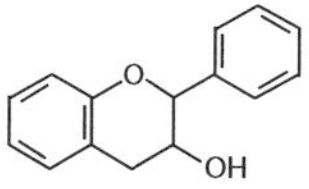		Tea, cacao	(+)-Catechin	3,5,7,3',4'-OH	2.40[a]; 3.22[b]	–	51.0[f]
			(−)-EC	3,5,7,3',4'-OH	2.50[a]; 3.52[b]	–	30.0[f]
			(−)-ECG	5,7,3',4'-OH; 3-gallate	4.93[a]; 6.12[b]	–	10.0[f]
			(−)-EGC	3,5,7,3',4',5'-OH	3.82[a]; 3.61[b]	–	16.0[f]
			(−)-EGCG	5,7,3',4',5'-OH; 3-gallate	4.75[a]; 6.01[b]	–	11.0[f]
Flavanones 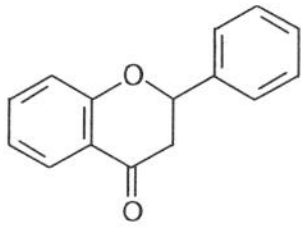		Citrus fruits and juices	Hesperetin	5,7,3'-OH; 4'-OMe	1.37[a]	–	–
			Hesperidin	5,3'-OH; 4'-OMe; 7-rutinose	1.08[a]	0.04[d]	–
			Naringenin	5,7,4'-OH	1.53[a]	2.67[d]	>100[f]
			Naringin	5,4'-OH; 7-neohesperidose	0.24[a]	0.37[d]	–
			Eriodictyol	5,7,3',4'-OH	1.80[a]	3.41[d]	–

(continued)

TABLE 14.3 (Continued)
Chemical Structure, Dietary Sources, and Antioxidant Activity of Selected Flavonoids in TEAC, ORAC, and LPO Assays

Flavonoid Class	Dietary Source	Main Representatives	Substitution Pattern	TEAC (pH 7.4) Trolox Equiv. (mM)	ORAC$_{ROO·}$ Trolox Equiv./comp. (µM/µM)	LPO IC$_{50}$ (µM)
Isoflavones	Soybean	Genistein	5,7,4'-OH	2.90[a]	2.38[d]	–
		Genistin	5,4'-OH; 7-glucose	1.24[a]	–	–
		Daidzein	7,4'-OH	1.25[a]	1.65[d]	>100[f]
		Daidzin	4'-OH; 7-glucose	1.15[a]	–	>100[f]
Anthocyanidins, anthocyanins	Apple, pear, tomato	Pelargonidin	3,5,7,4'-OH	1.30[c]; 1.23[c]	1.54[e]	–
		Pelargonidin-3-glucoside	5,7,4'-OH; 3-glucose	–	1.56[e]	–
		Cyanidin	3,5,7,3',4'-OH	4.42[a]; 4.12[c];	2.24[e]	–
		Cyanidin-3-glucoside	5,7,3',4'-OH; 3-glucose	2.94[c]	3.49[e]	–
		Delphinidin	3,5,7,3',4',5'-OH	4.44[a]; 5.11[c]	1.81[e]	–
		Delphinidin-3-glucoside	5,7,3',4',5'-OH; 3-glucose	2.61[c]	–	–
		Malvidin	3,5,7,4'-OH; 3',5'-OMe	2.06[a]; 2.71[c]	2.01[e]	–
		Malvidin-3-glucoside	5,7,4'-OH; 3',5'-OMe; 3-glucose	1.78[a]; 1.89[e]	1.40[e]	–

Source: Shahidi, F. and M. Naczk, *Phenolics in Food and Nutraceuticals.* Boca Raton, FL: CRC Press, 2004.

[a] Rice-Evans et al. 1995, 1996.
[b] Muzolf et al. 2008.
[c] Borkowski et al. 2005.
[d] Cao et al. 1997.
[e] Wang et al. 1997.
[f] Yang et al. 2001.

Quercetin is the main flavonol present in our diet. It occurs mainly as glycosides (e.g., rutin, isoquercitrin) in a wide variety of fruits, vegetables, and beverages. Quercetin (Table 14.3) is one of the most extensively studied flavonols because it fulfills all structural requirements for a good antioxidant and prooxidant. Other important dietary flavonids comprise kaempferol, myricetin, and their glycosides, belonging to flavonols and flavones (e.g., chrysin, luteolin, and apigenin). It has been estimated that average flavonol consumption in the United States, Denmark, and Holland is 20–25 mg/day with the main sources being onions, cabbage, and broccoli (Hertog et al. 1993; Justesen et al. 1997; Sampson et al. 2002). In Italy, the consumption of flavonols ranges from 5 to 125 mg/day, with an average of 35 mg/day (Pietta et al. 1996), which is related to the presence of large amounts of vegetables in the Mediterranean diet. Citrus fruits and their products are especially rich in flavanones. They are present in the glycoside and aglycone forms. Among the aglycones, naringenin and hesperetin are the most important. There are two types of flavanone glycosides: neohesperidosides (rhamnosyl-α-1,2-glucose residue) and rutinosides (rutinose; rhamnosyl-α-1,6-glucose residue). The 7-O-glycosylflavones are the most abundant in nature. The most important neohesperidose flavanones are naringin, neohesperidin, neoeriocitrin, and rutinosides—hesperidin, narirutin, and didymin (Tripoli et al. 2007). It was estimated that, for those eating the flesh of a whole orange (200 g) or drinking orange juice (250 mL), the daily intake of flavanones (as aglycones) could be as high as 125–375 and 25–60 mg, respectively (Tomas-Barberan and Clifford 2000).

The potent ability of flavonols, flavones, and flavanones to scavenge ROS, singlet oxygen, peroxynitrite, and radicals of different origin has been confirmed in various *in vitro* systems (Tournaire et al. 1993; Hanasaki et al. 1994; Haenen et al. 1997; Aherne and O'Brien 1999; Yamamoto et al. 1999; Horakova et al. 2001; Choi et al. 2002). It was found that both aglycones (quercetin, kaempferol, myricetin, and luteolin) and glycosides (quercitrin, isoquercitrin) protect against oxidative DNA damage both *in vitro* and *ex vivo* in the Comet assay, which is a widely used technique for measuring and analyzing DNA breakage in individual cells in *in vitro*, *ex vivo*, and *in vivo* systems (Cemeli et al. 2009). Protection of flavonols against H_2O_2-induced oxidative DNA damage was confirmed in Caco-2, HepG2 cells (O'Brien et al. 2000), human leukemia cell lines (Horvathova et al. 2003, 2004), and human lymphocytes (Norozi et al. 1998). Rutin, quercetin, and naringin were found to protect against the genotoxicity of UVA on mouse fibroblasts (Yeh et al. 2005).

Catechins (flavan-3-ols) are important components of the human diet because of a relatively high daily intake with the main sources being tea, chocolate, fruits and fruit juices, and red wine (Beecher 2003; Auger et al. 2004; Manach et al. 2005). It has been estimated that the average daily catechin consumption amounts to approximately 158 mg in US adults, which constitutes approximately 83.5% of the total flavonoid intake (Chun et al. 2007). In food, they are present as monomers, oligomers, or polymers. Green tea especially contains considerable amounts of catechins, namely, catechin (C), epicatechin (EC), and epigallocatechin (EGC) and their gallate esters: epicatechin gallate (ECG) and epigallocatechin gallate (EGCG) (Figure 14.1) (Higdon and Frei 2003; Belitz et al. 2009). Moreover, tea polyphenols include theaflavins and thearubigins as products of flavan-3-ol oxidation and condensation.

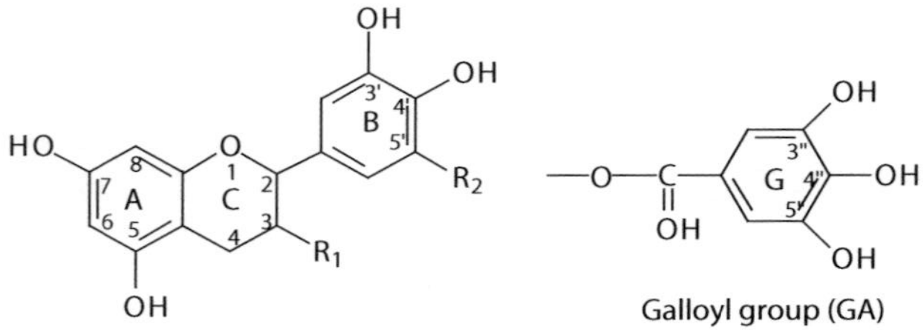

Tea catechins	R₁	R₂
(+)-Catechin (C)	OH	H
(−)-Epicatechin (EC)	OH	H
(−)-Epigallocatechin (EGC)	OH	OH
(−)-Epicatechin gallate (ECG)	GA	H
(−)-Epigallocatechin gallate (EGCG)	GA	OH

FIGURE 14.1   Structures of various tea catechins.

White and green teas mainly contain flavan-3-ols, whereas, in fermented black tea, significant amounts of theaflavins and thearubigins are present. The content of catechins in green tea accounts for approximately 90% of the polyphenol fraction (nearly 30% of the dry weight of green tea; the content is higher in young leaves), whereas, in black tea, the content does not exceed 20% (Belitz et al. 2009). Theaflavins and thearubigins in dry weight of black tea are up to 2% and 10%–20%, respectively (Balentine et al. 1997).

Among all catechins present in food, EGCG and ECG are the most abundant, biologically active, and comprehensively studied (Higdon and Frei 2003; Belitz et al. 2009). Their antioxidant activities are one of the highest among flavonoids (Table 14.3) (Nanjo et al. 1996; Rice-Evans et al. 1996; Yang et al. 2001; Muzolf et al. 2008). Theaflavins and thearubigins also exhibit antioxidant activity. Theaflavins present in black tea may possess at least the same antioxidant potency as the catechins present in green tea (Leung et al. 2001).

Anthocyanins, glycosides, and acyl-glycosides and their aglycones (anthocyanidins) are one of the major groups of natural pigments widely distributed in higher plants. They are responsible for the red, blue, or purple colors of fruits, vegetables, and flowers. The differences between the more than 600 anthocyanins found in nature result from diverse hydroxyl and methoxyl substitution of the 2-phenylbenzopyrylium (flavylium) chromophore and also from the nature, the number, and the position of the sugar moieties attached to the molecule (Kong et al. 2003; Torskangerpoll and Andersen 2005). The most commonly occurring anthocyanins are 3-O-glycosidic or 3,5-O-diglycosidic derivatives of cyanidin. Cyanidin 3-O-glucoside and cyanidin are effective antioxidants capable of inhibiting oxidation in LDL, liposomes, rabbit erythrocyte membranes, and rat liver microsomal systems (Tsuda et al. 1994; Heinonen et al. 1998). These compounds may scavenge ·OH, O_2^- (Tsuda et al. 1996), ROO· (Wang et al. 1997), and nitric oxide (van Acker et al. 1995). The protective effects of cyanidin 3-O-glucoside, cyanidin, and its degradation product protocatechuic acid against H_2O_2-induced oxidative stress in a human neuronal cell line (SH-SY5Y) were also reported (Tarozzi et al. 2007). The radical-scavenging capacity of anthocyanins, determined by the trolox equivalent antioxidant capacity (TEAC) assay, is pH-dependent. In the physiological pH range, the radical-scavenging activity of cyanidin is similar to that of quercetin, a flavonol with a similar substitution pattern (Borkowski et al. 2005).

Anthocyans are of great scientific and nutritional interest as natural pigments alternative to the synthetic colorants used in the food industry and because of their beneficial health effects. However, they are unstable compounds and in aqueous solutions undergo pH-dependent structural and color changes. They exist in a mixture of essentially four molecular species: the flavylium cation, which predominates at pH 1–3; the carbinol pseudobase, which is formed at pH 4–5; the quinoidal base isomers formed at pH 6–7; and the chalcons formed at pH 7–8 (Lapidot et al. 1999). The relative amounts of flavylium cations and other forms at equilibrium vary with both pH and the structure of the anthocyanins. The stability of the anthocyanin color can be improved by their copigmentation with other flavonoids (Baranac et al. 1996, 1997a,b,c; Wilska-Jeszka and Korzuchowska 1996; Dimitric-Markovic et al. 2000; Boulton 2001; Bakowska et al. 2003; Mazzaracchio et al. 2004; Oszmiański et al.

2004; Rein and Heinonen 2004; Mollov et al. 2007; Awika 2008). Although the bioavailability of anthocyanins is poor, these compounds are considered promising candidates as dietary compounds with a potential beneficial role in human health associated with their constant and high consumption estimated to be 180–215 mg/day in the United States (Kühnau 1976), which is much higher than the intake (23 mg/day) of other flavonoids, including quercetin, luteolin, apigenin, kaempferol, and myricetin (Hertog et al. 1993).

Isoflavones differ structurally from other classes of flavonoids by having the phenyl ring (B-ring) attached at the 3- instead of the 2-position of the heterocyclic ring C (Table 14.3). The main sources of isoflavones, present mainly as glycosylated forms, in food are soybeans and soy-based products. Dietary intake of isoflavones in Southeast Asian countries was estimated to be 20–50 mg/day with a maximum intake of approximately 100 mg/day. The dietary isoflavone intake of European and North American populations and vegetarians is much lower (<1–2 and 3–12 mg/day, respectively) (van Erp-Bart et al. 2003; Bakker 2004; Manach et al. 2004). Isoflavones are phytoestrogens; they are able to mimic or block the action of the human estrogens, although they are much less potent. Epidemiological studies suggest that a relatively high intake of soy is associated with a lower risk of osteoporosis. The positive effects of isoflavones on menopausal symptoms and the cardiovascular and immune systems have been reported, but the results are not unequivocal. Although most animal studies have shown cancer-preventive effects, a few studies suggest that soy phytoestrogens may stimulate breast cancer cell growth under certain circumstances (Kurzer 2003).

Table 14.3 presents the antioxidant activities of the most abundant flavonoids measured in the TEAC, oxygen radical absorbance capacity (ORAC), and lipid peroxidation (LPO) assays. It has been established that the position and the degree of hydroxylation are of primary importance in the antioxidant activity of flavonoids. Flavonoids with catechol or pyrogallol moiety in the B-ring, such as quercetin, myricetin, EGC, cyanidin, and delphinidin, have relatively high radical-scavenging and antioxidant activities in lipid systems. The absence of the hydroxyl group at the C3 position in flavanones and flavones decreases their antioxidant activity. As members of the group of flavonoids, flavan-3-ols contain the diphenylpropane skeleton ($C_6C_3C_6$), but they do not possess a 4-oxo function, and they do have a saturated heterocyclic C-ring. These structural features cause a lack of electron delocalization between the A and B rings, enabling stabilization of the phenoxyl radical formed upon the electron-donating action. This delocalization is generally considered a factor that enhances the antioxidant activity of flavonoids. Therefore, it was concluded that the potent radical-scavenging antioxidant capacity of catechins is rather a result of a high number of OH groups in their structures (Rice-Evans et al. 1996). Structure–activity relationships with the most biologically active flavan-3-ols, such as EGCG, indicate that a linear increase in the rate constants for the reaction of EGCG with OH• radicals correlates with the number of reactive hydroxyl groups, suggesting that the galloyl moiety attached to the flavan-3-ol is important for the antioxidant activity of EGCG (Moyers and Kumar 2004). It is of interest to note that the catechins with a galloyl moiety are comparable or even more effective radical scavengers and inhibitors of lipid peroxidation than flavonols. This seems to be important in view of the fact that catechins are ubiquitous in tea, which is the most commonly consumed beverage worldwide after water. The TEAC values of catechins and anthocyanins reported by Rice-Evans et al. (1996) are generally lower than those published by Muzolf et al. (2008) for catechins and Borkowski et al. (2005) for anthocyanins; nevertheless, significant correlations between appropriate results were reported (Borkowski et al. 2005; Muzolf et al. 2008). Alteration of the flavonoid structure by glycosylation, either at the C3 or C7 positions; methylation; or sulfation usually decreases the antioxidant activity of flavonoids (Table 14.3) (Rice-Evans et al. 1996; Heim et al. 2002; Lemańska et al. 2004; Shahidi and Naczk 2004), although a higher hepatic metabolic stability and intestinal absorption of the methylated flavonoids than those of unmethylated forms was reported (Wen and Walle 2006).

Metal chelation by flavonoids is considered to be one of the mechanisms of the antioxidant activity of flavonoids. The interaction of flavonoids with metal ions may change the antioxidant properties and some biological effects of the flavonoid. It has been reported that the flavonoid–metal complexes are more effective antioxidants than the free flavonoids (Souza et al. 2003; Souza and De Giovani 2005; Chen et al. 2009).

It was also found that the antioxidant activity of food flavonoids, as measured in the TEAC assay, is strongly pH-dependent (Tyrakowska et al. 1999; Lemańska et al. 2001, 2004; Borkowski et al. 2005; Muzolf et al. 2008) in contrast to ascorbic acid and α-tocopherol, for which the TEAC values are unaffected over the wide pH range (Gliszczyńska-Świgło and Muzolf 2007). A comparison of the pK_a values to the pH-dependent TEAC profiles of polyphenols led the authors to the conclusion that a significant increase in the TEAC value of these compounds with increasing pH is related to the deprotonation of their most acidic hydroxyl moiety. Upon deprotonation of this OH group, phenolic compounds become better free radical scavengers (Tyrakowska et al. 1999; Lemańska et al. 2001, 2004; Borkowski et al. 2005; Muzolf et al. 2008). This effect is especially of interest because the pH range of different human body fluids and food, in which antioxidants are present or to which they are added, is known to vary from acidic to basic. Moreover, the pH-dependent changes in the radical-scavenging activity of flavonoids suggest that the possible health effects of these compounds, associated with their radical-scavenging activity, will vary with the tissue under investigation.

In recent years, flavonoids have been widely used as natural antioxidants in plant and animal fats and meat against lipid oxidation as well as supplements for animal feeds both to improve animal health and to protect animal products. Usually, they are found to be more potent than α-tocopherol or synthetic antioxidants, such as butylhydroxyanisole (BHA), butylhydroxytoluene (BHT), and *tert*-butylhydroquinone (TBHQ). Moreover, they are proposed as antimicrobial agents in foodstuffs and as health-functional ingredients in various foods and dietary supplements (Ramanathan and Das 1992, 1993; Shahidi et al. 1993; Chen and Chan 1996; He and Shahidi 1997; McCarthy et al. 2001; Pokorny 2001; Tang et al. 2001a,b; Hassan and Fan 2005; Mason et al. 2005; Yilmaz 2006; Gramza-Michałowska et al. 2007; DeJong and Lanari 2009).

14.2.2.3 Tannins

Tannins comprise a group of compounds with a wide diversity in structure, which can be classified into three groups: condensed tannins (proanthocyanidins), hydrolyzable tannins, and complex tannins (Vermerris and Nicholson 2006). Proanthocyanidins are the most abundant group of natural phenolics after lignin. They are oligomeric or polymeric flavonoid compounds composed of flavan-3-ol (catechin) subunits. Their presence in foods, including fruits, vegetables, cereals, and wines, affects their color and taste. There is a variety of different classes of proanthocyanidins, depending on the substitution pattern of the monomer flavan-3-ol unit. The most abundant in plants are procyanidins, which exclusively consist of (epi)catechin units (Hümmer and Schreier 2008). Examples of condensed tannins are procyanidin B1 [epicatechin-(4β→8)-catechin] and procyanidin B2 [epicatechin-(4β→8)-epicatechin]. Procyanidins are present, especially in grapes (*Vitis vinifera*), strawberries (*Fragaria x ananassa*), apples, and red wine (Monagas et al. 2003; Sanchez-Moreno et al. 2003; Oszmiański and Wojdyło 2009; Oszmiański et al. 2009). It was suggested that strawberry proanthocyanidins can be used as markers for gray mold resistance and predictability of strawberry shelf life (Hebert et al. 2002). They play a role in long-term red wine color stability and influence its astringency. The proanthocyanidins present in foods are also of interest in nutrition and medicine because of their much more potent antioxidant properties than those of monomeric phenolics and their possible effects on reducing the risk of chronic diseases, such as cardiovascular disease and cancer (Hagerman et al. 1998; Santos-Buelga and Scalbert 2000).

14.2.2.4 Lignans

Lignans are biologically active antioxidants belonging to the group of phytoestrogens (Schottner et al. 1998; Hallund et al. 2006). Particularly rich sources of lignans include seeds, especially flaxseed (*Linum usitatissimum* L.), and whole grains, although coffee, tea, vegetables, and fruits supply substantial amounts as well. The major flaxseed lignan is secoisolariciresinol (SECO) present in the form of diglucoside (SDG). SDG is linked to 3-hydroxy-3-methylglutaric acid, which can be attached to more than one unit of lignan-forming oligomers (Kamal-Eldin et al. 2001). In mammals, SECO is metabolized by intestinal microflora into enterolactone and enterodiol, the so-called mammalian lignans or enterolignans. Antioxidant activities of SDG, SECO, and mammalian lignans have been demonstrated in several *in vitro* assays in both the lipid and aqueous phases (Prasad 1997, 2000a; Kitts et al. 1999; Niemeyer and Metzler 2003; Hosseinian et al. 2006, 2007; Hu et al. 2007). It was also found that lignans possess a variety of biological activities, including reduction of the risk of diabetes and cardiovascular disease and prevention of the progression of breast, prostate, and colon cancers (Thompson et al. 1996; Prasad 1999, 2000b; Westcott and Muir 2003; McCann et al. 2004; Clavel et al. 2007), which may be partially attributed to their antioxidant properties (Kitts et al. 1999; Hosseinian et al. 2007; Hu et al. 2007).

14.2.2.5 Phenolics of Herbs and Spices

Recently, most of the interest is focusing on phenolic antioxidants of herbal and spice origin. Herb and spice extracts are more often used as food antioxidants, especially because consumers have questioned the use of the synthetic antioxidants BHT and BHA in food products and because a lot of studies demonstrated that herbal and spice extracts are as efficient as synthetic antioxidants. The main compounds responsible for the high antioxidant effect of these extracts are phenol monoterpenes and

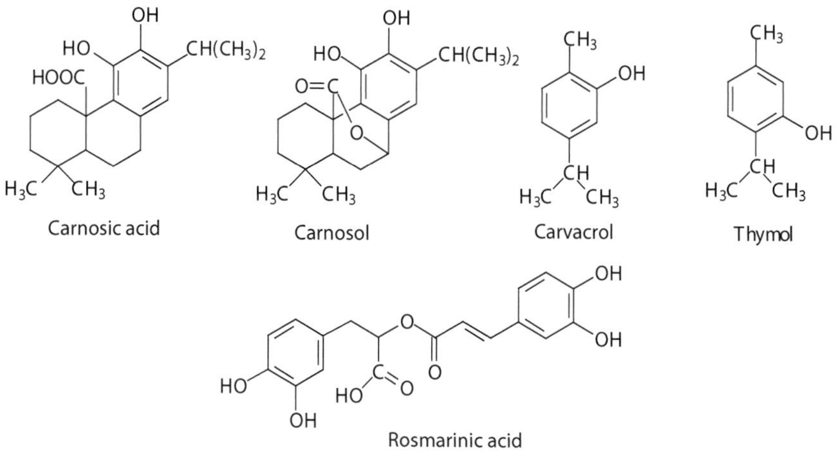

FIGURE 14.2 Structures of main antioxidant phenolic compounds of rosemary, sage, oregano, and thyme.

diterpenes, such as carnosic acid and carnosol from rosemary (*Rosmarinus officinalis*) and sage (*Salvia officinalis* L.), carvacrol and thymol from oregano (*Origanum vulgare*), and thymol from thyme (*Thymus vulgaris*). The caffeic acid derivative rosmarinic acid from oregano, rosemary, and sage contributes to the antioxidant activity of extracts from these plants (Figure 14.2). Flavonoids, mainly flavones and flavonols, and cinnamic acids as well as certain components of essential oils are of less significance (Lu and Foo 2001). Thyme and rosemary extracts have been found to have high antioxidant activities in the TEAC, 1,1-diphenyl-2-picrylhydrazyl (DPPH), and ferric reducing antioxidant power (FRAP) assays followed by oregano and sage (Wojdyło et al. 2007). These extracts and their main compounds can inhibit lipid peroxidation in a wide variety of food products, including meat, bulk oils, and lipid emulsions (Aruoma et al. 1992; Frankel et al. 1996; Zegarska et al. 1996; Botsoglou et al. 1997; Vareltzis et al. 1997; Gramza-Michałowska et al. 2007).

14.2.3 Prooxidant Action of Flavonoids

The role of flavonoids in food is generally considered to be beneficial to consumer health, and several flavonoids have recently been marked as herbal medicines and/or dietary supplements. However, plant polyphenols have also been reported to exert prooxidant and mutagenic activity leading to the formation of ROS and/or reactive and mutagenic electrophile-type metabolites (MacGregor and Jurd 1978; Nagano et al. 1981; Laughton et al. 1989; Jurado et al. 1991; Galati et al. 1999, 2001; Cao et al. 1997; Awad et al. 2000, 2001, 2002, 2003; Moridani et al. 2001b). Formation of oxidation products of flavonoids may occur during the actual antioxidant action. Different mechanisms of prooxidant activity of flavonoid compounds have been proposed.

It was reported that flavonoids with a phenol-type substitution pattern in their B-ring, such as apigenin and naringenin, in the presence of glutathione (GSH) and peroxidases generate ROS (Galati et al. 1999, 2001). The mechanism of prooxidant chemistry of phenol-type flavonoids may be as follows: the enzymatic and/or chemical (auto)oxidation of flavonoid generates the flavonoid semiquinone radical, which may be regenerated to the parent flavonoid by GSH. The thiyl radical (GS˙) formed may react with GSH, generating a disulfide radical anion (GSSG˙⁻), which rapidly reduces molecular oxygen to superoxide radicals (Figure 14.3) (Galati et al. 1999; Rietjens et al. 2002). The same mechanism has been proposed for the peroxidase-catalyzed metabolic activation of resveratrol belonging to stilbenes (Galati et al. 2002).

Phenol-type flavonoids were found to generate increased lipid peroxidation and to act as a prooxidant at concentrations where other flavonoids were still active as antioxidants. The high one-electron oxidation potential of phenol-type flavonoid phenoxyl radicals seems to be important in determining the oxidation products formed upon their prooxidant activity (Galati et al. 1999).

Flavonoids containing a catechol or pyrogallol-type substitution pattern in their B-ring do not oxidize GSH probably as a result of the lower one-electron oxidation potentials of their semiquinone radicals (Galati et al. 1999, 2001). For this type of flavonoids, another mechanism of their prooxidant activity has been proposed (Figure 14.4). The presence of an intrinsic catechol moiety in the molecule of flavonoids provides the possibility of efficient autoxidation and/or enzymatic one- or two-electron oxidation of the compound, resulting in the formation of semiquinone and reactive electrophilic o-quinones/quinone methides, capable of forming adducts with reduced glutathione (GSH), amino acids, proteins, RNA, and DNA (Awad et al. 2003; Walle et al. 2003; van der Woude et al. 2005, 2006). The role of quinone/quinone methide chemistry is thought to be involved in the mechanism underlying the toxic effects, including cytotoxicity, immunotoxicity, and carcinogenesis of 3′,4′-dihydroxyflavonoids and catechol-type metabolites of estrogens and polycyclic aromatic hydrocarbons (Bolton et al. 1998, 2000; Penning et al. 1999; Gliszczyńska-Świgło et al. 2003; van der Woude et al. 2003; Galati et al. 2006; Cavalieri et al. 2004). Moreover, the formation of various ROS, especially through redox cycling of quinones, may cause oxidative stress that may contribute to the cytotoxicity of the parent flavonoid. It was also proposed that the prooxidant action of polyphenols may be an important mechanism of their anticancer and apoptosis-inducing properties (Hadi et al. 2000; Azam et al. 2004).

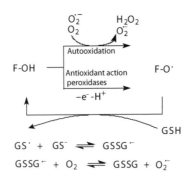

FIGURE 14.3 Prooxidant chemistry of fenol-type flavonoids.

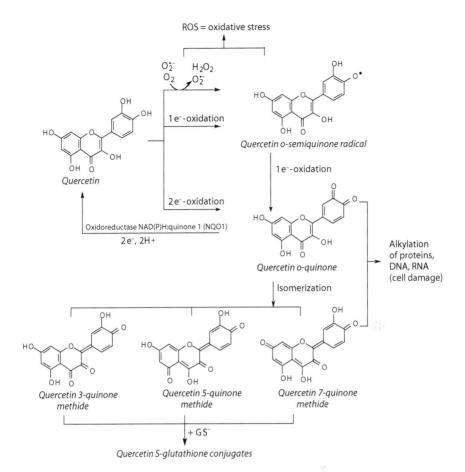

FIGURE 14.4 Prooxidant chemistry of quercetin as an example of catechol-type flavonoid as described in literature. (From MacGregor, J.T. and L. Jurd, *Mutat Res* 54, 297–309, 1978; Awad, H.M. et al., *Arch Biochem Biophys* 378, 224–233, 2000; Awad, H.M. et al., *Chem Res Toxicol* 14, 398–408, 2001; Boersma, M.G. et al., *Chem Res Toxicol* 13, 185–191, 2000; Gliszczyńska-Świgło, A. et al., *Toxicol in Vitro* 17, 423–431, 2003.)

It was found that quercetin, luteolin, fisetin, and some catechins undergo both one- or two-electron oxidation catalyzed by tyrosinase or horseradish peroxidase (HRP)/H_2O_2 (Boersma et al. 2000; Awad et al. 2001; Galati et al. 2001, 2006; Sang et al. 2005, 2007; Muzolf-Panek et al. 2008), resulting in the formation of electrophilic, toxic quinone-type metabolites, which were efficiently scavenged by glutathione (GSH) by conjugate formation. Similar quinoids and hydroxylated products were detected in the case of enzymatically oxidized dihydroxycinnamic acids, such as caffeic, dihydrocaffeic, and chlorogenic acids (Moridani et al. 2001a).

Quercetin is one of the most prominent dietary flavonoids ubiquitously present in vegetables, fruits, tea, and wine, as well as in food supplements. Oxidation of quercetin yields a quercetin quinone, which has four tautomeric forms, that is, an *o*-quinone and three quinone methides (Figure 14.4). It has been well documented that oxidation products, such as semiquinone radicals and quinones, display various toxic effects resulting from their ability to arylate protein thiols. This thiol reactivity of quinones manifests by the preferential reaction with GSH, and this reaction cannot be prevented by ascorbate (Boots et al. 2003). It has been also shown that, as long as the GSH concentration is high, it will protect against quinone metabolites by trapping it as GS-conjugates. However, when the concentration of GSH is low, the GSH–quinone adduct dissociates, and quinone will react with other thiol groups, such as protein thiols (Boots et al. 2005). It has been shown that quercetin efficiently protects against H_2O_2-induced DNA damage in rat lung epithelial cells, but toxic changes resulting in a reduction in the GSH level and an increase in LDH leakage as well as an increase in the cytosolic free calcium concentration are induced by the oxidation products of quercetin formed during this protection (Boots et al. 2007). This may imply that quinone conjugation by GSH will not offer complete protection against quinones; GSH protects against quinones by scavenging them at the time and site of formation, but ultimately, GSH will transfer the quinone to other thiols (Boots et al. 2005, 2007). This may lead to toxic effects, such as increased membrane permeability (Yen et al. 2003), and altered functioning of enzymes containing SH-groups (Ito et al. 1988; Boots et al. 2002, 2003, 2008; van Zanden et al. 2003). The study by Choi et al. (2003) revealed the protective effect of quercetin against lipid peroxidation in the liver of rats, but the concentration of glutathione and glutathione reductase significantly decreased, indicating the prooxidant activity of quercetin. This protective-toxic effect of quercetin has recently been defined as the quercetin paradox, and it might also apply for other free radical-scavenging antioxidants (Boots et al. 2007, 2008).

It was also reported that catechol-O-methylation of quercetin does not eliminate although considerably attenuates the formation of GSH-adducts (van der Woude et al. 2006). Formation of quercetin quinone/quinone methide metabolites reflected by the formation of the glutathionyl quercetin adducts as metabolites was also observed in an *in vitro* cell model (B16F-10 melanoma and HL-60 cells) by Awad et al. (2002) and van der Woude et al. (2005). Moreover, the EGCG–quinone–glutathionyl conjugate formation was observed in Hepa1c1c7 cells stably transfected with a luciferase reporter gene under the control of the EpRE derived from the human NQO1 gene (EpRE-LUX cells) (Muzolf-Panek et al. 2008). Studies by Sang et al. (2005, 2007) revealed the formation of EGCG–thiol conjugates both *in vitro* and in mice exposed i.p. to high toxic doses of EGCG (200 and 400 mg/kg of body weight) with the 2′-thiol-EGCG being the major conjugate. These adducts were no longer observed when the mice were given lower i.p. or oral doses, but this could be a result of the low bioavailability of EGCG upon oral dosing in combination with the detection limit of the method applied because it is most likely that the related chemistry will be ongoing also at lower dose levels (Muzolf-Panek et al. 2008).

Moreover, evidence for covalent binding of quercetin and its catechol-O-methylated metabolites to cellular protein and DNA has been also reported (Walle et al. 2003; van der Woude et al. 2005, 2006).

Phenolic compounds have the potential to act as prooxidants in systems containing oxygen and transition metal ions, such as copper and iron. These metals catalyze the redox cycling of phenolics, leading to the formation of ROS and other organic radicals that can damage DNA, lipids, and other biological molecules (Rahman et al. 1989; Li and Trush 1994; Cao et al. 1997; Yamanaka et al. 1997; Yoshino et al. 1999;

Azam et al. 2004; Galati and O'Brien 2004; Zheng et al. 2008). It has been suggested that the interaction of polyphenols with metal ions may result in a spectrum of DNA lesions, including oxidative base modifications, strand breaks, and formation of DNA adducts leading to carcinogenesis (Li and Trush 1994; Yoshino et al. 1999; Sakihama et al. 2002; Furukawa et al. 2003). The reactive species responsible for DNA damage is probably ($^{\bullet}$OH) radical or a species with similar oxidative potential (Li and Trush 1994). The mechanism of its formation in the presence of Cu(II) or Fe(III) can be as follows (Sakihama et al. 2002; Furukawa et al. 2003):

$$F-OH + Cu(II) \rightarrow F-O^{\bullet} + Cu(I) + H^{+} \tag{14.1}$$

$$F-O^{\bullet} + O_2 \rightarrow F=O + O_2^{\bullet-} \tag{14.2}$$

$$F-OH + O_2^{\bullet-} \rightarrow F-O^{\bullet} + H_2O_2 \tag{14.3}$$

$$2O_2^{\bullet-} + 2H^{+} \rightarrow H_2O_2 + O_2 \tag{14.4}$$

$$O_2^{\bullet-} + Cu(II) \rightarrow O_2 + Cu(I) \tag{14.5}$$

$$Cu(I) + H_2O_2 \rightarrow Cu(II) + {}^{\bullet}OH + {}^{-}OH$$
$$\downarrow \tag{14.6}$$
$$\text{e.g., DNA damage}$$

Cu(II) or Fe(III) oxidizes the phenolic compound (F–OH) to a semiquinone radical (F–O$^{\bullet}$) (reaction 14.1), which may subsequently react with oxygen with the formation of $O_2^{\bullet-}$ and flavonoid quinone (F = O) (reaction 14.2); $O_2^{\bullet-}$ may oxidize F–OH to F–O$^{\bullet}$ and form H_2O_2 (reaction 14.3) and reduce Cu(II) to Cu(I) (reaction 14.5). H_2O_2 can also form by the disproportionation of $O_2^{\bullet-}$ (reaction 14.4). In a Fenton reaction, H_2O_2 oxidizes Cu(I) to Cu(II) with the formation of $^{\bullet}$OH (reaction 14.6). A similar mechanism has been proposed by Furukawa et al. (2003) for oxidative damage of isolated and cellular DNA by EGCG in the presence of Fe(III) but different in the presence of Cu(II) where the Cu(I)-hydroperoxo complex formed (reaction 14.7) participates in Cu(II)-mediated DNA damage by EGCG:

$$Cu(I) + H_2O_2 \rightarrow Cu(I)OOH + H^{+} \tag{14.7}$$

According to Furukawa et al. (2003), in view of the very tightly controlled physiological uptake and turnover of copper and iron, it is difficult to consider any presence of free copper and iron ions available for the postulated reactions. Therefore, it is possible that DNA and/or other natural complexes with these metals might participate in carcinogenesis *in vivo*.

14.2.4 CONTRIBUTION OF ANTIOXIDANT AND PROOXIDANT ACTIVITY OF FLAVONOIDS TO HEALTH-PROMOTING ACTIVITY

A relatively high level of flavonoids in the human diet has been reported to be correlated with the reduced risk of common chronic diseases. The results of many studies indicate that flavonoids may reduce the risk of coronary heart disease through modulation of arterial vasomotion or inhibition of platelet aggregation or provide endothelial protection (Colantuoni et al. 1991; Morazzoni et al. 1991; Duffy et al. 2001; Youdim et al. 2002; Cooper et al. 2005a,b; Cabrera et al. 2006; Barbosa 2007; Tripoli et al. 2007). Moreover, they have been reported to be anticarcinogenic and anti-inflammatory, antibacterial, antiviral, and/or antibiotic compounds (Lietti et al. 1976; Kandaswami et al. 1991; Kamei et al. 1995; Bomser et al. 1996; Mabe et al. 1999; H. Wang et al. 1999; Meiers et al. 2001; Galvano et al. 2004; Navarro-Martinez et al. 2005; Prior and Gu 2005; Song et al. 2005). The broad range of flavonoid-mediated biological activities is often, at least in part, related to their antioxidant properties (Middleton and Kandaswami 1993; Formica and Regelson 1995; Duthie and Crosier 2000; Pietta 2000; Rietvield and Wiseman 2003; Cooper et al. 2005a,b; Tripoli et al. 2007).

Recent results with flavonoids revealed that these compounds induce an electrophile-responsive element (EpRE)-mediated expression of enzymes involved in chemoprevention, such as NAD(P)H-quinone oxidoreductase (NQO1) and glutathione S-transferases (GSTs) (Chou et al. 2003; Yang et al. 2006; Lee-Hilz et al. 2006, 2008; Muzolf-Panek et al. 2008), the major defense enzymes against electrophilic toxicants and oxidative stress. An EpRE-mediated expression of these enzymes by polyphenols is assumed to involve the release of the transcription factor nuclear factor erythroid 2-related factor 2 (Nrf2) from a complex with Kelch-like erythroid cell-derived protein with CNC homology-associating protein 1 (Keap1) (Dinkova-Kostova et al. 2005). A possible mechanism for the polyphenol-induced release of Nrf2 from Keap1 includes their oxidation to reactive electrophilic quinones that may generate oxidative stress through redox cycling, thereby activating Nrf2 release from Keap1 and EpRE-mediated gene expression (Dinkova-Kostova et al. 2005). The induction of EpRE-mediated gene expression by the prooxidant activity of flavonoids points to a beneficial effect of a supposed toxic chemical reaction.

Formation of ROS and quinoid-type metabolites by flavonoids has been postulated to be an important mechanism responsible for some of the observed anticancer and apoptosis-inducing properties of flavonoids (Azam et al. 2004; Galati et al. 2004; Hou et al. 2005; Vargas and Burd 2010).

14.3 ANTIOXIDANT ACTIVITY OF BETALAINS

Betalains are natural water-soluble colorants present in plants of most families of the plant order *Caryophyllales* (with the exception of *Caryophyllaceae* and *Moluginaceae*) and in some higher fungi (Frank et al. 2005). Among the numerous natural sources of betalains, red and yellow beets (*Beta vulgaris*), prickly pear, colored Swiss chard, grain amaranth (*Amaranthus*), and cactus fruits (*Opuntia*) are edible sources of these compounds (Cai et al. 2001; Kanner et al. 2001; Stintzing and

Carle 2004; Frank et al. 2005). The main groups of betalains are the red-violet beta-cyanins (e.g., betanin and isobetanin) and the yellow betaxanthins (e.g., vulgaxan-thin I and II). The betacyanins (betanin and isobetanin) are water-soluble immonium conjugates of betalamic acid with 3,4-dihydroxyphenylalanine (cyclo-DOPA), which may be glucosylated, while yellow betaxanthins contain different amino acids, for example, glutamate and glutamic acid (Figure 14.5).

The best-known betacyanin is betanin, which is a betanidin 5-O-β-glucoside (Figure 14.5). The isobetanin is the C15-epimer of betanin. These compounds con-tain a phenolic and a cyclic amine group, both of which are very good electron donors, acting as antioxidants (Kanner et al. 2001). Red beetroots contain a large concentration of betanin, 300–600 mg/kg (75%–95% of the total coloring matter found in the beet) and lower concentrations of isobetanin, betanidin, and betaxan-thins (Kanner et al. 2001). The prickly pear (*Opuntia ficus indica*) contains approxi-mately 50 mg/kg of betanin and 26 mg/kg of indicaxanthin (Butera et al. 2002). The pigment mixture of betacyanins in the form of beet juice concentrate or beet powder is an approved additive for use in food, drugs, and cosmetic products (E162).

Several studies have shown that betalains are effective free radical scavengers and that they prevent active oxygen-induced and free radical-mediated oxidation of biological molecules (Escribaño et al. 1998; Zakharova and Petrova 1998; Pedreno and Escribaño 2000, 2001; Kanner et al. 2001; Butera et al. 2002; Pavlov et al. 2002; Wettasinghe et al. 2002; Cai et al. 2003; Tesoriere et al. 2004, 2005; Allegra et al. 2005; Frank et al. 2005; Stintzing et al. 2005; Gliszczyńska-Świgło et al. 2006). For instance, in a study by Kanner et al. (2001), linoleate peroxidation by cytochrome c was inhibited by betanin, betanidin, catechin, and α-tocopherol with IC_{50} values of 0.4, 0.8, 1.2, and 5.0 μM, respectively. The IC_{50} values for the inhibition of soy-bean lipoxygenase by betanidin, betanin, and catechin were found to be 0.3, 0.6, and 1.2 μM, respectively. The TEAC value of betanin and betanidin is very high (approx-imately 8 mM) in comparison to some flavonoids (Table 14.3). The TEAC value of indicaxanthin (2.7 mM), which is not a phenol compound, is also relatively high (Gandia-Herrero 2010). It is worthwhile to notice that the free radical-scavenging activity of betanin measured in the TEAC assay at pH 7.4 and that in the DPPH

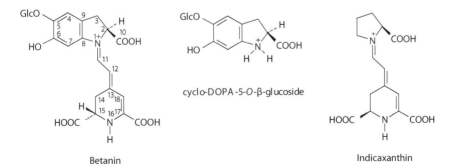

FIGURE 14.5 Chemical structures and atom numbering system of betanidin 5-O-β-D-glucoside (betanin), cyclo-DOPA-5-O-β-D-glucoside, and indicaxanthin.

assay is approximately 7.5-fold and 3-fold higher, respectively, than that of vitamin C (Cai et al. 2003; Gliszczyńska-Świgło 2006). Moreover, the antioxidant activity of betanin and betanidin is pH-dependent, and at a pH above 4, it is much higher than the most abundant natural colorant cyanidin-3-O-glucoside and its aglycone cyanidin (Figure 14.6). It was suggested that the exceptionally high radical-scavenging activities of betanin and betanidin are associated with an increase in its H-donation and/or electron-donation ability when going from a cationic state to monodeprotonated, dideprotonated, and trideprotonated states present at a different pH of the environment (Gliszczyńska-Świgło et al. 2006; Gliszczyńska-Świgło and Szymusiak 2007c).

pH-dependent changes in the antiradical activity of betalains and anthocyanins suggest that possible beneficial health effects of these natural dyes will vary with the tissue under investigation and that betanin at a pH higher than 4 could be an even better free radical scavenger than the extensively studied flavonoids.

In food processing, betalains are less commonly used than water-soluble anthocyanins, although the color of betalains is more stable between pH 3 and 7 (they retain their tinctorial strength and color shade). At pH values lower than 3, the color turns more violet, and at a pH higher than 7, it becomes more yellowish-brown (Roy et al. 2004). The stability of betalains may be highly promoted by its encapsulation in a maltodextrin matrix (Gandia-Herrero et al. 2010). Anthocyanins have the greatest color intensity at pH values less than 4 where they exist in the form of a flavylium cation. At pH 4–5, a colorless carbinol pseudobase is formed upon deprotonation and hydration of the flavylium cation (Lapidot et al. 1999). Thus, betalains are well suited for coloring acidic and slightly acidic foods, whereas anthocyanins are used as a source for food colors in applications that have an acidic pH, such as beverages and dessert products (Strack et al. 2003; Roy et al. 2004).

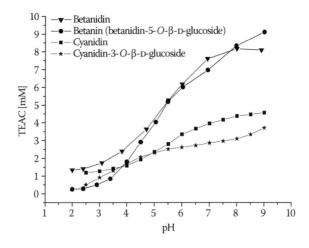

FIGURE 14.6 pH-dependent TEAC profile of betacyanins (betanidin and betanin) and anthocyanins (cyanidin and cyanidin-3-O-β-D-glucoside) as examples.

The bioavailability of betalains is at least as high as flavonoids, which are well-accepted natural antioxidants. Plasma concentrations of betalains in humans after ingestion are sufficiently high to bind to LDL and prevent its oxidation. Moreover, indicaxanthin shows a synergistic interaction with vitamin E, which adds a remarkable potential to indicaxanthin in LDL protection (Tesoriere et al. 2003). Betalains, as natural antioxidants, may provide protection against oxidative stress-related disorders (Kanner et al. 2004; Tesoriere et al. 2005). Therefore, consumers may benefit from regular consumption of products rich in betalains, such as red beet juice and other products made of red beets or foods colored with betalains as safe natural colorants.

14.4 ANTIOXIDANT AND PROOXIDANT ACTIVITY OF VITAMINS (SEE ALSO CHAPTER 11)

14.4.1 Vitamin C

Vitamin C (L-ascorbic acid) is a water-soluble vitamin with high reductive potential. It is considered to be a most important water-soluble antioxidant, protecting extracellular and intracellular spaces in most biological systems and reducing tocopherol radicals back to their active form at the cellular membranes (Kaur and Kapoor 2001). It can directly scavenge superoxide anion radicals, singlet oxygen, hydrogen peroxide, and hydroxyl radicals. It also plays a role as a coenzyme of oxidation enzymes and, in this way, is involved in the metabolism of neurotransmitters, lipids, and collagen (Kojo 2004). Plasma vitamin C levels are about 40 μmol/L in healthy humans, ranging from 20 to 150 μmol/L. A high level of ascorbate was found in the pituitary and adrenal glands (30–400 mg/100 g of tissue), in the brain, spleen, pancreas, liver, and eye lens (10–50 mg/100 g of tissue) (Stahl et al. 2002).

Currently, ascorbic acid is the most widely used vitamin/antioxidant supplement worldwide available as a single or in multicompound preparations. It is added to processed food to fortify it, to restore vitamin C lost, or as an antioxidant either as ascorbic acid and its salts or as a fatty acid ester, ascorbyl palmitate (E300–304). The major sources of vitamin C in the human diet are fruits, vegetables, and their products. Both ascorbic acid and its oxidation product, dehydroascorbic acid, have vitamin C activity.

The antioxidant chemistry of vitamin C in the human body and in most foods is the chemistry of the ascorbate anion because, at physiological pH, 99.9% of ascorbic acid ($pKa_1 = 4.17$) is present as ascorbate anion (AH^-) and only very small proportions as ascorbic acid (AH_2; 0.05%) and A^{2-} (0.004%) (Valko et al. 2006). AH^- reacts with radicals to produce an ascorbate free radical ($AH^{\bullet}$), which is not protonated ($pKa = -0.86$) but is present in the form of a poorly reactive semidehydroascorbate radical (ascorbyl radical; $A^{\bullet-}$) (Figure 11.1). Both ascorbate and the ascorbyl radical have a low reduction potential and can react with most other biologically relevant radicals and oxidants. Moreover, the ascorbyl radical reactivity is low as a result of the resonance stabilization of the unpaired electron; it dismutates to ascorbate and dehydroascorbic acid. In addition, ascorbate can be regenerated from both the ascorbyl radical and dehydroascorbic acid by enzyme-dependent and independent pathways (Carr and Frei 1999).

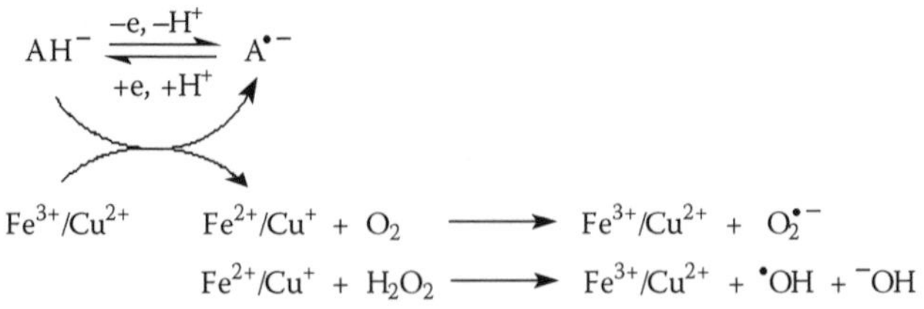

$$AH^- \underset{+e, +H^+}{\overset{-e, -H^+}{\rightleftharpoons}} A^{\bullet-}$$

$$Fe^{3+}/Cu^{2+}$$

$$Fe^{2+}/Cu^+ + O_2 \longrightarrow Fe^{3+}/Cu^{2+} + O_2^{\bullet-}$$

$$Fe^{2+}/Cu^+ + H_2O_2 \longrightarrow Fe^{3+}/Cu^{2+} + {}^{\bullet}OH + {}^-OH$$

FIGURE 14.7 Prooxidant chemistry of ascorbic acid.

Vitamin C, depending on conditions, may also interact with transition metal ions, such as copper and iron. It reduces redox-active transition metals in the active sites of specific biosynthetic enzymes, such as hydroxylases and oxygenases, enzymes involved in the biosynthesis of procollagen, carnitine, and neurotransmitters. The reduction of transition metal ions by ascorbate may also contribute to the oxidative damage of lipids, proteins, and DNA through the formation of ROS, such as hydroxyl radicals (Figure 14.7). *In vitro* induction of lipid peroxidation by an ascorbate–iron system is a standard test for inducing ROS via Fenton reaction and testing antioxidant activity of other antioxidants. In this reaction, ascorbate converts Fe^{3+} to Fe^{2+}; this subsequently reacts with oxygen or hydrogen peroxide resulting in the formation of superoxide or hydroxyl radicals (Figure 14.7). The role of vitamin C, both in the presence or absence of metal ions, in oxidative DNA, lipids, and protein damage was investigated in many *in vitro* and *in vivo* studies. Reduction in markers of oxidative DNA, lipid, and protein damage, even in the presence of iron, has been shown in a majority of physiologically relevant *in vitro* systems and in animal and human *in vivo* studies (Collis et al. 1997; Carr and Frei 1999; Yang et al. 1999; K. Chen et al. 2000; Suh et al. 2003). Moreover, the relevance of the metal-catalyzed prooxidant activity of vitamin C *in vivo* has been questioned, the main point of contention being the availability of free catalytic metal ions *in vivo* (Halliwell and Gutteridge 1986).

14.4.2 VITAMIN E

The term "vitamin E" refers to a group of compounds occurring naturally in plants, all deriving from 6-chromanol with a 2-phytyl substituent. The structures of tocol-related compounds, tocopherols, and tocotrienols are shown in Figure 14.8. Tocopherols are vitamin E compounds with a saturated phytyl chain, and tocotrienols have three double bonds at the positions 3′, 7′, and 11′ of the alkyl side chain. The α-, β-, γ-, δ-tocopherols and tocotrienols are differentiated in the number and location of methyl substituents in the chroman ring (Figure 14.8). α-Tocopherol is the most biologically active form of vitamin E in humans and is a powerful biological antioxidant. It is considered the most effective lipid-soluble chain-breaking antioxidant, protecting cell membranes against peroxyl radicals and mutagenic nitrogen oxide species (van Acker et al. 1993; Christen et al. 1997; Wang and Quinn 1999). Plasma or serum concentrations of α-tocopherol are approximately 20–35 μmol/L (4.5–6.0 μmol α-tocopherol/mmol cholesterol). γ-Tocopherol concentrations are approximately 5%–15% of those of α-tocopherol; the concentrations of γ-tocotrienol

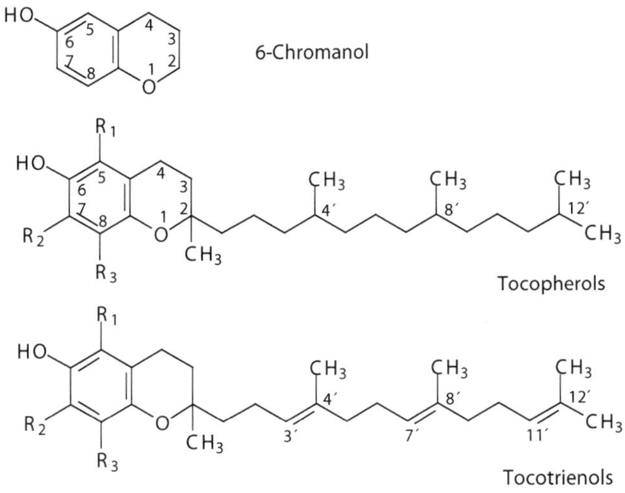

Name	R_1	R_2	R_3	Biological activity (%)
α-Tocopherol	CH_3	CH_3	CH_3	100
β-Tocopherol	CH_3	H	CH_3	15–40
γ-Tocopherol	H	CH_3	CH_3	3–20
δ-Tocopherol	H	H	CH_3	<2
α-, β-, γ-, δ-Tocotrienol	Like tocopherols			1–25
Tocol	H	H	H	–

FIGURE 14.8 Structures of 6-chromanol, tocopherols, and tocotrienols and biological activity of vitamin E derivatives. (From Friedrich, W., *Vitamins*. Berlin, New York: Walter de Gruyter, 1988.)

remain below 1 μmol/L (Stahl et al. 2002). The order of reactivity of tocopherols toward singlet oxygen is $\alpha > \beta > \gamma > \delta$, and antioxidant potency is in the reverse order (Gregory 2008). Synthetic α-tocopheryl acetate is widely used in food fortification. The presence of the acetate ester improves the stability of the compound by blocking the phenolic hydroxyl group and, thus, eliminating its radical-quenching activity (Gregory 2008).

α-Tocopherol acting as an antioxidant is converted to an α-tocopherol radical, which can be reduced to the parent form by ascorbic acid (Kojo 2004) or reduced glutathione (Bast and Haenen 2002). Increasing only the level of α-tocopherol, may, especially under conditions of oxidative stress, result in increased levels of α-tocopherol radicals, which can no longer be effectively detoxified by the co-antioxidants. This provides the possibility for the prooxidant toxicity of the α-tocopherol radical (Rietjens et al. 2002). The prooxidant activity of tocopherol, similarly to that of vitamin C, can also be caused by the reducing power of tocopherol that is responsible for the reduction of transition metals. This prooxidant effect was reported to be involved in the increase in fatal myocardial infarctions observed in a clinical study with vitamin E supplements (Halliwell 2000; Bast and Haenen 2002).

Increased vitamin E intake has been inversely associated with a lower risk of cardiovascular and coronary heart diseases (Rimm et al. 1993; Stampfer et al. 1993; Losonczy et al. 1996). The protective role of vitamin E against atherosclerosis, cardiovascular diseases, cataract, neural tube defects, and cancer has been the subject of extensive studies (Azzi and Stocker 2000). α-Tocopherol exhibits the greatest activity in the prevention of vitamin E deficiency abnormalities, whereas γ-tocopherol was found to be a potent NO(X) radical scavenger (Christen et al. 1997) with major implications in chronic inflammation (Pignatelli et al. 1998; Jiang et al. 2000) and steroid hormone (Yoshie and Ohshima 1998) associated carcinogenesis. Major dietary sources of vitamin E are vegetable oils and food containing oils. Grains, nuts, dairy products, and legumes may also contribute to the total vitamin E intake.

14.4.3 CAROTENOIDS

Carotenoids are fat-soluble pigments with a 40-carbon polyene chain derived from isoprene. They act as antioxidants, and some of them possess vitamin A activity. Based on their composition, carotenoids are divided into two classes: carotenes containing only carbon and hydrogen atoms, and oxocarotenoids (xanthophylls), which carry at least one oxygen atom. The most common carotenoids in the human diet are β-carotene, lycopene, lutein, β-cryptoxanthin, and zeaxanthin (Figure 14.9). In industrialized countries, fruits and vegetables provide an estimated 1.7–3.0 mg/day of provitamin A carotenoids, of which β-carotene is the principle component. β-Carotene is primarily found in red palm oil, palm fruits, leafy green vegetables, carrot, sweet potatoe, mature squash, pumpkin, mango, and papaya. Other sources of β-carotene include food additives (1–2 mg/person/day) and supplements (Rietjens et al. 2005). Lutein is predominantly present in dark green leafy vegetables, such as spinach and kale, whereas its isomer zeaxanthin is in corn, squash, pea, cabbage, pepper, orange, kiwi, and grape (Ho et al. 2008). Lycopene is especially present in tomato, watermelon, papaya, apricot, orange, and pink grapefruit. Its bioavailability is rather poor but is significantly improved by the thermal processing of food.

The polyene backbone of carotenoids consists of conjugated double bonds, which allows the carotenoids to take up excess energy from other molecules through a nonradiative energy transfer mechanism (Palozza and Krinsky 1992; Ho et al. 2008). This feature may be responsible for their well-documented antioxidant and radical-scavenging activities, as well as quenching of singlet oxygen (Miller et al. 1996; Woodal et al. 1997; Stahl et al. 1998; Stahl and Sies 2003; Müller et al. 2011). Most of the carotenoids show ferric-reducing activity, measured in the FRAP assay. They also effectively scavenge the ABTS·+ radical cation and peroxyl radicals. Their antioxidant activities are even much higher than the activity of α-tocopherol (Müller et al. 2011) (Table 14.4). Matos et al. (2006) reported that lycopene and β-carotene protect *in vivo* iron-induced oxidation damage in the rat prostate tissue. Among the various radicals that are formed under oxidative conditions in the organism, carotenoids

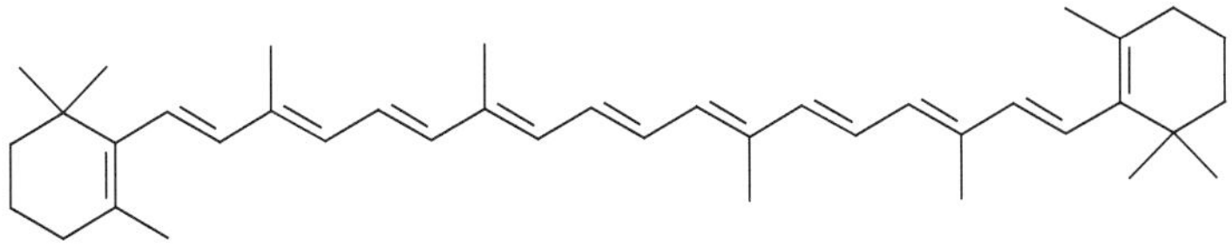

β-Carotene

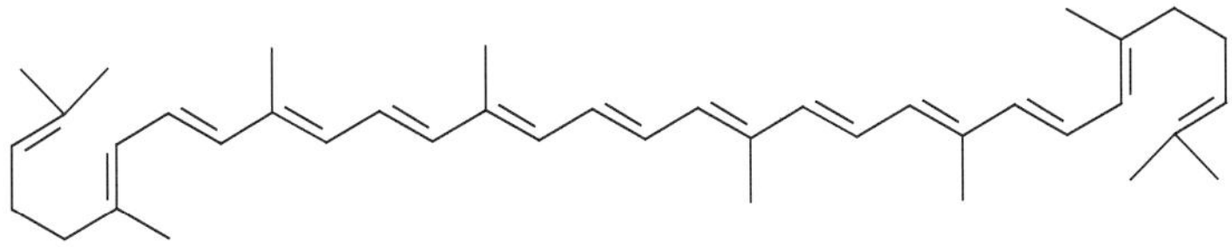

Lycopene

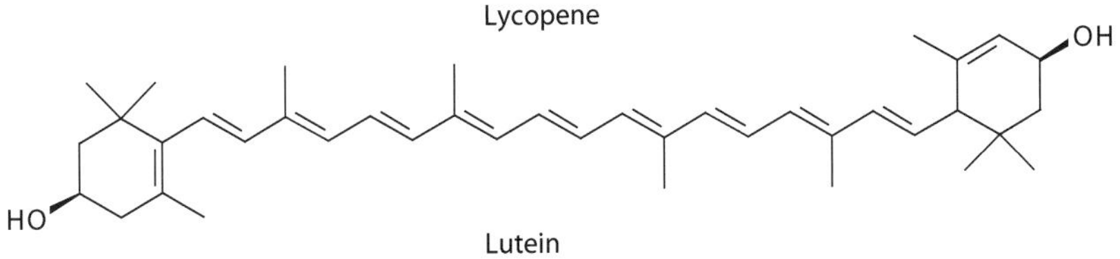

Lutein

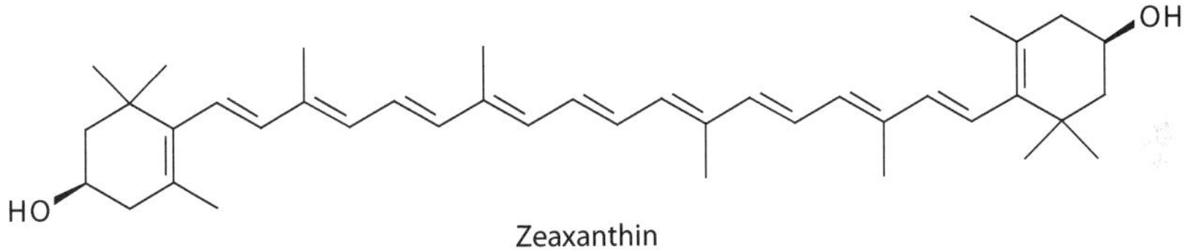

Zeaxanthin

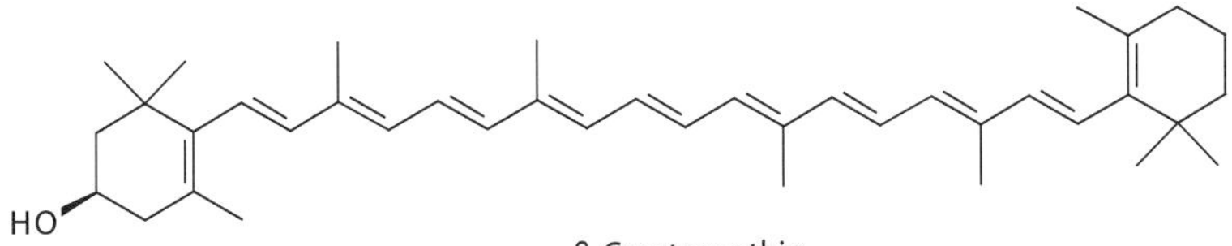

β-Cryptoxanthin

FIGURE 14.9 Chemical structure of main food carotenoids.

most efficiently react with peroxyl radicals generated in the process of lipid peroxidation. Because of their lipophilicity and specific properties to scavenge peroxyl radicals, carotenoids are thought to play an important role in the protection of cellular membranes and lipoproteins against oxidative damage (Sies and Stahl 1995; Stahl and Sies 2003). The antioxidant activity of carotenoids regarding the deactivation of peroxyl radicals likely depends on the formation of radical adducts forming a resonance-stabilized carbon-centered radical (Stahl and Sies 2003).

In addition to antioxidant activities, other health benefits of carotenoid intake include enhancement of immune function, protection from sunburn, decrease in the risk of age-related macular degeneration and cataract formation, and inhibition of development of certain forms of cancer (Peto et al. 1981; Ziegler 1991; Mayne 1996; Burrie 1997). Numerous studies suggest a reduced risk of a variety of cancers and cardiovascular disease resulting from the higher consumption of tomato-based products rich in lycopene (Ho et al. 2008). Beneficial health effects of lycopene

TABLE 14.4

Antioxidant Activities of Carotenoids as Compared to α-Tocopherol

	FRAP	TEAC	LPSC	LPO
Carotenoid	mol α-tocopherol equiv./mol			% of control
β-Carotene	0	3.1	19.1	73 ± 9
Lycopene	2.1	3.9	13.3	25 ± 10
Lutein	2.1	2.0	19.6	77 ± 9
Zeaxanthin	2.0	1.9	20.3	73 ± 9
β-Cryptoxanthin	2.1	3.2	19.3	55 ± 8
α-Tocopherol	1.0	1.0	1.0	43 ± 7

Source: Stahl, W. et al., *FEBS Lett* 427, 305–308, 1998; Müller, L. et al., *Food Chem* 129, 139–148, 2011.

Note: LPSC—luminal-chemiluminescence peroxyl radical scavenging capacity.

are believed to be related to its antioxidant activity, although other mechanisms of action, such as hormone and immune system modulation, are also suggested (Roa and Agarwal 1999; Ho et al. 2008).

The antioxidant activity of carotenoids depends on the oxygen tension present in the system (Burton and Ingold 1984; Palozza 1998). At low partial pressures of oxygen, such as those found in most tissues under physiological conditions, β-carotene was found to inhibit the oxidation. At higher oxygen tension, a prooxidant effect is observed (Burton and Ingold 1984). The concentration of carotenoids also influences their antioxidant or prooxidant properties; at high carotenoid concentrations, there is a propensity for prooxidant behavior (Valko et al. 2006). While epidemiological evidence shows that people who ingest more dietary carotenoids exhibit a reduced risk for cancer, results from intervention trials indicate that supplemental β-carotene, either alone or in combination with vitamin A or E, enhances lung cancer incidence and mortality among smokers and asbestos workers (The Alpha-Tocopherol Beta Carotene Cancer Prevention Study Group 1994; Omenn et al. 1996; Paolini et al. 1999). Baron et al. (2003) reported an increased risk of colon cancer in cigarette smokers with a high intake of β-carotene. A possible mechanism that can explain the dual role of β-carotene as both a beneficial and a harmful agent in cancer as well as in other chronic diseases is its ability to modulate intracellular redox status. β-Carotene may serve as an antioxidant or as a prooxidant, depending on its intrinsic properties and concentration as well as on the redox potential of the biological environment in which it acts (Palozza et al. 2003). The exact mechanism by which β-carotene increases lung cancer risk in both smokers and asbestos workers is unclear, although some hypotheses have been reported. One possible mechanism is a co-carcinogenic effect of β-carotene through stimulation of phase I bioactivating enzymes: an induction of CYP activity by β-carotene, which may result in increased formation of genotoxic metabolites of cigarette smoke constituents in cigarette smokers. Another possible explanation suggests the alteration of retinoid signaling by the formation of reactive oxidative cleavage products of β-carotene that are able to interfere with normal retinoid signaling (Rietjens et al. 2005). The high oxygen pressure in the lungs may favor this oxidative degeneration of β-carotene (Palozza et al. 1995). Toxic β-carotene oxidized metabolites may also result from the interaction between β-carotene with ROS derived from tobacco smoke or induced in the lung upon asbestos exposure (Mayne et al. 1996; Omaye et al. 1997; Lotan 1999; X.-D. Wang et al. 1999). Induction of CYP and enhanced retinoic acid catabolism in the lung may also reduce retinoid signaling by cigarette smoke and high doses of β-carotene (Liu et al. 2003; Rietjens et al. 2005).

14.4.4 FOLATES

Folates are a class of compounds having a chemical structure and nutritional activity similar to that of folic acid (FA; vitamin B9; Figure 14.10). FA (pteroyl-L-glutamic acid, folate, vitamin B9) is made up of a 2-amino-4-hydroxypteridine (purine and pyrazine parts fused together to give a pterin moiety) that is linked to the *p*-amino-benzoic acid coupled to the monoglutamate or polyglutamate residue via its α-amino group (Figure 14.10). FA is *in vivo* reduced to 7,8-dihydrofolate (DHF), which is

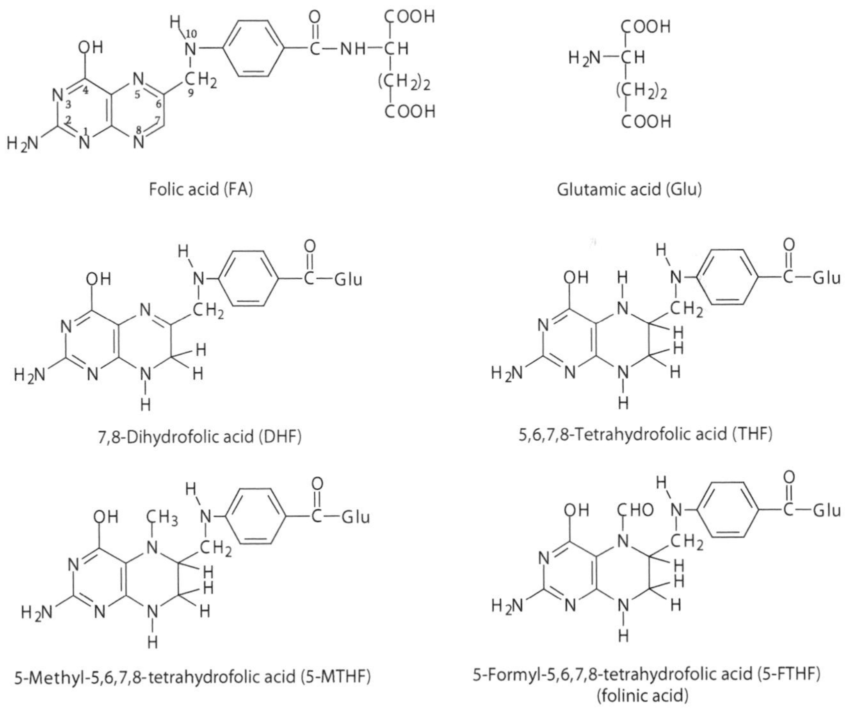

FIGURE 14.10 Chemical structures and atom numbering system of FA and its reduced forms.

subsequently reduced to 5,6,7,8-tetrahydrofolate (THF) and then enzymatically converted into 5-methyltetrahydrofolate (5-MTHF); in both latter structures, two double bonds of a pterin ring system are reduced (Figure 14.10). Reduced forms of FA are cofactors in the transfer and utilization of one-carbon units, such as methyl, formyl, and hydroxymethyl groups; they donate a one-carbon group in the biosynthesis of purine, pyrimidine, and DNA and play a key role in the regeneration of methionine (Stanger 2002).

Folates are found in both vegetable and animal foods. Citrus fruits, grains, yeasts, mushrooms, liver, pork meat, eggs, and leafy green vegetables, such as spinach, lettuce, and asparagus, are especially rich in folates. FA is used, in many countries, in nutritional supplements or for fortification of cereals and their products. It is also used in vitamin pills. Proper metabolism and sufficient intake of dietary FA before conception and during early pregnancy decrease the risk of a baby developing neural tube defects, which include spina bifida (Daly et al. 1995; Olney and Mulinare 2002). Moreover, FA deficiency has been associated with neurological and neuropsychiatric disorders (Manzoor and Runcie 1976; Alpert and Fava 2003) and a megaloblastic anemia. 5-Formyltetrahydrofolic acid (5-FTHF), known also as folinic acid, citrovorum factor, or leucovorin, is one of the coenzyme forms of FA, which is produced commercially. It is used in combination with other chemotherapy drugs to enhance the anticancer effects of fluorouracil or to help prevent or lessen the toxic effect of methotrexate (Friedrich 1988).

Some literature data suggest that folates may act as antioxidants. It was shown that FA can efficiently scavenge such free radicals as $CCl_3O_2^{\cdot}$, $N_3^{\cdot}$, $SO_4^{\cdot-}$, $Br_2^{\cdot-}$, $^{\cdot}OH$, and $O_2^{\cdot-}$. Moreover, FA can also scavenge and repair thiyl radicals at physiological pH (Joshi et al. 2001). Its physiological reduced forms (DHF, THF, and 5-MTHF) are peroxynitrite scavengers and inhibitors of lipid peroxidation (Nakano et al. 2001; Rezk et al. 2003). The antioxidant activities of folates were also observed in the TEAC, DPPH, and FRAP assays (Gliszczyńska-Świgło 2007; Gliszczyńska-Świgło and Muzolf 2007). Activity of FA against the radical-mediated oxidative damage in human whole blood was reported by Stocker et al. (2003). Their antioxidant activities are comparable to or even higher than the activity of ascorbic acid and α-tocopherol (Table 14.5).

It was also reported that the radical-scavenging activities of folates, measured in the TEAC assay, are strongly pH-dependent (Figure 14.11), but their pH-dependent TEAC profiles are generally quite different than those observed for flavonoids and betacyanins (Figure 14.6). FA is a better radical-scavenger at acid and basic pH than at neutral pH. Reduced forms of FA are better radical scavengers at acid than at neutral and basic pH values with the exception of 5-FTHF for which, at a pH higher than 5, an increase of radical-scavenging activity with increasing pH of the medium is observed (Gliszczyńska-Świgło and Muzolf 2007).

Structurally related to folates, tetrahydrobiopterin (BH_4), which is a physiologically reduced form of biopterin, exhibits a similarly pH-dependent TEAC profile to those of DHF and THF (Gliszczyńska-Świgło and Szymusiak 2007a). Biopterin as tetrahydrobiopterin (BH_4) is the cofactor of some hydroxylases (e.g., phenylalanine, tyrosine, and tryptophan hydroxylases), which use molecular oxygen to incorporate hydroxyl groups into aromatic rings. Animals have lost the ability to biosynthesize FA, but they have retained the enzyme systems for the synthesis of BH_4 (Friedrich 1988).

TABLE 14.5
Antioxidant Activities of Folic Acid and Its Reduced Forms as Compared to Ascorbic Acid and α-Tocopherol

Compound	TEAC[a] (mM)	FRAP[a] (mM)	DPPH[a] IC$_{50}$ (μM)	PON[b] IC$_{50}$ (μM)	LPO[b] IC$_{50}$ (μM)	% Inhibition[c] Vitamin Concentration 10^{-6} M	10^{-5} M
KF	0.06 ± 0.01	0.04 ± 0.01	374 ± 31	>100	>500	11	83
DHF	0.98 ± 0.01	2.85 ± 0.19	107 ± 6	2.4 ± 0.3	>500	–	–
THF	1.24 ± 0.11	2.27 ± 0.09	24.1 ± 1.7	1.5 ± 0.2	189 ± 26	–	–
5-MTHF	0.77 ± 0.04	1.75 ± 0.06	50.5 ± 4.3	0.9 ± 0.1	>500	–	–
5-FTHF	0.55 ± 0.02	0.76 ± 0.01	>500	–	–	–	–
Ascorbic acid	0.99 ± 0.05	1.98 ± 0.05	21.8 ± 1.6	–	–	18	32
α-Tocopherol	0.97 ± 0.03	1.95 ± 0.20	18.2 ± 1.1	–	–	13	43

[a] Gliszczyńska-Świgło 2007, 2010; Gliszczyńska-Świgło 2007, 2010; Gliszczyńska-Swigło and Muzolf 2007.

[b] Rezk et al. 2003.

[c] Inhibition of radical-mediated oxidative damage in human whole blood (Stocker et al. 2003).

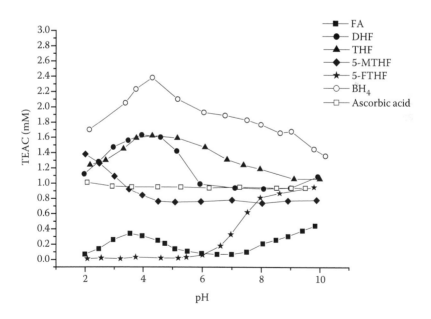

FIGURE 14.11 Effect of pH on the TEAC values of FA, its physiological reduced forms, ascorbic acid, and BH$_4$. (From Gliszczyńska-Świgło, A. and M. Muzolf, *J Agric Food Chem* 55, 8237–8242, 2007a; Gliszczyńska-Świgło, A. and H. Szymusiak, 2007.)

Several reports indicate a clear association between folate intake and cardio-vascular diseases (Doshi et al. 2002; Verhaar et al. 2002; Moat et al. 2004). FA is considered to be potentially protective against cardiovascular diseases because of its homocysteine-lowering potential (Boushey et al. 1995). However, it has also been suggested that folates may enhance endothelial function via the mechanisms independent of homocysteine lowering (Doshi et al. 2002), including a direct anti-oxidant role *in vivo*. Plausible mechanisms include the role of 5-MTHF in the redox cycling of the inactive quinoid dihydrobiopterin (BH_2) or in the chemical stabiliza-tion of tetrahydrobiopterin (BH_4) (Doshi et al. 2002; Verhaar et al. 2002), which is an essential cofactor of endothelial NO synthase (eNOS). The depletion of BH_4 results in the uncoupling of eNOS activity and a switch from the production of NO to the generation of a superoxide (Vásquez-Vivar et al. 1998). Folates may also act as direct antioxidants against superoxides. The last mechanism suggested is the direct effect of folates on eNOS, in which 5-MTHF reduces superoxide generation and increases NO synthesis in a BH_4-dependent manner (Doshi et al. 2002; Verhaar et al. 2002) (Figure 14.12).

There is also evidence that a deficiency of folates can cause damage to DNA that may lead to cancer (Duthie et al. 2002). It was proposed that the presumed protective effects of folates in the pathogenesis of different diseases, such as neu-ral tube defects, megaloblastic anemia, cardiovascular disease, and certain forms of cancer, could be associated, at least in part, with their antioxidant activity (Nakano et al. 2001). Physiological concentrations of folates are much lower than the level of vitamin C, the main biological water-soluble antioxidant. On the other hand, blood concentrations of folates as well as some polyphenols and carotenoids can reach similar level in humans following their habitual or supplemented diets (Mackey and Picciano 1999; Erlund et al. 2002; Manach et al. 2005; Lamers et al. 2006). The role of folates as biological antioxidants is still uncertain, however, cannot be excluded.

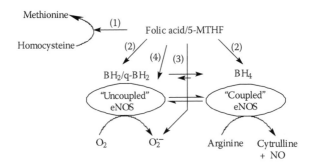

FIGURE 14.12   Possible mechanisms for beneficial effects of folates on vascular endothelial function: (1) 5-MTHF as methyl donor in conversion of homocysteine to methionine (homo-cysteine-lowering effect), (2) chemical stabilization and regeneration of BH_4 from BH_2 by 5-MTHF, (3) direct scavenging of superoxide radicals, (4) direct effect on enzymatic activity of uncoupled eNOS and reduction of superoxide generation and increase of NO synthesis in BH_4-dependent manner. (From Verhaar, M.C. et al., *Arterioscler Thromb Vasc Biol* 22, 6–13, 2002; Moat, S.J. et al., *J Nutr Biochem* 15, 64–79, 2004.)

14.4.5 OTHER VITAMINS

The activity of pyridoxine, one of the forms of vitamin B6, against the radical-mediated oxidative damage in human whole blood was reported by Stocker et al. (2003). Thiamine (vitamin B1) has been found to protect against lead-induced lipid peroxidation in rat liver and kidneys (Senapati et al. 2000). It may scavenge $O_2^{\cdot-}$ and $\cdot OH$ directly and thus affect the cellular response to oxidative stress (Jung and Kim 2003). It was also reported that thiamine deficiency results in selective neuronal death in animal models. The neuronal death was associated with increased free radical production, suggesting that oxidative stress processes may play an important early role in the brain damage associated with thiamine deficiency; however, the mechanism of the possible antioxidant activity of thiamine is unknown (Todd and Butterworth 1999). It was also reported that thiamine and vitamin B6 forms (pyridoxine, pyridoxal, pyridoxamine, and their metabolite pyridoxic acid) are able to scavenge the ABTS$^{\cdot+}$ radical cation, although they react with it relatively slowly (Gliszczyńska-Świgło 2006). The radical-scavenging activity of water-soluble vitamins in the TEAC assay is also pH-dependent and increases at pH higher than 6 (Gliszczyńska-Świgło and Szymusiak 2007b).

14.5 OTHER FOOD ANTIOXIDANTS: THIOL ANTIOXIDANTS

Glutathione, the tripeptide γ-glutamylcysteinylglycine (Figure 14.13), is the major thiol nonenzymatic intracellular antioxidant maintaining protein thiols in a reduced state. It exists either in reduced (GSH) or oxidized (glutathione disulfide, GSSG) form and participates in redox reactions by the reversible oxidation of its active thiol residue. Under normal cellular conditions, glutathione is in its reduced form and is

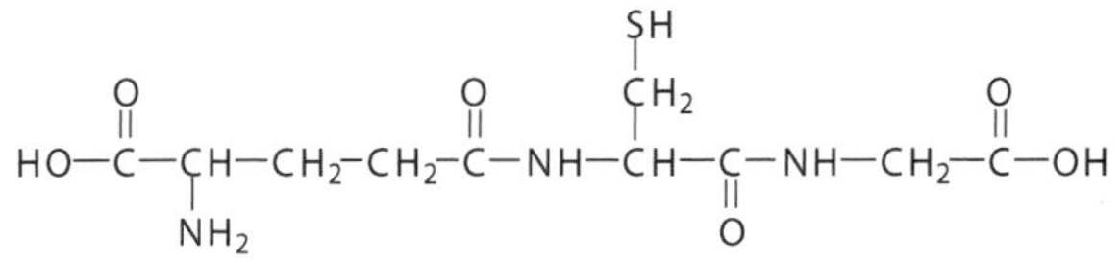

Glutathione (GSH)

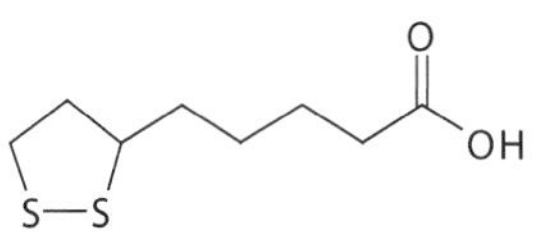

Lipoic acid (LA)

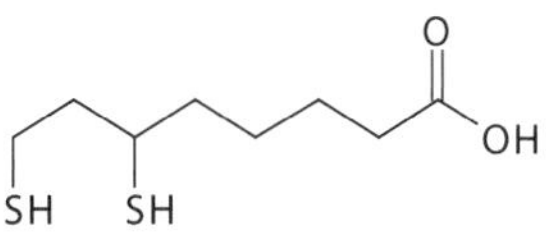

Dihydrolipoic acid (DHLA)

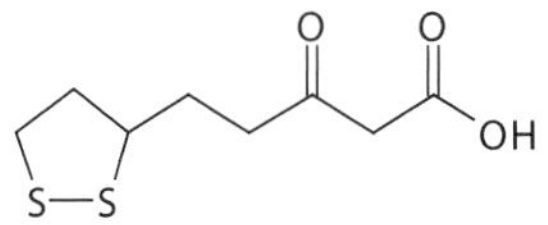

3-Ketolipoic acid

FIGURE 14.13 Chemical structures of thiol antioxidants.

present in millimolar concentrations in the cytosol (1–11 mM), nuclei (3–15 mM), and mitochondria (5–11 mM) (Valko et al. 2006). Cellular GSH concentrations are mainly influenced by the dietary availability of cysteine. GSH concentration in human plasma is low and may reach only 20 µM (Lash and Jones 1989) with an average of 8 µM (Davis et al. 2006). Deficiency of glutathione was observed in symptom-free HIV-seropositive and diabetic patients and with alcoholic liver disease (Buhl et al. 1989; Samiec et al. 1998; Albano 2002). The low ratio of GSH/GSSG is a good indicator of oxidative stress in organism.

GSH directly scavenges hydroxyl radicals and singlet oxygen or acts as a substrate for glutathione peroxidase and glutathionyl transferase during the detoxification of hydrogen peroxide, lipid peroxides, and electrophilic compounds. It is able to regenerate vitamins C and E. In these ways, GSH exerts a protective role against oxidative stress (Masella et al. 2005; Valko et al. 2006).

Glutathione is present in all foods, although food is not a good source of glutathione. Avocado has been noted as a particularly rich fruit source of GSH (Stahl et al. 2002). Much of the ingested glutathione is converted into its constituent amino acids in the intestinal lumen; thus, food may only serve as a safe source of amino acid precursors of GSH synthesized in the human liver (Stahl et al. 2002).

α-Lipoic acid (LA) or 6,8-thioctic acid is a disulfide derivative of octanoic acid. It is both water- and fat-soluble and, therefore, is distributed in both cellular membranes and the cytosol. It is readily absorbed from food and reduced in many tissues to dihydrolipoic acid (DHLA) (Figure 14.13). In the human diet, lipoic acid is present at parts-per-million levels (mg/kg) in milk, wheat germ, wheat flour, yeast, chicken eggs, and animal organs (Drinda and Baltes 1999). Both LA and DHLA are effective antioxidants, scavenging ROS, such as singlet oxygen, hydroxyl radicals, hypochlorous acid, superoxide anion radicals, peroxyl radicals, and hydrogen peroxide. It regenerates vitamins C and E and glutathione, chelates transition metals, and repairs oxidized proteins (Valko et al. 2006). The reduced form has an antioxidant function because of the two SH-moieties that may result in the 1,2-thiolane group upon oxidation. Dihydrolipoic acid can also function as a prooxidant. Similar to vitamins E and C, this prooxidant action of lipoic acid is probably mediated by the reduction of transition metals (Bast and Haenen 2002).

Relatively high concentrations of 3-ketolipoic acid (Figure 14.13) as a major metabolite of lipoic acid were detected in the plasma of male volunteers after the oral administration of 1 g of R-lipoic acid. Its structural characteristics suggest that it is still an antioxidant. This metabolite is probably formed during the beta-oxidation of lipoic acid. It may largely contribute to the therapeutic activity of lipoic acid (Bast and Haenen 2002).

Lipoic acid is used as a potent detoxication agent for heavy metal poisoning and has been implicated as a means to improve age-associated cognitive decline. It is a useful agent for treatment of complications associated with diabetes mellitus (Rahimi et al. 2005).

14.6 SUMMARY

It is commonly accepted that antioxidant-rich fruits and vegetables protect against chronic diseases. Many dietary antioxidants, including flavonoids, are candidates for drugs used in chemoprevention or cancer treatment. The effect of flavonoids on cell proliferation and the viability of various carcinoma cell lines were extensively studied. In the majority of studies, an inhibition of proliferation at the higher flavonoid concentrations was observed (Scambia et al. 1990; Kuo 1996; So et al. 1996, 1997; Kawaii et al. 1999; Damianaki et al. 2000; Knowles et al. 2000; Casagrande and Darbon 2001; van der Woude et al. 2003), but a dualistic influence of, for example, quercetin on the colon carcinoma cell lines HCT-29 and HT29 and the mammary adenocarcinoma cell line MCT-7 was also reported. At lower physiologically relevant concentrations, a subtle but significant stimulation of cell proliferation was observed (van der Woude et al. 2003). Moreover, either high doses or chronic exposure to phytochemicals might cause genotoxicity or cytotoxicity to normal cells, limiting their maximum exposure doses. There is no evidence that normal dietary intake of antioxidants is harmful, whereas therapeutic administration and very high dose supplements can be harmful or even toxic (Galati et al. 2004; Stevenson and Hurst 2007; Finley et al. 2011). It was reported that EGCG doses of 10^{-8}–10^{-5} M protected the DNA of lymphocytes against oxidative damage, whereas high doses of 10^{-3} M caused an increase in DNA lesions (Kanadzu et al. 2006). Hepatotoxicity related to the consumption of high doses of green tea phenolics and tea-based dietary supplements was also reported (Bonkowsky 2006; Galati et al. 2006). Quercetin administered orally to rats caused a significant reduction of glutathione and glutathione reductase concentrations (Choi et al. 2003). High tannin supplementation of chicken feed reduced the absorption of essential minerals, such as calcium, magnesium, iron, potassium, sodium, and phosphorus (Hassan et al. 2003). Male rats dosed with large amounts of a kiwi fruit extract showed suppression of testosterone levels and sperm count (Panjeh-Shahin et al. 2005). High doses of β-carotene caused an increased risk for lung and colon cancers in certain populations (The Alpha-Tocopherol Beta Carotene Cancer Prevention Study Group 1994; Baron et al. 2003). Similar results have been reported for vitamin E (Dotan et al. 2009). The incorporation of high amounts of flaxseed into the rat diet caused a significant reduction in the vitamin E level and an elevation of urinary thiobarbituric reacting substances (Ratnayake et al. 1992). The results of Frank et al. (2004) revealed that SDG and its oligomers supplemented to rats caused an increase in liver cholesterol and a twofold reduction in the levels of α- and γ-tocopherols in rat plasma and liver. Reduced levels of vitamin E, especially of γ-tocopherol, have been associated with an increased risk for cardiovascular disease (Hensley et al. 2004). More examples of adverse effects of dietary antioxidants can be found in the literature.

Still, little is known about the interactions of dietary antioxidants with other food compounds or with drugs and about consequences of these interactions. Genetic polymorphisms in the different enzyme systems may also influence the risk of toxicity. Moreover, elimination of too much ROS/RNS can be also harmful because they play either a harmful or beneficial role in biological systems. Beneficial effects include physiological roles in several cellular signaling pathways and in cellular responses against infectious agents. In the context of the increased number of compounds or plant extracts that humans might be exposed to, it must be remembered that dietary antioxidant compounds are able to exert both beneficial as well as potentially harmful effects, depending on physiological conditions and the dosage used.

Already approximately 500 years ago, Paracelsus stated that toxicity of the compound is a matter of dose; it means that adverse health effects upon either acute or chronic exposure to phytochemicals may occur.

REFERENCES

Abd El Mohsen, M.M., Kuhnle, G., Rechner, A.R., Schroeter, H., Rose, S., Jenner, P. and C.A. Rice-Evans. 2002. Uptake and metabolism of epicatechin and its access to the brain after oral ingestion. *Free Radic Biol Med* 33: 1693–1702.

Aherne, S.A. and N.M. O'Brien. 1999. Protection by the flavonoids myricetin, quercetin, and rutin against hydrogen peroxide-induced DNA damage in Caco-2 and Hep G2 cells. *Nutr Cancer* 34: 160–166.

Albano, E. 2002. Free radical mechanisms in immune reactions associated with alcoholic liver disease. *Free Radic Biol Med* 32: 110–114.

Allegra, M., Furtmueller, P.G., Jantschko, W., Zederbauer, M., Tesoriere, L., Livrea, M.A. and C. Obinger. 2005. Mechanism of interaction of betanin and indicaxanthin with human myeloperoxidase and hypochlorous acid. *Biochem Biophys Res Commun* 332: 837–844.

Alpert, J.E. and M. Fava. 2003. Nutrition and depression: The role of folate. *Nutr Rev* 55: 145–149.

Andreason, M.F., Kroon, P., Williamson, G. and M.T. Garcia-Conesa. 2001. Esterase activity able to hydrolyse dietary antioxidant hydroxycinnamates is distributed along the intestine of mammals. *J Agric Food Chem* 49: 5679–5684.

Arts, I.C. and P.C. Hollman. 2005. Polyphenols and disease risk in epidemiologic studies. *Am J Clin Nutr* 81: 317S–325S.

Aruoma, O.I., Halliwell, B., Aeschbach, R. and J. Löligers. 1992. Antioxidant and pro-oxidant properties of active rosemary constituents: Carnosol and carnosic acid. *Xenobiotica* 22: 257–268.

Auger, C., Al-Awwadi, N., Bornet, A., Rouanet, J.-M., Grasc, F., Cros, G. and P.-L. Teissedre. 2004. Catechins and procyanidins in Mediterranean diets. *Food Res Int* 37: 233–245.

Awad, H.M., Boersma, M.G., Boeren, S., van Bladeren, P., Vervoort, J. and I.M.C.M. Rietjens. 2001. Structure-activity study on the quinone/quinone methide chemistry of flavonoids. *Chem Res Toxicol* 14: 398–408.

Awad, H.M., Boersma, M., Boeren, S., van Bladeren, P.J., Vervoort, J. and I.M.C.M. Rietjens. 2003. Quenching of quercetin quinone/quinone methides by different thiolate scavengers: Stability and reversibility of conjugate formation. *Chem Res Toxicol* 16: 822–831.

Awad, H.M., Boersma, M.G., Boeren, S., van der Woude, H., van Zanden, J., van Bladeren, P., Vervoort, J. and I.M.C.M. Rietjens. 2002. Identification of o-quinone/quinone methide metabolites of quercetin in a cellular *in vitro* system. *FEBS Lett* 520: 30–34.

Awad, H.M., Boersma, M.G., Vervoort, J. and I.M.C.M. Rietjens. 2000. Peroxidase-catalysed formation of quercetin quinone methide glutathione adducts. *Arch Biochem Biophys* 378: 224–233.

Awika, J.M. 2008. Behavior of 3-deoxyanthocyanidins in the presence of phenolic copigments. *Food Res Int* 41: 532–538.

Azam, S., Hadi, N., Khan, N.U. and S.M. Hadi. 2004. Prooxidant property of green tea polyphenols epicatechin and epigallocatechin-3-gallate: Implications for anticancer properties. *Toxicol in Vitro* 18: 555–561.

Azzi, A. and A. Stocker. 2000. Vitamin E: Non-antioxidant roles. *Progr Lipid* 39: 231–255.

Bakker, M.I. 2004. Dietary intake of phytoestrogens. *RIVM Report* 320103002/2004.

Bakowska, A., Kucharska, A.Z. and J. Oszmiański. 2003. The effects of heating, UV irradiation, and storage on stability of the anthocyanin-polyphenol copigment complex. *Food Chem* 81: 349–355.

Balentine, D.A., Wiseman, S.A. and L.C.M. Bouwens. 1997. The chemistry of tea flavonoids. *Crit Rev Food Sci Nutr* 37: 693–704.

Baranac, J.M., Petranovic, N.A. and J.M. Dimitric-Markovic. 1996. Spectrophotometric study of anthocyanin copigmentation reactions. *J Agric Food Chem* 44: 1333–1336.

Baranac, J.M., Petranovic, N.A. and J.M. Dimitric-Markovic. 1997a. Spectrophotometric study of anthocyanin copigmentation reactions. 3. Malvin and the nonglycosidized flavone morin. *J Agric Food Chem* 45: 1698–1700.

Baranac, J.M., Petranovic, N.A. and J.M. Dimitric-Markovic. 1997b. Spectrophotometric study of anthocyan copigmentation reactions. 2. Malvin and the nonglycosidized flavone quercetin. *J Agric Food Chem* 45: 1694–1697.

Baranac, J.M., Petranovic, N.A. and J.M. Dimitric-Markovic. 1997c. Spectrophotometric study of anthocyanin copigmentation reactions. 4. Malvin and apigenin 7-glucoside. *J Agric Food Chem* 45: 701–703.

Barbosa, D.S. 2007. Green tea polyphenolic compounds and human health. *J Verbr Lebensm* 2: 407–413.

Baron, A.B., Cole, B.F., Mott, L., Haile, R., Grau, M., Church, T.R., Beck, G.J. and E.R. Greenberg. 2003. Neoplastic and antineoplastic effects of β-carotene on colorectal adenoma recurrence: Results of a randomized intervention trial. *J Natl Cancer Inst* 95: 717–722.

Bast, A. and G.R.M.M. Haenen. 2002. The toxicity of antioxidants and their metabolites. *Environ Toxicol Pharmacol* 11: 251–258.

Beecher, G.R. 2003. Overview of dietary flavonoids: Nomenclature, occurrence and intake. *J Nutr* 133: 3248S–3254S.

Belitz, H.-D., Grosch, W. and P. Schieberle. 2009. *Food Chemistry*. Berlin: Springer.

Boersma, M.G., Vervoort, J., Szymusiak, H., Lemanska, K., Tyrakowska, B., Cenas, N., Segura-Aguilar, J. and I.M.C.M. Rietjens. 2000. Regioselectivity and reversibility of the glutathione conjugation of quercetin quinone methide. *Chem Res Toxicol* 13: 185–191.

Bolton, J.L., Pisha, E., Zhang, F. and S. Qiu. 1998. Role of quinoids in estrogen carcinogenesis. *Chem Res Toxicol* 11: 1113–1126.

Bolton, J.L., Trush, M.A., Penning, T.M., Dryhurst, G. and T.J. Monks. 2000. Role of quinones in toxicology. *Chem Res Toxicol* 13: 135–160.

Bomser, J., Madhavi, D.L., Singletary, K. and M.A. Smith. 1996. *In vitro* anticancer activity of fruit extracts from *Vaccinium* species. *Planta Med* 62: 212–216.

Bonkovsky, H.L. 2006. Hepatotoxicity associated with supplements containing Chinese green tea (*Camellia sinensis*). *Ann Int Med* 144: 68–71.

Boots, A.W., Balk, J.M., Bast, A. and G.R.M.M. Haenen. 2005. The reversibility of the glutathionyl-quercetin adduct spread oxidized quercetin-induced toxicity. *Biochem Biophys Res Commun* 338: 923–929.

Boots, A.W., Haenen, G.R.M.M. and A. Bast. 2008. Health effects of quercetin: From antioxidant to nutraceutical. *Eur J Pharm* 585: 325–337.

Boots, A.W., Haenen, G.R.M.M., den Hartog, G.J.M. and A. Bast. 2002. Oxidative damage shifts from lipid peroxidation to thiol arylation by catechol-containing antioxidants. *Biochim Biophys Acta* 1583: 279–284.

Boots, A.W., Kubben, N., Haenen, G.R.M.M. and A. Bast. 2003. Oxidized quercetin reacts with thiols rather than with ascorbate: Implication for quercetin supplementation. *Biochem Biophys Res Commun* 308: 560–565.

Boots, A.W., Li, H., Schins, R.P., Duffin, R., Heemskerk, J.W., Bast, A. and G.R.M.M. Haenen. 2007. The quercetin paradox. *Toxicol Appl Pharmacol* 222: 89–96.

Borkowski, T., Szymusiak, H., Gliszczyńska-Świgło, A., Rietjens, I.M.C.M. and B. Tyrakowska. 2005. Radical scavenging capacity of wine anthocyanins is strongly pH-dependent. *J Agric Food Chem* 53: 5526–5534.

Bors, W., Hellen, W., Michel, C. and M. Saran. 1990. Flavonoids as antioxidants: Determination of radical-scavenging efficiencies. *Methods Enzymol* 186: 343–355.

Botsoglou, N.A., Yannakopoulos, A.L., Fletouris, D.J., Tserveni-Goussi, A.S. and P.D. Fortomaris. 1997. Effect of dietary thyme on the oxidative stability of egg yolk. *J Agric Food Chem* 45: 3711–3716.

Boulton, R. 2001. The copigmentation of anthocyanins and its role in the color of red wine: A critical review. *Am J Enol Vitic* 52: 67–87.

Boushey, C.J., Beresford, S.A., Omenn, G.S. and A.G. Motulsky. 1995. A quantitative assessment of plasma homocysteine as a risk factor for vascular disease: Probable benefits of increasing folic acid intakes. *J Am Med Assoc* 274: 1049–1057.

Buettner, G.R. 1993. The pecking order of free radicals and antioxidants: Lipid peroxidation, alpha-tocopherol, and ascorbate. *Arch Biochem Biophys* 300: 535–543.

Buhl, R., Jaffe, H.A., Holroyd, K.J., Wells, F.B., Mastrangeli, A., Saltini, C., Cantin, A.M. and R.G. Crystal. 1989. Systemic glutathione deficiency in symptom-free HIV-seropositive individuals. *Lancet* 2: 1294–1298.

Burrie, B.J. 1997. β-Carotene and human health: A review of currant research. *Nutr Res* 17: 547–580.

Burton, G.W. and K.U. Ingold. 1984. β-Carotene: An unusual type of lipid antioxidant. *Science* 224: 569–573.

Butera, D., Tesoriere, L., Di Gaudio, F., Bongiorno, A., Allegra, M., Pintaudi, A.M., Kohen, R. and M.A. Livrea. 2002. Antioxidant activities of Sicilian prickly pear (*Opuntia ficus indica*) fruit extracts and reducing properties of its betalains: Betanin and indicaxanthin. *J Agric Food Chem* 50: 6895–6901.

Cabrera, C., Artach, R. and R. Jimenez. 2006. Beneficial effects of green tea: A review. *J Am Coll Nutr* 25: 79–99.

Cai, Y., Sun, M. and H. Corke. 2003. Antioxidant activity of betalains from plants of the Amaranthaceae. *J Agric Food Chem* 51: 2288–2294.

Cao, G., Muccitelli, H.U., Sánchez-Moreno, C. and R.L. Prior. 2001. Anthocyanins are absorbed in glycated forms in elderly women: A pharmacokinetic study. *Am J Clin Nutr* 73: 920–926.

Cao, G., Sofic, E. and R.L. Prior. 1997. Antioxidant and prooxidant behavior of flavonoids: Structure-activity relationships. *Free Radic Biol Med* 22: 749–760.

Carr, A. and B. Frei. 1999. Does vitamin C act as a pro-oxidant under physiological conditions? *FASEB J* 13: 1007–1024.

Casagrande, F. and J.-M. Darbon. 2001. Effects of structurally related flavonoids on cell cycle progression of human melanoma cells: Regulation of cyclin-dependent kinases CDK2 and CDK1. *Biochem Pharmacol* 61: 1205–1215.

Cemeli, E., Baumgartner, A. and D. Anderson. 2009. Antioxidants and the Comet assay. *Mutat Res* 681: 51–67.

Chang, H.C., Churchwell, M.I., Delclos, K.B., Newbold, R.R. and D.R. Doerge. 2000. Mass spectrometric determination of genistein tissue distribution in diet-exposed Sprague–Dawley rats. *J Nutr* 130: 1963–1970.

Chen, C., Yu, R., Owuor, E.D. and A.-N. Kong. 2000. Activation of antioxidant-response element (ARE), mitogen-activated protein kinases (MAPKs) and caspases by major green tea polyphenol components during cell survival. *Arch Pharm Res* 23: 605–621.

Chen, K., Suh, J., Carr, A.C., Morrow, J.D., Zeind, J. and B. Frei. 2000. Vitamin C suppresses oxidative lipid damage *in vivo*, even in the presence of iron overload. *Am J Physiol Endocrinol Metab* 279: E1406–E1412.

Chen, W., Sun, S., Cao, W., Liang, Y. and J. Song. 2009. Antioxidant property of quercetin-Cr(III) complex: The role of Cr(III) ion. *J Mol Struct* 918: 194–197.

Chen, Z.Y. and P.T. Chan. 1996. Antioxidative activity of green tea catechins in canola oil. *Chem PhysLipids* 82: 163–172.

Choi, E.J., Chee, K.-M. and B.H. Lee. 2003. Anti- and prooxidant effects of chronic quercetin administration in rats. *Eur J Pharm* 482: 281–285.

Choi, J.S., Chung, H.Y., Kang, S.S., Jung, M.J., Kim, J.W., No, J.K. and H.A. Jung. 2002. The structure-activity relationship of flavonoids as scavengers of peroxynitrite. *Phytother Res* 16: 232–235.

Christen, S., Woodall, A.A., Shigenaga, M.K., Southwell-Keely, P.T., Duncan, M.W. and B.N. Ames. 1997. γ-Tocopherol traps mutagenic electrophiles such as NOx and complements α-tocopherol: Physiological implications. *Proc Natl Acad Sci USA* 94: 3217–3222.

Chun, O.K., Chung, S.J. and W.O. Song. 2007. Estimated dietary flavonoid intake and major food sources of U.S. adults. *J. Nutr* 137: 1244–1252.

Clavel, T., Lippman, R., Gavini, F., Doré, J. and M. Blaut. 2007. *Clostridium saccharogumia* sp. nov. and *Lactonifactor longoviformis* gen. nov., sp. nov., two novel human faecal bacteria involved in the conversion of the dietary phytoestrogen secoisolariciresinol diglucoside. *Syst Appl Microbiol* 30: 16–26.

Clifford, M.N. 1999. Chlorogenic acids and other cinnamates, occurrence and dietary burden. *J Sci Food Agric* 79: 362–372.

Clifford, M.N. 2004. Diet-derived phenols in plasma and tissues and their implications for health. *Planta Med* 70: 1103–1114.

Colantuoni, A., Bertuglia, S., Magistretti, M.J. and L. Donato. 1991. Effects of Vaccinium Myrtillus anthocyanosides on arterial vasomotion. *Arzneimittelforschung* 41: 905–909.

Coldham, N.G. and M.J. Sauer. 2000. Pharmacokinetics of [(14)C]genistein in the rat: Gender-related differences, potential mechanisms of biological action, and implications for human health. *Toxicol Appl Pharmacol* 164: 206–215.

Collis, C.S., Yang, M., Diplock, A.T., Hallinan, T. and C.A. Rice-Evans. 1997. Effects of co-supplementation of iron with ascorbic acid on antioxidant-pro-oxidant balance in the guinea pig. *Free Radic Res* 27: 113–121.

Cook, N.C. and S. Samman. 1996. Flavonoids: Chemistry, metabolism, cardioprotective effects, and dietary sources. *Nutr Biochem* 7: 66–76.

Cooper, R., Morré, J. and D. Morré. 2005a. Medicinal benefits of green tea: Part I. Review of noncancer health benefits. *J Altern Complement Med* 5: 521–528.

Cooper, R., Morré, J. and D. Morré. 2005b. Medicinal benefits of green tea: Part II. Review of anticancer properties. *J Altern Complemen Med* 11: 639–652.

Crespy, V., Morand, C., Besson, C., Manach, C., Demigne, C. and C. Remesy. 2002. Quercetin, but not its glycosides, is absorbed from the rat stomach. *J Agric Food Chem* 50: 618–621.

Crespy, V. and G. Williamson. 2004. A review of the health effects of green tea catechins in *in vivo* animal models. *J Nutr* 134: 3431S–3440S.

Daly, L.E., Kirke, P.N., Molloy, A., Weir, D.G. and J.M. Scott. 1995. Folate levels and neural tube defects: Implications for prevention. *J Am Med Assoc* 274: 1698–1702.

Damianaki, A., Bakogeorgou, E., Kampa, M., Notas, G., Hatzoglou, A., Panagiotou, S., Gemetzi, C., Kouroumalis, E., Martin, P.M. and E. Castanas. 2000. Potent inhibitory action of red wine polyphenols on human breast cancer cells. *J Cell Biochem* 78: 429–441.

Datla, K.P., Christidou, M., Widmer, W.W., Rooprai, H.K. and D.T. Dexter. 2001. Tissue distribution and neuroprotective effects of citrus flavonoid tangeretin in a rat model of Parkinson's disease. *Neuroreport* 12: 3871–3875.

Davis, S.R., Quinlivan, E.P., Stacpoole, P.W. and J.F. Gregory III. 2006. Plasma glutathione and cystathionine concentrations are elevated but cysteine flux is unchanged by dietary vitamin B6 restriction in young men and women. *J Nutr* 136: 373–378.

Day, A.J., DuPont, M.S., Ridley, S., Rhodes, M., Rhodes, M.J., Morgan, M.R. and G. Williamson. 1998. Deglycosylation of flavonoid and isoflavonoid glycosides by human small intestine and liver beta-glucosidase activity. *FEBS Lett* 436: 71–75.

de Boer, V.C.J., Dihal, A.A., van der Woude, H., Arts, I.C.W., Wolfram, S., Alink, G.M., Rietjens, I.M.C.M., Keijer, J. and P.C.H. Hollman. 2005. Tissue distribution of quercetin in rats and pigs. *J Nutr* 135: 1718–1725.

DeJong, S. and M.C. Lanari. 2009. Extracts of olive polyphenols improve lipid stability in cooked beef and pork: Contribution of individual phenolics to the antioxidant activity of the extract. *Food Chem* 116: 892–897.

Dimitrovic-Markovic, J.M., Petranovic, N.A. and J.M. Baranac. 2000. A spectrophotometric study of the copigmentation of malvin with caffeic and ferulic acids. *J Agric Food Chem* 48: 5530–5536.

Dinkova-Kostova, A.T., Holtzclaw, W.D. and T.W. Kensler. 2005. The role of Keap1 in cellular protective responses. *Chem Res Toxicol* 18: 1779–1791.

Doshi, S.N., McDowell, I.F.W., Moat, S.J., Payne, N., Durrant, H.J., Lewis, M.J. and J. Goodfellow. 2002. Folic acid improves endothelial function in coronary artery disease via mechanism largely independent of homocysteine lowering. *Circulation* 105: 22–26.

Dotan, Y., Pinchuk, I., Lichtenberg, D. and M. Leshno. 2009. Decision analysis supports the paradigm that indiscriminate supplementation of vitamin E does more harm than good. *Arterioscler Thromb Vasc Biol* 29: 1304–1309.

Drinda, H. and W. Baltes. 1999. Antioxidant properties of lipoic and dihydrolipoic acid in vegetable oils and lard. *Z Lebensm Unters Forsch A* 208: 270–276.

Duffy, S.J., Keaney, J.F., Holbrook, M., Gokce, N., Swerdloff, P.L., Frei, B. and J.A. Vita. 2001. Short- and long-term black tea consumption reverses endothelial dysfunction in patients with coronary artery disease. *Circulation* 104: 151–156.

Duthie, G. and A. Crosier. 2000. Plant-derived phenolic antioxidants. *Curr Opin Clin Nutr Metab Care* 3: 447–451.

Duthie, S.J., Narayanan, S., Brand, G.M., Pirie, L. and G. Grant. 2002. Impact of folate deficiency on DNA stability. *J Nutr* 132: 2444S–2449S.

Erlund, I., Silaste, M.L., Alfthan, G., Rantala, M., Kesäniemi, Y.A. and A. Aro. 2002. Plasma concentrations of the flavonoids hesperetin, naringenin and quercetin in human subjects following their habitual diets, and diets high or low in fruit and vegetables. *Eur J Clin Nutr* 56: 891–898.

Escribaño, J., Pedreno, M.A., Garcia-Carmona, F. and R. Munoz. 1998. Characterization of the antiradical activity of betalains from *Beta vulgaris* L. roots. *Phytochem Anal* 9: 124–127.

Felgines, C., Talavéra, S., Gonthier, M.P., Texier, O., Scalbert, A., Lamaison, J.L. and C. Rémésy. 2003. Strawberry anthocyanins are recovered in urine as glucuro- and sulfo-conjugates in humans. *J Nutr* 133: 1296–1301.

Finley, J.W., Kong, A.-N., Hintze, K.J., Jeffery, E.H., Ji, L.L. and X.G. Lei. 2011. Antioxidants in foods: State of the science important to the food industry. *J Agric Food Chem* 59: 6837–6846.

Fleschhut, J., Kratzer, F., Rechkemmer, G. and S.E. Kulling. 2006. Stability and biotransformation of various dietary anthocyanins *in vitro*. *Eur J Nutr* 45: 7–18.

Formica, J.V. and W. Regelson. 1995. Review of the biology of quercetin and related bioflavonoids. *Food Chem Toxicol* 33: 1061–1080.

Frank, J., Eliasson, C., Leroy-Nivard, D., Budek, A., Lundh, T., Vessby, B., Aman P. and A. Kamal-Eldin. 2004. Dietary secoisolariciresinol diglucoside and its oligomers with 3-hydroxy-3-methyl glutaric acid decrease vitamin E levels in rats. *Br J Nutr* 92: 169–176.

Frank, T., Stintzing, F.C., Carle, R., Bitsch, I., Quas, D., Straβ, G., Bitsch, R. and M. Netzel. 2005. Urinary pharmacokinetics of betalains following consumption of red beet juice in healthy humans. *Pharmacol Res* 52: 290–297.

Frankel, E.N., Huang, S.-W., Aeschbach, R. and E. Prior. 1996. Antioxidant activity of a rosemary extract and its constituents, carnosic acid, carnosol, and rosmarinic acid, in bulk oil and oil-in-water emulsion. *J Agric Food Chem* 44: 131–135.

Frei, B. and J.V. Higdon. 2003. Antioxidant activity of tea polyphenols *in vivo*: Evidence from animal studies. *J Nutr* 133: 3275S–3284S.

Friedrich, W. 1988. *Vitamins*. Berlin, New York: Walter de Gruyter.

Furukawa, A., Oikawa, S., Murata, M., Hiraku, Y. and S. Kawanishi. 2003. (-)-Epigallocatechin gallate causes oxidative damage to isolated and cellular DNA. *Biochem Pharmacol* 66: 1769–1778.

Galati, G., Chan, T., Wu, B. and P.J. O'Brien. 1999. Glutathione-dependent generation of reactive oxygen species by the peroxidase-catalyzed redox cycling of flavonoids. *Chem Res Toxicol* 12: 521–525.

Galati, G., Lin, A., Sultan, A.M. and P.J. O'Brien. 2006. Cellular and *in vivo* hepatotoxicity caused by green tea phenolic acids and catechins. *Free Radic Biol Med* 40: 570–580.

Galati, G., Moridani, M.Y., Chan, T.S. and P.J. O'Brien. 2001. Peroxidative metabolism of apigenin and naringenin versus luteolin and quercetin: Glutathione oxidation and conjugation. *Free Radic Biol Med* 30: 370–382.

Galati, G. and P.J. O'Brien. 2004. Potential toxicity of flavonoids and other dietary phenolics: Significance for their chemopreventive and anticancer properties. *Free Radic Biol Med* 37: 287–303.

Galati, G., Sabzevari, O., Wilson, J.X. and P.J. O'Brien. 2002. Prooxidant activity and cellular effects of the phenoxyl radicals of dietary flavonoids and other polyphenolics. *Toxicol* 177: 91–104.

Galvano, F., La Fauci, L., Lazzarino, G., Fogliano, V., Ritieni, A., Ciappellano, S., Battistini, N.C., Tavazzi, B. and G. Galvano. 2004. Cyanidins: Metabolism and biological properties. *J Nutr Biochem* 15: 2–11.

Gandia-Herrero, F., Jimenez-Atienzar, M., Cabanes, J., Garcia-Carmona, F. and J. Escribano. 2010. Stabilization of the bioactive pigment of opuntia fruits through maltodextrin encapsulation. *J Agric Food Chem* 58: 10646–10652.

Gee, J.M., DuPont, M.S., Rhodes, M.J. and I.T. Johnson. 1998. Quercetin glucosides interact with the intestinal glucose transport pathway. *Free Radic Biol Med* 25: 19–25.

Gliszczyńska-Świgło, A. 2006. Antioxidant activity of water soluble vitamins in the TEAC (trolox equivalent antioxidant capacity) and the FRAP (ferric reducing antioxidant power) assays. *Food Chem* 96: 131–136.

Gliszczyńska-Świgło, A. 2007. Folates as antioxidants. *Food Chem* 101: 1497–1500.

Gliszczyńska-Świgło, A. and M. Muzolf. 2007. pH-dependent radical scavenging activity of folates. *J Agric Food Chem* 55: 8237–8242.

Gliszczyńska-Świgło, A. and H. Szymusiak. 2007a. Factors affecting radical-scavenging activity of folic acid and biopterin. *Acta Toxicol* 15: 13–18.

Gliszczyńska-Świgło, A. and H. Szymusiak. 2007b. Vitamin B6 and its metabolite reveal radical scavenging activity at basic pH. *Polish J Food Nutr Sci* 57: 163–167.

Gliszczyńska-Świgło, A. 2010. *Antioxidant and prooxidant properties of selected food components as its quality determinants* (in Polish). Poznań: The Poznań University of Economics Publishing House.

Gliszczyńska-Świgło, A. and H. Szymusiak. 2007c. Molecular insight in the pH-dependent radical-scavenging activity of betanidin. *Polish J Natural Sci Suppl* 4: 17–24.

Gliszczyńska-Świgło, A., Szymusiak, H. and P. Malinowska. 2006. Betanin, the main pigment of red beet: Molecular origin of its exceptionally high free radical scavenging activity. *Food Addit Contam* 11: 1079–1087.

Gliszczyńska-Świgło, A. and B. Tyrakowska. 2003. Quality of commercial apple juices evaluated on the basis of the polyphenol content and the TEAC antioxidant activity. *J Food Sci* 68: 1844–1849.

Gliszczyńska-Świgło, A., van der Woude, H., de Haan, L., Tyrakowska, B., Aarts, J.M.M.J.G. and I.M.C.M. Rietjens. 2003. The role of quinone reductase (NQO1) and quinone chemistry in quercetin cytotoxicity. *Toxicol in Vitro* 17: 423–431.

Godfrey, D. and D. Richardson. 2002. Vitamins and minerals for health. *Br Food J* 104: 913–933.

Gramza-Michałowska, A., Korczak, J. and J. Reguła. 2007. Use of plant extracts in summer and winter season butter oxidative stability improvement. *Asia Pac J Clin Nutr* 16 (Suppl. 1): 85–88.

Gregory III, J.F. 2008 Vitamins. In: *Fennema's Food Chemistry*, eds. S. Damodaran, K.L. Parkin and O.R. Fennema, 439–521. Boca Raton, FL: CRC Press.

Hadi, S.M., Asad, S.F., Singh, S. and A. Ahmad. 2000. Putative mechanism for anticancer and apoptosis inducing properties of plant-derived polyphenolic compounds. *IUBMB Life* 50: 167–171.

Haenen, G.R.M.M., Paquay, J.B.G., Korthouwer, R.E.M. and A. Bast. 1997. Peroxynitrite scavenging by flavonoids. *Biochem Biophys Res Commun* 236: 591–593.

Hagerman, A.E., Riedl, K.M., Jones, A., Sovik, K.N., Ritchard, N.T., Hartfeld, P.W. and T.L. Riechel. 1998. High molecular weight plant polyphenolics (tannins) as biological antioxidants. *J Agric Food Chem* 46: 1887–1892.

Halliwell, B. 2000. The antioxidant paradox. *Lancet* 355: 1179–1180.

Halliwell, B. 2007. Dietary polyphenols: Good, bad, or indifferent for your health? *Cardiovascular Res* 73: 341–347.

Halliwell, B. and J.M.C. Gutteridge. 1986. Oxygen free radicals and iron in relation to biology and medicine: Some problems and concepts. *Arch Biochem Biophys* 246: 501–514.

Hallund, J., Ravn-Haren, G., Bügel, S., Tholstrup, T. and I. Tetens. 2006. A lignan complex isolated from flaxseed does not affect plasma lipid concentrations or antioxidant capacity in healthy postmenopausal women. *J Nutr* 136: 112–116.

Hanasaki, Y., Ogawa, S. and S. Fukui. 1994. The correlation between active oxygens scavenging and antioxidative effects of flavonoids. *Free Radic Biol Med* 16: 845–850.

Harborne, J.B. and N.W. Simmonds. 1964. *Biochemistry of phenolic compounds*. London: Academic Press.

Hassan, I.A.G., Elzubeir, E.A. and A.H. El Tinay. 2003. Growth and apparent absorption of minerals in broiler chicks fed diets with low or high tannin contents. *Trop Anim Health Prod* 35: 189–196.

Hassan, O. and L.S. Fan. 2005. The anti-oxidation potential of polyphenol extract from cocoa leaves on mechanically deboned chicken meat (MDCM). *Lebensm-Wiss Technol* 38: 315–321.

He, Y. and F. Shahidi. 1997. Antioxidant activity of green tea and its catechins in a model fish system. *J Agric Food Chem* 45: 4262–4266.

Hebert, C., Charles, M.T., Willemot, C., Gauthier, L., Khanizadeh, S. and J. Cousineau. 2002. Strawberry proanthocyanidins: Biochemical markers for *Botrytis cinerea* resistance and shelf-life predictability. *Acta Horticulture* 567: 659–662.

Heim, K.E., Tagliaferro, A.R. and D.J. Bobilya. 2002. Flavonoid antioxidants: Chemistry, metabolism and structure-activity relationships. *J Nutr Biochem* 13: 572–584.

Heinonen, I.M., Meyer, A.S. and E.N. Frankel. 1998. Antioxidant activity of berry phenolics on human low-density lipoprotein and liposome oxidation. *J Agric Food Chem* 46: 4107–4112.

Hensley, K., Benaksas, E.J., Bolli, R., Comp, P., Grammas, P., Hamdheydari, L., Mou, S., Pye, Q.N., Stoddard, M.F., Wallis, G., Williamson, K.S., West, M., Wechter, W.J. and R.A. Floyd. 2004. New perspectives on vitamin E: Gamma-tocopherol and carboxyethylhydroxychroman metabolites in biology and medicine. *Free Radic Biol Med* 36: 1–15.

Hertog, M.G.L., Hollman, P.C.H., Katan, M.B. and D. Kromhout. 1993. Intake of potentially anticarcinogenic flavonoids and their determinants in adults in the Netherlands. *Nutr Cancer* 20: 21–29.

Higdon, J.V. and B. Frei. 2003. Tea catechins and polyphenols: Health effects, metabolism, and antioxidant functions. *Crit Rev Food Sci Nutr* 43: 89–143.

Ho, C.-T., Rafi, M.M. and G. Ghai. 2008. Bioactive substances: Nutraceuticals and toxicants. In *Fennema's Food Chemistry*, eds. S. Damodaran, K.L. Parkin, and O.W. Fennema, 751–779. Boca Raton, FL: CRC Press.

Holt, R.R., Lazarus, S.A., Sullards, M.C., Zhu, Q.Y., Schramm, D.D., Hammerstone, J.F., Fraga, C.G., Schmitz, H.H. and C.L. Keen. 2002. Procyanidin dimer B2 [epicatechin-(4beta-8)-epicatechin] in human plasma after the consumption of a flavanol-rich cocoa. *Am J Clin Nutr* 76: 798–804.

Horakova, K., Sovcikova, A., Seemannova, Z., Syrova, D., Busanyova, K., Drobna, Z. and M. Ferencik. 2001. Detection of drug-induced, superoxide-mediated cell damage and its prevention by antioxidants. *Free Radic Biol Med* 30: 650–664.

Horvathova, K., Novotny, L., Tothova, D. and A. Vachalkova. 2004. Determination of free radical scavenging activity of quercetin, rutin, luteolin and apigenin in H_2O_2-treated human ML cells K562. *Neoplasma* 51: 395–399.

Horvathova, K., Novotny, L. and A. Vachalkova. 2003. The free radical scavenging activity of four flavonoids determined by the comet assay. *Neoplasma* 50: 291–295.

Hosseinian, F.S., Muir, A.D., Westcott, N.D. and E.S. Krol. 2006. Antioxidant capacity of flaxseed lignans in two model systems. *J Am Oil Chem Soc* 83: 835–840.

Hosseinian, F.S., Muir, A.D., Westcott, N.D. and E.S. Krol. 2007. AAPH-mediated antioxidant reactions of secoisolariciresinol and SDG. *Org Biomol Chem* 5: 644–654.

Hou, Z., Sang, S., You, H., Lee, M.J., Hong, J., Chin, K.V. and C.S. Yang. 2005. Mechanism of action of (-)-epigallocatechin-3-gallate: Auto-oxidation-dependent inactivation of epidermal growth factor receptor and direct effects on growth inhibition in human esophageal cancer KYSE 150 cells. *Cancer Res* 65: 8049–8056.

Hu, C., Yuan, Y.V. and D.D. Kitts. 2007. Antioxidant activities of the flaxseed lignan secoisolariciresinol diglucoside, its aglycone secoisolariciresinol and the mammalian lignans enterodiol and enterolactone *in vitro*. *Food Chem Toxicol* 45: 2219–2227.

Huang, D., Ou, B. and R. Prior. 2005. The chemistry behind antioxidant capacity assays. *J Agric Food Chem* 53: 1841–1856.

Hümmer, W. and P. Schreier. 2008. Analysis of proanthocyanidins. *Mol Nutr Food Res* 52: 1381–1398.

Imai, Y., Tsukahara, S., Asada, S. and Y. Sugimoto. 2004. Phytoestrogens/flavonoids reverse breast cancer resistance protein/ABCG2-mediated multidrug resistance. *Cancer Res* 64: 4346–4352.

Ito, S., Kato, T. and K. Fujita. 1988. Covalent binding of catechols to proteins through the sulphydryl group. *Biochem Pharmacol* 37: 1707–1710.

Jenner, A.M., Rafter, J. and B. Halliwell. 2005. Human fecal water content of phenolics: The extent of colonic exposure to aromatic compounds. *Free Radic Biol Med* 38: 763–772.

Jiang, Q., Elson-Schwab, I., Courtemanche, C. and B.N. Ames. 2000. Gamma-tocopherol and its major metabolite, in contrast to alphatocopherol, inhibit cyclooxygenase activity in macrophages and epithelial cells. *Proc Natl Acad Sci USA* 97: 11494–11499.

Joshi, R., Adhikari, S., Patro, B.S., Chattopadhyay, S. and T. Mukherjee. 2001. Free radical scavenging behavior of folic acid: Evidence for possible antioxidant activity. *Free Radic Biol Med* 30: 1390–1399.

Jung, I.L. and J.G. Kim. 2003. Thiamine protects against paraquat-induced damage: Scavenging activity of reactive oxygen species. *Environ Toxicol Pharmacol* 15: 19–26.

Jurado, J., Alejandre-Duran, E., Alonso-Moraga, A. and C. Pueyo. 1991. Study on the mutagenic activity of 13 bioflavonoids with the Salmonella Ara test. *Mutagenesis* 6: 289–295.

Justesen, U., Knuthsen, P. and T. Leth. 1997. Determination of plant polyphenols in Danish foodstuffs by HPLC-UV and LC-MS detection. *Cancer Lett* 114: 165–167.

Kamal-Eldin, A., Peerlkamp, N., Johnsson, P., Andersson, R., Andersson, R.E., Lundgren, L.N. and P. Aman. 2001. An oligomer from flaxseed composed of secoisolariciresinol diglucoside and 3-hydroxy-3-methyl glutaric acid residues. *Phytochem* 58: 587–590.

Kamei, H., Kojima, T., Hasegawa, M., Koide, T., Umeda, T., Yukawa, T. and K. Terabe. 1995. Suppression of tumor cell growth by anthocyanins *in vitro*. *Cancer Invest* 13: 590–594.

Kanadzu, M., Lu, Y. and K. Morimoto. 2006. Dual function of (-)-epigallocatechin gallate (EGCG) in healthy human lymphocytes. *Cancer Lett* 241: 250–255.

Kandaswami, C., Perkins, E., Soloniuk, D.S., Drzewiecki, G. and E. Middleton. 1991. Antiproliferative effects of citrus flavonoids on a human squamous cell carcinoma *in vitro. Cancer Lett* 56: 147–152.

Kanner, J., Harel, S. and R. Granit. 2001. Betalains: A new class of dietary cationized antioxidants. *J Agric Food Chem* 49: 5178–5185.

Kaur, C. and H.C. Kapoor. 2001. Antioxidants in fruits and vegetables: The millennium's health. *Int J Food Sci Technol* 36: 703–725.

Kawaii, S., Tomono, Y., Katase, E. and K. Ogawa. 1999. Antiproliferative activity of flavonoids on several cancer cell lines. *Biosci Biotechnol Biochem* 63: 896–899.

Kay, C.D., Mazza, G.J. and B.J. Holub. 2005. Anthocyanins exist in the circulation primarily as metabolites in adult men. *J Nutr* 135: 2582–2588.

Kay, C.D., Mazza, G., Holub, B.J. and J. Wang. 2004. Anthocyanin metabolites in human urine and serum. *Br J Nutr* 91: 933–942.

Khan, S.G., Katiyar, S.K., Agarwal, R. and H. Mukhtar. 1992. Enhancement of antioxidant and phase II enzymes by oral feeding of green tea polyphenols in drinking water to SKH-1 hairless mice: Possible role in cancer chemoprevention. *Cancer Res* 52: 4050–4052.

Kim, S.B., Lee, M.J., Hong, J.I., Li, C., Smith, T.J., Yang, G.-Y., Seril, D.N. and C.S. Yang. 2000. Plasma and tissue levels of tea catechins in rats and mice during chronic consumption of green tea polyphenols. *Nutr Cancer* 37: 41–48.

Kitts, D.D., Yuan, Y.V., Wijewickreme, A.N. and L.U. Thompson. 1999. Antioxidant activity of the flaxseed lignan secoisolariciresinol diglycoside and its mammalian lignan metabolites enterodiol and enterolactone. *Mol Cell Biochem* 202: 91–100.

Knowles, L.M., Zigrossi, D.A., Tauber, R.A., Hightower, C. and J.A. Milner. 2000. Flavonoids suppress androgen-independent human prostate tumor proliferation. *Nutr Cancer* 38: 116–122.

Kojo, S. 2004. Vitamin C: Basic metabolism and its function as an index of oxidative stress. *Curr Medic Chem* 11: 1041–1064.

Kong, J.-M., Chia, L.-S., Goh, N.-K., Chia, T.-F. and R. Brouillard. 2003. Analysis and biological activities of anthocyanins. *Phytochem* 64: 923–933.

Kris-Etherton, P.M., Hecker, K.D., Bonanome, A., Coval, S.M., Binkoski, A.E., Hilpert, K.F., Griel, A.E. and T.D. Etherton. 2002. Bioactive compounds in food: Their role in the prevention of cardiovascular disease and cancer. *Am J Med* 113: 71S–88S.

Kühnau, J. 1976. The flavonoids. A class of semi-essential food components: Their role in human nutrition. *World Rev Nutr Diet* 24: 117–191.

Kuo, S.M. 1996. Antiproliferative potency of structurally distinct dietary flavonoids on human colon cancer cells. *Cancer Lett* 110: 41–48.

Kurzer, M.S. 2003. Phytoestrogen supplement use by women. *J Nutr* 133: 1983S–1986S.

Lamers, Y., Prinz-Langenohl, R., Brämswig, S. and K. Pietrzik. 2006. Red blood cell folate concentrations increase more after supplementation with [6S]-methyltetrahydrofolate than with folic acid in women of childbearing age. *Am J Clin Nutr* 84: 156–161.

Lapidot, T., Harel, S., Akiri, B., Granit, R. and J. Kanner. 1999. pH-dependent forms of red wine anthocyanins as antioxidants. *J Agric Food Chem* 47: 67–70.

Lapidot, T., Harel, S., Granit, R. and J. Kanner. 1998. Bioavailability of red wine anthocyanins as detected in human urine. *J. Agric Food Chem* 46: 4297–4302.

Lash, L.H. and D.P. Jones. 1986. Renal glutathione transport: Characteristics of the sodium-dependent system in basal-lateral membrane. *Arch Biochem Biophys* 247: 120–130.

Laughton, M.J., Halliwell, B., Evans, P.J. and J.R.S. Hoult. 1989. Antioxidant and pro-oxidant actions of the plant phenolics quercetin, gossypol and myricetin. *Biochem Pharmacol* 38: 2859–2865.

Lee-Hilz, Y.Y., Boerboom, A.M., Westphal, A.H., Berkel, W.J.H., Aarts, J.M. and I.M.C.M. Rietjens. 2006. Pro-oxidant activity of flavonoids induces EpRE-mediated gene expression. *Chem Res Toxicol* 19: 1499–1505.

Lee-Hilz, Y.Y., ter Borg, S., Berkel, W.J.H., Rietjens, I.M.C.M. and J.M.M.J.G. Aarts. 2008. Shifted concentration dependency of EpRE- and XRE-mediated gene expression points at monofunctional EpRE-mediated induction by flavonoids at physiologically relevant concentrations. *Toxicol in Vitro* 22: 921–926.

Lemańska, K., Szymusiak, H., Tyrakowska, B., Zieliński, R., Soffers, A.E.M.F. and I.M.C.M. Rietjens. 2001. The influence of pH on antioxidant properties and the mechanism of antioxidant action of hydroxyflavones. *Free Radic Biol Med* 31: 869–881.

Lemańska, K., van der Woude, H., Szymusiak, H., Boersma, M.G., Gliszczyńska-Świgło, A., Rietjens, I.M.C.M. and B. Tyrakowska. 2004. The effect of catechol O-methylation on radical scavenging characteristic of quercetin and luteolin: A mechanistic insight. *Free Radic Res* 38: 639–647.

Leung, L.K., Su, Y., Chen, R., Zhang, Z., Huang, Y. and Z.-Y. Chen. 2001. Theaflavins in black tea and catechins in green tea are equally effective antioxidants. *J Nutr* 131: 2248–2251.

Li, Y. and M.A. Trush. 1994. Reactive oxygen-dependent DNA damage resulting from the oxidation of phenolic compounds by a copper-redox cycle mechanism. *Cancer Res* 54: 1895S–1898S.

Lietti, A., Cristoni, A. and M. Picci. 1976. Studies on *Vaccinium myrtillus* anthocyanosides. I. Vasoprotective and antiinflammatory activity. *Arzneimittelforschung* 26: 829–832.

Liu, C., Russel, R.M. and X.-D. Wang. 2003. Exposing ferrets to cigarette smoke and a pharmacological dose of β-carotene supplementation enhance *in vitro* retinoic acid catabolism in lungs via induction of cytochrome P450 enzymes. *J Nutr* 133: 171–179.

Losonczy, K.G., Harris, T.B. and R.J. Havlik. 1996. Vitamin E and vitamin C supplement use and risk of all-cause and coronary heart disease mortality in older persons: The established populations for epidemiologic studies of the elderly. *Am J Clin Nutr* 64: 190–196.

Lotan, R. 1999. Lung cancer promotion by β-carotene and tobacco smoke: Relationship to suppression of retinoic acid receptor-b and increased activator protein-1? *J Natl Cancer Inst* 91: 7–9.

Lu, Y. and L.Y. Foo. 2001. Antioxidant activity of polyphenols from sage (*Salvia officinalis*). *Food Chem* 75: 197–202.

Ma, X., Li, H., Dong, J. and W. Qian. 2011. Determination of hydrogen peroxide scavenging activity of phenolic AIDS by employing gold nanoshells precursor composites as nanoprobes. *Food Chem* 126: 698–704.

Mabe, K., Yamada, M., Oguni, I. and T. Takahashi. 1999. *In vitro* and *in vivo* activities of tea catechins against *Helicobacter pylori*. *Antimicrob Agents Chemother* 43: 1788–1791.

MacGregor, J.T. and L. Jurd. 1978. Mutagenicity of plant flavonoids: Structural requirements for mutagenic activity in *Salmonella typhimurium*. *Mutat Res* 54: 297–309.

Mackey, A.D. and M.F. Picciano. 1999. Maternal folate status during extended lactation and the effect of supplemental folic acid. *Am J Clin Nutr* 69: 285–292.

Manach, C., Scalbert, A., Morand, C., Rémésy, C. and L. Jiménez. 2004. Polyphenols: Food sources and bioavailability. *Am J Clin Nutr* 79: 727–747.

Manach, C., Williamson, G., Morand, C., Scalbert, A. and C. Rémésy. 2005. Bioavailability and bioefficacy of polyphenols in humans. I. Review of 97 bioavailability studies. *Am J Clin Nutr* 81: 230S–242S.

Manzoor, M. and J. Runcie. 1976. Folate-responsive neuropathy: Report of 10 cases. *Brit Med J* 1: 1176–1178.

Masella, R., Di Benedetto, R., Vari, R., Filesi, C. and C. Giovannini. 2005. Novel mechanisms of natural antioxidant compounds in biological systems: Involvement of glutathione and glutathione-related enzymes. *J Nutr Biochem* 16: 577–586.

Mason, L.M., Hogan, S.A., Lynch, A., O'Sullivan, K., Lawlor, P.G. and J.P. Kerry. 2005. Effects of restricted feeding and antioxidant supplementation on pig performance and quality characteristics of longissimus dorsi muscle from Landrace and Duroc pigs. *Meat Sci* 70: 307–317.

Matos, H.R., Marques, S.A., Gomes, O.F., Silva, A.A., Heimann, J.C., Di Mascio, P. and M.H.G. Medeiros. 2006. Lycopene and ß-carotene protect *in vivo* iron-induced oxidative stress damage in rat prostate. *Braz J Med Biol Res* 39: 203–210.

Matsumoto, H., Inaba, H., Kishi, M., Tominaga, S., Hirayama, M. and T. Tsuda. 2001. Orally administered delphinidin 3-rutinoside and cyanidin 3-rutinoside are directly absorbed in rats and humans and appear in the blood as the intact forms. *J Agric Food Chem* 49: 1546–1551.

Mayne, S.T. 1996. β-Carotene, carotenoids, and disease prevention in humans. *FASEB J* 10: 690–701.

Mayne, S.T., Handelman, G.J. and G. Beecher. 1996. β-Carotene and lung cancer promotion in heavy smokers: A plausible relationship? *J Natl Cancer Inst* 88: 1513–1515.

Mazzaracchio, P., Pifferi, P., Kindt, M., Munyaneza, A. and G. Barbiroli. 2004. Interactions between anthocyanins and organic food molecules in model systems. *Int J Food Sci Technol* 39: 53–59.

McCann, S.E., Muti, P., Vito, D., Edge, S.B., Trevisan, M. and J.L. Freudenheim. 2004. Dietary lignan intakes and risk of pre- and postmenopausal breast cancer. *Int J Cancer* 111: 440–443.

McCarthy, T.L., Kerry, J.P., Kerry, J.F., Lynch, P.B. and D.J. Buckley. 2001. Evaluation of the antioxidant potential of natural food/plant extracts as compared with synthetic antioxidants and vitamin E in raw and cooked pork patties. *Meat Sci* 57: 45–52.

Medina, I., Gallardo, J.M., Gonzalez, M.J., Lois, S. and N. Hedges. 2007. Effect of molecular structure of phenolic families as hydroxycinnamic acids and catechins on their antioxidant effectiveness in minced fish muscle. *J Agric Food Chem* 55: 3889–3895.

Meiers, S., Kemény, M., Weyand, U., Gastpar, R., von Angerer, E. and D. Marko. 2001. The anthocyanidins cyanidin and delphinidin are potent inhibitors of the epidermal growth-factor receptor. *J Agric Food Chem* 49: 958–962.

Middleton, E. Jr. and C. Kandaswami. 1993. The impact of plant flavonoids on mammalian biology: Implications for immunity, inflammation and cancer. In *The Flavonoids: Advances in Research since 1986*, ed. J.B. Harborne, 619–652. London: Chapman & Hall.

Miller, N.J., Sampson, J., Candeias, L.P., Bramley, P.M. and C.A. Rice-Evans. 1996. Antioxidant activities of carotenes and xanthophylls. *FEBS Lett* 384: 240–242.

Miranda, C.L., Stevens, J.F., Ivanow, V., McCall, M., Frei, B., Deinzer, M.L. and D.R. Buhler. 2000. Antioxidant and prooxidant action of prenylated and nonprenylated chalcones and flavanones *in vitro*. *J Agric Food Chem* 48: 3876–3884.

Miyazawa, T., Nakagawa, K., Kudo, M., Muraishi, K. and K. Someya. 1999. Direct intestinal absorption of red fruit anthocyanins, cyanidin-3-glucoside and cyanidin-3,5-diglucoside, into rats and humans. *J Agric Food Chem* 47: 1083–1091.

Moat, S.J., Lang, D., McDowell, I.F.W., Clarke, Z.L., Madhavan, A.K., Lewis, M.J. and J. Goodfellow. 2004. Folate, homocysteine, endothelial function and cardiovascular disease. *J Nutr Biochem* 15: 64–79.

Mohsen, M.A.E., Mark, J., Kuhnle, G., Moore, K., Debnam, E., Srai, S.K., Rice-Evans, C. and J.P.E. Spencer. 2006. Absorption, tissue distribution and excretion of pelargonidin and its metabolites following oral administration to rats. *Brit J Nutr* 95: 51–55.

Mollov, P., Mihalev, K., Shikov, V., Yoncheva, N. and V. Karagyozov. 2007. Colour stability improvement of strawberry beverage by fortification with polyphenolic copigments naturally occurring in rose petals. *Innov Food Sci Emerg Technol* 8: 318–321.

Monagas, M., Gomez-Cordoves, C., Bartolome, B., Laureano, O. and J.M. Ricardo da Silva. 2003. Monomeric, oligomeric, and polymeric flavan-3-ol composition of wines and grapes from *Vitis vinifera* L. Cv. Graciano, Tempranillo, and Cabernet Sauvignon. *J Agric Food Chem* 51: 6475–6481.

Morazzoni, P., Livio, S., Scilingo, A. and S. Malandrino. 1991. *Vaccinium myrtillus* anthocyanosides pharmacokinetics in rats. *Arzneim Forsch* 41: 128–131.

Moridani, M.Y., Scobie, H., Jamshidzadeh, A., Salehi, P. and P.J. O'Brien. 2001a. Caffeic acid, chlorogenic acid, and dihydrocaffeic acid metabolism: Glutathione conjugate formation. *Drug Metab Dispos* 29: 1432–1439.

Moridani, M.Y., Scobie, H., Salehi, P. and P.J. O'Brien. 2001b. Catechin metabolism: Glutathione conjugate formation catalyzed by tyrosinase, peroxidase, and cytochrome P450. *Chem Res Toxicol* 14: 841–848.

Moyers, S.B. and N.B. Kumar. 2004. Green tea polyphenols and cancer chemoprevention: Multiple mechanisms and endpoints for phase II trials. *Nutr Rev* 62: 204–211.

Mullen, W., Graf, B.A., Caldwell, S.T., Hartley, R.C., Duthie, G.G., Edwards, C.A., Lean, M.E. and A. Crozier. 2002. Determination of flavonol metabolites in plasma and tissues of rats by HPLC-radiocounting and tandem mass spectrometry following oral ingestion of [2-(14)C]quercetin-4′-glucoside. *J Agric Food Chem* 50: 6902–6909.

Müller, L., Fröchlich, K. and V. Böhm. 2011. Comparative antioxidant activities of carotenoids measured by ferric reducing antioxidant power (FRAP), ABTS blenching assays (αTEAC), DPPH assay and peroxyl radical scavenging assay. *Food Chem* 129: 139–148.

Muzolf, M., Szymusiak, H., Gliszczyńska-Świgło, A., Rietjens, I.M.C.M. and B. Tyrakowska. 2008. pH-Dependent radical scavenging capacity of green tea catechins. *J Agric Food Chem* 56: 816–823.

Muzolf-Panek, M., Gliszczyńska-Świgło, A., de Haan, L., Aarts, J.M.M.J.G., Szymusiak, H., Vervoort, J.M., Tyrakowska, B. and I.M.C.M. Rietjens. 2008. A role of catechin quinones in the induction of EpRE-mediated gene expression. *Chem Res Toxicol* 21: 2352–2360.

Nagano, M., Morita, N., Yahagi, T., Shimizu, M., Kuroyanagi, M., Fukuoka, M., Yoshihira, K., Natori, S., Fujino, T. and T. Sugimura. 1981. Mutagenicities of 61 flavonoids and 11 related compounds. *Environ Mutagen* 3: 401–419.

Nakano, E., Higgins, J.A. and H.J. Powers. 2001. Folate protects against oxidative modification of human LDL. *Br J Nutr* 86: 637–639.

Nanjo, F., Mori, M., Goto, K. and Y. Hara. 1996. Radical scavenging activity of tea catechins and their related compounds. *Biosci Biotechnol Biochem* 63: 1621–1623.

Nardini, M. and A. Ghiselli. 2004. Determination of free and bound phenolic acids in beer. *Food Chem* 84: 137–143.

Navarro-Martinez, M.D., Navarro-Peran, E., Cabezas-Herrera, J., Ruiz-Gomez, J., Garcia-Canovas, F. and J.N. Rodriguez-Lopez. 2005. Antifolate activity of epigallocatechin gallate against *Stenotrophomonas maltophilia. Antimicrob Agents Chemother* 49: 2914–2920.

Niemeyer, H.B. and M. Metzler. 2003. Differences in the antioxidant activity of plant and mammalian lignans. *J Food Eng* 56: 255–256.

Noroozi, M., Angerson, W.J. and M.E. Lean. 1998. Effects of flavonoids and vitamin C on oxidative DNA damage to human lymphocytes. *Am J Clin Nutr* 67: 1210–1218.

O'Brien, N.M., Woods, J.A., Aherne, S.A. and Y.C. O'Callaghan. 2000. Cytotoxicity, genotoxicity and oxidative reactions in cell-culture models: Modulatory effects of phytochemicals. *Biochem Soc Trans* 28: 22–26.

Olney, R.S. and J. Mulinare. 2002. Trends in neural tube defect prevalence, folic acid fortification, and vitamin supplement use. *Sem Perinat* 26: 277–285.

Omaye, S.T., Krinsky, N.I., Kagan, V.E., Mayne, S.T., Liebler, D.C. and W.R. Bidlack. 1997. β-Carotene: Friend or foe? *Fundam Appl Toxicol* 40: 163–174.

Omenn, G.S., Goodman, G.E., Thornquist, M.D., Balmes, J., Cullen, M.R., Glass, A., Keogh, J.P., Meyskens, F.L., Valanis, B., Williams, J.H., Barnhart, S. and S. Hammar. 1996. Effects of a combination of β-carotene and vitamin A on lung cancer and cardiovascular disease. *N Engl J Med* 334: 1150–1155.

Oszmiański, J., Bakowska, A. and S. Piacente. 2004. Thermodynamic characteristics of copigmentation reaction of acylated anthocyanin isolated from blue flowers of *Scutellaria baicalensis* Georgi with copigments. *J Sci Food Agric* 84: 1500–1506.

Oszmiański, J. and A. Wojdyło. 2009. Comparative study of phenolic content and antioxidant activity of strawberry puree, clear, and cloudy juices. *Eur Food Res Technol* 228: 623–631.

Oszmiański, J., Wojdyło, A. and J. Kolniak. 2009. Effect of L-ascorbic acid, sugar, pectin and freeze-thaw treatment on polyphenol content of frozen strawberries. *LWT – Food Sci Technol* 42: 581–586.

Palozza, P. 1998. Prooxidant actions of carotenoids in biologic systems. *Nutr Rev* 56: 257–265.

Palozza, P., Calviello, G. and G.M. Bartoli. 1995. Prooxidant activity of β-carotene under 100% oxygen pressure in rat liver microsomes. *Free Radic Biol Med* 19: 887–892.

Palozza, P. and N.I. Krinsky. 1992. Antioxidant effects of carotenoids *in vivo* and *in vitro*: An overview. *Methods Enzymol* 213: 403–420.

Palozza, P., Serini, S., Di Nicuolo, F., Piccioni, E. and G. Calviello. 2003. Prooxidant effects of β-carotene in cultured cells. *Mol Asp Med* 24: 353–362.

Panjeh-Shahin, M.-R., Panahi, Z., Dehghani, F. and T. Talaei-Khozani. 2005. The effects of hydroalcoholic extract of *Actinidia chinensis* on sperm count and mortality, and on the blood levels of estradiol and testosterone in male rats. *Archiv Iran Med* 8: 211–216.

Paolini, M., Cantelli-Forti, G., Perocco, P., Pedulli, G.F., Abdel-Rahman, S.Z. and M.S. Legator. 1999. Co-carcinogenic effect of β-carotene. *Nature* 398: 760–761.

Passamonti, S., Vrhovsek, U., Vanzo, A. and F. Mattivi. 2003. The stomach as a site for antho-cyanins absorption from food. *FEBS Lett* 544: 210–213.

Passamonti, S., Vrhovsek, U., Vanzo, A. and F. Mattivi. 2005. Fast access of some grape pig-ments in the brain. *J Agric Food Chem* 53: 7029–7034.

Pavlov, A., Kovatcheva, P., Georgiev, V., Koleva, I. and M. Ilieva. 2002. Biosynthesis and radical scavenging activity of betalains during the cultivation of red beet (*Beta vulgaris*) hairy root cultures. *Z Naturforsch* 57c: 640–644.

Pedreño, M.A. and J. Escribano. 2000. Studying the oxidation and the antiradical activity of betalain from beetroot. *J Biol Educ* 35: 49–51.

Pedreño, M.A. and J. Escribano. 2001. Correlation between antiradical activity and stability of betanine from *Beta vulgaris* L roots under different pH, temperature and light condi-tions. *J Sci Food Agric* 81: 627–631.

Penning, T.M., Burczyński, M.E., Hung, C.F., McCoull, K.D., Palackal, N.T. and L.S. Tsuruda. 1999. Dihydrodiol dehydrogenases and polycyclic aromatic hydrocarbon acti-vation: Generation of reactive and redox-active o-quinones. *Chem Res Toxicol* 12: 1–18.

Peto, R., Doll, R., Buckley, J.D. and M. Sporn. 1981. Can dietary β-carotene materially reduce human cancer rates? *Nature* 290: 201–208.

Pietta, P.G. 2000. Flavonoids as antioxidants. *J Nat Prod* 63: 1035–1042.

Pietta, P., Simonetti, P., Roggi, C., Brusamolino, A., Pellegrini, N., Maccarini, L. and G. Testolin. 1996. Dietary flavonoids and oxidative stress. In *Natural Antioxidants and Food Quality in Atherosclerosis and Cancer Prevention*, eds. J.T. Kumpulainen and J.T. Salonen, 249–255. London: Royal Society of Chemistry.

Pignatelli, B., Bancel, B., Esteve, J., Malaveille, C., Calmels, S., Correa, P., Patricot, L.M., Laval, M., Lyandrat, N. and H.J. Ohshima. 1998. Inducible nitric oxide synthase, anti-oxidant enzymes and *Helicobacter pylori* infection in gastritis and gastric precancerous lesions in humans. *Eur J Cancer Prev* 7: 439–447.

Plumb, G.W., Garcia Conesa, M.T., Kroon, P.A., Rhodes, M., Ridley, S. and G. Williamson. 1999. Metabolism of chlorogenic acid by human plasma, liver, intestine and gut micro-flora. *J Sci Food Agric* 79: 390–392.

Pokorny, J., Trojakova, L. and M. Takacsova. 2001. The use of natural antioxidants in food products of plant origin. In *Antioxidants in Food*, ed. J. Pokorny, N. Yanishlieva and M. Gordon, 355–368. Boca Raton, FL: CRC Press.

Prasad, K. 1997. Hydroxyl radical-scavenging property of secoisolariciresinol diglucoside (SDG) isolated from flaxseed. *Mol Cell Biochem* 168: 117–123.

Prasad, K. 1999. Reduction of serum cholesterol and hypercholesterolemic atherosclerosis in rabbits by secoisolariciresinol diglucoside isolated from flaxseed. *Circulation* 99: 1355–1362.

Prasad, K. 2000a. Antioxidant activity of secoisolariciresinol diglucoside-derived metabolites, secoisolariciresinol, enterodiol, and enterolactone. *Int J Angiol* 9: 220–225.

Prasad, K. 2000b. Oxidative stress as a mechanism of diabetes in diabetic BB prone rats: Effect of secoisolariciresinol diglucoside (SDG). *Mol Cell Biochem* 209: 89–96.

Prior, R.L. and L. Gu. 2005. Occurrence and biological significance of proanthocyanidins in the American diet. *Phytochem* 66: 2264–2280.

Rahimi, R., Nikfar, S., Larijani, B. and M. Abdollahi. 2005. A review on the role of antioxidants in the management of diabetes and its complications. *Biomed Pharmacother* 59: 365–373.

Rahman, A., Shahabuddin, H.S.M., Parish, J.H. and K. Ainley. 1989. Strand scission in DNA induced by quercetin and Cu(II): Role of Cu(I) and oxygen free radicals. *Carcinogenesis* 10: 1833–1839.

Ramanathan, L. and N.P. Das. 1992. Studies on the control of lipid oxidation in ground fish by some polyphenolic natural products. *J Agric Food Chem* 40: 17–21.

Ramanathan, L. and N.P. Das. 1993. Natural products inhibit oxidative rancidity in salted cooked ground fish. *J Food Sci* 58: 318–320.

Ratnayake, W.M.N., Behrens, W.A., Fischer, P.W.F., L'Abbé, M.R., Mongeau, R. and. J.L. Beare-Rogersa. 1992. Chemical and nutritional studies of flaxseed (variety Linott) in rats. *J Nutr Biochem* 3: 232–240.

Rein, M.J. and M. Heinonen. 2004. Stability and enhancement of berry juice color. *J Agric Food Chem* 52: 3106–3114.

Rezk, B.M., Haenen, G.R.M.M., van der Vijgh, W.J.F. and A. Bast. 2003. Tetrahydrofolate and 5-methyltetrahydrofolate are folates with high antioxidant activity: Identification of the antioxidant pharmacophore. *FEBS Lett* 555: 601–605.

Rice-Evans, C.A., Miller, N.J., Bolwell, P.G., Bramley, P.M. and J.B. Pridham. 1995. The relative antioxidant activities of plant-derived polyphenolic flavonoids. *Free Radic Res* 22: 375–383.

Rice-Evans, C., Miller, N.J. and G. Paganga. 1996. Structure-antioxidant activity relationships of flavonoids and phenolic acids. *Free Radic Biol Med* 20: 933–956.

Rietjens, I.M.C.M., Boersma, M.G., de Haan, L., Spenkelink, B., Awad, H.M., Cnubben, N.H.P., van Zanden, J.J., van der Woude, H., Alink, G.M. and J.H. Koeman. 2002. The pro-oxidant chemistry of the natural antioxidants vitamin C, vitamin E, carotenoids and flavonoids. *Environ Toxicol Pharmacol* 11: 321–333.

Rietjens, I.M.C.M., Martena, M.J., Boersma, M.G., Spiegelenberg, W. and G.M. Alink. 2005. Molecular mechanism of toxicity of important food-borne phytotoxins. *Mol Nutr Food Res* 49: 131–158.

Rietvield, A. and S. Wiseman. 2003. Antioxidant effects of tea: Evidence from human clinical trials. *J Nutr* 133: 3285–3292.

Rimm, E.B., Stempfer, M.J., Ascherio, A., Giovanucci, E., Colditz, G.A. and W.C. Wilett. 1993. Vitamin E consumption and the risk of coronary heart disease in men. *New Engl J Med* 328: 1450–1456.

Roa, A.V. and S. Agarwal. 1999. Role of lycopene as antioxidant carotenoid in the prevention of chronic diseases: A review. *Nutr Res* 19: 305–323.

Rothwell, J.A., Day, A.J. and M.R. Morgan. 2005. Experimental determination of octanol-water partition coefficients of quercetin and related flavonoids. *J Agric Food Chem* 53: 4355–4360.

Roy, K., Gullapalli, S., Roy, U. and R. Chakraborty. 2004. The use of a natural colorant based on betalain in the manufacture of sweet products in India. *Int J Food Sci Technol* 39: 1087–1091.

Sakihama, Y., Cohen, M.F., Grace, S.C. and H. Yamasaki. 2002. Plant phenolic antioxidant and prooxidant activities: Phenolics-induced oxidative damage mediated by metals in plants. *Toxicol* 177: 67–80.

Samiec, P.S., Drews-Botsch, C., Flagg, E.W., Kurtz, J.C., Sternberg Jr. P., Reed, R.L. and D.P. Jones. 1998. Glutathione in human plasma: Decline in association with aging, age-related macular degeneration, and diabetes. *Free Radic Biol Med* 24: 699–704.

Sampson, L., Rimm, E., Hollman, P.C., de Vries, J.I.I. and M.B. Katan. 2002. Flavonol and flavone intakes in US health professionals. *J Am Diet Assoc* 102: 1414–1420.

Sanchez-Moreno, C., Cao, G., Ou, B. and R.L. Prior. 2003. Anthocyanin and proanthocyanidin content in selected white and red wines: Oxygen radical absorbance capacity comparison with nontraditional wines obtained from highbush blueberry. *J Agric Food Chem* 51: 4889–4896.

Sang, S., Lambert, J.D., Hong, J., Tian, S., Lee, M.-J., Stark, R.E., Ho, C.-T. and C.S. Yang. 2005. Synthesis and structure identification of thiol conjugates of (-)-epigallocatechin gallate and their urinary levels in mice. *Chem Res Toxicol* 18: 1762–1769.

Sang, S., Yang, I., Buckley, B., Ho, C.-T. and C.S. Yang. 2007. Autoxidative quinone formation *in vitro* and metabolite formation *in vivo* from tea polyphenol (-)-epigallocatechin gallate: Studied by real-time mass spectrometry combined with tandem mass ion mapping. *Free Radic Biol Med* 43: 362–371.

Sano, A., Yamakoshi, J., Tokutake, S., Tobe, K., Kubota, Y. and M. Kikuchi. 2003. Procyanidin B1 is detected in human serum after intake of procyanidin-rich grape seed extract. *Biosci Biotechnol Biochem* 67: 1140–1143.

Santos-Buelga, C. and A. Scalbert. 2000. Proanthocyanidins and tanninlike compounds: Nature, occurrence, dietary intake and effects on nutrition and health. *J Sci Food Agric* 80: 1094–1117.

Scalbert, A. and G. Williamson. (2000) Dietary intake and bioavailability of polyphenols. *J Nutr* 130: 2073S–2085S.

Scambia, G., Ranelletti, F.O., Benedetti Panici, P., Piantelli, M., Rumi, C., Battaglia, F., Larocca, L.M., Capelli, A. and S. Mancuso. 1990. Type-II estrogen binding sites in a lymphoblastoid cell line and growth-inhibitory effect of estrogen, anti-estrogen and bioflavonoids. *Int J Cancer* 46: 1112–1116.

Schottner, M., Spiteller, G. and D. Gansser. 1998. Lignans interfering with 5 alphadihydrotestosterone binding to human sex hormone-binding globulin. *J Nat Prod* 61: 119–121.

Seeram, N.P., Bourquin, L.D. and M.G. Nair. 2001. Degradation products of cyanidin glucosides from tart cherries and their bioactivities. *J Agric Food Chem* 49: 4924–4929.

Senapati, S.K., Dey, S., Dwivedi, S.K., Patra, R.C. and D. Swarup. 2000. Effect of thiamine hydrochloride on lead induced lipid peroxidation in rat liver and kidney. *Vet Human Toxicol* 42: 236–237.

Sesink, A.L., Arts, I.C., de Boer, V.C., Breedveld, P., Schellens, J.H., Hollman, P.C. and F.G. Russel. 2005. Breast cancer resistance protein (Bcrp1/Abcg2) limits net intestinal uptake of quercetin in rats by facilitating apical efflux of glucuronides. *Mol Pharmacol* 67: 1999–2006.

Shahidi, F. and M. Naczk. 2004. *Phenolics in Food and Nutraceuticals*. Boca Raton, FL: CRC Press.

Shahidi, F., Zheng, Y. and Z.Q. Saleemi. 1993. Stabilization of meat lipids with flavonoids and flavonoid-related compounds. *J Food Lipids* 1: 69–78.

Sies, H. and W. Stahl. 1995. Vitamins E and C, beta-carotene, and other carotenoids as antioxidants. *Am J Clin Nutr* 62: 1315S–1321S.

So, F.V., Guthrie, N., Chambers, A.F. and K.K. Carroll. 1997. Inhibition of proliferation of estrogen receptor-positive MCF-7 human breast cancer cells by flavonoids in the presence and absence of excess estrogen. *Cancer Lett* 112: 127–133.

So, F.V., Guthrie, N., Chambers, A.F., Moussa, M. and K.K. Carroll. 1996. Inhibition of human breast cancer cell proliferation and delay of mammary tumorigenesis by flavonoids and citrus juices. *Nutr Cancer* 26: 167–181.

Song, J.-M., Lee, K.-H. and B.-L. Seong. 2005. Antiviral effect of catechins in green tea on influenza virus. *Antiviral Res* 68: 66–74.

Souza, R.F.V. and W.F. De Giovani. 2005. Synthesis, spectral and electrochemical properties of Al(III) and Zn(II) complexes with flavonoids. *Spectrochim Acta Part A: Mol Biomol Spectroscopy* 61: 1985–1990.

Souza, R.F.V., Sussuchi, E.M. and W.F. De Giovani. 2003. Synthesis, electrochemical, spectral, and antioxidant properties of complexes of flavonoids with metal ions. *Synth React Inorg Met-Org Chem* 33: 1125–1144.

Stahl, W., Junghans, A., De Boer, B., Driomina, E.S., Briviba, K. and H. Sies. 1998. Carotenoid mixtures protect multilamellar liposomes against oxidative damage: Synergistic effects of lycopene and lutein. *FEBS Lett* 427: 305–308.

Stahl, W. and H. Sies. 2003. Antioxidant activity of carotenoids. *Mol Aspects Med* 24: 345–351.

Stahl, W., van den Berg, H., Arthur, J., Bast, A., Dainty, J., Faulks, R.M., Gärtner, C., Haenen, G., Hollman, P., Holst, B., Kelly, F.J., Polidori, M.C., Rice-Evans, C., Southon, S., van Vliet, T., Viña-Ribes, J., Williamson, G. and S.B. Astley. 2002. Bioavailability and metabolism. *Mol Aspects Med* 23: 39–100.

Stampfer, M.J., Hennekens, C.H., Manson, J.E., Colditz, G.A., Rosner, B. and W.C. Willett. 1993. Vitamin E consumption and the risk of coronary disease in women. *New Engl J Med* 328: 1444–1449.

Stanger, O. 2002. Physiology of folic acid in health and disease. *Curr Drug Metab* 3: 211–223.

Stevenson, D.E. and R.D. Hurst. 2007. Polyphenolic phytochemicals: Just antioxidants or much more? *Cell Mol Life Sci* 64: 2900–2916.

Stintzing, F.C. and R. Carle. 2004. Functional properties of anthocyanins and betalains in plants, food, and in human nutrition. *Trends Food Sci Technol* 15: 19–38.

Stintzing, F.C., Herbach, K.M., Mosshammer, M.R., Carle, R., Yi, W., Sellappan, S., Akoh, C.C., Bunch, R. and P. Felker. 2005. Color, betalain pattern, and antioxidant properties of cactus pear (Opuntia spp.) clones. *J Agric Food Chem* 53: 442–451.

Stocker, P., Lesgards, J.F., Vidal, N., Chalier, F. and M. Prost. 2003. ESR study of a biological assay on whole blood: Antioxidant efficiency of various vitamins. *Biochim Biophys Acta* 1621: 1–8.

Strack, D., Vogt, T. and W. Schlieman. 2003. Recent advances in betalain research. *Phytochem* 62: 247–269.

Suganuma, M., Okabe, S., Oniyama, M., Tada, Y., Ito, H. and H. Fujiki. 1998. Wide distribution of [3H](-)-epigallocatechin gallate, a cancer preventive tea polyphenol, in mouse tissue. *Carcinogenesis* 19: 1771–1776.

Suh, J., Zhu, B.-Z. and B. Frei. 2003. Ascorbate does not act as a pro-oxidant towards lipids and proteins in human plasma exposed to redox-active transition metals ions and hydrogen peroxide. *Free Radic Biol Med* 34: 1306–1314.

Talavéra, S., Felgines, C., Texier, O., Besson, C., Gil-Izquierdo, A., Lamaison, J.L. and C. Rémésy. 2005. Anthocyanin metabolism in rats and their distribution to digestive area, kidney, and brain. *J Agric Food Chem* 53: 3902–3908.

Talavéra, S., Felgines, C., Texier, O., Besson, C., Lamaison, J.-L. and C. Rémésy. 2003. Anthocyanins are efficiently absorbed from the stomach in anesthetized rats. *J Nutr* 133: 4178–4182.

Talavéra, S., Felgines, C., Texier, O., Besson, C., Manach, C., Lamaison, J.L. and C. Rémésy. 2004. Anthocyanins are efficiently absorbed from the small intestine in rats. *J Nutr* 134: 2275–2279.

Tang, S.Z., Kerry, J.P., Sheehan, D., Buckley, D.J. and P.A. Morrissey. 2001a. Antioxidative effect of dietary tea catechins on lipid oxidation of long-term frozen stored chicken meat. *Meat Sci* 57: 331–336.

Tang, S., Kerry, J.P., Sheehan, D., Buckley, D.J. and P.A. Morrissey. 2001b. Antioxidative effect of added tea catechins on susceptibility of cooked red meat, poultry and fish patties to lipid oxidation. *Food Res Int* 34: 651–657.

Tarozzi, A., Morroni, F., Hreli, S., Angeloni, C., Marchesi, A., Cantelli-Forti, G. and P. Hreli. 2007. Neuroprotective effects of anthocyanins and their *in vivo* metabolites in SH-SY5Y cells. *Neurosci Lett* 424: 36–40.

Tesoriere, L., Allegra, M., Butera, D. and M.A. Livrea. 2004. Absorption, excretion, and distribution of dietary antioxidant betalains in LDLs: Potential health effects of betalains in humans. *Am J Clin Nutr* 80: 941–945.

Tesoriere, L., Butera, D., Allegra, M., Fazzari, M. and M.A. Livrea. 2005. Distribution of betalain pigments in red blood cells after consumption of cactus pear fruits and increased resistance of the cells to *ex vivo* induced oxidative hemolysis in humans. *J Agric Food Chem* 53: 1266–1270.

The Alpha-Tocopherol Beta Carotene Cancer Prevention Study Group. 1994. The effect of vitamin E and beta carotene on the incidence of lung cancer and other cancers in male smokers. 1999. *N Engl J Med* 330: 1029–1035.

Thompson, L.U., Seidl, M.M., Rickard, S.E., Orcheson, L.J. and H.H.S. Fong. 1996. Antitumorigenic effect of a mammalian lignan precursor from flaxseed. *Nutr Cancer Int J* 26: 159–165.

Todd, K. and R.F. Butterworth. 1999. Mechanisms of selective neuronal cell death due to thiamine deficiency. *Ann NY Acad Sci* 893: 404–411.

Tomas-Barberan, F.A. and M.N. Clifford. 2000. Flavonoids, chalcones and dihydrochalcones: Nature, occurrence and dietary burden. *J Sci Food Agric* 80: 1073–1080.

Torskangerpoll, K. and Ø.M. Andersen. 2005. Colour stability of anthocyanins in aqueous solution at various pH values. *Food Chem* 89: 427–440.

Tournaire, C., Croux, S., Maurette, M.T., Beck, I., Hocquaux, M., Braun, A.M. and E. Oliveros. 1993. Antioxidant activity of flavonoids: Efficiency of singlet oxygen (1 delta g) quenching. *J Photochem Photobiol B* 19: 205–215.

Tripoli, E., La Guardia, M., Giammanco, S., Di Majo, D. and M. Giammanco. 2007. Citrus flavonoids: Molecular structure, biological activity and nutritional properties: A review. *Food Chem* 104: 466–479.

Tsuda, T., Horio, F. and T. Osawa. 1999. Absorption and metabolism of cyanidin 3-O-β-D-glucoside in rats. *FEBS Lett* 449: 179–182.

Tsuda, T., Shiga, K., Oshima, K., Kawakishi, S. and T. Osawa. 1996. Inhibition of lipid peroxidation and the active oxygen radical scavenging effect of anthocyanin pigments isolated from *Phaseolus vulgaris* L. *Biochem Pharmacol* 52: 1033–1039.

Tsuda, T., Watanabe, M., Ohshima, K., Narinobu, S., Choi, S.W., Kawakishi, S. and T. Osawa. 1994. Antioxidative activity of the anthocyanin pigments cyanidin 3-O-β-D-glucoside and cyanidin. *J Agric Food Chem* 42: 2407–2410.

Tyrakowska, B., Soffers, A.E.M.F., Szymusiak, H., Boeren, S., Boersma, M.G., Lemańska, K., Vervoort, J. and I.M.C.M. Rietjens. 1999. TEAC antioxidant activity of 4-hydroxybenzoates. *Free Radic Biol Med* 27: 1427–1436.

Valko, M., Rhodes, C.J., Moncol, J., Izakovic, M. and M. Mazur. 2006. Free radicals, metals and antioxidants in oxidative stress-induced cancer. *Chem Biol Interact* 160: 1–40.

van Acker, S.A.B.E., Koymans, L.M.H. and A. Bast. 1993. Molecular pharmacology of vitamin E: Structural aspects of antioxidant activity. *Free Radic Biol Med* 15: 311–328.

van Acker, S.A.B.E., Tromp, M.N.J.L., Haenen, G.R.M.M., van der Vijgh, W.J.F. and A. Bast. 1995. Flavonoids as scavengers of nitric oxide radical. *Biochem Biophys Res Commun* 214: 755–759.

van der Woude, H., Alink, G.M., van Rossum, B.E.J., Walle, K., van Steeg, H., Walle, T. and I.M.C.M. Rietjens. 2005. Formation of transient covalent protein and DNA adducts by quercetin in cells with and without oxidative enzyme activity. *Chem Res Toxicol* 18: 1907–1916.

van der Woude, H., Boersma, M.G., Alink, G.M., Vervoort, J. and I.M.C.M. Rietjens. 2006. Consequences of quercetin methylation for its covalent glutathione and DNA adduct formation. *Chem Biol Int* 160: 193–203.

van der Woude, H., Gliszczyńska-Świgło, A., Struijs, K., Smeets, A., Alink, G.M. and I.M.C.M. Rietjens. 2003. Biphasic modulation of cell proliferation by quercetin at concentrations physiologically relevant in humans. *Cancer Lett* 200: 41–47.

van Erp-Baart, M.A., Brants, H.A., Kiely, M., Mulligan, A., Turrini, A., Sermoneta, C., Kilkkinen, A. and L.M. Valsta. 2003. Isoflavone intake in four different European countries: The VENUS approach. *Br J Nutr* 89: S25–30.

van Zanden, J.J., Ben Hamman, O., van Iersel, M.L., Boeren, S., Cnubben, N.H., Lo Bello, M., Vervoort, J., van Bladeren, P.J. and I.M.C.M. Rietjens. 2003. Inhibition of human glutathione S-transferase P1-1 by the flavonoid quercetin. *Chem. Biol. Interact* 145: 139–148.

Vareltzis, K., Koufidis, D., Gavriilidou, E., Papavergou, E. and S. Vasiliadou. 1997. Effectiveness of a natural rosemary (*Rosmarinus officinalis*) extract on the stability of filleted and minced fish during frozen storage. *Z Lebensm Unters Forsch A* 205: 93–96.

Vargas, A.J. and R. Burd. 2010. Hormesis and synergy: Pathway and mechanisms of quercetin in cancer prevention and management. *Nutr Rev* 68: 418–428.

Vásquez-Vivar, J., Kalyanaraman, B., Martásek, P., Hogg, N., Masters, B.S., Karoui, H., Tordo, P. and K.A. Pritchard. 1998. Superoxide generation by endothelial nitric oxide synthase: The influence of cofactors. *Proc Natl Adad Sci USA* 95: 9220–9225.

Verhaar, M.C., Stroes, E. and T.J. Rabelink. 2002. Folates and cardiovascular disease. *Arterioscler Thromb Vasc Biol* 22: 6–13.

Vermerris, W. and R. Nicholson. 2006. *Phenolic Compound Biochemistry.* Dordrecht, The Netherlands: Springer.

Vitrac, X., Desmouliere, A., Brouillaud, B., Krisa, S., Deffieux, G., Barthe, N., Rosenbaum, J. and J.-M. Mérillon. 2003. Distribution of [14C]-*trans*-resveratrol, a cancer chemopreventive polyphenol, in mouse tissues after oral administration. *Life Sci* 72: 2219–2233.

Walgren, R.A., Lin, J.T., Kinne, R.K. and T. Walle. 2000. Cellular uptake of dietary flavonoid quercetin 4′-β-glucoside by sodium-dependent glucose transporter SGLT1. *J Pharmacol Exp Ther* 294: 837–843.

Walle, T., Otake, Y., Walle, U.K. and F.A. Wilson. 2000. Quercetin glucosides are completely hydrolyzed in ileostomy patients before absorption. *J Nutr* 130: 2658–2661.

Walle, T., Vincent, T.S. and U.K. Walle. 2003. Evidence of covalent binding of the dietary flavonoid quercetin to DNA and protein in human intestinal and hepatic cells. *Biochem Pharmacol* 65: 1603–1610.

Walle, T. and U.K. Walle. 2003. The beta-D-glucoside and sodium-dependent glucose transporter 1 (SGLT1)-inhibitor phloridzin is transported by both SGLT1 and multidrug resistance-associated proteins 1/2. *Drug Metab Dispos* 31: 1288–1291.

Walle, U.K., French, K.L., Walgren, R.A. and T. Walle. 1999. Transport of genistein-7-glucoside by human intestinal CACO-2 cells: Potential role for MRP2. *Res Commun Mol Pathol Pharmacol* 103: 45–56.

Wang, H., Cao, G. and R.L. Prior. 1997. Oxygen radical absorbing capacity of anthocyanins. *J Agric Food Chem* 45: 304–309.

Wang, H., Nair, M.G., Strasburg, G.M., Chang, Y.C., Booren, A.M., Gray, J.I. and D.L. DeWitt. 1999. Antioxidant and anti-inflammatory activities of anthocyanins and their aglycon, cyanidin, from tart cherries. *J Nat Prod* 62: 294–296.

Wang, X.-D., Liu, C., Bronson, R.T., Smith, D.E., Krinsky, N.I. and R.M. Russell. 1999. Retinoid signaling and activator protein-1 expression in ferrets given β-carotene supplements and exposed to tobacco smoke. *J Natl Cancer Inst* 91: 60–66.

Wang, X.Y. and P.J. Quinn. 1999. Vitamin E and its function in membranes. *Progr Lipid Res* 38: 309–336.

Wen, X. and T. Walle. 2006. Methylated flavonoids have greatly improved intestinal absorption and metabolic stability. *Drug Metab Dispos* 34: 1786–1792.

Westcott, N.D. and A.D. Muir. 2003. Flaxseed lignan in disease prevention and health promotion. *Phytochem* 2: 401–417.

Wettasinghe, M., Bolling, B., Plhak, L., Xiao, H. and K. Parkin. 2002. Phase II enzyme-inducing and antioxidant activities of beetroot (*Beta vulgaris* L.) extracts from phenotypes of different pigmentation. *J Agric Food Chem* 50: 6704–6709.

Williamson, G., DuPont, M.S., Wanigatunga, S., Heaney, R.K., Musk, S.R.R., Fenwick, G.R. and M.J.C. Rhodes. 1997. Induction of glutathione-S-transferase activity in hepG2 cells by extracts from fruits and vegetables. *Food Chem* 60: 157–160.

Williamson, G. and C. Manach. 2005. Bioavailability and bioefficiency of polyphenols in humans. II. Review of 93 intervention studies. *Am J Clin Nutr* 81: 243S–255S.

Wilska-Jeszka, J. and A. Korzuchowska. 1996. Anthocyanins and chlorogenic acid copigmentation: Influence on the color of strawberry and chokeberry juices. *Z Lebensmit–Forsch A* 203: 38–42.

Wojdyło, A., Oszmiański, J. and R. Czemerys. 2007. Antioxidant activity and phenolic compounds in 32 selected herbs. *Food Chem* 105: 940–949.

Woodal, A.A., Lee, S.W.M., Weesie, R.J., Jackson, M.J. and G. Britton. 1997. Oxidation of carotenoids by free radicals: Relationship between structure and reactivity. *Biochem Biophys Acta* 1336: 33–42.

Wu, X., Cao, G. and R.L. Prior. 2002. Absorption and metabolism of anthocyanins in elderly women after consumption of elderberry or blueberry. *J Nutr* 132: 1865–1871.

Yamamoto, N., Moon, J.H., Tsushida, T., Nagao, A. and J. Terao. 1999. Inhibitory effect of quercetin metabolites and their related derivatives on copper ion-induced lipid peroxidation in human low-density lipoprotein. *Arch Biochem Biophys* 372: 347–354.

Yamanaka, N., Oda, O. and S. Nagao. 1997. Green tea catechins such as (-)-epicatechin and (-)-epigallocatechin accelerate Cu2+-induced low-density lipoprotein oxidation in propagation phase. *FEBS Lett* 401: 230–234.

Yang, B., Kotani, A., Arai, K. and F. Kusu. 2001. Estimation of the antioxidant activities of flavonoids from their oxidation potentials. *Analyt Sci* 17: 599–604.

Yang, M., Collis, C.S., Kelly, M., Diplock, A.T. and C. Rice-Evans. 1999. Do iron and vitamin C co-supplementation influence platelet function or LDL oxidizability in healthy volunteers? *Eur J Clin Nutr* 53: 367–374.

Yeh, S.L., Wang, W.Y., Huang, C.H. and M.L. Hu. 2005. Pro-oxidative effect of beta-carotene and the interaction with flavonoids on UVA-induced DNA strand breaks in mouse fibroblast C3H10T1/2 cells. *J Nutr Biochem* 16: 729–735.

Yen, G.C., Duh, P.D., Tsai, H.L. and S.L. Huang. 2003. Pro-oxidative properties of flavonoids in human lymphocytes. *Biosci Biotechnol Biochem* 67: 1215–1222.

Yilmaz, Y. 2006. Novel uses of catechins in foods. *Trends Food Sci Technol* 17: 64–71.

Yoshie, Y. and H. Ohshima. 1998. Synergistic induction of DNA strand breakage by catechol-estrogen and nitric oxide: Implications for hormonal carcinogenesis. *Free Radic Biol Med* 24: 341–348.

Yoshino, M., Haneda, M., Naruse, M. and K. Murakami. 1999. Prooxidant activity of flavonoids: Copper-dependent strand breaks and the formation of 8-hydroxy-2'-deoxyguanosine in DNA. *Mol Gen Metab* 68: 468–472.

Youdim, K.A., McDonald, J., Kalt, W. and J.A. Joseph. 2002 Potential role of dietary flavonoids in reducing microvascular endothelium vulnerability to oxidative and inflammatory insults. *J Nutr Biochem* 13: 282–288.

Yu, R., Jiao, J.J., Duh, J.L., Gudehithlu, K., Tan, T.H. and A.N. Kong. 1997. Activation of mitogen-activated protein kinases by green tea polyphenols: Potential signaling pathways in the regulation of antioxidant-responsive element-mediated phase II enzyme gene expression. *Carcinogenesis* 18: 451–456.

Zakharova, N.S. and T.A. Petrova. 1998. Relationship between the structure and antioxidant activity of various betalains. *Priklady Biokhim Mikrobiol* 34: 199–202.

Zegarska, A., Amarowicz, R., Karmac, R. and R. Rafalowski. 1996. Antioxidative effect of rosemary ethanolic extract on butter. *Milchwissenschaft* 51: 195–198.

Zhang, J., Melton, L.D., Adaim, A. and M.A. Skinner. 2008. Cytoprotective effects of poly-phenolics on H2O2-induced cell death in SH-SY5Y cells in relation to their antioxidant activities. *Eur Food Res Technol* 228: 123–131.

Zheng, L.F., Dai, F., Zhou, B., Yang, L. and Z.-L. Liu. 2008. Prooxidant activity of hydroxy-cinnamic acids on DNA damage in the presence of Cu(II) ions: Mechanism and structure-activity relationship. *Food Chem Toxicol* 46: 149–156.

Zhou, B., Wu, L.-M., Yang, L. and Z.-L. Liu. 2005. Evidence for α-tokoferol regeneration reaction of green tea polyphenols in SDS micelles. *Free Radic Biol Med* 38: 78–84.

Ziegler, R.G. 1991. Vegetables, fruits and carotenoids and the risk of cancer. *Am J Clin Nutr* 53: 251S–259S.

15 Bioavailability and Antioxidant Activity of Curcuminoids and Carotenoids in Humans

Alexa Kocher, Christina Schiborr, Daniela Weber, Tilman Grune, and Jan Frank

CONTENTS

15.1   INTRODUCTION

Curcuminoids and carotenoids are dietary phytochemicals that, although having been known for decades, attracted the attention of nutritionists, food scientists, medical researchers, and scientists from many other fields in recent years. They have been—and still are—studied for their potential health-beneficial properties, among which their antioxidant effects in humans as well as model systems, foods, and other mammals have been prominent (Stahl and Sies 2003; Bengmark 2006).

Phytochemicals are compounds that are generated in the secondary metabolism of plants and, therefore, are sometimes also called "secondary plant metabolites." They are divided into classes according to their chemical structures. An important and intensively studied subclass of the phytochemicals is the group of polyphenols. Polyphenols share one defining common feature, namely, one or more aromatic rings with at least one hydroxyl substituent, and may vary greatly in complexity from simple phenols to the highly polymerized tannins and lignins. The structural diversity of plant phenolic compounds results in a plethora of phytochemicals ingested by man (Bravo 1998). In this chapter, we focus on two polyphenol subgroups, curcuminoids and carotenoids, and describe their release from the food matrix, gastrointestinal stability, absorption, biotransformation, and excretion, which determine their resulting plasma and tissue concentrations and, ultimately, their antioxidant activities in humans.

15.1.1   Oxidative Stress and Disease

A multiplicity of disorders, including atherosclerosis, stroke, heart disease, cancer, Alzheimer's disease, diabetes mellitus types I and II, and obesity, to name only a few prominent examples, have been suggested as being caused by or resulting in an excess formation of free radicals (Ames et al. 1993; Davies 1995; Keaney et al. 2003; Maritim 2003). It was suggested that the consumption of dietary antioxidants, which are capable of inactivating free radical species, might be helpful in the prevention and treatment of these diseases, but human intervention trials with antioxidant supplements have largely disappointed the expectations of researchers and resulted in inconclusive and often contradictory findings [reviewed in Frank and Rimbach (2009) and Gutteridge and Halliwell (2010)]. Epidemiological studies, on the other hand, suggest a positive correlation of dietary antioxidant intake with better health. In US American adults, for example, persons in the lowest quartile for total carotenoid, α-carotene, and lycopene plasma concentrations had the highest all-cause mortality risk of the studied population (Shardell et al. 2011).

Investigating the potential health-beneficial effects of dietary antioxidants is much more complex than studying the effects of drugs that are not naturally present in the organism or the habitual diet. The antioxidant activity of a nutrient or phytochemical, when absent from the diet, may be replaced by that of other food antioxidants. Furthermore, the subjects in the control groups of clinical trials ingest at least small amounts of the respective dietary antioxidant under investigation, and thus, the contribution of a single dietary antioxidant to health is often difficult to determine [see Frank and Rimbach (2009) for further details on the problems of studying antioxidants in nutrition intervention trials]. The *in vivo* antioxidant activities of dietary polyphenols are furthermore limited, among other things, by their restricted absorption, rapid conversion to often non-antioxidant metabolites, swift excretion, and the resulting low plasma and tissue concentrations, or, to describe this with one term conceptually uniting these processes, their "bioavailability." The bioavailability of a given dietary antioxidant may furthermore underlie great interindividual variation, which additionally complicates research into its antioxidant activity in humans.

15.1.2 BIOAVAILABILITY

The term "bioavailability"—short for "biological availability"—and the underlying concept were originally introduced in the field of pharmacology, where bioavailability was defined as "the rate and extent to which a drug reaches its site of action." Because of the problems in the quantification of a compound at its site of action, this concept was modified to account for the fraction of an oral dose of a substance or its metabolites that reaches the systemic circulation (Stahl et al. 2002). Bioavailability can be determined in a single-dose experiment by measuring the peak blood concentration (C_{max}), the time to reach the peak concentration (t_{max}), and the area under the blood concentration time curve (AUC). The AUC is the most reliable measure of bioavailability because it takes into account the entire response over time, whereas C_{max}, which is used by some researchers to describe the "fold-increase in bioavailability," measures only one point in time and is, therefore, less robust. In a multiple-dose study, the compound of interest is given for at least five times its half-life ($t_{1/2}$) in the tissue intended for analysis (e.g., the blood or liver) to reach the steady-state concentration, which is the most important parameter in this type of bioavailability study.

The bioavailability of dietary antioxidants is influenced by a multitude of factors, including liberation from the food matrix (bioaccessibility), absorption, distribution, metabolism, and excretion—a concept termed "LADME"—which, in turn, are governed by a large number of parameters themselves (Holst and Williamson 2004). In the specific case of curcuminoids and carotenoids, bioavailability may be affected by their release from the food matrix; the secretion of digestive enzymes, particularly bile acids and pancreatic enzymes; the amount and type of concurrently ingested fat; the dose and composition of curcuminoids and carotenoids consumed; the action of membrane transporters; metabolic conversion and excretion; the exposure to oxidative stress or other processes consuming antioxidants; the presence of regenerating co-antioxidants (e.g., ascorbate); and many other processes (Stahl et al. 2002; Holst and Williamson 2004).

15.2 CURCUMINOIDS

Curcuminoids (Figure 15.1) are lipophilic phenolic substances with a characteristic yellow color and are derived from the rhizome of the plant turmeric (*Curcuma longa*). Curcumin, the major curcuminoid in turmeric, is commonly used as a food additive (E100) for coloring and flavoring in many parts of the world and particularly on the Indian subcontinent (Strimpakos and Sharma 2008). Curcumin is a *bis*-α,β-unsaturated β-diketone with two ferulic acid moieties joined by a methylene bridge. The curcumin derivatives demethoxy- and *bis*-demethoxy-curcumin (Figure 15.1) are present in

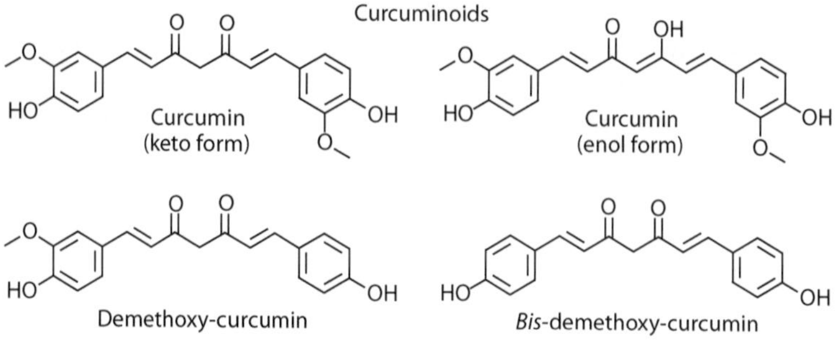

FIGURE 15.1 Chemical structures of curcuminoids from *Curcuma longa* Linnaeus and keto- and enol-conformations of the major curcuminoid curcumin.

turmeric and its extracts in smaller quantities. The mean daily dietary consumption of curcumin was estimated to be 0.4–1.5 mg/kg bodyweight (bw) in India (Srinivasan and Satyanarayana 1988) and 0.48 mg/kg bw in France (Verger et al. 1998).

Studies in humans showed that curcumin is generally recognized as safe (GRAS) and well tolerated even at very high doses. A phase I clinical trial showed that oral doses up to 8 g/day for 3 months were not toxic (Cheng et al. 2001). The acceptable daily intake of curcumin as a food additive, as set by the World Health Organization (WHO), is 0–1 mg/kg bw (World Health Organization 2000).

15.2.1 BIOTRANSFORMATION OF CURCUMINOIDS

In contrast to the extensive research on the potential anti-inflammatory, antioxidant, and anticarcinogenic activities of curcuminoids (Leu and Maa 2002; Aggarwal et al. 2003; Bengmark 2006; Bengmark et al. 2009), detailed information on their biotransformation in mammals is scarce (Ireson et al. 2001, 2002). During phase I metabolism in rodents, reductases in the intestinal mucosa and liver convert curcuminoids (curcumin, demethoxy-curcumin, *bis*-demethoxy-curcumin) into dihydrocurcumin (DHC), tetrahydrocurcumin (THC), hexahydrocurcumin (HHC), and octahydrocurcumin (OHC; Figures 15.2 and 15.3) (Holder et al. 1978; Ravindranath and Chandrasekhara 1981b; Pan et al. 1999; Asai and Miyazawa 2000; Ireson et al. 2001, 2002). During phase II metabolism, the curcuminoids and their reductive metabolites are conjugated with glucuronic acid (from uridine-5'-diphospho-glucuronic acid) and sulfate (from 3'-phosphoadenosine-5'-phosphosulfate; Figures 15.2 and 15.4), which renders them more hydrophilic and, thus, more readily excretable (Ravindranath and Chandrasekhara 1980; Pan et al. 1999; Asai and Miyazawa 2000; Hoehle et al. 2006). This conjugation reaction is catalyzed by enzymes, such as uridine-5'-diphospho-glucuronosyltransferases (UGT), that are localized on the luminal side of the endoplasmic reticulum. Seventeen functional human UGT isoforms have been characterized and are classified into two subfamilies, UGT1 and UGT2 (Mackenzie et al. 2005), of which the UGT1 subfamily appears to be more important for curcuminoid metabolism than the UGT2 (see below).

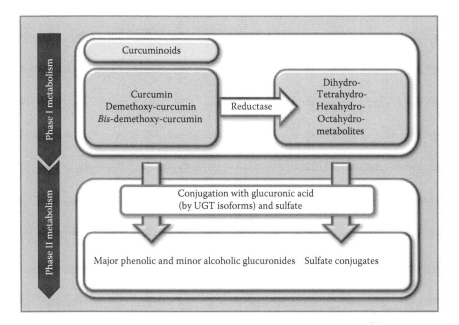

FIGURE 15.2 Schematic presentation of metabolic conversion of curcuminoids. During phase I metabolism in the intestinal mucosa and liver, curcuminoids are reduced to dihydro-, tetrahydro-, hexahydro-, and octahydro-metabolites. In the course of phase II metabolism, curcuminoids and their reductive metabolites are then conjugated with glucuronic acid and sulfate.

Two distinct monoglucuronides are formed upon incubation of curcumin with human liver microsomes, one carrying the glucuronic acid at the phenolic and the other at the alcoholic hydroxyl group. All curcuminoids are preferentially conjugated with glucuronic acid at the phenolic hydroxyl group (Figure 15.4). The hexahydro-metabolites, however, are conjugated with glucuronic acid only at the phenolic hydroxyl group (Pfeiffer et al. 2007). Incubation of curcuminoids with

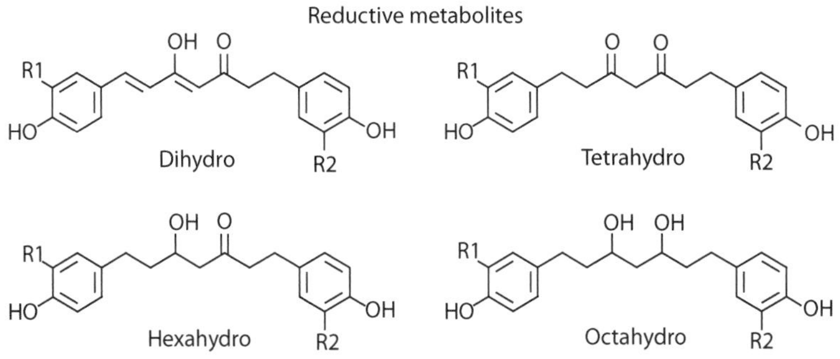

FIGURE 15.3 Chemical structures of reductive metabolites of curcuminoids: -curcumin ($R1 = OCH_3$, $R2 = OCH_3$), -demethoxy-curcumin ($R1 = OCH_3$, $R2 = H$), and -*bis*-demethoxy-curcumin ($R1 = H$, $R2 = H$).

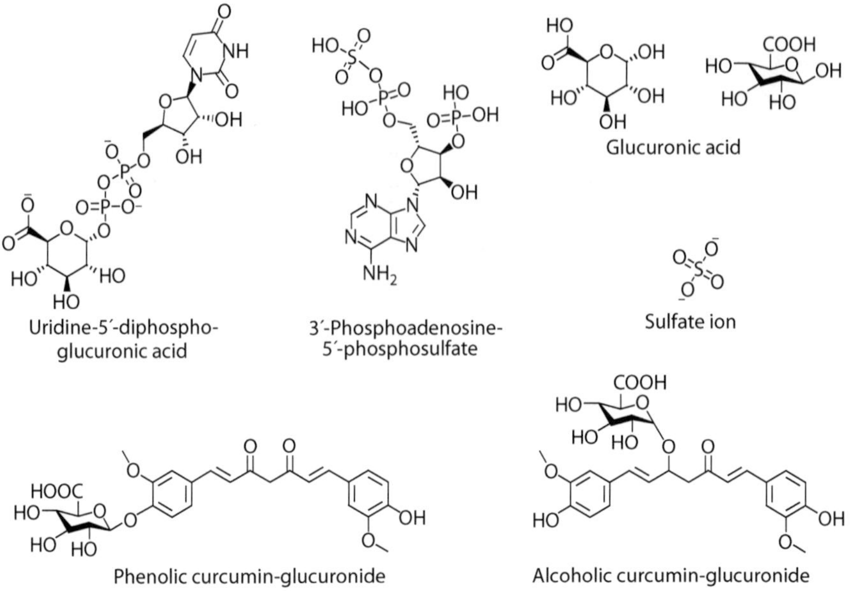

FIGURE 15.4 Chemical structures of phenolic and alcoholic glucuronides of curcumin, of glucuronic acid and sulfate ion, as well as their metabolic precursors uridine-5′-diphospho-glucuronic acid and 3′-phosphoadenosine-5′-phosphosulfate.

human intestinal microsomes resulted in the generation of phenolic glucuronides only. Compared to the liver microsomes, glucuronidation of curcuminoids by intestinal microsomes was approximately threefold higher, whereas hexahydro-metabolites were converted to a similar extent by hepatic and intestinal microsomes (Pfeiffer et al. 2007). These observations suggest that the gastrointestinal tract plays an important role in the first-pass metabolism of dietary curcuminoids and that their low systemic bioavailability might be explained by their rapid transformation by UGT and subsequent rapid elimination (Pfeiffer et al. 2007).

The specific UGT involved in the glucuronidation of curcumin and its metabolites were studied in human hepatic and intestinal microsomes, and UGT1A1, 1A3, 1A7, 1A8, 1A9, 1A10, and 2B7 were identified as being involved in the conjugation reactions (Hoehle et al. 2007). Curcumin and demethoxy-curcumin were mainly glucuronidated by UGT1A1, 1A8, and 1A10 (Hoehle et al. 2007), which are predominantly expressed in the gastrointestinal tract and show little or no activity in the liver (Strassburg et al. 1999; Tukey and Strassburg 2000). *Bis*-demethoxy-curcumin was a less favorable substrate than other curcuminoids for all UGT investigated, and hexahydro-curcuminoids were most actively conjugated by UGT1A8, 1A9, and 2B7. Hexahydro-*bis*-demethoxy-curcumin was only marginally glucuronidated by UGT1A1, 1A9, and 2B7. Similar glucuronidation patterns were observed for the UGT from hepatic and intestinal microsomes; all UGT isoforms except UGT1A9 generated exclusively phenolic curcuminoid glucuronides, and UGT1A9 formed both the phenolic and the alcoholic glucuronide (Hoehle et al. 2007). The formation of the alcoholic glucuronides may play an important role in the kidneys where UGT1A9 mRNA expression in humans is threefold higher than in the liver (Sutherland et al. 1993).

Dietary curcumin is partially absorbed in the intestine (Ravindranath and Chandrasekhara 1981a), but the majority of the ingested curcumin reaches the cecum and colon with its wide range of bacteria. *Escherichia coli* from human feces metabolizes curcumin via a NADPH-dependent curcumin-converting enzyme that is involved in the reduction of curcumin to dihydrocurcumin and tetrahydrocurcumin (Hassaninasab et al. 2011).

15.2.2 Gastrointestinal Stability of Curcuminoids and Their Metabolites

The three natural curcuminoids and their major glucuronides differ in their chemical stability and appear to be chemically less stable than their hexahydro-metabolites (Hoehle et al. 2006). Curcumin itself degrades in aqueous solutions at pH above 7. The degradation products have been identified as vanillin, vanillic acid, ferulic acid, ferulic aldehyde, and *trans*-6-(4′-hydroxy-3′-methoxyphenyl)-4-dioxo-5-hexenal (Wang et al. 1997; Appiah-Opong et al. 2007). Both curcumin and its phenolic glucuronide rapidly degraded in aqueous solutions (phosphate buffer at pH 7.4 and 37°C) by more than 90% within 1 h with the glucuronide being less stable than the parent compound. The decomposition of *bis*-demethoxy-curcumin at these conditions was less pronounced than that of its phenolic glucuronide. Hexahydro-curcumin and its glucuronide, on the other hand, were completely stable in the phosphate buffer. The aqueous solutions of the curcumin- and *bis*-demethoxy-curcumin-glucuronides did not contain the unconjugated parent compounds after 1 and 2 h, and none of the known degradation products of curcumin could be detected, suggesting that degradation of the curcuminoid glucuronides is probably not a simple hydrolysis of the glycosidic bond (Pfeiffer et al. 2007).

15.2.3 Bioavailability of Curcuminoids: Absorption, Tissue Distribution, and Excretion

A limited number of human trials (Table 15.1) have been published that deal with the absorption, distribution, and excretion of curcuminoids (see below). In order to describe these phenomena in sufficient detail, data from both animal models and human studies are presented and discussed.

In one of the first comprehensive experiments investigating the absorption and excretion of curcumin in rats, approximately 75% of an oral dose of 1 g curcumin/kg bw were excreted with feces while only traces were detected in urine (<0.006% of the dose) within 72 h after administration. Plasma concentrations of curcumin in these rats were very low (close to zero) when curcumin was administered by oral gavage. Upon intravenous injection, curcumin concentrations dropped from 270 nmol/L to zero within 60 min. Biliary concentrations of curcumin were higher than plasma concentrations, and biliary excretion of conjugated curcumin was approximately 10 times higher than that of the free compound (Wahlström and Blennow 1978). In another study with Wistar rats, only 40% of a single oral dose of 400 mg curcumin was excreted unchanged in the feces over a period of 5 days. Curcumin

TABLE 15.1

Pharmacokinetic Parameters and Maximum Plasma or Serum Concentrations of Curcumin in Humans upon Oral Ingestion of Capsules Containing Curcumin or Curcuma Extracts

Subjects	Formulation	Dose (mg)	Treatment	AUC (nmol/L*h)	C_{max} (nmol/L)	T_{max} (min)	Comments	Ref.
Patients with precancerous lesions	Curcumin (99.3%)	4000	Daily oral dose for 3 months	2550 ± 1760	510 ± 110	100 ± 35	Serum levels peaked at 1 to 2 h and declined within 12 h, no curcumin was detected in urine	Cheng et al. 2001
		6000		4800 ± 4490	630 ± 60	120 ± 104		
		8000		13,740 ± 5630	1770 ± 1870	105 ± 21		
Healthy volunteers		2000	Single oral dose	11	16 ± 14	60		Shoba et al. 1998
Colorectal cancer patients	Curcuma extract (curcumin, 90%; demethoxy-curcumin, 10%)	36	Daily oral dose for 4 months		n.d.[a]		No curcumin in blood and urine; 144–519 and 64–1054 nmol curcumin/g dried feces, respectively, in day 29 fecal samples of patients consuming 144 or 180 mg/day curcumin	Sharma et al. 2001
		72			n.d.			
		108			n.d.			
		144			n.d.			
		180			n.d.			
Colorectal cancer patients	Curcumin, 90%; demethoxy-curcumin, 8%; bis-demethoxy-curcumin, 2%	450	Daily oral dose for 4 months		n.d.		Urinary concentrations in subjects consuming the highest dose: curcumin, 100–1300; curcumin sulfate, 19–45; curcumin glucuronide, 210–510 nmol/L; curcumin recovered in feces in all groups	Sharma et al. 2004
		900			n.d.			
		1800			n.d.			
		3600			11 ± 1[b]			

Subjects	Formulation	Dose (mg)	Regimen	Result		Comments	Reference
Healthy volunteers	Curcumin, 75%; demethoxycurcumin, 23%; bis-demethoxycurcumin, 2%	500 1000 2000 4000 6000 8000 10,000 12,000	Single oral dose	n.d. n.d. n.d. n.d. n.d. n.d. Traces Traces			Lao et al. 2006
Patients with hepatic metastatic disease from primary colorectal adenocarcinomas	Purified turmeric extract (curcumin, 90%; demethoxycurcumin, 6%; bis-demethoxycurcumin, 4%)	450 1800 3600	Daily oral dose for 1 week	n.d. n.d. Traces		Concentrations below LLOQ[a] and near LOD (~3 nmol/L) in patients receiving the highest dose	Garcea et al. 2005
Healthy human subjects	Powder extract (curcumin, 75%; demethoxycurcumin, 23%; bis-demethoxycurcumin, 2%)	10,000 12,000	Single oral dose	8 ± 1[c] 5 ± 2[c]	260 220	Free curcumin was detected in the plasma of only one subject 30 min after ingestion of the 10 g dose	Vareed et al. 2008

[a] n.d., not detected; LLOQ, lower limit of quantification; LOD, limit of detection.

[b] Mean concentration of curcumin for three patients consuming 3.6 g curcumin 1 h after intake on day 1.

[c] Curcumin conjugates.

glucuronides and sulfates, but no free curcumin, were detected in urine for up to 7 days. No curcumin was present in the heart blood with only traces in the portal blood and negligible amounts in the liver and kidneys from 15 min to 24 h after administration (Ravindranath and Chandrasekhara 1980).

In our own experiments, no curcumin could be detected in the plasma, liver, or brain in mice within 1 h of administration of 50 mg curcumin/kg bw by oral gavage. However, when curcumin was injected intraperitoneally (100 mg/kg bw), concentrations in the brain reached 4.16, 5.01, and 4.84 µg/g tissue after 20, 30, and 40 min, respectively (Schiborr et al. 2010). In another mouse study, C_{max} in plasma after an oral dose of 1 g curcumin/kg bw was 0.22 µg/mL at 1 h and declined within 6 h. Intraperitoneal (i.p.) injection of 0.1 g curcumin/kg bw resulted in 10 times higher peak plasma concentrations of 2.25 µg/mL within the first 15 min and returned to zero within 1 h. Curcumin concentrations 1 h after i.p. administration were 177, 26, 27, and 8 µg/g in the intestines, spleen, liver, and kidneys, respectively, while only traces (0.41 µg/g) were detected in the brain. The major metabolites were curcumin glucuronide, dihydrocurcumin glucuronide, tetrahydrocurcumin glucuronide, and tetrahydrocurcumin (Pan et al. 1999).

The above-described animal experiments demonstrate the importance of the gastrointestinal tract for the poor absorption of orally ingested curcumin and its rapid metabolism, which is mirrored in the low blood concentrations of curcumin and its metabolites usually observed in human studies (see next paragraph for details).

In eight healthy 20–26 year-old male volunteers, serum concentrations of curcumin were either undetectable or very low (C_{max}, 0.006 µg/mL) even after an oral dose of 2 g (Shoba et al. 1998). In agreement with this, curcumin was only found in feces but not in the blood or urine from colorectal cancer patients after an oral administration of 36–180 mg/day for up to 4 months (Sharma et al. 2001). In healthy humans (six subjects per dose) receiving a single oral dose of 10 or 12 g curcumin, concentrations of curcumin glucuronide and sulfate at T_{max} were 2.04 ± 0.31 and 1.06 ± 0.40 µg/mL at the lower dose and 1.40 ± 0.74 and 0.87 ± 0.44 µg/mL at the higher dose and returned to zero within 24 h. Free curcumin was detected in only one person receiving a 10 g dose and in none of those ingesting 12 g of curcumin (Vareed et al. 2008). Similarly, oral intake of curcumin at doses of 10 and 12 g resulted in low serum curcumin concentrations in only 2 of the 24 subjects studied in another human trial (Lao et al. 2006). Because of the poor absorption of curcumin, one study investigated its concentrations in colon tissue. Patients with colorectal cancer ingested 0.45, 1.80, or 3.60 g curcumin/day for 7 days. Only traces of curcumin were detected in the peripheral circulation of patients receiving the highest dose 1 h after the last intake of curcumin. Curcumin concentrations in normal and malignant colorectal tissue were 12.7 ± 5.7 and 7.7 ± 1.8 nmol/g, respectively, 6 to 7 h after the last intake of 3.6 g curcumin. Furthermore, curcumin conjugates were found in the tissue of these patients (Garcea et al. 2005). Absorbed curcumin may undergo hydrophobic interactions with and therefore be associated with albumin in the blood from where it may be taken up into target cells (Pulla Reddy et al. 1999). There, the polyphenol assembles in membranous structures, such as the plasma membrane, the endoplasmic reticulum, and the nuclear envelope (Jaruga et al. 1998).

In summary, oral administration of curcumin results in very low systemic concentrations and rapid excretion even in humans (Table 15.1). Because the majority of curcumin remains in the gastrointestinal tract, it is here that health benefits appear most likely. Nevertheless, biological activities in other organs have been described (Bengmark et al. 2009). Therefore, solutions to overcome the low bioavailability of curcumin are currently studied to facilitate its use in the prevention or treatment of diseases.

15.2.4 STRATEGIES FOR ENHANCED BIOAVAILABILITY OF CURCUMIN IN ANIMALS AND HUMANS

A number of different strategies, such as the formulation with liposomes, phospholipids, micelles, or nanoparticles, have been investigated for their potential to improve the bioavailability of curcumin in animal models and humans.

Mice were given a single oral dose of curcumin (50 mg/kg/bw), liposome-encapsulated curcumin (50 mg/kg bw), or liposome-encapsulated curcumin plus resveratrol (25 mg/kg bw, each). Liposome-encapsulated curcumin resulted in higher serum C_{max} (100 ng/mL) compared to native curcumin (50 ng/mL), and the combination with resveratrol amplified this effect (252 ng/mL). Serum T_{max} of native curcumin was 1.5 h and concentrations declined immediately, whereas they remained elevated up to 4 h after administration of the liposome formulations (Narayanan et al. 2009). Curcumin has also been conjugated with phospholipids and formulated into complexes known as phytosomes. Phytosomes differ from liposomes in that a phytosome is an aggregate of a phytochemical (e.g., curcumin) bonded to a phospholipid (e.g., phosphatidylcholine), whereas a liposome is an aggregate of phospholipid molecules that can embed phytochemicals in its core but without specifically binding to them (Kidd 2009). The bioavailability of a curcumin-phosphatidylcholine phytosome was compared to that of unformulated curcumin (340 mg/kg) given orally to rats. Peak plasma concentrations and AUC for the phytosomes (33.4 ± 7.1 nmol/L) were fivefold higher than that of native curcumin (6.5 ± 4.5 nmol/L). Liver concentrations of curcumin and its metabolites curcumin sulfate, curcumin glucuronide, tetrahydrocurcumin, and hexahydrocurcumin were higher and those in the gastrointestinal mucosa lower upon ingestion of the phytosome complex compared to the native curcumin (Marczylo et al. 2007).

The absorption of curcumin incorporated into micelles was also studied in the everted rat intestinal sack model. Rat everted intestinal sacks were incubated with micellar curcumin at concentrations from 14 to 271 µmol/L, and absorption had plateaued already at concentrations of 27 µmol/L. Micellar in comparison to native curcumin resulted in a 7% higher absorption. In an *in vivo* study, curcumin micelles were intravenously injected into rats, and curcumin was still detectable in plasma after 24 h, whereas unformulated curcumin was completely eliminated within 6 h; the $t_{1/2}$ of micellar curcumin was 60 h and that of unformulated curcumin was 0.57 h (Ma et al. 2007).

Curcumin-loaded solid lipid nanoparticles (approximately 92% curcuminoids of which 95% was curcumin and 5% demethoxy- and *bis*-demethoxy-curcumin) with a mean diameter of 135 nm were prepared (Kakkar et al. 2011) and administered to rats by oral gavage at a dose of 50 mg curcumin/kg bw. Blood samples were drawn over 24 h, and curcumin pharmacokinetics were compared to that of an equal dose of native curcumin. Curcumin from nanoparticles was less rapidly absorbed (T_{max}, 0.5 vs. 0.25 h, respectively) but reached significantly higher C_{max} (14.3 vs. 0.3 µg/mL, respectively) and AUC (42 vs. 1 µg/mL × h) (Kakkar et al. 2010).

Bioavailability-enhancing strategies were also investigated in human trials. One such strategy that has been tested in humans is to apply adjuvants that can block the metabolic degradation of curcumin. In eight healthy males, combined administration of curcumin (2 g) with piperine (20 mg), an inhibitor of intestinal and hepatic phase II metabolism (mainly glucuronidation), increased serum C_{max} from 0.006 ± 0.005 µg/mL, when curcumin was given alone, to 0.18 ± 0.16 µg/mL when administered together with piperine (Shoba et al. 1998).

Another promising formulation is a nanoparticle colloidal dispersion termed theracurmin. In contrast to curcumin powder, which has a mean particle size of 22.75 µm, theracurmin has a mean particle size of 190 nm and is water soluble and heat- and UV-stable. In a human trial with 14 volunteers who took either 30 mg native curcumin ($n = 7$) or the same amount of theracurmin (300 mg formulation; $n = 7$), the maximum plasma concentration of total curcumin (free and conjugated) was 1.8 ± 2.8 ng/mL and peaked 6 h after ingestion of curcumin powder and 29.5 ± 12.9 ng/mL at 1 h after the intake of theracurmin. The AUC of theracurmin was 27-fold higher than that of native curcumin (Sasaki et al. 2011).

The improved bioavailability of solid lipid curcumin particles (curcumin content, 20%–30%) compared to curcumin from native curcuma extract has been studied in six healthy volunteers. After an oral dose of 650 mg, no curcumin was detectable in blood after more than 8 h when native curcumin was given, whereas a C_{max} of 22 ng/mL was achieved with the solid lipid curcumin particles (Gota et al. 2010).

15.2.5 Antioxidant Activities of Curcuminoids in Humans

Despite the large number of *in vitro*, cell culture, and animal studies that report on the antioxidant activities of curcuminoids [reviewed in Bengmark (2006) and Strimpakos and Sharma (2008)], surprisingly few randomized controlled human trials have been performed. Performing a PubMed search with the terms "curcumin" and "antioxidant" retrieves 1382 publications; limiting the search results to "clinical trial" or "randomized controlled trial" reduces the number to 15 and 7, respectively (PubMed search performed on December 22, 2011).

Sharma et al. (2001, 2004) performed two comparable studies with increasing doses of curcuma extracts and isolated curcuminoids in patients with colorectal adenocarcinomas who ingested capsules containing curcuma extracts (440–2200 mg containing 36–180 mg curcumin) or a mixture of curcuminoids (500–4000 mg; each capsule containing curcumin 450 mg, demethoxy-curcumin 40 mg, and *bis*-demethoxy-curcumin 10 mg) every morning after a 2 h-fast for up to 29 days. There was no effect on the leukocyte concentrations of the DNA oxidation product M_1G (a deoxyguanosine adduct) in subjects consuming the curcuma extracts or the curcuminoids, respectively. In a single-blind, placebo-controlled study with patients suffering from tropical pancreatitis, subjects were randomized to take either one capsule containing curcumin (500 mg) and piperine (5 mg, $n = 8$) or a placebo capsule ($n = 7$) three times per day after a meal for 6 weeks. Treatment with curcumin and piperine reduced the concentrations of the lipid peroxidation marker malondialdehyde [placebo 11, curcumin + piperine, 6 nmol/g hemoglobin (Hb)] but not of the antioxidant glutathione in erythrocytes (Durgaprasad et al. 2005). Thirty-four Chinese Alzheimer's disease patients, of which 27 completed the study, were randomized to receive a placebo or 1 or 4 g of curcumin once per day as capsules to take after a meal or powder to be mixed with food. All subjects also ingested one capsule containing 120 mg of a standardized ginkgo leaf extract per day. Concentrations of vitamin E and the lipid peroxidation biomarker F2-isoprostane were quantified after 0, 1, and 6 months of treatment. Curcumin treatment modestly increased vitamin E but had no effect on F2-isoprostane plasma concentrations after 1 and 6 months of intervention (Baum et al. 2008). Thalassemia is a hereditary disease resulting in increased blood concentrations of free iron and ultimately oxidative stress. Parameters of antioxidant status and oxidative stress were determined in 21 β-thalassemia/Hb E patients relative to 26 healthy controls. Thalassemia patients were given 500 mg curcuminoids (96% curcumin) daily for 12 months. Erythrocyte malondialdehyde concentrations decreased from 1596 ± 45 nmol/g Hb at baseline to 1101 ± 46 nmol/g Hb after 6 months and 1134 ± 1 nmol/g Hb after 12 months, and erythrocyte glutathione increased from 1.62 (baseline) to 1.76 (6 months) and 1.78 mmol/L (12 months), respectively. The activities of the antioxidant enzymes glutathione peroxidase and superoxide dismutase, however, also decreased relative to baseline during curcuminoid treatment (Kalpravidh et al. 2010). Today, the largest intervention study addressing the antioxidant activity of curcumin was performed in 286 healthy Indian volunteers (women and men ages 25–55 years) living in villages where the groundwater is contaminated with arsenic, and therefore, increased oxidative DNA damage is prevalent. Half of the volunteers received capsules with 500 mg of a mixture of curcumin and piperine (20:1) or placebo capsules twice daily for 3 months. The authors observed a time-dependent decrease in DNA single-strand breaks in isolated lymphocytes under curcumin/piperine treatment as early as after 1 month of treatment. DNA damage in the arsenic-exposed curcumin/piperine group after 3 months of intervention was similar to that in a control population ($n = 100$) exposed to arsenic-free water, while that in the arsenic-exposed placebo group remained unchanged. Similarly, the concentrations of reactive oxygen species (ROS), malondialdehyde, and protein carbonyls (a biomarker for protein oxidation) in plasma decreased during curcumin and piperine supplementation. The concentrations of protein carbonyls, however, were significantly reduced after 3 months of intervention only, whereas ROS and malondialdehyde reacted more quickly and dropped already after 1 month of treatment with the phytochemicals. The improved antioxidant status under curcumin and piperine treatment was explained by increased activities of the antioxidant enzymes catalase, superoxide dismutase, glutathione peroxidase, glutathione reductase, and glutathione S-transferase and elevated concentrations of the nonenzymatic antioxidant glutathione relative to baseline and the placebo group at each time point (Biswas et al. 2010).

15.3 CAROTENOIDS

Carotenoids are a class of approximately 600 pigments found primarily in plants, algae, microorganisms, bacteria, and fungi but also in animals (e.g., in eggs, shrimp, lobster, and salmon) whose diets include the aforementioned sources of carotenoids. Of the more than 600 carotenoids that have been characterized so far, approximately 35 are present in the human diet and 20 in the human circulatory system (Figure 15.5) in relevant (measurable) concentrations.

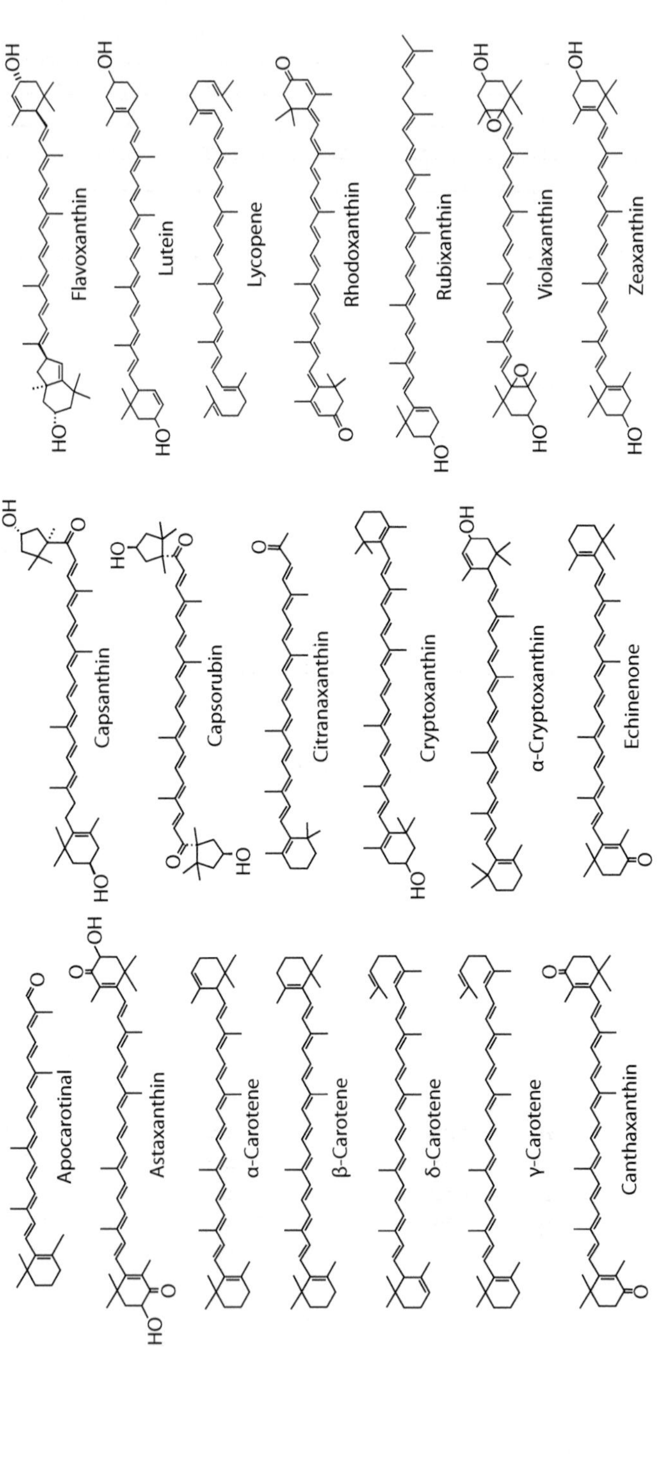

FIGURE 15.5 Chemical structures of the 20 most common carotenoids found in human diet and organism.

Because humans and animals cannot synthesize carotenoids, all carotenoids in these mammals are derived from the diet. Because of their lipophilicity, carotenoids accumulate in lipid compartments, such as cell membranes or lipoproteins. Several factors affect the content of carotenoids in plant foods, for example, variety, genotype, season, geographic location/climate, stage of maturity, and growing conditions. Carotenoids are ingested mainly from fruits, vegetables, and the above-mentioned sources but are also added to the human diet in the forms of colorants, spices (saffron, paprika, and annatto), and flavors (Table 15.2).

TABLE 15.2
E Numbers, Trivial Names, Colors, Dietary Sources, and/or Use of Carotenoids as Food Additives

E Number	Trivial Name	Color	Dietary Sources and/or Uses
		Carotenes (E160)	
E160a	α-, β-, γ-carotene	Orange-yellow	Carrots, green leafy vegetables, tomatoes, fruits, juices, squash, cakes, desserts, butter, and margarine
E160b	Annatto, bixin, norbixin	Red	Widely used as colorant for foodstuffs, fabric, soap
E160c	Capsanthin, capsorubin, paprika extract	Red to orange	Eggs, meat products, spices derived from pods and seeds of the red pepper
E160d	Lycopene	Red	Tomato, tomato products (ketchup, soup, sauce, juice), watermelon, papaya
E160e	β-apo-8′-carotenal (C30)	Synthetic yellow-red	Processed cheese
E160f	Esters of β-apo-8′-carotenic acid (C30)	Orange-yellow (derivative of E160e)	Processed cheese
		Xanthophylls (E161)	
E161a	Flavoxanthin	Natural yellow	Part of a normal diet
E161b	Lutein	Yellow-red	Egg yolks (fed to poultry to enhance yolk color), naturally found in green leaves and marigolds
E161c	β-Cryptoxanthin	Natural yellow	Citrus fruits, potatoes, tomatoes, in egg yolks and butter
E161d	Rubixanthin	Natural yellow	Rosehip, part of a normal diet
E161e	Violoxanthin	Natural yellow	Yellow pansies
E161f	Rhodoxanthin	Natural yellow	Yew tree seeds
E161g	Canthaxanthin	Natural orange	Mushrooms, crustaceans, fish, sauces, preserves, sweets
E161h	Zeaxanthin	Natural yellow-orange	Corn, spinach
E161i	Citranaxanthin	Natural yellow but mainly prepared synthetically	Mainly used as colorant for animal feeds

Carotenoids are intensely yellow-, red-, and orange-colored molecules. In plants, however, the color is sometimes masked by the green of chlorophyll. Carotenoids consist of a C_{40} carbon skeleton, which can be modified by the cyclization of either or both of the ends, and differ in the degree of hydrogenation (saturation) and the presence of additional functional groups (mainly oxygen). Two major classes of carotenoids can be distinguished based on the absence or presence of oxygen in the molecule: carotenes and xanthophylls, respectively. The general chemical formula of carotenoids is $C_{40}H_{56}O_n$ ($n =$ 0–6). Carotenoids with fewer than 40 carbon atoms are considered apo-carotenoids. Because of the presence of conjugated double bonds in the chemical structure, carotenoids appear as *cis-* and *trans*-isomers. The *trans*-isomers are more common in foods and are thermodynamically more stable because of the lack of bends in their structure that arise from *cis*-formation. These structural features render carotenoids susceptible to oxidation, heat, pH, and light (Scott 1992; Shi and Le Maguer 2000).

The trivial names of carotenoids are often derived from the natural sources of the corresponding carotenoid, for example, *carota* (Latin for carrot), from which carotene was first isolated. The most common carotenes, which do not contain oxygen, are α- and β-carotene and lycopene. The most prominent xanthophylls, which are also called oxocarotenoids because of the presence of oxygen, are lutein, zeaxanthin, and cryptoxanthin. The xanthophylls, compared to carotenes, are less lipophilic and more polar. Approximately 90% of the carotenoids in the human diet and body are made up of α-carotene, β-carotene, lycopene, lutein, and β-cryptoxanthin (Gerster 1997).

15.3.1 RELEASE OF CAROTENOIDS FROM FOOD MATRIX

In plants, carotenoids are generally localized in subcellular compartments named plastids (e.g., chloroplasts and chromoplasts) in free, esterified, or protein-bound forms. In green leafy plants, for example, carotenoids in chloroplasts are bound to proteins and serve as accessory pigments in photosynthesis. In chromoplasts, they are found in semicrystalline membrane-bound solids (e.g., in carrots and tomatoes), in dissolved form (in many fruits), or as esters in oil droplets (Castenmiller and West 1998; van het Hof et al. 1998). β-Carotene shows a better absorption from fruits, where it is present in oil droplets, compared to green vegetables or carrots, where the bound forms first need to be released from the matrix. During mastication, foods are ground and mixed with saliva, which contains enzymes that help to release carotenoids from the food matrix. Other factors that affect carotenoid release (bioaccessibility) and absorption (bioavailability) are mechanical processing and heating as well as the presence of fat in the food. In the gastrointestinal tract, carotenoid esters are hydrolyzed by the pancreatic carboxylic ester hydrolase prior to absorption (Stahl et al. 2002).

15.3.2 BIOAVAILABILITY OF CAROTENOIDS: ABSORPTION, TISSUE DISTRIBUTION, AND EXCRETION

The fat-soluble carotenoids are absorbed similarly to other dietary lipids. The steps of carotenoid absorption include emulsification, solubilization in mixed micelles, diffusion across the unstirred water layer, and permeation through the brush border membrane of the enterocyte into the cytoplasm (Figure 15.6) (Borel 2003).

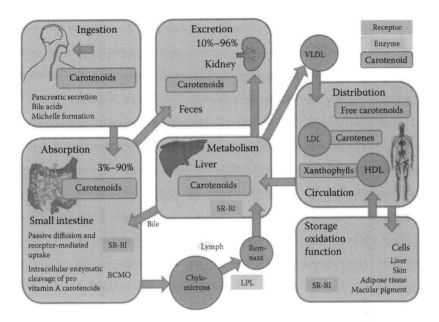

FIGURE 15.6 Schematic overview over absorption, distribution, and elimination of carotenoids in humans. During mastication and digestion, carotenoids are released from food matrix and, under aid of bile acids, incorporated into mixed micelles together with other dietary lipids. At the brush border membrane of small intestinal cells, carotenoids are taken up by simple diffusion or transporter-mediated (SR-BI) processes. Carotenoids are packed into chylomicrons and secreted into lymph and eventually reach the liver. There they are packed into lipoproteins and distributed to various tissues for storage, oxidation, or functional purposes. Abbreviations: LPL, lipoprotein lipase; SR-BI, scavenger receptor class B type I; BCMO, β,β-15,15′-dioxygenase; LDL, low-density lipoprotein; HDL, high-density lipoprotein; VLDL, very low-density lipoprotein.

In the stomach and duodenum, carotenoids separate from the food matrix and dissolve in the lipid phase. In the stomach, they are transferred to the fat phase of a meal and are incorporated into lipid droplets (solubilization). Polar xanthophylls are located at the surface of the droplet, whereas apolar carotenoids are located in the core (Borel et al. 1996). Factors that influence the transfer of carotenoids from lipid droplets to micelles include the pH, the concentration of bile salts, and the hydrophobicity of the carotenoids (Tyssandier et al. 2001). In the duodenum, the lipid phase interacts with bile salts and pancreatic lipases, forming multilamellar lipid vesicles termed "mixed micelles." Carotenoids are mainly absorbed in the small intestine via a passive diffusion process. Additionally, there is evidence that the scavenger receptor class B type I (SR-BI) might be involved in the receptor-mediated uptake of carotenoids into the intestinal mucosa cells (Reboul et al. 2005; van Bennekum et al. 2005). Lipophilic apolar carotenoids diffuse more easily through the lipid bilayer of cell membranes than the more polar ones. Carotenoids are transported through the enterocytes and packed into chylomicrons, which pass from the lymphatic system via the thoracic duct and the subclavian vein into the circulatory system. Endothelial lipoprotein lipase hydrolyzes triacylglycerols and thus releases free fatty acids from chylomicrons. The chylomicrons thus become chylomicron remnants, which continue to the liver where they are taken up and release their content, including carotenoids. The carotenoids are then incorporated into lipoproteins and released into the circulatory system (Figure 15.6) (Stahl et al. 2002).

Carotenoids are distributed differently among lipoprotein classes. In the plasma of fasting subjects, very low density lipoprotein (VLDL), low-density lipoprotein (LDL), and high-density lipoprotein (HDL) particles contained 14%, 55%, and 31%, respectively, of the total carotenoids present. Furthermore, carotenes are mainly located in LDL, whereas the more polar xanthophylls are primarily present in HDL (Clevidence and Bieri 1993). The major sites for the storage of carotenoids are adipose tissue and the liver (Chung et al. 2009). Significant amounts of carotenoids can also be stored in skin when large quantities are ingested; consequently, some carotenoids will be lost by the sloughing-off of keratinized skin cells (Olson 1994).

Not all carotenoids consumed are taken up into the body. Unabsorbed carotenoids are excreted in the feces together with the biliary metabolites of carotenoids and those present in the residues of mucosal cells. Polar metabolites of carotenoids, probably in conjugated form, are most likely excreted in the urine. A relatively minor part (<5%) of carotenoids is assumed to be oxidized, in whole or in part, to carbon dioxide (Glover 1960).

A number of factors affect the absorption of carotenoids and the resulting plasma concentrations. Importantly, the fat content of a meal determines the rate of absorption of dietary carotenoids. The presence of dietary fat stimulates the secretion of bile salts and thus increases their luminal concentration, which aid the formation of mixed micelles. β-Carotene dissolved in oil is more easily absorbed than without oil. The minimum amount of fat required for an optimal absorption of carotenoids is about 3 g per meal (Roodenburg et al. 2000).

Not all β-carotene taken up into enterocytes is left intact for secretion with chylomicrons. Instead, some is enzymatically cleaved by the cytosolic, nonmembrane bound enzyme β,β-15,15′-dioxygenase in the gut tissue, which is the key enzyme that centrally cleaves β-carotene into two molecules of retinal (Lakshman 2004). Eccentric cleavage is also possible, leading to only one molecule retinal and apo-carotenal. The maximum amount of β-carotene an adult intestine can cleave in a day is approximately 2.5 mg (During et al. 2001).

The simultaneous consumption of dietary fiber impairs the absorption of carotenoids. This may, in part, result from their sequestering of bile acids, which enhances fecal excretion of bile acids and leads to an overall decrease in the absorption of fat-soluble micronutrients. The bioaccessibility (liberation) of carotenoids from dietary fiber-rich fruit and vegetable matrices is low because fiber and polysaccharides may bind carotenoids in the upper intestine, and, thus, enzymatic hydrolysis would be required for absorption. Enzymatic hydrolysis, however, is restricted by the action of dietary fiber matrices formed in the chyme. Dietary fiber furthermore slows the emptying of the stomach and shortens the duration of gut passage and thereby limits absorption. However, all unabsorbed carotenoids reaching the large intestine remain in the colonic lumen where they may contribute to a healthy antioxidant environment (Palafox-Carlos et al. 2011).

The stereochemistry of the carotenoids accounts for some of the differences in their absorption. The naturally occurring and predominant *trans*-β-carotene seems to be preferentially absorbed over the *cis*-isomers, which are converted to *trans*-β-carotene before they enter the bloodstream (You et al. 1996). Furthermore, the *cis*-isomer of lycopene is better solubilized in the fat phase than the *trans*-isomer (Stahl and Sies 1992).

Under normal dietary habits, a mixture of carotenoids, rather than individual ones, is ingested. These carotenoids may interact with each other during intestinal absorption, although the underlying mechanisms are still unknown. When adults were given the same doses of β-carotene and lutein simultaneously, β-carotene significantly reduced the serum AUC of lutein to 54%–61% of those observed when β-carotene was ingested alone. Lutein, on the other hand, reduced β-carotene AUC in five subjects but enhanced it in three (Kostic et al. 1995). In another study with simultaneous administration of β-carotene with either lutein or lycopene, lutein but not lycopene significantly reduced the absorption of β-carotene (66% compared with 101%, respectively) (van den Berg and van Vliet 1998). Co-ingested α-carotene, on the other hand, had no effect on β-carotene absorption (van het Hof et al. 1999).

Food processing, most of all cooking, and mechanical disintegration appear to improve the bioavailability of carotenoids from foods. A number of studies observed better absorption of carotenoids from cooked than from raw ground carrots (Livny et al. 2003), from cooked and pureed carrots than from raw and sliced carrots or spinach (Rock et al. 1998), from tomato paste than from fresh tomato (Gärtner et al. 1997), from thermally processed than from unprocessed tomato juice (Stahl and Sies 1992), from tomato soup than from tomato juice (Cohn et al. 2004), and from canned tomatoes that were severely homogenized than from mildly or nonhomogenized canned tomatoes (van het Hof et al. 2000).

Alcohol intake and smoking are negatively correlated with serum carotenoid concentrations, which might be a result of lower intake of carotenoid-rich plant foods, impaired absorption, or enhanced oxidative decay (Forman et al. 1995; Albanes et al. 1997; van der Gaag et al. 2000; Wallstrom et al. 2001).

15.3.3 CAROTENOID CONCENTRATIONS IN HUMANS

Being lipid-soluble molecules, carotenoids are preferentially stored in the liver and in adipose tissue but have also been found in the testes, adrenal glands, prostate, breasts, and the skin (Kaplan et al. 1990; Stahl et al. 1992). Mean plasma and serum concentrations of carotenoids in fasted human subjects are commonly in the range of 0.1–1.5 μmol/L (Table 15.3). The concentrations of lutein and zeaxanthin in human lenses were at 13.8 ± 0.9 ng/g wet weight; other carotenoids were not detectable in this tissue (Yeum et al. 1995). In human subcutaneous adipose tissue samples taken from the upper buttock, abdomen, and thigh of 25 healthy subjects, carotenoids were measured in concentrations of 0.1–6.0 μmol/g (Table 15.4) (Chung et al. 2009).

TABLE 15.3
Concentrations (μmol/L) of Carotenoids in Serum or Plasma of Fasted Human Subjects[a]

Subjects	Matrix	Age/Sampling	α-Carotene	β-Carotene	β-Cryptoxanthin	Lutein	Zeaxanthin	Lycopene	Reference
			μmol/L ± SD						
Men, $n = 9$	Plasma	20–40 years	0.09 ± 0.01	0.44 ± 0.07	0.34 ± 0.03	0.22 ± 0.02	0.03 ± 0.00	n.d.	Yeum et al. 1996
Women, $n = 9$	Plasma	20–40 years	0.18 ± 0.04	0.80 ± 0.17	0.54 ± 0.09	0.28 ± 0.03	0.04 ± 0.01	n.d.	Yeum et al. 1996
Men, $n = 9$	Plasma	60–80 years	0.27 ± 0.07	1.51 ± 0.41	1.04 ± 0.24	0.38 ± 0.05	0.05 ± 0.01	n.d.	Yeum et al. 1996
Women, $n = 9$	Plasma	60–80 years	0.20 ± 0.04	0.78 ± 0.10	0.54 ± 0.11	0.25 ± 0.03	0.03 ± 0.00	n.d.	Yeum et al. 1996
Men, $n = 201$	Plasma	68–91 years	0.08 ± 0.05	0.33 ± 0.23	0.20 ± 0.12	0.52 ± 0.23	+	0.64 ± 0.38	Tucker et al. 1999
Women, $n = 346$	Plasma	67–93 years	0.12 ± 0.09	0.51 ± 0.34	0.27 ± 0.17	0.56 ± 0.27	+	0.61 ± 0.36	Tucker et al. 1999
Women, $n = 168$	Plasma	50–65 years, winter	–	0.44 ± 0.25		0.40 ± 0.12	–	0.27 ± 0.3	Scott et al. 1996
Women, $n = 168$	Plasma	50–65 years, spring	–	0.39 ± 0.22		0.374 ± 0.15	–	0.25 ± 0.12	Scott et al. 1996
Women, $n = 168$	Plasma	50–65 years, summer	–	0.69 ± 0.40		0.493 ± 0.18	–	0.39 ± 0.20	Scott et al. 1996
Women, $n = 168$	Plasma	50–65 years, autumn	–	0.65 ± 0.36		0.438 ± 0.16	–	0.37 ± 0.14	Scott et al. 1996
Adults	Plasma	≥65 years, Northern England	0.06 ± 0.00[b]	0.30 ± 0.01[c]	0.11 ± 0.01[d]	0.318 ± 0.01[e]	–	0.21 ± 0.01[f]	Elia and Stratton 2005

Adults	Plasma	0.07 ± 0.01^b	0.33 ± 0.01^c	0.13 ± 0.01^d	0.388 ± 0.01^e	–	0.22 ± 0.01^f	Elia and Stratton 2005
≥65 years, Central England								
Adults	Plasma	0.08 ± 0.00^b	0.40 ± 0.01^c	0.16 ± 0.01^d	0.386 ± 0.01^e	–	0.28 ± 0.01^f	Elia and Stratton 2005
≥65 years, Southern England								
Adults, $n = 468$	Serum	0.05 ± 0.00	0.24 ± 0.01	0.14 ± 0.01	0.31 ± 0.01	+	0.41 ± 0.02	Dixon et al. 2001
20–59 years, from food-insufficient families								
Adults, $n = 6007$	Serum	0.08 ± 0.00	0.35 ± 0.01	0.16 ± 0.00	0.36 ± 0.01	+	0.47 ± 0.00	Dixon et al. 2001
20–59 years, from food-sufficient families								
Adults, $n = 131$	Serum	0.10 ± 0.02	0.41 ± 0.07	0.14 ± 0.01	0.41 ± 0.05	+	0.31 ± 0.04	Dixon et al. 2001
≥60 years, from food-insufficient families								
Adults, $n = 3559$	Serum	0.10 ± 0.00	0.49 ± 0.01	0.18 ± 0.01	0.43 ± 0.01	+	0.34 ± 0.01	Dixon et al. 2001
≥60 years, from food-sufficient families								
Adults, $n = 5742$	Serum	0.07 ± 0.1	0.30 ± 0.3	0.20 ± 0.15	0.40 ± 0.25	+	0.45 ± 0.21	McKeever et al. 2004
17–59 years								
Children, $n = 4271$	Serum	0.06 ± 0.05	0.29 ± 0.17	0.22 ± 0.12	0.36 ± 0.15	+	0.45 ± 0.19	McKeever et al. 2004
6–16 years								

a All values are mean ± standard deviation and expressed in μmol/L; n.d., not detected; +, zeaxanthin values are included in concentrations for lutein; –, zeaxanthin was not determined.

b $n = 936$.

c $n = 946$.

d $n = 931$.

e $n = 946$.

f $n = 939$

TABLE 15.4

Concentrations of Carotenoids (nmol/g ± Standard Error) in Adipose Tissues Sampled from Different Sites in 25 Healthy Subjects (12 Women and 13 Men)

	Abdomen	Buttocks	Thigh
Carotenoid Concentration		nmol/g ± SE	
α-Carotene	280.5 ± 74.3	166.7 ± 18.6	127.3 ± 23.4
β-Carotene	939.2 ± 175.7	709.2 ± 87.6	557.0 ± 90.7
β-Cryptoxanthin	418.6 ± 46.8	399.2 ± 54.8	256.3 ± 27.0
Lutein	295.8 ± 38.9	170.8 ± 24.5	181.3 ± 26.9
Zeaxanthin	183.4 ± 32.3	127.5 ± 24.1	101.0 ± 15.6
Lycopene	3329.6 ± 448.1	2472.0 ± 275.8	2055.8 ± 280.6
Total carotenoids	5938.7 ± 678.5	4426.7 ± 400.1	3507.0 ± 387.9

Source: Chung, H. Y. et al., *Am J Clin Nutr* 90, 533–539, 2009.

15.3.4 Antioxidant Activities of Carotenoids

The chemical structure of carotenoids allows these molecules to absorb light, to physically quench singlet oxygen ($^1O_2$), and to scavenge free radical species, such as peroxyl radicals.

15.3.4.1 Physical Quenching of Singlet Oxygen

The major antioxidant activity of carotenoids lies in their ability to physically quench singlet oxygen ($^1O_2$) (Young and Lowe 2001). As shown in reaction 15.1, carotenoids (CAR) can directly absorb energy from singlet oxygen:

$$^1O_2 + CAR \rightarrow {}^3O_2 + {}^3CAR^* \tag{15.1}$$

A carotenoid in the triplet-state ($^3CAR^*$) can then easily return to the ground state (CAR), dissipating the energy as heat. In this quenching reaction, the carotenoid remains intact and may subsequently quench additional $^1O_2$. The quenching efficiency of a given carotenoid increases and the energy of its excited state decreases with the number of conjugated double bonds in the molecule (Conn et al. 1991). Carotenoids with less than five conjugated double bonds show no quenching activity at all (Stahl and Sies 1993). Additionally, epoxide groups might increase the quenching ability of carotenoids (Conn et al. 1991). The carotenoid with the highest quenching efficiency is lycopene because of its open ring structure (Figure 15.5). The triplet state of a carotenoid is of such low energy that it is unable to generate other reactive species by energy transfer and instead dissipates its excitation energy harmlessly to its surroundings (Britton 1995). Thus, the carotenoid acts as a catalyst, deactivating $^1O_2$ (Edge et al. 1997).

15.3.4.2 Free Radical Scavenging

The reaction of a carotenoid with a radical will lead to an electron transfer reaction in which either a hydrogen atom is abstracted from the carotenoid (reaction 15.2), an unpaired electron is moved to the carotenoid (reaction 15.3), or an adduct is formed with the radical (reaction 15.4):

$$R^{\bullet} + CAR(H) \rightarrow RH + CAR^{\bullet} \tag{15.2}$$

$$R^{\bullet} + CAR \rightarrow R^{-} + CAR^{\bullet+} \tag{15.3}$$

$$R^{\bullet} + CAR \rightarrow R-CAR^{\bullet} \tag{15.4}$$

Such an electron transfer leads to the formation of an anion (reaction 15.2), cation (reaction 15.3), or alkyl radical (reaction 15.4) of the respective carotenoid.

The scavenging of peroxyl radicals is the second most important antioxidant activity of carotenoids and depends on the formation of adducts with a resonance-stabilized carbon center, which inhibits lipid peroxidation by stopping the chain reaction. This chemical reaction leads to the destruction of the carotenoid, which itself can be observed as bleaching (loss of color).

β-Carotene inhibits oxidation at a low partial pressure of oxygen, such as under physiological conditions. However, at high oxygen pressures (>150 mm Hg, 20% O_2) combined with high carotenoid concentrations, β-carotene exhibits prooxidant activity (Tapiero et al. 2004). The water-soluble ascorbic acid can reduce (regenerate) the radical cation of carotenoids, but because of their different solubilities, carotenoids (and their radical forms) and ascorbic acid are located in different cellular compartments, making it more difficult for ascorbic acid to efficiently regenerate the lipophilic carotene radicals (Truscott 1996; Bohm et al. 1998).

15.3.5 Provitamin A Activity of Carotenoids

Some carotenoids may act as precursors of vitamin A; these include α- and β-carotene and β-cryptoxanthin (Simpson 1983). Preformed vitamin A is present only in animal foods, such as meat, liver, kidneys, fatty fish, dairy products, and eggs. Populations that exclude certain types of food, even in developed countries, might be at risk of vitamin A insufficiency. Therefore, provitamin A carotenoids from plants are an additional and important dietary source of vitamin A for most of the world's population (Bendich and Olson 1989). Compared with preformed vitamin A, β-carotene and other provitamin A carotenoids are relatively poor, yet important sources of vitamin A.

β-Carotene can be centrally cleaved by β,β-15,15'-dioxygenase to yield two molecules of retinal and ultimately vitamin A (retinol) or eccentrically by β-carotene-9,10'-oxygenase to yield only one molecule of retinal and eventually retinol (Kiefer et al. 2001). In practice, however, more than one molecule of β-carotene is required to substitute for the activity of one molecule retinol. The recently accepted conversion factors for β-carotene, β-cryptoxanthin, and α-carotene are 12, 24, and 24, respectively, such that 12 µg of β-carotene or 24 µg of β-cryptoxanthin or α-carotene, respectively, are thought to exert the activity of 1 µg vitamin A. The retinol activity of carotenoids is given as retinol activity equivalents (RAE). In 2001, the US Institute of Medicine introduced this new conversion factor for β-carotene, replacing the former equivalent of 1 µg retinol (retinol equivalent, RE) = 6 µg β-carotene. The currently accepted conversion factors are 1 RAE = 1 µg retinol = 12 µg β-carotene = 24 µg α-carotene = 24 µg β-cryptoxanthin (Food and Nutrition Board of the Institute of Medicine 2001).

15.4 SUMMARY

The biological activities and availabilities of curcuminoids and carotenoids have been studied extensively in the test tube and in animal models and, to a lesser extent, in humans. The number of properly controlled human studies investigating the pharmacokinetics and biological effects of curcuminoids in humans, however, is surprisingly small. Nevertheless, the poor bioavailability of curcuminoids observed in animal studies has been confirmed in humans, and maximum plasma concentrations upon oral consumption, even of very high doses, typically remain in the nanomolar range.

The bioavailability of carotenoids is, in part, determined by their liberation from the food in the gastrointestinal tract, which can be enhanced by mechanical disintegration and thermal processing (heating) of the food matrix and can be improved when ingested together with fat, something that it also believed to improve the absorption of the lipid-soluble curcuminoids. Carotenoids are more bioavailable than curcuminoids and can reach micromolar plasma concentrations in humans comparable to those of lipid-soluble antioxidant vitamins. Furthermore, some carotenoids can accumulate in human tissues. Carotenoids are thus more likely to be able to function as direct antioxidants, quenching $^1O_2$ or scavenging reactive species, than curcuminoids, which appear to exert their antioxidant activity mainly by induction of antioxidant enzymes.

The limited absorption and rapid excretion of curcuminoids have led to attempts to improve their bioavailability by enhancing their uptake and/or inhibiting their metabolic conversion in the intestine and liver, thus enhancing their retention in the body. Such strategies may then lead to higher concentrations of the curcuminoids at their "site of action," which is hoped to enhance their health-promoting biological activities.

Overall, curcuminoids and carotenoids are important dietary phytochemicals that may promote health when regularly ingested as part of a balanced diet rich in vegetables and hold promise to aid in the prevention and treatment of human diseases.

ACKNOWLEDGMENTS

Dr. Grune and Dr. Frank are financially supported by the German Federal Ministry of Education and Research, which sponsors an interdisciplinary research network coordinated by Dr. Frank that is aimed at developing novel strategies to enhance the bioavailability of curcumin and, thereby, its beneficial effects on human health (http://www.nutrition-research.de/bmbf.html).

REFERENCES

Aggarwal, B. B., A. Kumar and A. C. Bharti (2003). Anticancer potential of curcumin: Preclinical and clinical studies. *Anticancer Res* 23(1A): 363–398.

Albanes, D., J. Virtamo, P. R. Taylor, M. Rautalahti, P. Pietinen and O. P. Heinonen (1997). Effects of supplemental beta-carotene, cigarette smoking, and alcohol consumption on serum carotenoids in the Alpha-Tocopherol, Beta-Carotene Cancer Prevention Study. *Am J Clin Nutr* 66(2): 366–372.

Ames, B. N., M. K. Shigenaga and T. M. Hagen (1993). Oxidants, antioxidants, and the degenerative diseases of aging. *Proc Natl Acad Sci U S A* 90(17): 7915–7922.

Appiah-Opong, R., J. N. Commandeur, B. van Vugt-Lussenburg and N. P. Vermeulen (2007). Inhibition of human recombinant cytochrome P450s by curcumin and curcumin decomposition products. *Toxicology* 235(1–2): 83–91.

Asai, A. and T. Miyazawa (2000). Occurrence of orally administed curcuminoid as glucuronide and glucuronide/sulfate conjugates in rat plasma. *Life Sci* 67(23): 2785–2793.

Baum, L., C. W. Lam, S. K. Cheung, T. Kwok, V. Lui, J. Tsoh, L. Lam, V. Leung, E. Hui, C. Ng, J. Woo, H. F. Chiu, W. B. Goggins, B. C. Zee, K. F. Cheng, C. Y. Fong, A. Wong, H. Mok, M. S. Chow, P. C. Ho, S. P. Ip, C. S. Ho, X. W. Yu, C. Y. Lai, M. H. Chan, S. Szeto, I. H. Chan and V. Mok (2008). Six-month randomized, placebo-controlled, double-blind, pilot clinical trial of curcumin in patients with Alzheimer disease. *J Clin Psychopharmacol* 28(1): 110–113.

Bendich, A. and J. A. Olson (1989). Biological actions of carotenoids. *FASEB J* 3(8): 1927–1932.

Bengmark, S. (2006). Curcumin, an atoxic antioxidant and natural NFkappaB, cyclooxygenase-2, lipooxygenase, and inducible nitric oxide synthase inhibitor: A shield against acute and chronic diseases. *J Parenter Enteral Nutr* 30(1): 45–51.

Bengmark, S., M. D. Mesa and A. Gil (2009). Plant-derived health: The effects of turmeric and curcuminoids. *Nutricion hospitalaria: organo oficial de la Sociedad Espanola de Nutricion Parenteral y Enteral* 24(19721899): 273–281.

Biswas, J., D. Sinha, S. Mukherjee, S. Roy, M. Siddiqi and M. Roy (2010). Curcumin protects DNA damage in a chronically arsenic-exposed population of West Bengal. *Human and Experimental Toxicology* 29(6): 513–524.

Bohm, F., R. Edge, D. J. McGarvey and T. G. Truscott (1998). Beta-carotene with vitamins E and C offers synergistic cell protection against NOx. *FEBS Lett* 436(3): 387–389.

Borel, P. (2003). Factors affecting intestinal absorption of highly lipophilic food microconstituents (fat-soluble vitamins, carotenoids and phytosterols). *Clin Chem Lab Med* 41(8): 979–994.

Borel, P., P. Grolier, M. Armand, A. Partier, H. Lafont, D. Lairon and V. Azais-Braesco (1996). Carotenoids in biological emulsions: Solubility, surface-to-core distribution, and release from lipid droplets. *J Lipid Res* 37(2): 250–261.

Bravo, L. (1998). Polyphenols: Chemistry, dietary sources, metabolism, and nutritional significance. *Nutr Rev* 56(11): 317–333.

Britton, G. (1995). Structure and properties of carotenoids in relation to function. *FASEB J* 9(15): 1551–1558.

Castenmiller, J. J. and C. E. West (1998). Bioavailability and bioconversion of carotenoids. *Annu Rev Nutr* 18: 19–38.

Cheng, A. L., C. H. Hsu, J. K. Lin, M. M. Hsu, Y. F. Ho, T. S. Shen, J. Y. Ko, J. T. Lin, B. R. Lin, W. Ming-Shiang, H. S. Yu, S. H. Jee, G. S. Chen, T. M. Chen, C. A. Chen, M. K. Lai, Y. S. Pu, M. H. Pan, Y. J. Wang, C. C. Tsai and C. Y. Hsieh (2001). Phase I clinical trial of curcumin, a chemopreventive agent, in patients with high-risk or pre-malignant lesions. *Anticancer Res* 21(4B): 2895–2900.

Chung, H. Y., A. L. Ferreira, S. Epstein, S. A. Paiva, C. Castaneda-Sceppa and E. J. Johnson (2009). Site-specific concentrations of carotenoids in adipose tissue: Relations with dietary and serum carotenoid concentrations in healthy adults. *Am J Clin Nutr* 90(3): 533–539.

Clevidence, B. A. and J. G. Bieri (1993). Association of carotenoids with human plasma lipoproteins. *Methods Enzymol* 214: 33–46.

Cohn, W., P. Thurmann, U. Tenter, C. Aebischer, J. Schierle and W. Schalch (2004). Comparative multiple dose plasma kinetics of lycopene administered in tomato juice, tomato soup or lycopene tablets. *Eur J Nutr* 43(5): 304–312.

Conn, P. F., W. Schalch and T. G. Truscott (1991). The singlet oxygen and carotenoid interaction. *J Photochem Photobiol B* 11(1): 41–47.

Davies, K. J. (1995). Oxidative stress: The paradox of aerobic life. *Biochem Soc Symp* 61: 1–31.

Dixon, L. B., M. A. Winkleby and K. L. Radimer (2001). Dietary intakes and serum nutrients differ between adults from food-insufficient and food-sufficient families: Third National Health and Nutrition Examination Survey, 1988–1994. *J Nutr* 131(4): 1232–1246.

Durgaprasad, S., C. G. Pai, Vasanthkumar, J. F. Alvres and S. Namitha (2005). A pilot study of the antioxidant effect of curcumin in tropical pancreatitis. *Indian J Med Res* 122(4): 315–318.

During, A., M. K. Smith, J. B. Piper and J. C. Smith (2001). Beta-carotene 15,15′-dioxygenase activity in human tissues and cells: Evidence of an iron dependency. *J Nutr Biochem* 12(11): 640–647.

Edge, R., D. J. McGarvey and T. G. Truscott (1997). The carotenoids as anti-oxidants: A review. *J Photochem Photobiol B* 41(3): 189–200.

Elia, M. and R. J. Stratton (2005). Geographical inequalities in nutrient status and risk of malnutrition among English people aged 65 y and older. *Nutrition* 21(11–12): 1100–1106.

Food and Nutrition Board of the Institute of Medicine (2001). *Dietary Reference Intakes for Vitamin A, Vitamin K, Arsenic, Boron, Chromium, Copper, Iodine, Iron, Manganese, Molybdenum, Nickel, Silicon, Vanadium, and Zinc*. Washington, DC: National Academy Press.

Forman, M. R., G. R. Beecher, E. Lanza, M. E. Reichman, B. I. Graubard, W. S. Campbell, T. Marr, L. C. Yong, J. T. Judd and P. R. Taylor (1995). Effect of alcohol consumption on plasma carotenoid concentrations in premenopausal women: A controlled dietary study. *Am J Clin Nutr* 62(1): 131–135.

Frank, J. and G. Rimbach (2009). Vitamin E in disease prevention: A critical appraisal of vitamin E supplementation trials. *Aktuel Ernaehr Med* 34: 131–140.

Garcea, G., D. P. Berry, D. J. Jones, R. Singh, A. R. Dennison, P. B. Farmer, R. A. Sharma, W. P. Steward and A. J. Gescher (2005). Consumption of the putative chemopreventive agent curcumin by cancer patients: Assessment of curcumin levels in the colorectum and their pharmacodynamic consequences. *Cancer Epidemiol Biomarkers Prev* 14(1): 120–125.

Gärtner, C., W. Stahl and H. Sies (1997). Lycopene is more bioavailable from tomato paste than from fresh tomatoes. *Am J Clin Nutr* 66(1): 116–122.

Gerster, H. (1997). The potential role of lycopene for human health. *J Am Coll Nutr* 16(2): 109–126.

Glover, J. (1960). The conversion of beta-carotene into vitamin A. *Vitam Horm* 18: 371–386.

Gota, V. S., G. B. Maru, T. G. Soni, T. R. Gandhi, N. Kochar and M. G. Agarwal (2010). Safety and pharmacokinetics of a solid lipid curcumin particle formulation in osteosarcoma patients and healthy volunteers. *J Agric Food Chem* 58(4): 2095–2099.

Gutteridge, J. M. and B. Halliwell (2010). Antioxidants: Molecules, medicines, and myths. *Biochem Biophys Res Commun* 393(4): 561–564.

Hassaninasab, A., Y. Hashimoto, K. Tomita-Yokotani and M. Kobayashi (2011). Discovery of the curcumin metabolic pathway involving a unique enzyme in an intestinal microorganism. *Proc Natl Acad Sci USA* 108(16): 6615–6620.

Hoehle, S. I., E. Pfeiffer and M. Metzler (2007). Glucuronidation of curcuminoids by human microsomal and recombinant UDP-glucuronosyltransferases. *Mol Nutr Food Res* 51(8): 932–938.

Hoehle, S. I., E. Pfeiffer, A. M. Solyom and M. Metzler (2006). Metabolism of curcuminoids in tissue slices and subcellular fractions from rat liver. *J Agric Food Chem* 54(3): 756–764.

Holder, G. M., J. L. Plummer and A. J. Ryan (1978). The metabolism and excretion of curcumin (1,7-bis-(4-hydroxy-3-methoxyphenyl)-1,6-heptadiene-3,5-dione) in the rat. *Xenobiotica* 8(12): 761–768.

Holst, B. and G. Williamson (2004). Methods to study bioavailability of phytochemicals. *Phytochecmials in Health and Disease*. Y. Bao and R. Fenwick. New York, Marcel Dekker: 25–56.

Ireson, C. R., D. J. Jones, S. Orr, M. W. Coughtrie, D. J. Boocock, M. L. Williams, P. B. Farmer, W. P. Steward and A. J. Gescher (2002). Metabolism of the cancer chemopreventive agent curcumin in human and rat intestine. *Cancer Epidemiol Biomarkers Prev* 11(1): 105–111.

Ireson, C., S. Orr, D. J. Jones, R. Verschoyle, C. K. Lim, J. L. Luo, L. Howells, S. Plummer, R. Jukes, M. Williams, W. P. Steward and A. Gescher (2001). Characterization of metabolites of the chemopreventive agent curcumin in human and rat hepatocytes and in the rat in vivo, and evaluation of their ability to inhibit phorbol ester-induced prostaglandin E2 production. *Cancer Res* 61(3): 1058–1064.

Jaruga, E., S. Salvioli, J. Dobrucki, S. Chrul, J. Bandorowicz-Pikula, E. Sikora, C. Franceschi, A. Cossarizza and G. Bartosz (1998). Apoptosis-like, reversible changes in plasma membrane asymmetry and permeability, and transient modifications in mitochondrial membrane potential induced by curcumin in rat thymocytes. *FEBS Lett* 433(3): 287–293.

Kakkar, V., S. Singh, D. Singla and I. P. Kaur (2011). Exploring solid lipid nanoparticles to enhance the oral bioavailability of curcumin. *Mol Nutr Food Res* 55(3): 495–503.

Kakkar, V., S. Singh, D. Singla, S. Sahwney, A. S. Chauhan, G. Singh and I. P. Kaur (2010). Pharmacokinetic applicability of a validated liquid chromatography tandem mass spectroscopy method for orally administered curcumin loaded solid lipid nanoparticles to rats. *J Chromatogr B Analyt Technol Biomed Life Sci* 878(32): 3427–3431.

Kalpravidh, R. W., N. Siritanaratkul, P. Insain, R. Charoensakdi, N. Panichkul, S. Hatairaktham, S. Srichairatanakool, C. Phisalaphong, E. Rachmilewitz and S. Fucharoen (2010). Improvement in oxidative stress and antioxidant parameters in beta-thalassemia/Hb E patients treated with curcuminoids. *Clin Biochem* 43(4–5): 424–429.

Kaplan, L. A., J. M. Lau and E. A. Stein (1990). Carotenoid composition, concentrations, and relationships in various human organs. *Clin Physiol Biochem* 8(1): 1–10.

Keaney, J. F., Jr., M. G. Larson, R. S. Vasan, P. W. Wilson, I. Lipinska, D. Corey, J. M. Massaro, P. Sutherland, J. A. Vita and E. J. Benjamin (2003). Obesity and systemic oxidative stress: Clinical correlates of oxidative stress in the Framingham Study. *Arterioscler Thromb Vasc Biol* 23(3): 434–439.

Kidd, P. M. (2009). Bioavailability and activity of phytosome complexes from botanical polyphenols: The silymarin, curcumin, green tea, and grape seed extracts. *Altern Med Rev* 14(3): 226–246.

Kiefer, C., S. Hessel, J. M. Lampert, K. Vogt, M. O. Lederer, D. E. Breithaupt and J. von Lintig (2001). Identification and characterization of a mammalian enzyme catalyzing the asymmetric oxidative cleavage of provitamin A. *J Biol Chem* 276(17): 14110–14116.

Kostic, D., W. S. White and J. A. Olson (1995). Intestinal absorption, serum clearance, and interactions between lutein and beta-carotene when administered to human adults in separate or combined oral doses. *Am J Clin Nutr* 62(3): 604–610.

Lakshman, M. R. (2004). Alpha and omega of carotenoid cleavage. *J Nutr* 134(1): 241S–245S.

Lao, C. D., M. T. T. Ruffin, D. Normolle, D. D. Heath, S. I. Murray, J. M. Bailey, M. E. Boggs, J. Crowell, C. L. Rock and D. E. Brenner (2006). Dose escalation of a curcuminoid formulation. *BMC Complement Altern Med* 6: 10.

Leu, T. H. and M. C. Maa (2002). The molecular mechanisms for the antitumorigenic effect of curcumin. *Curr Med Chem Anticancer Agents* 2(3): 357–370.

Livny, O., R. Reifen, I. Levy, Z. Madar, R. Faulks, S. Southon and B. Schwartz (2003). Beta-carotene bioavailability from differently processed carrot meals in human ileostomy volunteers. *Eur J Nutr* 42(6): 338–345.

Ma, Z., A. Shayeganpour, D. R. Brocks, A. Lavasanifar and J. Samuel (2007). High-performance liquid chromatography analysis of curcumin in rat plasma: Application to pharmacokinetics of polymeric micellar formulation of curcumin. *Biomed Chromatogr* 21(5): 546–552.

Mackenzie, P. I., K. W. Bock, B. Burchell, C. Guillemette, S. Ikushiro, T. Iyanagi, J. O. Miners, I. S. Owens and D. W. Nebert (2005). Nomenclature update for the mammalian UDP glycosyltransferase (UGT) gene superfamily. *Pharmacogenet Genomics* 15(10): 677–685.

Marczylo, T. H., R. D. Verschoyle, D. N. Cooke, P. Morazzoni, W. P. Steward and A. J. Gescher (2007). Comparison of systemic availability of curcumin with that of curcumin formulated with phosphatidylcholine. *Cancer Chemother Pharmacol* 60(2): 171–177.

Maritim, A. C., R. A. Sanders and J. B. Watkins III (2003). Diabetes, oxidative stress, and antioxidants: A review. *J Biochem Mol Toxicol* 17(1): 24–38.

McKeever, T. M., S. A. Lewis, H. Smit, P. Burney, J. Britton and P. A. Cassano (2004). Serum nutrient markers and skin prick testing using data from the Third National Health and Nutrition Examination Survey. *J Allergy Clin Immunol* 114(6): 1398–1402.

Narayanan, N. K., D. Nargi, C. Randolph and B. A. Narayanan (2009). Liposome encapsulation of curcumin and resveratrol in combination reduces prostate cancer incidence in PTEN knockout mice. *Int J Cancer* 125(1): 1–8.

Olson, J. A. (1994). Absorption, transport, and metabolism of carotenoids in humans. *Pure and Appl Chem* 66(5): 1011–1016.

Palafox-Carlos, H., J. F. Ayala-Zavala and G. A. Gonzalez-Aguilar (2011). The role of dietary fiber in the bioaccessibility and bioavailability of fruit and vegetable antioxidants. *J Food Sci* 76(1): R6–R15.

Pan, M. H., T. M. Huang and J. K. Lin (1999). Biotransformation of curcumin through reduction and glucuronidation in mice. *Drug Metab Dispos* 27(4): 486–494.

Pfeiffer, E., S. I. Hoehle, S. G. Walch, A. Riess, A. M. Solyom and M. Metzler (2007). Curcuminoids form reactive glucuronides in vitro. *J Agric Food Chem* 55(2): 538–544.

Pulla Reddy, A. C., E. Sudharshan, A. G. Appu Rao and B. R. Lokesh (1999). Interaction of curcumin with human serum albumin: A spectroscopic study. *Lipids* 34(10): 1025–1029.

Ravindranath, V. and N. Chandrasekhara (1980). Absorption and tissue distribution of curcumin in rats. *Toxicology* 16(3): 259–265.

Ravindranath, V. and N. Chandrasekhara (1981a). In vitro studies on the intestinal absorption of curcumin in rats. *Toxicology* 20(2–3): 251–257.

Ravindranath, V. and N. Chandrasekhara (1981b). Metabolism of curcumin: Studies with [3H] curcumin. *Toxicology* 22(4): 337–344.

Reboul, E., L. Abou, C. Mikail, O. Ghiringhelli, M. Andre, H. Portugal, D. Jourdheuil-Rahmani, M. J. Amiot, D. Lairon and P. Borel (2005). Lutein transport by Caco-2 TC-7 cells occurs partly by a facilitated process involving the scavenger receptor class B type I (SR-BI). *Biochem J* 387(Pt 2): 455–461.

Rock, C. L., J. L. Lovalvo, C. Emenhiser, M. T. Ruffin, S. W. Flatt and S. J. Schwartz (1998). Bioavailability of beta-carotene is lower in raw than in processed carrots and spinach in women. *J Nutr* 128(5): 913–916.

Roodenburg, A. J., R. Leenen, K. H. van het Hof, J. A. Weststrate and L. B. Tijburg (2000). Amount of fat in the diet affects bioavailability of lutein esters but not of alpha-carotene, beta-carotene, and vitamin E in humans. *Am J Clin Nutr* 71(5): 1187–1193.

Sasaki, H., Y. Sunagawa, K. Takahashi, A. Imaizumi, H. Fukuda, T. Hashimoto, H. Wada, Y. Katanasaka, H. Kakeya, M. Fujita, K. Hasegawa and T. Morimoto (2011). Innovative preparation of curcumin for improved oral bioavailability. *Biol Pharm Bull* 34(5): 660–665.

Schiborr, C., G. P. Eckert, G. Rimbach and J. Frank (2010). A validated method for the quantification of curcumin in plasma and brain tissue by fast narrow-bore high-performance liquid chromatography with fluorescence detection. *Anal Bioanal Chem* 397(5): 1917–1925.

Scott, K. J. (1992). Observations on some of the problems associated with the analysis of carotenoids in foods by HPLC. *Food Chemistry* 45(5): 357–364.

Scott, K. J., D. I. Thurnham, D. J. Hart, S. A. Bingham and K. Day (1996). The correlation between the intake of lutein, lycopene and beta-carotene from vegetables and fruits, and blood plasma concentrations in a group of women aged 50–65 years in the UK. *Br J Nutr* 75(3): 409–418.

Shardell, M. D., D. E. Alley, G. E. Hicks, S. S. El-Kamary, R. R. Miller, R. D. Semba and L. Ferrucci (2011). Low-serum carotenoid concentrations and carotenoid interactions predict mortality in US adults: The Third National Health and Nutrition Examination Survey. *Nutrition Research* 31(3): 178–189.

Sharma, R. A., S. A. Euden, S. L. Platton, D. N. Cooke, A. Shafayat, H. R. Hewitt, T. H. Marczylo, B. Morgan, D. Hemingway, S. M. Plummer, M. Pirmohamed, A. J. Gescher and W. P. Steward (2004). Phase I clinical trial of oral curcumin: Biomarkers of systemic activity and compliance. *Clin Cancer Res* 10(20): 6847–6854.

Sharma, R. A., H. R. McLelland, K. A. Hill, C. R. Ireson, S. A. Euden, M. M. Manson, M. Pirmohamed, L. J. Marnett, A. J. Gescher and W. P. Steward (2001). Pharmacodynamic and pharmacokinetic study of oral curcuma extract in patients with colorectal cancer. *Clin Cancer Res* 7(7): 1894–1900.

Shi, J. and M. Le Maguer (2000). Lycopene in tomatoes: Chemical and physical properties affected by food processing. *Crit Rev Biotechnol* 20(4): 293–334.

Shoba, G., D. Joy, T. Joseph, M. Majeed, R. Rajendran and P. S. Srinivas (1998). Influence of piperine on the pharmacokinetics of curcumin in animals and human volunteers. *Planta Med* 64(4): 353–356.

Simpson, K. L. (1983). Relative value of carotenoids as precursors of vitamin A. *Proc Nutr Soc* 42(1): 7–17.

Srinivasan, M. R. and M. N. Satyanarayana (1988). Influence of capsaicin, eugenol, curcumin and ferulic acid on sucrose-induced hypertriglyceridemia in rats. *Nutr Rep Int* 38(3): 571–581.

Stahl, W., W. Schwarz, A. R. Sundquist and H. Sies (1992). Cis-trans isomers of lycopene and beta-carotene in human serum and tissues. *Arch Biochem Biophys* 294(1): 173–177.

Stahl, W. and H. Sies (1992). Uptake of lycopene and its geometrical isomers is greater from heat-processed than from unprocessed tomato juice in humans. *J Nutr* 122(11): 2161–2166.

Stahl, W. and H. Sies (1993). Physical quenching of singlet oxygen and cis-trans isomerization of carotenoids. *Ann N Y Acad Sci* 691: 10–19.

Stahl, W. and H. Sies (2003). Antioxidant activity of carotenoids. *Mol Aspects Med* 24(6): 345–351.

Stahl, W., H. van den Berg, J. Arthur, A. Bast, J. Dainty, R. M. Faulks, C. Gartner, G. Haenen, P. Hollman, B. Holst, F. J. Kelly, M. C. Polidori, C. Rice-Evans, S. Southon, T. van Vliet, J. Vina-Ribes, G. Williamson and S. B. Astley (2002). Bioavailability and metabolism. *Mol Aspects Med* 23(1–3): 39–100.

Strassburg, C. P., N. Nguyen, M. P. Manns and R. H. Tukey (1999). UDP-glucuronosyltransferase activity in human liver and colon. *Gastroenterology* 116(1): 149–160.

Strimpakos, A. S. and R. A. Sharma (2008). Curcumin: Preventive and therapeutic properties in laboratory studies and clinical trials. *Antioxid Redox Signal* 10(3): 511–545.

Sutherland, L., T. Ebner and B. Burchell (1993). The expression of UDP-glucuronosyltransferases of the UGT1 family in human liver and kidney and in response to drugs. *Biochem Pharmacol* 45(2): 295–301.

Tapiero, H., D. M. Townsend and K. D. Tew (2004). The role of carotenoids in the prevention of human pathologies. *Biomed Pharmacother* 58(2): 100–110.

Truscott, T. G. (1996). Beta-carotene and disease: A suggested pro-oxidant and anti-oxidant mechanism and speculations concerning its role in cigarette smoking. *J Photochem Photobiol B* 35(3): 233–235.

Tucker, K. L., H. Chen, S. Vogel, P. W. Wilson, E. J. Schaefer and C. J. Lammi-Keefe (1999). Carotenoid intakes, assessed by dietary questionnaire, are associated with plasma carotenoid concentrations in an elderly population. *J Nutr* 129(2): 438–445.

Tukey, R. H. and C. P. Strassburg (2000). Human UDP-glucuronosyltransferases: Metabolism, expression, and disease. *Annu Rev Pharmacol Toxicol* 40: 581–616.

Tyssandier, V., B. Lyan and P. Borel (2001). Main factors governing the transfer of carotenoids from emulsion lipid droplets to micelles. *Biochim Biophys Acta* 1533(3): 285–292.

van Bennekum, A., M. Werder, S. T. Thuahnai, C. H. Han, P. Duong, D. L. Williams, P. Wettstein, G. Schulthess, M. C. Phillips and H. Hauser (2005). Class B scavenger receptor-mediated intestinal absorption of dietary beta-carotene and cholesterol. *Biochemistry* 44(11): 4517–4525.

van den Berg, H. and T. van Vliet (1998). Effect of simultaneous, single oral doses of beta-carotene with lutein or lycopene on the beta-carotene and retinyl ester responses in the triacylglycerol-rich lipoprotein fraction of men. *Am J Clin Nutr* 68(1): 82–89.

van der Gaag, M. S., R. van den Berg, H. van den Berg, G. Schaafsma and H. F. Hendriks (2000). Moderate consumption of beer, red wine and spirits has counteracting effects on plasma antioxidants in middle-aged men. *Eur J Clin Nutr* 54(7): 586–591.

van het Hof, K. H., B. C. de Boer, L. B. Tijburg, B. R. Lucius, I. Zijp, C. E. West, J. G. Hautvast and J. A. Weststrate (2000). Carotenoid bioavailability in humans from tomatoes processed in different ways determined from the carotenoid response in the triglyceride-rich lipoprotein fraction of plasma after a single consumption and in plasma after four days of consumption. *J Nutr* 130(5): 1189–1196.

van het Hof, K. H., C. Gartner, A. Wiersma, L. B. Tijburg and J. A. Weststrate (1999). Comparison of the bioavailability of natural palm oil carotenoids and synthetic beta-carotene in humans. *J Agric Food Chem* 47(4): 1582–1586.

van het Hof, K. H., G. A. Kivits, J. A. Weststrate and L. B. Tijburg (1998). Bioavailability of catechins from tea: The effect of milk. *Eur J Clin Nutr* 52(5): 356–359.

Vareed, S. K., M. Kakarala, M. T. Ruffin, J. A. Crowell, D. P. Normolle, Z. Djuric and D. E. Brenner (2008). Pharmacokinetics of curcumin conjugate metabolites in healthy human subjects. *Cancer Epidemiol Biomarkers Prev* 17(6): 1411–1417.

Verger, P., M. Chambolle, P. Babayou, S. Le Breton and J. L. Volatier (1998). Estimation of the distribution of the maximum theoretical intake for ten additives in France. *Food Addit Contam* 15(7): 759–766.

Wahlström, B. and G. Blennow (1978). A study on the fate of curcumin in the rat. *Acta Pharmacol Toxicol (Copenh)* 43(2): 86–92.

Wallstrom, P., E. Wirfalt, P. H. Lahmann, B. Gullberg, L. Janzon and G. Berglund (2001). Serum concentrations of beta-carotene and alpha-tocopherol are associated with diet, smoking, and general and central adiposity. *Am J Clin Nutr* 73(4): 777–785.

Wang, Y. J., M. H. Pan, A. L. Cheng, L. I. Lin, Y. S. Ho, C. Y. Hsieh and J. K. Lin (1997). Stability of curcumin in buffer solutions and characterization of its degradation products. *J Pharm Biomed Anal* 15(12): 1867–1876.

World Health Organization (2000). Evaluation of Certain Food Additives: 51st Report of the Joint FAO/WHO Expert Committee on Food Additives. *WHO Technical Report Series 891*. Geneva, World Health Organization.

Yeum, K. J., S. L. Booth, J. A. Sadowski, C. Liu, G. Tang, N. I. Krinsky and R. M. Russell (1996). Human plasma carotenoid response to the ingestion of controlled diets high in fruits and vegetables. *Am J Clin Nutr* 64(4): 594–602.

Yeum, K. J., A. Taylor, G. Tang and R. M. Russell (1995). Measurement of carotenoids, retinoids, and tocopherols in human lenses. *Invest Ophthalmol Vis Sci* 36(13): 2756–2761.

You, C. S., R. S. Parker, K. J. Goodman, J. E. Swanson and T. N. Corso (1996). Evidence of cis-trans isomerization of 9-cis-beta-carotene during absorption in humans. *Am J Clin Nutr* 64(2): 177–183.

Young, A. J. and G. M. Lowe (2001). Antioxidant and prooxidant properties of carotenoids. *Arch Biochem Biophys* 385(1): 20–27.

16 Case Studies on Selected Natural Food Antioxidants

Miguel Herrero, José A. Mendiola,
Alejandro Cifuentes, and Elena Ibáñez

CONTENTS

16.1 INTRODUCTION

As seen in previous chapters, antioxidants play an important role in food technology because of their usefulness against lipid oxidation and other oxidation processes. Moreover, plant antioxidants, derived from fruits and vegetables, have been associated with lower risks of coronary heart disease and cancer (Brigelius-Flohe et al. 2002; Harris et al. 2002). Many antioxidant compounds from natural origins have synergistic effects with some endogenous enzymes, such as superoxide dismutase or glutathione peroxidase; antioxidants enhance their inhibitory effect against the degenerative processes of cells. For instance, some natural antioxidants, such as tocopherols, have demonstrated higher activities than their synthetic forms (Brigelius-Flohe et al. 2002; National Institute for Health 2002).

Therefore, the interest in finding natural sources of antioxidants is increasing, and the search for new natural sources is also becoming more important. The main families of compounds with proven antioxidant activity are phenolic compounds, carotenoids, and tocopherols, which are readily available in the vegetable kingdom. On the other hand, there is, at present, a huge interest in the potential use of marine natural sources to obtain these bioactives—mainly considering their huge diversity in terms of the number of different species that might potentially be used, their sometimes unique chemical structures, and their ability to work as natural bioreactors potentiating the synthesis of valuable compounds, depending on the cultivation conditions.

16.2 NOVEL AND GREEN EXTRACTION METHODS

One important aspect that has to be closely considered when searching for natural food antioxidants is how these potential functional ingredients are obtained. In this regard, the need for appropriate, selective, cost-effective, and environmentally friendly extraction procedures to isolate these interesting compounds from natural sources has to be combined with the requirement of using food-grade solvents and processes. The use of new advanced extraction techniques, such as supercritical fluid extraction (SFE), pressurized liquid extraction (PLE), pressurized hot water extraction (PHWE), ultrasound-assisted extraction (UAE), and microwave-assisted extraction (MAE), among others, can effectively overcome these problems.

16.2.1 SUPERCRITICAL FLUID EXTRACTION

SFE is based on the use of solvents at temperatures and pressures above their critical points. This technique has been already employed to extract a wide variety of interesting compounds from very different food-related materials (Mendiola et al. 2007).

SFE was first introduced in 1879 by Hannay and Hogarth. However, it was not until approximately 1960 that this extraction method started to be thoroughly investigated (Hosikian et al. 2010) as an alternative to conventional extraction methods, such as solid–liquid extraction (SLE) and liquid–liquid extraction (LLE), requiring large amounts of hazardous chemicals, such as chlorinated solvents.

One of the most valuable characteristics of SFE is the highly reduced (often to zero) employment of toxic organic solvents. In this sense, carbon dioxide is the solvent most commonly used to extract antioxidant compounds from natural sources. In fact, CO_2 has a series of interesting properties for antioxidant extraction: It is cheap, its critical conditions are easily attainable (30.9°C and 73.8 bar), and it is an environmentally friendly solvent that, besides, is considered to be generally recognized as safe (GRAS) for its use in the food industry.

At supercritical conditions, CO_2 has a high diffusivity while its solvent strength and density can be easily modified by tuning the temperature and pressure applied. Once the extraction procedure is finished, the depressurization of the system allows CO_2 to turn into gas and leave the matrix while the compounds extracted from the matrix and solubilized in the CO_2 at high pressures remained in the collector; therefore, solvent-free extracts are obtained. These properties are responsible for the extended use of supercritical CO_2 for the extraction of bioactive compounds. The main drawback of CO_2 is its low polarity, a problem that can be overcome employing low amounts (1%–10%) of polar modifiers, also called cosolvents, to change the polarity of the supercritical fluid and to increase its solvating power toward the analyte of interest.

16.2.2 Pressurized Liquid Extraction

In PLE, pressure is applied to allow the use of liquids at temperatures higher than their normal boiling point (Herrero et al. 2006a; Mendiola et al. 2007). PLE is also known as pressurized fluid extraction (PFE), enhanced solvent extraction (ESE), high-pressure solvent extraction (HPSE), or accelerated solvent extraction (ASE) (Nieto et al. 2010). This technique was described for the first time in 1996 by Richter et al.

PLE is broadly recognized as a green extraction technique, mainly because of its low organic solvent consumption. The combined use of high pressures and temperatures provides faster extraction processes that require small amount of solvents (e.g., 20 min using 10–50 mL of solvent in PLE can be compared with a traditional extraction procedure in which 10–48 h and up to 300 mL are required). Usually, as long as the pressure is enough to keep the solvent in a liquid or subcritical state, the effect of the pressure changes is not very noticeable.

On the other hand, the increase in the extraction temperature can promote higher analyte solubility by increasing both solubility and mass transfer rate. Besides, high temperatures decrease the viscosity and the surface tension of the solvents, helping to reach areas of the matrices more easily and thus improving the extraction rate. It could be said that instrumentation for PLE is quite simple, but nowadays, there are only a few commercial equipment options available.

16.2.3 Subcritical Water Extraction

Water has many advantages in terms of versatility and environmental impact and can be used in extraction processes to isolate functional ingredients from different raw materials, including plants and food waste. Subcritical water extraction (SWE), also known as PHWE, pressurized low polarity water (PLPW) extraction, or superheated water extraction (SHWE), is a particular use of PLE with water as the extracting solvent.

SWE is based on the use of water at temperatures above its atmospheric boiling point while keeping it as liquid by applying pressure, just like in PLE for other solvents. Under these conditions, the physical and chemical properties of water change dramatically; for instance, the dielectric constant of water decreases from approximately 80 at room temperature to approximately 33 at 200°C, that is, close to a polar organic solvent, such as ethanol (Herrero et al. 2005a; Turner and Ibañez 2012). Moreover, the viscosity and surface tension are both reduced with increasing temperature while diffusivity is increased, altogether enhancing the extraction process in terms of efficiency and speed. In addition, water's solubility parameter is also modified by temperature, thus favoring the solubility of different types of compounds and modifying its selectivity. Water is also the greenest solvent that can be used, perfectly complying with the rules of green chemistry and green engineering (Anastas and Zimmerman 2003).

When using pressurized hot water, it must be taken into account that extraction conditions should be lower than the supercritical point (374°C, 218 bar). Supercritical or near-critical conditions can be used for supercritical water oxidation, hydrolysis, and molecular transformations, such as biomass conversion, while in the subcritical region, extraction of antioxidant compounds can be performed.

16.2.4 Instrumentation for Compressed Fluids Extraction

Figure 16.1 shows the scheme of an extraction device for compressed fluids. As expected, a single device can be used, with some modifications, to work either with supercritical fluids or with pressurized liquids, such as water and ethanol.

A basic supercritical-fluid extractor consists of a tank for the mobile phase, usually CO_2; a pump to pressurize the gas; an oven containing the extraction vessel; a restrictor to maintain the high pressure inside the system; and a trapping vessel. When a solvent able to modify the supercritical fluid solubility is needed, a second pump (a high-pressure liquid pump) can be included in the system together with a mixing device (usually a coil) to heat the solvent mixture up to the needed temperature. After extraction, extracts are trapped by letting the solute-containing supercritical fluid decompress into an empty vial, through a solvent, or onto a solid or liquid material. An additional separator can be included in the system for fractional separation of the extracts at different precipitation conditions. Under these conditions, two different extracts can be obtained from each sample, each containing different compounds separated as a function of their solubility in the supercritical fluid at the conditions set in each separator. Pressurized liquid instrumentation is basically the same as for SFE but without the CO_2 pump. It consists of a solvent reservoir coupled

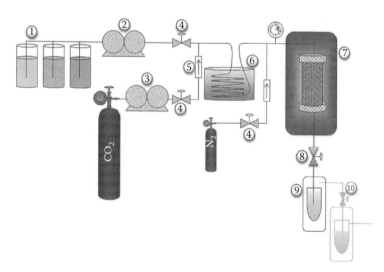

FIGURE 16.1 Multiple-purpose extraction device scheme that could be used for SFE, PLE, or SWE: liquid solvents (1); pump for liquids (2); CO_2 pump (3); on/off valves (4); check valves (5); preheating bath (6); oven and extraction cell (7); micrometering valve (8); extract collector (9); additional extract separator (10).

to a high-pressure pump to introduce the solvent into the system, an oven that contains the extraction vessel, and a restrictor or valve to keep the pressure inside the system. Extracts are collected in a vial placed at the end of the extraction system. In addition, the system can be equipped with a coolant device for rapid cooling of the resultant extract and with a N_2 gas line to purge the extraction cell and the whole system after extraction. The system device is the same independent of the solvent used, although some aspects should be considered depending on the maximum temperature used. For instance, working under supercritical conditions, maximum temperatures of approximately 100°C are used, while in PLE (or PHWE), temperatures are much higher (up to 200°C–250°C). This will influence the material used to build the extraction cell and the device employed for preheating the solvent (and its placement in the system). For further information on how to build your own system in PHWE, readers are referred to Turner and Ibáñez (2012).

Extractions with compressed fluids can be done under dynamic or static modes, or using a combination of both mechanisms. In a dynamic extraction, the fluid continuously flows through the sample into the extraction vessel and out the restrictor to the trapping vessel or vial. In the static mode, the fluid circulates in a loop containing the extraction vessel for some period of time before being released through the restrictor to the trapping vessel. In the combined mode, a static extraction is performed for some period of time, followed by a dynamic extraction. Additionally, when working at high temperatures in PLE, dynamic operation may avoid, to some extent, thermal degradation of the bioactive compounds because the liquid solvent flows continuously through the matrix at a certain flow rate, therefore improving the efficiency of the extraction and avoiding the excessive heating of the sample.

16.2.5 OTHER GREEN EXTRACTION METHODS: MICROWAVE- AND ULTRASOUND-ASSISTED EXTRACTION

Among green techniques for antioxidant extraction, UAE and MAE have enormous potential, although they have not been very frequently used for these purposes. Both techniques are fast, which is a key point to avoid degradation of labile compounds; use low amounts of solvents; and are cost-effective. Both methods are very versatile because of the possibility of using several solvents of different polarities; in fact, both can couple extraction and reaction at the same time.

UAE uses acoustic cavitation to cause disruption of cell walls, reduction of the particle size, and enhancement of contact between the solvent and the target compounds. When a liquid is irradiated by ultrasound, microbubbles form, grow, and oscillate extremely quickly, and eventually collapse powerfully if the acoustic pressure is high enough. These collapses, occurring near a solid surface, generate microjets and shock waves that result in cleaning, erosion, and fragmentation of the surface (Ötles 2009).

MAE was first described in 1986 (Ganzler et al. 1986); it uses microwave radiation that causes motion of polar molecules and rotation of dipoles to heat solvents and to promote transfer of target compounds from the sample matrix into the solvent. In general, samples for MAE are homogenized and mixed with a solvent and the suspension irradiated at higher than 2000 MHz for short periods of time. Heating is usually repeated several times with periods of cooling in between to prevent boiling. Techniques have also been developed using closed-system microwave heating—the most common nowadays—which lets the mixture of sample and solvent increase the pressure as a result of reaching the boiling point; therefore, the extraction takes place under a similar condition as PLE (Ötles 2009).

16.3 CASE STUDY 1: ROSEMARY ANTIOXIDANTS

Rosemary (*Rosmarinus officinalis* L.) is a medicinal plant from the order *Lamiales*, family *Lamiaceae*, and genus *Rosmarinus* L. Rosemary leaves contain essential oil (1.0%–2.5%), the composition of which depends on the origin, chemotype, and development stage of the plant at collection. The most characteristic compounds of the essential oil are 1,8-cineol (20%–50%), α-pinene (15%–25%), camphor (10%–25%), camphene (5%–10%), borneol (1%–6%), bornyl acetate (1%–5%), and α-terpineol (12%–24%). In the Mediterranean area there exist two main rosemary essential oils mainly differing in their content of 1,8-cineol: the one grown in Morocco and Tunisia with a high level and the one grown in Spain with a low content of this compound. Other important compounds found in rosemary extracts are phenolic diterpenes (carnosol and carnosic acid), polyphenols (caffeic and rosmarinic acid), flavonoids (apigenin and luteolin), and triterpenes (ursolic acid). Essential oil and extract composition will depend on the species and the type of plant and also on the growing conditions, the season, and the preprocessing after collection. All these factors, together with genetics, age, and origin, will influence the organoleptic characteristics and the bioactivity of plant extracts.

Hidalgo et al. (1998) determined that changes in the carnosic acid content of rosemary leaves were mainly a result of seasonal and environmental factors, such as leaf age, photoperiod, and temperature during growing. In general, younger leaves and those grown in summer months (more temperature and sunshine) contained a higher carnosic acid concentration. These results are in agreement with those of Celiktas et al. (2007) who studied the variability of the amounts of active constituents resulting from geographical location, growth, and seasonal variations; these authors also found that plants harvested in September possessed higher levels of active constituents. Nevertheless, other authors (Munné-Bosch et al. 2000) found that the highest concentrations of carnosic acid were produced during winter, and the lowest were produced in summer resulting from the highest heat and light stress of the plant.

Numerous works have been published on the influence on essential oil composition (Boyle et al. 1991; Mizrahi et al. 1991; Chalchat et al. 1993; Guillén et al. 1996).

In terms of bioactivity, the antioxidant capacity of rosemary plants was first reported in 1955 (Rac and Ostric-Matijasevic 1955) being its composition completely known at present. In 1964, carnosol was isolated (Brieskorn et al. 1964), and antioxidant properties were attributed to this compound. Its structure, together with carnosic acid, was confirmed in 1982 (Wu et al. 1982). Rosmanol, rosmarinic acid (Inatani et al. 1982), rosmadial (Inatani et al. 1983), epirosmanol, isorosmanol (Nakatani and Inatani 1984), rosmaridiphenol (Houlihan et al. 1984), and rosmariquinone (Houlihan et al. 1985) were further identified. Flavonoids with antioxidant activity have also been reported (Okamura et al. 1994); the chemical structures of some of the most important antioxidant compounds in rosemary are shown in Figure 16.2.

The main compound responsible for the antioxidant activity is carnosic acid (Aruoma et al. 1992; Cuvelier et al. 1996), a phenolic diterpene, which is also the most abundant compound in rosemary leaves. Carnosic acid is a lipophilic antioxidant able to neutralize oxygen and hydroxyl and peroxyl radicals, preventing the lipid oxidation and the damage in biological membranes (Aruoma et al. 1992; Haraguchi et al. 1995). The activity of carnosic acid against free radicals follows a mechanism similar to other known antioxidants, such as α-tocopherol, and is a result of the presence of two hydroxyl groups at the *ortho* position in the phenolic ring (positions C11 and C12; see Figure 16.2) (Richhelmer et al. 1999). Rosemary phenolic compounds act as primary antioxidants (Haraguchi et al. 1995; Frankel

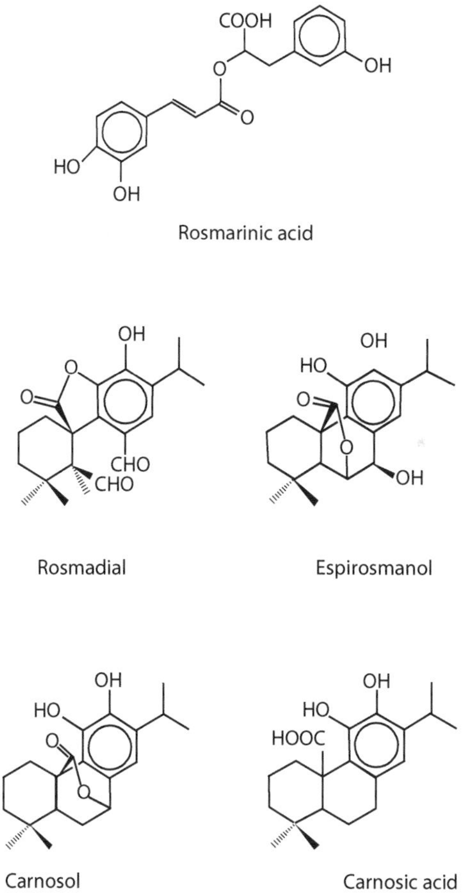

Rosmarinic acid

Rosmadial

Espirosmanol

Carnosol

Carnosic acid

FIGURE 16.2 Chemical structures of some of the most important antioxidants found in *Rosmarinus officinalis.*

et al. 1996; Basaga et al. 1997) and have shown synergies with other antioxidants, for instance, α-tocopherol (Wada and Fang 1992; Hopia et al. 1996) and the enzymes glutathione reductase and NADPH-quinone reductase. Some authors attributed the demonstrated protective effects against lung, liver, and stomach cancer in rats to these synergies with enzymes (Singletary and Rokusek 1997).

Although carnosic acid is, nowadays, recognized as the main antioxidant compound in rosemary leaves, carnosol can sometimes be detected as the main compound (up to 90%) coming from carnosic acid oxidation during the extraction process (Shwarz and Ternes 1992). During degradation, carnosic acid can be enzymatically dehydrogenated to carnosol (Munne-Bosch et al. 2000) and further oxidized to rosmanol and isorosmanol as a result of free radical attack (Luis 1991; Luis et al. 1994).

Therefore, the selection of the raw material and the processing conditions used to obtain the bioactive extract are important. As mentioned in the introduction, there is a need for developing new extraction processes able to keep the original bioactive properties while improving the whole process in terms of cost effectiveness, environmental impact, and health safety. Therefore, not only food-grade solvents should be used (including GRAS-approved solvents, such as ethanol, water, and carbon dioxide) but also sustainable processes providing a higher selectivity (extracting only the interesting compounds) and efficiency (extracting with high yields) at lower costs (economical and energy). In this case study, the techniques mentioned in the introduction (SFE, PLE, PHWE, UAE, and MAE) will be discussed in regard to their contribution to the extraction of antioxidants from rosemary.

SFE has been widely studied by several authors to obtain highly active rosemary antioxidant extracts. For instance, Topal et al. (2008) demonstrated that the antioxidant activity of supercritical extracts of different Turkish plants (rosemary among them) was higher than that obtained by steam distillation. Better results in terms of antioxidant activity were also achieved when compared to liquid solvent sonication (Tena et al. 1997).

Supercritical processing conditions will depend on the target product or products to be extracted. For instance, research has been conducted to optimize deodorization of rosemary extracts obtained by steam distillation and Soxhlet extraction; extracts with good antioxidant activity and 90% deodorization were achieved under relatively mild conditions (200 bar, 60°C, pure CO_2) (Lopez-Sebastian et al. 1998). Other authors reported 100 bar and 35°C as the best conditions to remove rosemary essential oil from crude extracts obtained using conventional processes (Hadolin et al. 2004). Sequential two-step extraction has been used to divide rosemary oleoresin into two fractions with different antioxidant activities and essential oil composition (Ibañez et al. 1999). In this paper, the authors reported not only the best conditions to obtain both fractions but also the effect of plant processing in the final composition of extracts. In this sense, conventional drying at ambient temperatures in a ventilated place seems to be the best processing condition. Different products were obtained under the following conditions: step 1—100 bar, 40°C, and essential oil fraction; step 2—400 bar, 60°C, and antioxidant fraction. Babovic et al. (2010) also studied the sequential extraction of rosemary in two different fractions with similar results and suggested the use of rosemary antioxidants as food additives to substitute synthetic antioxidants, such as Butylated hydroxyanisole (BHA) (Babovic et al. 2010).

Similar results could be obtained working under fractional separation after supercritical extraction. This approach allows for the extraction of a rosemary oleoresin that is further fractionated in two separators by stepwise decompression at different pressure and/or temperature conditions, leading to two different fractions with different antioxidant activities and composition. Señorans et al. (2000) studied the conditions to selectively recover one antioxidant fraction with almost no residual aroma in the first separator and an enriched essential oil fraction in the second separator; conditions leading to the best combination of extracts were as follows: extraction conditions—350 bar, 50°C, no modifier; fractionation conditions in separator 1—200 bar, 50°C; fractionation conditions in separator 2—atmospheric conditions. In a further study, the same authors studied both fractionation and extraction yields together with carnosic acid extraction as a function of experimental conditions and examined the correlation between carnosic acid and the antioxidant activity measured. Results obtained show that carnosic acid seemed to be the main compound responsible for the antioxidant activity of rosemary extracts, but also some other compounds present in the extract may affect, positively or negatively, the antioxidant activity of the final extracts (Cavero et al. 2005).

In an attempt to scale up the SFE of rosemary antioxidants, Carvalho et al. (2005) studied the kinetics of SFE in two different-scale extraction units and the fitting of the overall extraction curves (experimental values) to different mathematical models (Carvalho et al. 2005); kinetic and model parameters were obtained, and results showed that the models of Goto, Sovová, and Esquível provided the best results and can be used for process design. Based on these results, Garcia-Risco et al. (2011) studied the kinetic behavior of supercritical rosemary extract on a pilot scale (operated at 300 bar and 40°C with pure carbon dioxide) and the kinetics recovery of carnosic acid, and although the global extraction yield achieved was similar to that in analytical or low-scale experiments, the extraction time needed was higher; the authors suggested slower kinetics on a large scale because of the higher size of the solid particles used, which, in turn, makes it necessary for the process to be controlled by solute diffusion in the solid phase.

Antioxidant activity of rosemary extracts, together with other interesting bioactivities, has been studied under different supercritical conditions at different scales (analytical, pilot) by different authors. For instance, Leal et al. (2003) studied the antioxidant, anticancer, and antimycobacterial activities of different spices extracted under supercritical conditions, and Kuo et al. (2011) focused on the anti-inflammatory effects of both rosemary extracts and isolated carnosic acid; the authors demonstrated that at 345 bar and 80°C, higher yields, total phenolics, and the individual concentration of bioactive phenolics were obtained (Kuo et al. 2011). The same results were obtained under the same extraction conditions in terms of antioxidant activity (Chang et al. 2008).

As largely mentioned in this case study, all the reports published up to now associated the strong antioxidant activity of rosemary extracts with the presence of phenolic diterpenes, such as carnosic acid and carnosol, and therefore, there is a strong interest in isolating and purifying these compounds from a natural source, such as rosemary. Although fractional separation and/or two-step extraction can be considered as a first approach for concentrating the complex extracts in such important compounds, more sophisticated attempts have been made to truly isolate them using supercritical fluids. For instance, the pioneering works of Ramirez et al. (2004, 2005) demonstrated the ability of supercritical fluid chromatography (SFC) to isolate antioxidant compounds from rosemary supercritical extracts on an analytical scale on specially designed columns packed with coated particles and able to perform the expected separation using pure CO_2; these results were scaled up to a prep-SFC system with the columns built ad hoc and the separation and collection conditions optimized (Ramirez et al. 2006, 2007); important enrichment of antioxidant fractions was obtained using this procedure.

In a new approach by Braida et al. (2008), a new extraction–adsorption–desorption procedure using supercritical CO_2 as a solvent was developed using as a starting material a crude oleoresin obtained using organic solvents. In this new combination, different processes using supercritical CO_2 were employed as follows: First, a supercritical extraction of the oleoresin was carried out followed by an adsorption step with a commercial adsorbent (activated carbon); after adsorption, retained compounds were recovered in a desorption step under the same supercritical condition but using ethanol as a cosolvent. Even if it was possible to increase carnosic acid concentration, it was only to a lower extent because of the presence of nonsoluble compounds. A scheme of the experimental setup used can be seen in Figure 16.3.

Visentin et al. (2011) suggested the isolation of carnosic acid from a high viscous oleoresin extracted with ethanol by using supercritical fluid antisolvent fractionation. The advantages of the process include high concentrations of carnosic acid achieved and the possibility of carrying it out in a continuous or semicontinuous way, which can favor its scaling up to the industrial level.

Different green processes, other than SFE, have been also studied to extract bioactives from rosemary leaves. In a recent contribution by Herrero et al. (2010), the

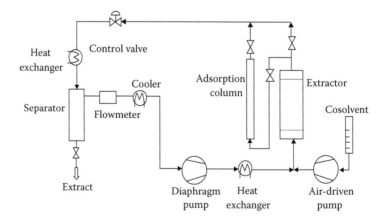

FIGURE 16.3 Schematic diagram of experimental set-up employed for the extraction–adsorption–desorption procedure. (From Braida, I. et al., *J. Supercrit. Fluids* 45, 195–199, 2008. With permission.)

performance of three different extraction procedures (PLE using water and ethanol as solvents, SFE using neat CO_2 and supercritical CO_2 modified with ethanol, and water extraction and particle formation online [WEPO]) toward the extraction of antioxidants from rosemary was studied. Different extraction conditions were tested, including extraction temperature, time, and pressure. PLE with both water and ethanol provided the best results in terms of extraction yield and quality of the antioxidants extracted. The best conditions were achieved using ethanol at 200°C or water at 100°C. The study confirmed the important effect of the extraction temperature on the selectivity of the process. Even if the WEPO process produced a lower extraction yield under not optimized conditions, recent results obtained in our research group (data not shown) demonstrated the potential of this new online process in which SWE is carried out in a dynamic mode, followed by a drying step in which supercritical CO_2 is mixed with the liquid extract and expanded into a precipitation chamber with a hot nitrogen current added (Ibáñez et al. 2009). Results obtained for SFE were similar to those previously mentioned.

Selectivity of hot water (or subcritical water) extraction toward extraction of antioxidants from rosemary was first reported by Ibañez et al. (2003). In this contribution, the effect of extraction temperature was studied for the first time to obtain extracts enriched in different polarity antioxidants. Results indicate the high selectivity of the subcritical water toward the most active compounds of rosemary, such as carnosol, rosmanol, carnosic acid, methyl carnosate, and some flavonoids, such as cirsimaritin and genkwanin. The antioxidant activity of the fractions obtained by extraction at different water temperatures was very high with values comparable to those achieved by SFE of rosemary leaves. Antioxidants were measured by using liquid chromatography-mass spectrometry (LC-MS) and capillary electrophoresis (CE) alone (Crego et al. 2004) or in combination with MS (Herrero et al. 2005b). In a recent paper, Plaza et al. (2010) demonstrated that no occurrence of Maillard reaction was observed in rosemary subcritical water extracts even considering the high extraction temperatures (up to 200°C). Although neoformation of antioxidants was observed in several natural raw materials extracted, mainly algae, no degradation of bioactive compounds or formation of new antioxidants could be observed for rosemary at 200°C.

MAE in the form of solvent-free microwave extraction (SFME) has been also used to extract essential oil from rosemary leaves. In a recent paper, Okoh et al. (2011) demonstrated the antioxidant activity of this essential oil, while Navarrete et al. (2011) used SFME to recover essential oil previous to antioxidant extraction of the residue by SLE with ethanol. After SFME, higher yields were obtained, mainly in carnosic acid and carnosol. This effect might be a result of modifications in the plant structure during treatment that lately favors the mass transfer of antioxidant compounds.

A few contributions can be found in the literature referring to the use of ultrasound to improve antioxidant extraction from rosemary leaves. For instance, Albu et al. (2004) studied the effect of solvent, leaf water content, and temperature on carnosic acid yields, considering sonication as the technique to increase the extraction efficiency. Recently, the same authors studied the scaling up of the ultrasonic extraction process using ethanol or methanol as extracting solvents and determined that the use of ultrasound provided a more effective extraction at lower temperatures with less dependence on the extraction solvent employed and that scale-up of the process was possible.

Other than *in vitro* assays to assess the bioactivity of supercritical rosemary extracts, some authors have also studied their *in vivo* effects in both aged and diabetic rats. Extracts containing 20% of carnosic acid showed an improvement of the oxidative stress status in aged rats (Posadas et al. 2009) and differences in the metabolites found in control and treated diabetic rats. Moreover, these extracts showed a low acute toxicity with oral lethal doses (LD_{50}) for male and female rats being greater than 2000 mg/kg of body weight (Anadon et al. 2008).

These results demonstrated the possibility of rosemary extracts enriched with phenolic diterpenes toward health enhancement. Nevertheless, more studies are needed to confirm these results and to further develop a functional ingredient able to act in the prevention or retardation of some diseases associated with oxidative stress or even aging. Initial steps have been taken to develop formulations to improve the digestion and bioavailability of rosemary supercritical extracts (Soler-Rivas et al. 2010).

Because of the above-mentioned demonstrated biological activities of rosemary supercritical extracts, at present, supercritical extraction with carbon dioxide is one of the processes used on the industrial scale to provide high-quality rosemary extracts. Companies such as Supercritical Fluid Technologies Inc., Natural Wisdom Holistic Beauty Ltd., Gaia Herbs, and Arkopharma are among those selling commercial rosemary extract obtained under supercritical conditions.

16.4 CASE STUDY 2: MICROALGAL ANTIOXIDANTS AND CAROTENOIDS

More than 60% of our planet is constituted by a marine environment, which offers a wide array of applications in biotechnology. The use of "blue biotechnology" is related to the application of molecular biological methods to marine and freshwater organisms. It involves the use of these organisms and their derivatives. Among those organisms, microalgae, especially those from marine origin, remain, to date, largely unexplored, so they represent a unique opportunity to discover novel metabolites and to produce known metabolites at lower costs (Guedes et al. 2011). In fact, current scientific consensus holds that significant amounts of oxygen (O_2) first appeared in the Earth's atmosphere some 2.4 billion years ago as a result of the photosynthetic activity of blue-green algae; therefore, marine microorganisms were the first to develop the antioxidant mechanism.

As mentioned, the interest in finding natural sources of antioxidants is increasing, and the search for new natural sources, such as algae or microalgae, is also becoming more important. Antioxidants can play a major role in food technology because of their usefulness against lipid oxidation. Moreover, plant antioxidants, derived from fruits and vegetables, have been associated with lower risks of coronary heart disease and cancer (Brigelius-Flohe et al. 2002). Natural antioxidants offer food, pharmaceutical, nutraceutical, and cosmetic manufacturers a "green" label, minimal regulatory interference with use, and the possibility of multiple actions that improve and extend food and pharmaceutical stabilization (Schaich 2006). Determining antioxidant capacity has become a very active research topic, and a plethora of antioxidant assay methods are currently in use.

Carotenoids are prominent for their distribution, structural diversity, and various functions. More than 600 different naturally occurring carotenoids are now known, excluding *cis* and *trans* isomers, all derived from the same basic C40 isoprenoid skeleton with some modifications, such as cyclization, substitution, elimination, addition, and rearrangement (Schubert et al. 2006). The beneficial effects of carotenoids have been well documented from numerous clinical and epidemiological studies in various populations, despite the fact that in certain circumstances, they could act as prooxidants (Palozza et al. 2008). Carotenoids play a key role in oxygenic photosynthesis as accessory pigments for harvesting light or as structural molecules that stabilize protein folding in the photosynthetic apparatus.

Green microalgae *Dunaliella salina* and *Haematococcus pluvialis* are among the most studied microalgae for their carotenoid content. Both microalgae have something important in common: They produce carotenoids in large amounts when they grow under stress conditions.

16.4.1 *DUNALIELLA SALINA*

The genus *Dunaliella* is one of the most reported for the production of carotenoids and belongs to the group of halotolerant unicellular microalgae. This microalga accumulates large amounts of β-carotene in chloroplasts. On average, it can produce 400 mg of β-carotene/m^2/day when cultured in open tanks, meaning 10%–14% of the dry weight (Dufossé et al. 2005; Ribeiro et al. 2011). Carotenoids from *Dunaliella salina* are produced on a commercial scale in open ponds in, for example, Australia and Israel. These systems seem to have reached their technical limits in the 1990s. High CO_2 consumption with low efficiency; impractical control of some environmental factors; contamination problems; and the requirement for high amounts of salt, water, land, and solar irradiance have probably limited the expansion of mass cultures of this microalga. The production of carotenoids from *D. salina* in photobioreactors has also been tested using different systems. The two most important were those developed by García-González et al. (2005) and Hejazi et al. (2004); these methods could reach higher yields than using open ponds. In Figure 16.4, different examples for the production of *D. salina* are summarized.

The required conditions to promote the carotenogenesis in *D. salina*, beyond the essential nutrients, are high salt concentration (up to 27% NaCl) and some light stress with photoperiod intervals of 12 h for 15 days. Different stress methods have also been studied and involve N and P suppression or the addition of organic nonpolar biocompatible solvents. In this case, if the solvent is highly nonpolar, a two-phase system is obtained, similar to what is occurring in the method developed by Hejazi et al. (2004), which used dodecane. Results showed that *D. salina* at a high light intensity remained viable over 45 days in the presence of dodecane; however, cell growth was very slow. β-Carotene could be continuously extracted to the organic phase, while the cells continued to produce β-carotene and the extracted molecules were continuously reproduced. β-Carotene extraction efficiency in this system was more than 55%, and productivity was much higher than that of commercial plants.

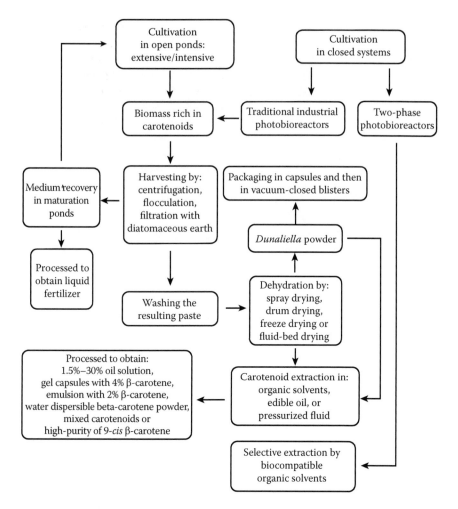

FIGURE 16.4 Flow chart of culturing and processing of *Dunaliella salina* in different culture systems. (From Hosseini Tafresi, A., Shariati, M., *J. Appl. Microbiol.* 107, 14–35, 2009. With permission.)

The β-carotene generated from stressing *Dunaliella* is a mixture of *cis* and *trans* isomers, which has 10% 15-*cis*-β-carotene, 41% 9-*cis*-β-carotene, 42% all *trans*-β-carotene, and 6% of other isomers, which accounts for approximately 80% of the total carotenoids produced with lutein being the second major carotene, comprising 15% of the total carotenoids (Ribeiro et al. 2011).

After culturing, *Dunaliella* is commonly sold after a drying step. But there are several studies on carotenoid extraction and purification. Among them, SFE could be considered to be the most promising as a result of the high solubility of β-carotene in CO_2 and the mild conditions needed, thus avoiding extract degradation. Some other novel techniques have been proposed to purify carotenoids from *D. salina* with promising results, among them UAE (Macias-Sanchez et al. 2009) and PLE (Herrero et al. 2006a). The supercritical extraction process is more selective for the recovery of carotenoids than the conventional techniques because it leads to higher values for the ratio of carotenoids to chlorophylls. Jaime et al. (2007) studied subcritical and supercritical CO_2 extraction of carotenoids from the freeze-dried *D. salina*. Higher yields were obtained at high pressures and low temperatures; that is, at higher CO_2 densities, with optimized extraction conditions equal to 9.8°C and 440 bar, maximum yields of 6.72% containing 52% of β-carotene were achieved. This work showed the strong influence of the supercritical extraction conditions in both the β-carotene isomer composition of the extracts and the antioxidant activity measured. Statistical analysis of all the data, considering yield, antioxidant activity, and relative concentration of carotenoids in the different extracts, suggested an important relationship among antioxidant activity and β-carotene isomeric relation, 9-*cis*/all-*trans*.

The antioxidant activity of *Dunaliella* has also been tested *in vivo*. The work developed by Murthy et al. (2005) shows a clear protective role of β-carotene-rich algae in the reduction of oxidative stress. Furthermore, it restores the activity of hepatic enzymes, such as catalase, peroxidase, and superoxide dismutase, which, in turn, protects vital organs against xenobiotic and other damage; results have shown a prevention of lipid oxidation, mainly peroxidation, to a greater extent. They treated three groups of rats with CCl_4, with CCl_4 and *Dunaliella*, and with CCl_4 and synthetic β-carotene. Treatment with CCl_4 decreased the activities of various antioxidant enzymes, such as catalase, superoxide dismutase, and peroxidase. While rats pretreated with synthetic β-carotene only partially avoided the decrease in enzymatic activities, rats pretreated with *Dunaliella* showed no alterations in superoxide dismutase and almost no reduction in the others. These results clearly indicated the beneficial effect of algal carotenoid compared to synthetic carotene as antioxidant.

16.4.2 *HAEMATOCOCCUS PLUVIALIS*

Haematococcus pluvialis is a ubiquitous freshwater green microalga that is known to synthesize and accumulate esters of the red ketocarotenoid astaxanthin (3,3′-dihydroxy-β,β-carotene-4,4′-dione) under stress conditions, such as nutrient deprivation, increased salinity, or light intensity (Collins et al. 2011).

Compared to other microbial sources, the green alga *Haematococcus pluvialis* produces the carotenoid astaxanthin in high concentrations (1.5%–4.0%). Astaxanthin is ubiquitous in nature, especially in the marine environment; it is well known because it is responsible for the pinkish-red color of lobster, salmon, and many other seafoods (Lorenz and Cysewski 2000; Grünewald et al. 2001).

The biosynthesis of astaxanthin is done through the isoprenoid pathway like many other lipid-soluble molecules, such as sterols; steroids; prostaglandins; hormones; and vitamins D, K, and E. *Haematococcus* primarily contains monoesters of astaxanthin linked to 16:0, 18:1, and 18:2 fatty acids. Fatty acids are esterified onto the hydroxyl group of astaxanthin after biosynthesis of the carotenoid, which increases its solubility and stability in the cellular lipid environment (Lorenz and Cysewski 2000). The carotenoid fraction of green vegetative cells consists mostly of lutein (75%) and β-carotene (18%), whereas in red cysts, astaxanthin accounts for approximately 80% of the whole carotenoid fraction (Grung et al. 1992).

Collins et al. (2011) recently investigated carotenogenesis in living *H. pluvialis* cells using resonance-enhanced confocal Raman microscopy and multivariate curve resolution (MCR) analysis. By mathematically isolating their spectral signatures, in turn, it was possible to locate astaxanthin and β-carotene along with chlorophyll in living cells of *H. pluvialis* in various stages of the life cycle. Chlorophyll emission was found only in the chloroplast, whereas astaxanthin was identified within globular and punctate regions of the cytoplasmic space. Moreover, they found evidence for β-carotene to be colocated with both the chloroplast and astaxanthin in the cytosol. These observations imply that β-carotene is a precursor for astaxanthin, and the synthesis of astaxanthin occurs outside the chloroplast.

H. pluvialis can be used as a whole biomass for animal feed and food purposes, as a pigment source, and as an antioxidant agent, but for many applications, astaxanthin should be extracted and purified. The main problem associated with astaxanthin extraction is its cell wall. *Haematococcus* has two distinct phases in its life cycle, the vegetative growth phase and the encysted secondary carotenoid accumulation phase. Hagen et al. (2002) studied the changes and composition of the cell wall. The motile biflagellated state exhibited a multilayered cell wall with a median tripartite crystalline layer. The transformation into the nonmotile cell state was characterized by formation of a new layer, a primary wall, within the extracellular matrix. Later, a trilaminar sheath is formed inside the primary wall, and the innermost and thickest part was an amorphous secondary mannan wall.

Before extracting the astaxanthin, it is important to set up a method for cell homogenization/disruption extraction or bioavailability. Different methods have been reported for extraction of astaxanthin using solvents, treatment with extracellular enzymes followed by solvent extraction, and cell disruption processes. All these methods result in loss of pigment to some extent and are difficult to apply on a large scale. Among them, those with a higher yield are those developed by Sarada et al. (2006) and Jaime et al. (2010). In the first one, the optimal conditions were reached using HCl at 70°C, cooled, centrifuged, washed with 2 mL of distilled water, and treated with acetone for 1 h; this procedure shows a 90% astaxanthin extractability. Treatment time, temperature, and concentration of the acid were found to be critical factors for maximum extractability. The treatment did not affect the astaxanthin ester profile, and the treated cells can be preserved until further use. Despite this method being highly interesting, it is difficult to apply on a large scale. In contrast, SFE and PLE have been proposed as useful green extraction techniques. Jaime et al. (2010) pretreated the alga by freezing and mashing it with liquid nitrogen in a ceramic mortar. The process was repeated three times in order to induce cell-wall lysis. After that, astaxanthin was extracted using different pressurized solvents (PLE). The best yields were obtained with ethanol at the higher extraction temperature (200°C), while the best antioxidant activity was also achieved using ethanol but at lower temperatures (50°C–100°C).

SFE has also been assayed to obtain astaxanthin from *H. pluvialis*, but results were not as good as using PLE. Although the astaxanthin molecule is considered to contain no strong polar moieties, its large molecule inhibited its solubility in pure SC-CO_2 because of its low volatility, making necessary the use of cosolvents, such as ethanol or vegetable oils, to increase the yield extraction. Nobre et al. (2006) studied

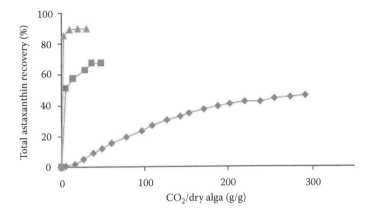

FIGURE 16.5 Recovery of total astaxanthin as a function of CO_2 amount with (■) and without (◆) ethanol as cosolvent, and CO_2 with ethanol doubling initial sample crushing time (▲) at 60°C and 300 bar. (From Nobre, B. et al., *Eur. Food Res. Technol.* 223, 787–790, 2006. With permission.)

the extraction of astaxanthin, astaxanthin esters, and other carotenoids from *H. pluvialis* using supercritical CO_2 in order to evaluate the best extraction conditions. The best recovery was achieved at 300 bar, 60°C, and 10% ethanol; under these conditions, all the carotenoids present in *H. pluvialis* (lutein, astaxanthin, β-carotene) were extracted with values higher than 90% (see Figure 16.5) with the exception of canthaxanthin (approximately 85%).

The antioxidant activity of *H. pluvialis* extracts has been measured using several methods. In the cited work published by Jaime et al. (2010), ABTS·+ (2,2-azinobis-3-ethyl-benzothiazoline-6-sulfonic acid) was used to measure the radical-scavenging activity. In general, ethanol extracts presented better antioxidant activity than hexane extracts at all temperatures tested. Antioxidant activity of *H. pluvialis* extracts seemed to be related to their free carotenoid content, which exists at higher concentrations in green cells showing higher TEAC values than red cells. Results demonstrated that the antioxidant activity of red cell extracts could be greatly improved after hydrolysis of the monoesters and diesters of astaxanthin, a reaction that seems to occur after ingestion of these products. Other authors used DPPH· to measure the antioxidant activity. DPPH· shows a maximum of absorption at 482 nm and others at 517 nm, and therefore, a clear interference with unreacted astaxanthin can be expected when measuring the antioxidant activities using this methodology.

16.5 CONCLUSIONS

In this chapter, different green extraction processes have been described to obtain food antioxidants from natural sources; the fundamentals of SFE, PLE, SWE, UAE, and MAE have been included together with a basic instrumentation device able to extract using compressed fluids. Two different case studies have been selected to illustrate the possibilities of plants and microalgae as natural sources of antioxidants and the benefits of the use of the mentioned green extraction processes. Overall, it can be concluded that some of the technologies are mature enough to be used to extract valuable compounds with antioxidant properties from different natural sources and that the possibility of application of such products will mainly depend on safety issues. In some cases, such as with rosemary antioxidants, the European Food Safety Authority (EFSA) already approved, in 2008, its use as a food additive (EFSA 2008). However, just recently rosemary antioxidants have received recognition as a safe and effective antioxidant for food preservation, including its range of applications, and can, therefore, be labeled as "antioxidant: extract of rosemary" and used in the different member states. More complex issues will need to be addressed if a different role, other than food preservation, wants to be played by antioxidants added to food; in this case, rigorous scientific demonstration will be needed in order to meet the requirements for a health claim involving antioxidants and their role in the prevention or retardation of certain diseases associated with oxidative stress.

REFERENCES

Albu, S., Joyce, E., Paniwnyk, L., Lorimer, J. P., Mason, T. J. 2004. Potential for the use of ultrasound in the extraction of antioxidants from *Rosmarinus officinalis* for the food and pharmaceutical industry. *Ultrason Sonochem* 11: 261–265.

Anadon, A., Martinez-Larranaga, M. R., Martinez, M. A., Ares, I., Garcia-Risco, M. R., Senorans, F. J., Reglero, G. 2008. Acute oral safety study of rosemary extracts in rats. *J Food Prot* 71: 790–795.

Anastas, P. T., Zimmerman, J. B. 2003. Design through the twelve principles of green engineering. *Environ Sci Technol* 37: 94A–101A.

Aruoma, O. I., Halliwell, B., Aeschbach, R., Loliger, J. 1992. Antioxidant and pro-oxidant properties of active rosemary constituents: Carnosol and carnosic acid. *Xenobiotica* 22: 257–268.

Babovic, N., Djilas, S., Jadranin, M., Vajs, V., Ivanovic, J., Petrovic, S., Zizovic, I. 2010. Supercritical carbon dioxide extraction of antioxidant fractions from selected *Lamiaceae* herbs and their antioxidant capacity. *Innov. Food Sci Emerg Technol* 11: 98–107.

Basaga, H., Tekkaya, C., Acikel, F. 1997. Antioxidative and free radical scavenging properties of rosemary extract. *Lebens Wissen Technol* 30: 105–108.

Boyle, T. H., Craker, L. E., Simon, J. E. 1991. Growing medium and fertilization regime influence growth and essential oil content of rosemary. *Hort Sci* 26: 33–34.

Braida, I., Mattea, M., Cardarelli, D. 2008. Extraction-adsorption-desorption process under supercritical condition as a method to concentrate antioxidants from natural sources. *J Supercrit Fluids* 45: 195–199.

Brieskorn, C., Fuchs, A., Bredenberg, J. B., McChesney, J. E. W. 1964. The structure of carnosol. *J Org Chem* 29: 2293–2298.

Brigelius-Flohe, R., Kelly, F. J., Salonen, J. T., Neuzil, J., Zingg, J.-M., Azzi, A. 2002. The European perspective on vitamin E: Current knowledge and future research. *Am J Clin Nutr* 76: 703–715.

Carvalho, R. N., Moura, L. S., Rosa, P. T. V., Meireles, M. A. A. 2005. Supercritical fluid extraction from rosemary (*Rosmarinus officinalis*): Kinetic data, extract's global yield, composition, and antioxidant activity. *J Supercrit Fluids* 35: 197–204.

Cavero, S., Jaime, L., Martin-Alvarez, P. J., Señorans, F. J., Reglero, G., Ibañez, E. 2005. *In vitro* antioxidant analysis of supercritical fluid extracts from rosemary (*Rosmarinus officinalis* L.). *Eur Food Res Technol* 221: 478–486.

Celiktas, O. Y., Bedir, E., Sukan, F. V. 2007. *In vitro* antioxidant activities of *Rosmarinus officinalis* extracts treated with supercritical carbon dioxide. *Food Chem* 101: 1457–1464.

Chalchat, J. C., Garry, R. P., Michet, A., Benjilali, B., Chabart, J. L. 1993. Essential oils of rosemary (*Rosmarinus officinalis* L.): The chemical composition of oils of various origins (Morocco, Spain, France). *J Essent Oil Res* 5: 613–618.

Chang, C. H., Chyau, C. C., Hsieh, C. L., Wu, Y. Y., Ker, Y. B., Tsen, H. Y., Peng, R. Y. 2008. Relevance of phenolic diterpene constituents to antioxidant activity of supercritical CO_2 extract from the leaves of rosemary. *Nat Prod Res* 22: 76–90.

Collins, A. M., Jones, H. D. T., Han, D., Hu, Q., Beechem, T. E., Timlin, J. A. 2011. Carotenoid distribution in living cells of *Haematococcus pluvialis* (chlorophyceae). *PLoS ONE* 6: e24302.

Crego, A. L., Ibañez, E., Garcia, E., De Pablos, R. R., Senorans, F. J., Reglero, G., Cifuentes, A. 2004. Capillary electrophoresis separation of rosemary antioxidants from subcritical water extracts. *Eur Food Res Technol* 219: 549–555.

Cuvelier, M. E., Richard, H., Berset, C. 1996. Antioxidative activity and phenolic composition of pilot-plant and commercial extracts of sage and rosemary. *J Am Oil Chem Soc* 73: 645–652.

Dufossé, L., Galaup, P., Yaron, A., Arad, S. M., Blanc, P., Murthy, K. N. C. et al. 2005. Microorganisms and microalgae as sources of pigments for food use: A scientific oddity or an industrial reality? *Trends Food Sci Technol* 16: 389–406.

EFSA. 2008. Use of rosemary extracts as a food additive 1. Scientific Opinion of the Panel on Food Additives, Flavourings, Processing Aids and Materials in Contact with Food, (Question No EFSA-Q-2003-140). *EFSA J* 721: 1–29.

Frankel, E. N., Shu, W. H., Aeschbatch, R., Prior, E. 1996. Antioxidant activity of a rosemary extract and its constituents carnosic acid, carnosol, and rosmarinic acid in bulk oil and oil-in-water emulsion. *J Agric Food Chem* 44: 131–135.

Ganzler, K., Salgó, A., Valkó, K. 1986. Microwave extraction: A novel sample preparation method for chromatography. *J Chromatogr A* 371: 299–306.

García-González, M., Moreno, J., Manzano, J. C., Florencio, F. J., Guerrero, M. G. 2005. Production of *Dunaliella salina* biomass rich in 9-cis-β-carotene and lutein in a closed tubular photobioreactor. *J Biotechnol* 115: 81–90.

Garcia-Risco, M. R., Hernandez, E. J., Vicente, G., Fornari, T., Señorans, F. J., Reglero, G. 2011. Kinetic study of pilot-scale supercritical CO_2 extraction of rosemary (*Rosmarinus officinalis*) leaves. *J Supercrit Fluids* 55: 971–976.

Grünewald, K., Hirschberg, J., Hagen, C. 2001. Ketocarotenoid biosynthesis outside of plastids in the unicellular green alga *Haematococcus pluvialis*. *J Biol Chem* 276: 6023–6029.

Grung, M., D'Souza, F. M. L., Borowitzka, M., Liaaen-Jensen, S. 1992. *Haematococcus pluvialis* aplanospores as a source of (3 S, 3′S)-astaxanthin esters. *J Appl Phycol* 4: 165–171.

Guedes, C. A., Amaro, H. M., Malcata, F. X. 2011. Microalgae as sources of high added-value compounds: A brief review of recent work. *Biotechnol Progress* 27: 597–613.

Guillén, M. D., Cabo, N., Burillo, J. 1996. Characterisation of the essential oils of some cultivated aromatic plants of industrial interest. *J Sci Food Agric* 70: 359–363.

Hadolin, M., Rizner Hras, A., Bauman, D., Knez, Z. 2004. Isolation and concentration of natural antioxidants with high-pressure extraction. *Innov Food Sci Emerg Technol* 5: 245–248.

Hagen, C., Siegmund, S., Braune, W. 2002. Ultrastructural and chemical changes in the cell wall of *Haematococcus pluvialis* (Volvocales, Chlorophyta) during aplanospore formation. *Eur J Phycol* 37: 217–226.

Haraguchi, H., Saito, T., Okamura, N., Yagi, A. 1995. Inhibition of lipid peroxidation and superoxide generation by diterpenoids from *Rosmarinus officinalis*. *Planta Medica* 61: 333–336.

Harris, A., Devaraj, S., Jialal, I. 2002. Oxidative stress, alpha-tocopherol therapy, and atherosclerosis. *Curr Atheroscler Rep* 4: 373–380.

Hejazi, M. A., Holwerda, E., Wijffels, R. H. 2004. Milking microalga *Dunaliella salina* for β-carotene production in two-phase bioreactors. *Biotechnol Bioeng* 85: 475–481.

Herrero, M., Arraez-Roman, D., Segura, A., Kenndler, E., Gius, B., Raggi, M. A., Ibanez, E., Cifuentes, A. 2005b. Pressurized liquid extraction-capillary electrophoresis-mass spectrometry for the analysis of polar antioxidants in rosemary extracts. *J Chromatogr A* 1084: 54–62.

Herrero, M., Cifuentes, A., Ibáñez, E. 2006a. Sub- and supercritical fluid extraction of functional ingredients from different natural sources: Plants, food-by-products, algae and microalgae: A review. *Food Chem* 98: 136–148.

Herrero, M., Jaime, L., Martin-Alvarez, P. J., Cifuentes, A., Ibanez, E. 2006b. Optimization of the extraction of antioxidants from *Dunaliella salina* microalga by pressurized liquids. *J Agric Food Chem* 54: 5597–5603.

Herrero, M., Martín-Álvarez, P. J., Señoráns, F. J., Cifuentes, A., Ibáñez, E. 2005a. Optimization of accelerated solvent extraction of antioxidants from *Spirulina platensis* microalga. *Food Chem* 93: 417–423.

Herrero, M., Plaza, M., Cifuentes, A., Ibanez, E. 2010. Green processes for the extraction of bioactives from rosemary: Chemical and functional characterization via ultra-performance liquid chromatography-tandem mass spectrometry and *in vitro* assays. *J Chromatogr A* 1217: 2512–2520.

Hidalgo, P. J., Ubera, J. L., Tena, M. T., Valcárcel, M. 1998. Determination of the carnosic acid content in wild and cultivated *Rosmarinus officinalis*. *J Agric Food Chem* 46: 2624–2627.

Hopia, A., Shu, W., Schwartz, K., German, J., Frankel, E. 1996. Effect of different lipid systems on antioxidant activity of rosemary constituents carnosol and carnosic acid with and without alpha-tocopherol. *J Agric Food Chem* 44: 2030–2036.

Hosikian, A., Lim, S., Halim, R., Danquah, M. K. 2010. Chlorophyll extraction from microalgae: A review on the process engineering aspects. *Int J Chem Eng* 2010: Article ID 391632.

Hosseini Tafresi, A., Shariati, M. 2009. *Dunaliella* biotechnology: Methods and applications. *J Appl Microbiol* 107: 14–35.

Houlihan, C., Ho, C., Chang, S. 1984. Elucidation of the chemical structure of a novel antioxidant, rosmaridiphenol, isolated from rosemary. *J Am Oil Chem Soc* 61: 1036–1039.

Houlihan, C., Ho, C., Chang, S. 1985. The structure of rosmariquinone: A new antioxidant isolated from *Rosmarinus officinalis* L. *J Am Oil Chem Soc.* 62: 96–98.

Ibáñez, E., Cifuentes, A., Rodríguez-Meizoso, I., Mendiola, J. A., Reglero, G., Señoráns, F. J., Turner, C. 2009. Device and procedure for the on-line extraction and drying of complex extracts. Patent: P200900164.

Ibañez, E., Kubatova, A., Senorans, F. J., Cavero, S., Reglero, G., Hawthorne, S. B. 2003. Subcritical water extraction of antioxidant compounds from rosemary plants. *J Agric Food Chem* 51: 375–382.

Ibañez, E., Oca, A., De Murga, G., Lopez-Sebastian, S., Tabera, J., Reglero, G. 1999. Supercritical fluid extraction and fractionation of different preprocessed rosemary plants. *J Agric Food Chem* 47: 1400–1404.

Inatani, R., Nakatani, N., Fuwa, H. 1983. Antioxidative effect of the constituents of rosemary and their derivatives. *Agric Biol Chem* 47: 521–528.

Inatani, R., Nakatani, N., Fuwa, H., Seto, H. 1982. Structure of a new antioxidative phenolic diterpene isolated from rosemary. *Agric Biol Chem* 46: 1661–1666.

Jaime, L., Mendiola, J. A., Ibáñez, E., Martin-Álvarez, P. J., Cifuentes, A., Reglero, G., Señoráns, F. J. 2007. β-Carotene isomer composition of sub- and supercritical carbon dioxide extracts: Antioxidant activity measurement. *J Agric Food Chem* 55: 10585–10590.

Jaime, L., Rodríguez-Meizoso, I., Cifuentes, A., Santoyo, S., Suarez, S., Ibáñez, E., Señorans, F. J. 2010. Pressurized liquids as an alternative process to antioxidant carotenoids' extraction from *Haematococcus pluvialis* microalgae. *LWT – Food Sci Technol* 43: 105–112.

Kuo, C. F., Su, J. D., Chiu, C. H., Peng, C. C., Chang, C. H., Sung, T. Y., Huang, S. H., Lee, W. C., Chyau, C. C. 2011. Anti-inflammatory effects of supercritical carbon dioxide extract and its isolated carnosic acid from *rosmarinus officinalis* leaves. *J Agric Food Chem* 59: 3674–3685.

Leal, P. F., Braga, M. E. M., Sato, D. N., Carvalho, J. E., Marques, M. O. M., Meireles, M. A. A. 2003. Functional properties of spice extracts obtained via supercritical fluid extraction. *J Agric Food Chem* 51: 2520–2525.

Lopez-Sebastian, S., Ramos, E., Ibanez, E., Bueno, J. M., Ballester, L., Tabera, J., Reglero, G. 1998. Dearomatization of antioxidant rosemary extracts by treatment with supercritical carbon dioxide. *J Agric Food Chem* 46: 13–19.

Lorenz, R. T., Cysewski, G. R. 2000. Commercial potential for *Haematococcus* microalgae as a natural source of astaxanthin. *Trends Biotechnol* 18: 160–167.

Luis, J. G. 1991. Chemistry, biogenesis, and chemotaxonomy of the diterpenoids of Salvia. In: *Ecological Chemistry and Biochemistry of Plant Terpenoids.* Eds., J. B. Harborne and F. A. Tomas-Barberan. Oxford: Clarendon Press.

Luis, J. G., Quiñones, W., Grillo, T. A., Kishi, M. P. 1994. Diterpenes from the aerial part of *Salvia columbariae. Phytochem* 35: 1373–1374.

Macías-Sánchez, M. D., Mantell, C., Rodríguez, M., Martínez de la Ossa, E., Lubián, L. M., Montero, O. 2009. Comparison of supercritical fluid and ultrasound-assisted extraction of carotenoids and chlorophyll a from *Dunaliella salina. Talanta* 77: 948–952.

Mendiola, J. A., Herrero, M., Cifuentes, A., Ibáñez, E. 2007. Use of compressed fluids for sample preparation: Food applications. *J Chromatogr A* 1152: 234–246.

Mizrahi, I., Juarez, M. A., Bandoni, A. L. 1991. The essential oil of *Rosmarinus officinalis* growing in Argentina. *J Essent Oil Res* 3: 11–16.

Munné-Bosch, S., Alegre, L., Schwarz, K. 2000. The formation of phenolic diterpenes in *Rosmarinus officinalis* L. under Mediterranean climate. *Eur Food Res Technol* 210: 263–267.

Murthy, K. N. C., Vanitha, A., Rajesha, J., Swamy, M. M., Sowmya, P. R., Ravishankar, G. A. 2005. *In vivo* antioxidant activity of carotenoids from *Dunaliella salina*—A green microalga. *Life Sci* 76: 1381–1390.

Nakatani, N., Inatani, R. 1984. Two antioxidative diterpenes from rosemary and a revised structure for rosmanol. *Agric Biol Chem* 48: 2081–2085.

National Institute for Health. 2002. *Facts about Dietary Suplements—Vitamin E.* Bethesda, MD: Warren Grant Magnuson Clinical Center.

Navarrete, A., Herrero, M., Martin, A., Cocero, M. J., Ibañez, E. 2011. Valorization of solid wastes from essential oil industry. *J Food Eng* 104: 196–201.

Nieto, A., Borrull, F., Pocurull, E., Marcé, R. M. 2010. Pressurized liquid extraction: A useful technique to extract pharmaceuticals and personal-care products from sewage sludge. *TrAC Trends Anal Chem* 29: 752–764.

Nobre, B., Marcelo, F., Passos, R., Beirão, L., Palavra, A., Gouveia, L., Mendes, R. 2006. Supercritical carbon dioxide extraction of astaxanthin and other carotenoids from the microalga *Haematococcus pluvialis. Eur Food Res Technol* 223: 787–790.

Okamura, N., Fujimoto, Y., Kuwabara, S., Yagi, A. 1994. High-performance liquid chromatographic determination of carnosic acid and carnosol in *Rosmarinus officinalis* and *Salvia officinalis. J Chromatogr A* 679: 381–386.

Okoh, O. O., Sadimenko, A. P., Afolayan, A. J. 2011. Antioxidant activities of *Rosmarinus officinalis* L. essential oil obtained by hydro-distillation and solvent free microwave extraction. *Afr J Biotechnol* 10: 4207–4211.

Ötles, S. 2009. *Handbook of Food Analysis Instruments.* 1st ed. Boca Raton, FL: CRC Press Taylor & Francis Group.

Palozza, P., Simone, R., Mele, M. C. 2008. Interplay of carotenoids with cigarette smoking: Implications in lung cancer. *Curr Med Chem* 15: 844–854.

Plaza, M., Amigo-Benavent, M., del Castillo, M. D., Ibañez, E., Herrero, M. 2010. Facts about the formation of new antioxidants in natural samples after subcritical water extraction. *Food Res Int* 43: 2341–2348.

Posadas, S. J., Caz, V., Largo, C., De la Gandara, B., Matallanas, B., Reglero, G., De Miguel, E. 2009. Protective effect of supercritical fluid rosemary extract, *Rosmarinus officinalis*, on antioxidants of major organs of aged rats. *Exp Gerontol* 44: 383–389.

Rac, M., Ostric-Matijasevic, B. 1955. The properties of rosemary as an antioxidant. *Rev Fr Corps Gras* 2: 796.

Ramirez, P., Fornari, T., Señorans, F. J., Ibañez, E., Reglero, G. 2005. Isolation of phenolic antioxidant compounds by SFC. *J Supercrit Fluids* 35: 128–132.

Ramirez, P., Garcia-Risco, M. R., Santoyo, S., Senorans, F. J., Ibanez, E., Reglero, G. 2006. Isolation of functional ingredients from rosemary by preparative-supercritical fluid chromatography (Prep-SFC). *J Pharm Biomed Anal* 41: 1606–1613.

Ramirez, P., Santoyo, S., Garcia-Risco, M. R., Senorans, F. J., Ibanez, E., Reglero, G. 2007. Use of specially designed columns for antioxidants and antimicrobials enrichment by preparative supercritical fluid chromatography. *J Chromatogr A* 114: 234–242.

Ramirez, P., Señorans, F. J., Ibanez, E., Reglero, G. 2004. Separation of rosemary antioxidant compounds by supercritical fluid chromatography on coated packed capillary columns. *J Chromatogr A* 1057: 241–245.

Ribeiro, B. D., Barreto, D. W., Coelho, M. A. Z. 2011. Technological aspects of β-carotene production. *Food Bioproc Technol* 4: 693–701.

Richhelmer, S. L., Bailey, D. T., Bernart, M. W., Kent, M., Vininski, J. V., Anderson, L. D. 1999. Antioxidant activity and oxidative degradation of phenolic compounds isolated from rosemary. *Recent Res Develop Oil Chem* 3: 45–58.

Richter, B. E., Jones, B. A., Ezzell, J. L., Porter, N. L., Avdalovic, N., Pohl, C. 1996. Accelerated solvent extraction: A technique for sample preparation. *Anal Chem* 68: 1033–1039.

Sarada, R., Vidhyavathi, R., Usha, D., Ravishankar, G. A. 2006. An efficient method for extraction of astaxanthin from green alga *Haematococcus pluvialis*. *J Agric Food Chem* 54: 7585–7588.

Schaich, K. M. 2006. Developing a rational basis for selection of antioxidant screening and testing methods. *Acta Hort* 709: 79–94.

Schubert, N., García-Mendoza, E., Pacheco-Ruiz, I. 2006. Carotenoid composition of marine algae. *J Phycol* 42: 1208–1216.

Schwarz, K., Ternes, W. 1992. Antioxidative constituents of *Rosmarinus officinalis* and *Salvia officinalis* II: Isolation of carnosic acid and formation of other phenolic diterpenes. *Z Lebensm Unters Forsch* 195: 99–103.

Señorans, F. J., Ibañez, E., Cavero, S., Tabera, J., Reglero, G. 2000. Liquid chromatographic-mass spectrometric analysis of supercritical-fluid extracts of rosemary plants. *J Chromatogr A* 870: 491–499.

Singletary, K. W., Rokusek, J. T. 1997. Tissue specific enhancement of xenobiotic detoxification enzymes in mice by dietary rosemary extract. *Plant Foods Human Nutr* 50: 47–53.

Soler-Rivas, C., Marin, F. R., Santoyo, S., Garcia-Risco, M. R., Senorans, J., Reglero, G. 2010. Testing and enhancing the *in vitro* bioaccessibility and bioavailability of *Rosmarinus officinalis* extracts with a high level of antioxidant abietanes. *J Agric Food Chem* 58: 1144–1152.

Tena, M. T., Valcarcel, M., Hidalgo, P. J., Ubera, J. L. 1997. Supercritical fluid extraction of natural antioxidants from rosemary: Comparison with liquid solvent sonication. *Anal Chem* 69: 521–526.

Topal, U., Sasaki, M., Goto, M., Otles, S. 2008. Chemical compositions and antioxidant properties of essential oils from nine species of Turkish plants obtained by supercritical carbon dioxide extraction and steam distillation. *Int J Food Sci Nutr* 59: 619–634.

Turner, C., Ibañez, E. 2012. Pressurized hot water extraction. In: *Enhancing Extraction Processes in the Food Industry*. Eds. Lebovka, N., Vorobiev, E., Chemat, F. Boca Raton, FL: CRC Press.

Visentin, A., Cismondi, M., Maestri, D. 2011. Supercritical CO_2 fractionation of rosemary ethanolic oleoresins as a method to improve carnosic acid recovery. *Innov Food Sci Emerg Technol* 12: 142–145.

Wada, S., Fang, X. 1992. The synergistic antioxidant effects of rosemary extract and a-tocopherol in sardine oil model system and frozen-crushed fish meat. *J Food Proc Pres* 16: 263–274.

Wu, J., Lee, M., Ho, C. T., Chang, S. S. 1982. Elucidation of the chemical structures of natural antioxidants isolated from rosemary. *J Am Oil Chem Soc* 59: 339–345.

17 Functional Antioxidant Foods

Manuel Viuda-Martos, Jose A. Pérez-Álvarez,
and Juana Fernández-López

CONTENTS

17.1 INTRODUCTION

Oxidative stress by free radicals or reactive oxygen species (ROS) is often associated with aging and the development of numerous chronic diseases, including cancer, multiple sclerosis, Parkinson's disease, autoimmune disease, and senile dementia (Ali et al. 2008; Caillet et al. 2011). Furthermore, stress, physical damage, viral infection, and cytotoxic or carcinogenic compounds resulting from chemical or biological aggression may cause the peroxidation of cell membrane lipids and the liberation of toxic substances, such as free radicals (Aruoma 1998). Indeed, oxidative stress, a major contributor to cardiovascular diseases (CVDs), is associated with lipid peroxidation in arterial macrophages and in lipoproteins. Oxidized low-density lipoprotein (Ox-LDL) has been shown to be atherogenic (Anoosh, Mojtab, and Fatemeh 2010). The simultaneous production of nitric oxide ($^{\bullet}$NO) and superoxide anions $\left(O_2^{\bullet-}\right)$ by vascular cells may explain peroxynitrite (ONOO$^-$) formation within the vascular wall. Peroxynitrite-modified LDL binds to scavenger receptors, leading to accumulation of the cholesteryl esters involved in the production of atherosclerotic lesions (Thomas, Davies, and Stocker 1998).

The consumption of fruits and vegetables, generally regarded as insufficient throughout the world, should be encouraged, and in this respect, it may be useful to enhance the concentrations of vitamins and secondary metabolites in fruits by genetic and/or environmental approaches (Poiroux-Gonord et al. 2010). It is widely accepted that a plant-based diet with a high intake of fruits, vegetables, and other nutrient-rich plant foods may reduce the risk of oxidative stress-related diseases (Stanner et al. 2004). Epidemiologic data have shown that persons with a high consumption of fruit and vegetables are at a lower risk of several types of cancer, CVD, and stroke than are persons with a low consumption (Hu 2003; Riboli and Norat 2003). This is because *de novo* antioxidant production is limited in animal cells, and oxidative damage is correspondingly higher. Furthermore, increased amounts of reactive oxygen and nitrogen species (ROS/RNS) are formed in animal cells as a consequence of disease processes (e.g., inflammation) and from tobacco smoke, environmental pollutants, food constituents, drugs, ethanol, and radiation (Griendling and FitzGerald 2003; Bandyopadhyay et al. 2004), and, if not eliminated by antioxidants, they may damage extracellular or cellular components (Sánchez-Quesada, Benitez, and Ordoñez-Llanos 2004).

Antioxidants are substances that can prevent or delay the oxidative damage to lipids, proteins, and nucleic acids caused by ROS, which include reactive free radicals, such as superoxide $\left(O_2^{\cdot-}\right)$, hydroxyl (HO$^\cdot$), peroxyl (ROO$^\cdot$), and alkoxyl, and nonradicals, such as hydrogen peroxide (H_2O_2), hypochlorous acid (HOCl), etc. (Lim, Lim, and Tee 2007). These substances can act in various ways, which include the complexation of redox-catalytic metal ions, the scavenging of free radicals, the reduction or decomposition of hydrogen peroxides, the quenching of superoxide and singlet oxygen, the inhibition of the initiation, and the breaking of chain propagation (Shi, Noguchi, and Niki 2001). Often, several mechanisms and mechanistic synergisms are involved, especially in food-related systems (e.g., extracts) and antioxidant activity studies (using multiple experimental approaches) allowing a complete screening of the putative chain-breaking capacity (Mello and Kubota 2007). The main source of exogenous antioxidants is the diet, and one of the healthiest dietary models is the Mediterranean diet. This diet is characteristically rich in fruits, vegetables, bread, cereals, potatoes, beans, nuts, seeds, olive oil, dairy products, and fish and is accompanied by the modest consumption of red wine (Pérez-Alvarez and Alesón-Carbonell 2003). These types of foods contain a great variety of phytochemicals, compounds produced by the plant kingdom for defense, protection, and cell-to-cell signaling and as attractants for pollinators (Kartal et al. 2007). They are bioactive nonnutrient plant compounds and can act as antioxidants.

17.2 BIOACTIVE COMPOUNDS WITH ANTIOXIDANT ACTIVITY

Phytochemicals can be defined, in the strictest sense, as bioactive compounds produced by plants; however, the term is generally used to describe chemicals from plants that may affect health but are not essential nutrients (El Gharras 2009). These bioactive compounds show a great diversity of structures, ranging from simple molecules to polymers.

17.2.1 Phenolic Acids

Phenolic acids are found in most plants, and in many cases, they contribute to their color and taste. Chemically, phenolic acids can be defined as substances that possess an aromatic ring bound to one or more hydrogenated substituents, including their functional derivates (Marin et al. 2001). There are two classes of phenolic acids (Figure 17.1): derivates of benzoic acid and derivates of cinnamic acid. Hydroxybenzoic acids are components of complex structures, such as hydrolyzable tannins [gallotannins (GTs) or ellagitannins (ETs)] (Manach et al. 2004), while the hydroxycinnamic acids are more common than the hydroxybenzoic acids and consist chiefly of *p*-coumaric, caffeic, ferulic, and sinapic acids (El Gharras 2009). The antioxidant activity of phenolic acids is widely demonstrated (Egüés, Sanchez, and Mondragon 2012; Porgali and Büyüktuncel 2012; Razali, Mat-Junit, and Abdul-Muthalib 2012).

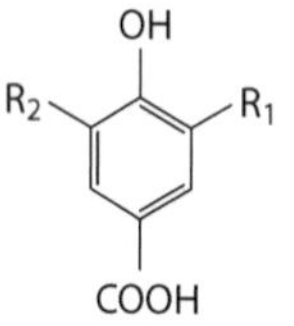

OH
R_2 ─ ⟨ring⟩ ─ R_1
COOH

OH
R_2 ─ ⟨ring⟩ ─ R_1
CH=CH-COOH

Derivates of benzoic acid				Derivates of cinnamic acid		
Compound	R_1	R_2		Compound	R_1	R_2
Vanillic acid	H	OCH_3		p-coumaric acid	H	H
Syringic acid	OCH_3	OCH_3		Ferulic acid	H	OCH_3
Gallic acid	OH	OH		Sinapic acid	OCH_3	OCH_3
p-hydroxy benzoic acid	H	H		Caffeic acid	OH	H
Dihydroxy benzoic acid	OH	H				

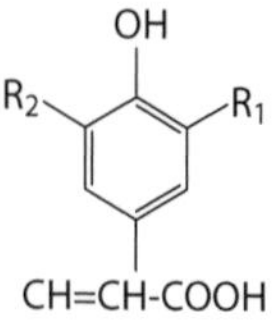

FIGURE 17.1 Phenolic acids as example of common natural antioxidants.

17.2.2 FLAVONOIDS

Flavonoids are naturally occurring substances in vegetables and fruits and are thought to have positive effects on human health (Ben Ammar et al. 2009). Flavonoids are low molecular weight compounds consisting of 15 carbon atoms arranged in a C_6–C_3–C_6 configuration. Essentially, the structure consists of two aromatic rings joined by a three-carbon bridge, usually in the form of a heterocyclic ring (Balasundram, Sundram, and Samman 2006; see Chapter 14). The flavonoids may themselves be divided into seven subclasses depending on the type of heterocycle involved: flavonols, flavones, isoflavones, flavanones, flavanols (Figure 17.2), anthocyanidins, and anthocyanins (Figure 17.3). The antioxidant activities of flavonoids and their forms have been extensively reviewed (Kilani-Jaziri et al. 2009). They can participate in protection against the harmful action of ROS and exhibit a wide range of biological effects, including antioxidant activity (Sreeramulu and Raghunath 2010). Flavonoids have also been found to inhibit a wide range of enzymes involved in oxidation systems, such as 5-lipoxygenase, cyclooxygenase, monooxygenase, or xanthine oxidase (Crespo et al. 2008).

17.2.3 CAROTENOIDS

Carotenoids are a family of more than 600 substances that are synthesized by higher plants and algae. They are a class of natural pigment, familiar to all through the orange-red to yellow colors of many fruits, vegetables, and flowers as well as for the provitamin A activity that some of them possess (Ribayo-Mercado et al. 2000). They are characterized by a linear polyisoprene structure with conjugated double bonds, either as such (lycopene) or as derived by cyclization of the two extremities with oxidation (xanthophylls, such as lutein and zeaxanthin) or without oxidation (carotenes). Carotenoid molecules, especially those without hydroxyl groups, are lipophilic (Noziere, Graulet, and Lucas 2006). Of the more than 600 naturally occurring carotenoids identified to date, 6 (β-carotene, β-cryptoxanthin, α-carotene, lycopene, lutein, and zeaxanthin) are commonly found in blood (Figure 15.5) (>95%

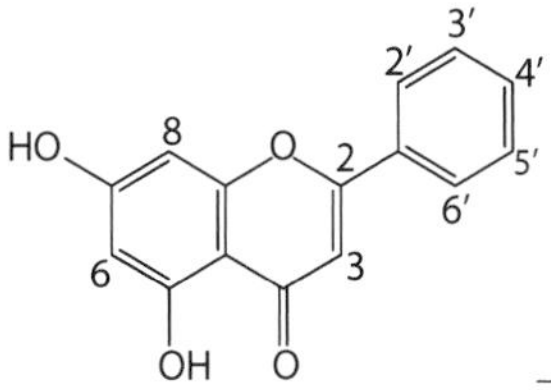

Flavones		
Compound	3'	4'
Apigenin	H	H
Chrysin	H	OH
Luteolin	OH	OH

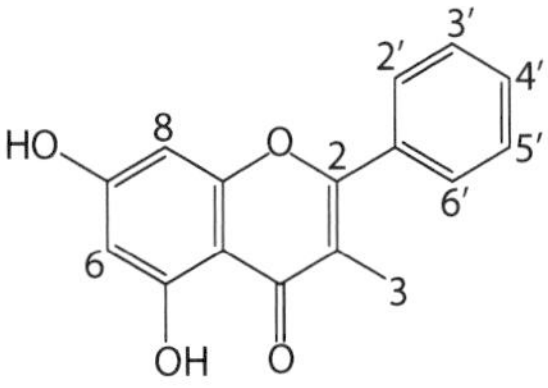

Flavonols				
Compound	2'	3'	4'	5'
Kaemperol	H	H	OH	H
Quercetin	H	OH	OH	H
Myricetin	H	OH	OH	OH
Datiscetin	OH	H	H	H
Morin	OH	H	OH	H
Rutin[Ψ]	H	OH	OH	H
Hesperidin[✱]	H	OH	COH$_3$	H

[Ψ] Rutin is a glycoside in which the C-3 position contains an o-rutinose.
[✱] Hesperidin contains a no-rutinose at the C-7 position.

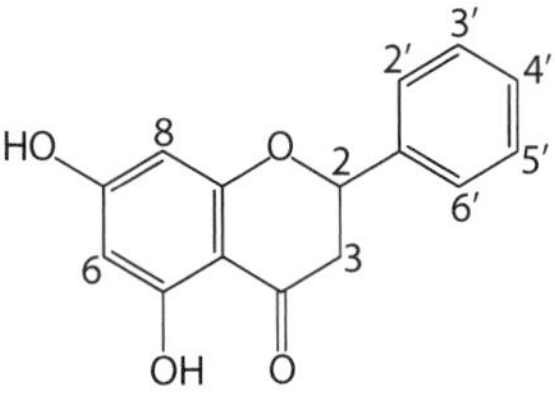

Flavanones			
Compound	3	3'	4'
Eriodictyol	H,H	OH	OH
Taxifolin	OH	OH	OH
Naringenin	H,H	H	OH
Naringin[Ψ]	ORh	H	OH

[Ψ] Naringin is a glycoside in which the C-3 position contains a rhamnoglucose unit.

FIGURE 17.2 Structure of flavones, flavonols, and flavanones and related compounds isolated from plant materials.

total blood carotenoids) (Maiani et al. 2009). Carotenoids have potential antioxidant properties because of their chemical structure consisting of abundant conjugated double bonds that interact with cellular membranes because of their fat-soluble nature (Riccioni 2009).

17.2.4 TANNINS

Tannins are high molecular weight plant compounds that can be divided into three chemically and biologically distinct groups: condensed tannins or proanthocyanidins (as found in tea, grapes, cranberries, and so on), hydrolyzable tannins or ETs (as in raspberries, strawberries, and so on), and GTs (Seeram et al. 2005). They differ from proanthocyanidins in their chemical structures. ETs are esters of hexahydroxydiphenic acid and a polyol, usually glucose or quinic acid (Clifford and Scalbert 2000). The

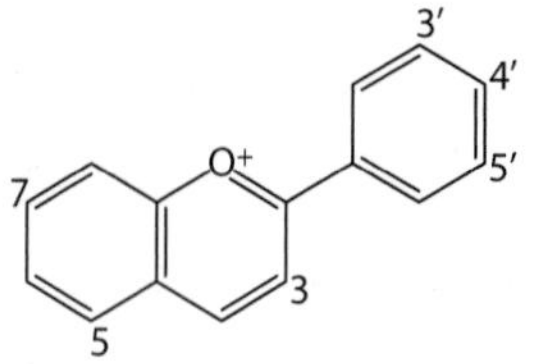

Anthocyanidins						
Compound	3	3'	4'	5'	5	7
Pelargonidin	OH	H	OH	H	OH	OH
Luteolidin	H	OH	OH	H	OH	OH
Cyanidin	OH	OH	OH	H	OH	OH
Apigenidin	H	H	OH	H	OH	OH
Malvidin	OH	OMe	OMe	OMe	OH	OH
Delphinidin	OH	OH	OH	OH	OH	OH
Petunidin	OH	OMe	OH	OH	OH	OH

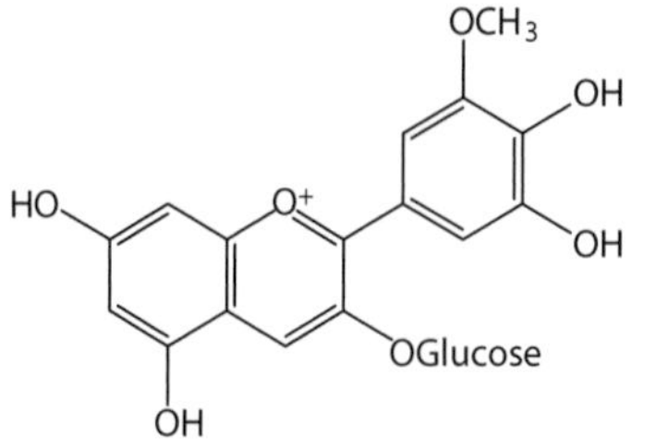

Petunidin 3-glucoside

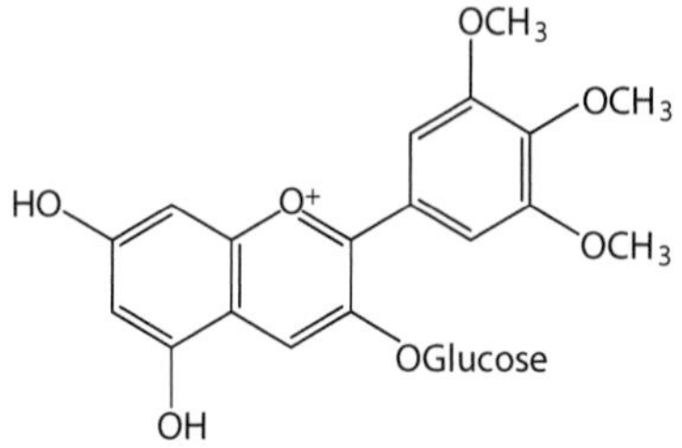

Malvidin 3-glucoside

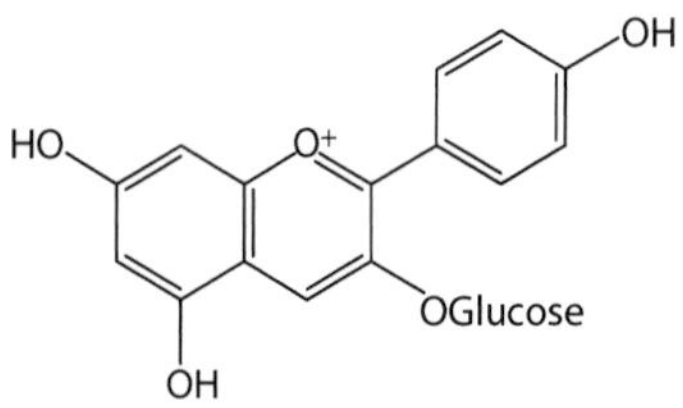

Pelargonidin 3-glucoside

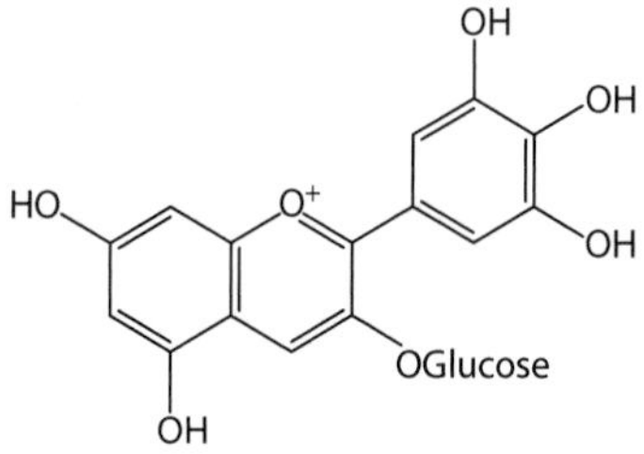

Delphidin 3-glucoside

FIGURE 17.3 Anthocyanidins and anthocyanins presents in fruits.

antioxidant activities of tannins have been widely demonstrated in the scientific literature (Osadee Wijekoon, Bhat, and Karim 2011; Zhou et al. 2011; Tian et al. 2012).

17.2.5 TERPENES

Terpenes are the name given to a substantial group of vegetal components with a common biosynthetic origin; they are the fundamental component of the essential oils from spices and aromatic herbs (Viuda-Martos et al. 2011). Despite their very different chemical structures, all result from the condensation of isoprenic units. Among their different forms are monoterpenes, diterpenes, and sesquiterpenes. They are extremely volatile and have been demonstrated to possess multiple functional properties, including antioxidant (Milan et al. 2008) and anticarcinogenic (Kim et al. 2003) capacities. Figure 17.4 shows several terpenes with demonstrated antioxidant activity.

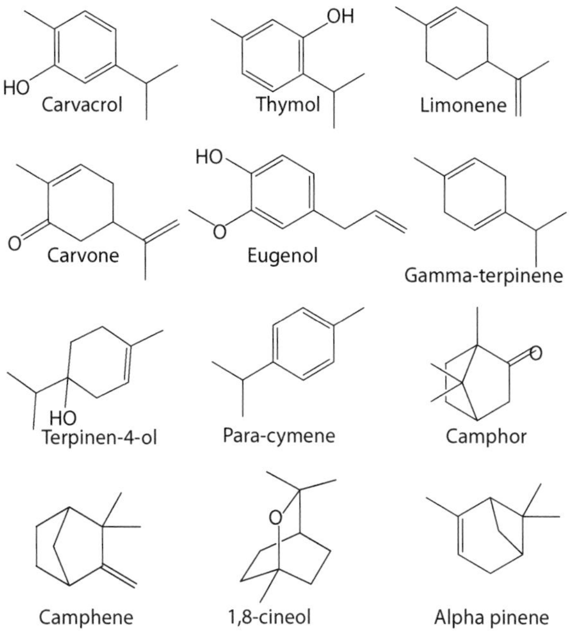

FIGURE 17.4 Main terpenes with antioxidant activity present in plants.

17.2.6 STEROLS AND STANOLS

Plant sterols are essential components of cell membranes and are present in all plants. They are structurally similar to cholesterol with differences in the side chain attached to the steroid ring (Carr and Jesh 2006). Human trials have established that plant sterols show lower total and LDL cholesterol uptake (Kritchevsky and Chen 2005). The most abundant sterols are β-sitosterol, campesterol, stigmastanol, and stigmasterol (Saura-Calixto and Goñi 2009). Stanols are saturated sterols and are much less abundant in nature than the corresponding sterols. Plant stanols comprise about 5%–10% of the total sterol/stanol mixture naturally present in the human diet (Valsta et al. 2004). Data comparing the impact of different sources of plant sterols on CVD risk factors and antioxidant levels are scarce, although some studies report the antioxidant activity of these compounds (Conforti et al. 2009; Heggen et al. 2010).

17.2.7 FIBER

Dietary fibers consist of a large group of substances that are not hydrolyzed by enzymes of the human small intestine. The main sources of dietary fiber in human nutrition are cereals, fruits, and vegetables (Dongowski 2007). The increased consumption of insoluble as well as soluble dietary fibers derived from some fruits and vegetables may promote a significant decrease in blood cholesterol concentrations (Chau, Huang, and Lin 2004). The exact mechanism by which dietary fibers lower serum LDL-cholesterol levels is not known. Evidence suggests that they may interfere with the lipid and/or bile acid metabolism. The hypocholesterolemic property of some dietary fiber is associated with the water-soluble fractions of fiber, such as uronic acid, glucomannans, and galactomannans (Trinidad et al. 2006). There are numerous scientific investigations that report the antioxidant activity of dietary fiber (Hassan et al. 2011; Navarro-González et al. 2011; Borchani et al. 2011).

17.3 FRUITS

Fruits and vegetables are important sources of various vitamins, minerals, and fibers for humans. However, they are different in many aspects, including the contents of vitamins, minerals, and fibers as well as their antioxidant capacities. It is well known that many fruits are rich in various antioxidants, including ascorbic acid, carotenoids, and polyphenolic compounds.

17.3.1 Pomegranate

Pomegranate (*Punica granatum* L.) fruits are globally consumed fresh and processed in the form of juice, jam, wine, and oil and in extract supplements (Gil et al. 2000). They contain high levels of a diverse range of phytochemicals of which polyphenols form a part, including punicalagin, ellagic acid, GTs, anthocyanins (cyanidin, delphinidin, and pelargonidin glycosides), and other flavonoids (quercetin, kaempferol, and luteolin glycosides) (Kim et al. 2002; Cerdá, Ceron, and Tomas-Barberan 2003). The health benefits of pomegranates, including their antioxidant and anti-atherosclerotic properties, have been attributed to this wide range of phytochemicals. Thus, Aviram, Rosenblat, and Gaitini (2004) investigated the effect of pomegranate juice consumption for 3 years on patients with carotid artery stenosis, finding that such consumption reduces common carotid intima-media thickness, blood pressure, and LDL oxidation. Anoosh, Mojtab, and Fatemeh (2010) analyzed the effect of pomegranate juice on plasma LDL-cholesterol in patients with hypercholesterolemia. These authors concluded that the consumption of pomegranate juice is beneficial for attenuating atherosclerosis development because it is associated with the reduced oxidation of LDL, the reduced uptake of oxidized LDL by macrophages, the reduced oxidative state of LDL, and reduced LDL aggregation. Sezer et al. (2007) compared the total phenol content and the antioxidant activity of pomegranate and red wines. The phenol levels of pomegranate and red wines (4850 mg/L gallic acid equivalents and 815 mg/L gallic acid equivalents, respectively) were in accordance with their total antioxidant activity (39.5% and 33.7%, respectively). Both wines decreased LDL-diene levels following a 30-min incubation period compared with controls (145 μmol/mg of LDL protein). However, pure pomegranate wine demonstrated a greater antioxidant effect on diene levels (110 μmol/mg of LDL protein) than red wine (124 μmol/mg of LDL protein). de Nigris et al. (2006) noted that pomegranate juice reduced the oxidized LDL down-regulation of endothelial nitric oxide synthase (NOSIII) in human coronary endothelial cells. Data suggested that pomegranate juice can exert beneficial effects on the evolution of clinical vascular complications, coronary heart disease, and atherogenesis in humans by enhancing NOSIII bioactivity. This is related to the positive effects of lowering blood pressure in hypertensive patients. Ignarro et al.

(2006) investigated the effects of pomegranate juice for its capacity to protect nitric oxide against oxidative destruction and enhance the biological actions of nitric oxide. The results demonstrate that pomegranate juice is a potent inhibitor of the superoxide anion-mediated disappearance of nitric oxide. These data suggest that pomegranate and pomegranate juice have considerable anti-atherosclerotic, anti-hypertensive, antioxidant, and anti-inflammatory effects in human subjects. The principal mechanism by which pomegranate juice acts may include decreasing systolic blood pressure, thus causing an overall positive effect on the progression of atherosclerosis and any ensuing potential development of coronary heart disease (Stowe 2011).

17.3.2 Açai

Açai berries (*Euterpe oleracea* Mart.) have recently gained popularity in North America and Europe as a new "super fruit" largely as a result of its extremely high antioxidant capacity and potential anti-inflammatory activities (Schauss et al. 2006a). The predominant chemical constituents of açai fruits are polyphenols, especially anthocyanins and flavonoids (Pacheco-Palencia, Duncan, and Talcott 2009). A complete nutrient analysis of freeze-dried açai fruit pulp/skin powder showed that it is very rich in polyphenols, especially anthocyanins (cyanidin 3-glucoside and cyanidin 3-rutinoside) and other compounds, such as unsaturated fatty acids (oleic and linoleic acids), phytosterols (β-sitosterol), and dietary fiber (Schauss et al. 2006b).

Using a range of biomarkers and serum lipid profiles, de Souza et al. (2010) investigated the *in vivo* antioxidant effects of açai pulp in rats that were given different (normal and hypercholesterolemic) diets, some of which were enriched with açai. Serum levels of carbonyl proteins and total, free, and protein sulfhydryl groups were reduced by açai ingestion in animals receiving the standard or hypercholesterolemic diet. Açai supplementation led to a significant reduction in superoxide dismutase activity, indicating an association between diet and açai treatment. Also, açai supplementation increased paraoxonase activity. These results suggest that the consumption of açai improves antioxidant status. Recently, Xie et al. (2011) investigated the athero-protective effects of a diet containing 5% of açai juice for 20 weeks in mice. The authors reported that biomarkers of lipid peroxidation, including F2-isoprostanes and isomers of hydroxyoctadecadienoic acids and hydroxyeicosatetraenoic acids, were significantly lower in serum and in the liver, and the expression of the two antioxidant enzyme genes, Gpx3 and Gsr, was significantly upregulated. Mertens-Talcott et al. (2008) showed that the consumption of açai juice or pulp by healthy human volunteers caused a significant increase in their plasma antioxidant capacity, which also indicates that açai fruits have antioxidant potential *in vivo*. Pozo-Insfran, Brenes, and Talcoot (2004) concluded that the anthocyanin content was the predominant contributing factor to the antioxidant capacity of açai, which was found to be higher than that of muscadine grape juice and of several berries, such as highbush blueberries, strawberries, raspberries, blackberries, and cranberries.

17.3.3 Berries

Berries from different species, such as strawberries (*Fragaria* x *ananasa*), blueberries (*Vaccinium corymbosum*), blackberries (*Rubus fruticosus*), black raspberries

(*Rubus occidentalis*), red raspberries (*Rubus idaeus*), and wolfberries (*Lycium barbarum*), have demonstrated a high antioxidant activity (Hassan and Yousef 2009; Lau, Joseph, and McDonald 2009; Hassan and Abdel-Aziz 2010), which can be attributed to the phytochemical compounds and antioxidant enzymes they contain. These phytochemicals include phenolics, such as anthocyanins, quercetin, proanthocyanidins, hydrolyzable tannins, and other flavonoid-related molecules (Seeram 2008). The main antioxidant enzymes in berries are glutathione peroxidase (GPx), superoxide dismutase (SOD), guaiacol peroxidase (G-POD), ascorbate peroxidase (AsA-POD), monodehydroascorbate reductase (MDAR), dehydroascorbate reductase (DHAR), and glutathione reductase (GR), and the major nonenzyme components are ascorbate (AsA) and glutathione (GSH) (Jiao and Wang 2000; Wang et al. 2005b; Wang and Ballington 2007). Berry phenolics are best known for their ability to act as antioxidants, but the biological activities exerted by berry phytochemicals *in vivo* extend beyond antioxidation. In fact, a large and growing body of evidence shows that berry phytochemicals regulate the activities of metabolizing enzymes; modulate nuclear receptors, gene expression, and subcellular signaling pathways; and repair DNA oxidative damage (Seeram 2006).

Jiao, Liu, and Wang (2005) reported that the total pigment extract from blackberries exhibited strong antioxidant activity against lipid peroxidation and scavenging capacities toward superoxide anion radicals and hydroxyl radicals. Szajdek and Borowska (2008) showed that blueberry juice constituents are noted for the ability to strengthen blood-vessel walls, improve blood-vessel elasticity, improve peripheral circulation, and inhibit LDL oxidation. Basu et al. (2010) reported that the screening of large populations of multiple berry species established a link between the antioxidant capacity of the berry types and the ability of the extracts to inhibit LDL oxidation.

17.3.4 DATE PALM

Date (*Phoenix dactylifera* L.) fruits are rich in phytochemicals, such as phenolics, flavonoids, sterols, carotenoids, procyanidins, and anthocyanins. The selenium present in dates is also reported to contribute to the antioxidant effects. Multiple studies have shown that this essential trace element exerts its antioxidant function mainly in the form of seleno-cysteine residues that are integral constituents of ROS-detoxifying seleno-enzymes (GPx, thioredoxin reductases, and possibly seleno-protein P) (Steinbrenner and Sies 2009). The amounts of these compounds contribute to the nutritional and organoleptic characteristics of the fruits (Hasan et al. 2010; Baliga et al. 2011). In addition, phytochemicals from dates have been shown to possess significant antioxidant capacities. Vayalil (2002) was the first to demonstrate that the aqueous extract of date fruit was a potent scavenger of superoxide and hydroxyl radicals and capable of inhibiting iron-induced lipid peroxidation and protein oxidation in a rat brain homogenate in a concentration-dependent manner. Studies conducted on the antioxidant activity and phenolic content of various fruits of *Phoenix dactylifera* cultivated in Iran, Algeria, and Bahrain demonstrated a linear relationship between antioxidant activity and the total phenolic content (TPC) of date fruit extract (Allaith 2005). Aqueous date extract was found to significantly inhibit lipid peroxidation and protein oxidation and also to exhibit a potent superoxide and hydroxyl radical-scavenging activity in a dose-dependent manner in an *in vitro* study (Dammak et al. 2007). Wasseem et al. (2009) analyzed the *in vivo* effect of Medjool or Hallawi date consumption on oxidative stress in healthy subjects. Both date varieties were seen to possess antioxidative properties *in vitro*. The susceptibility of serum to AAPH-induced lipid peroxidation decreased by 12% but only after Hallawi date consumption. In agreement with the above results, serum activity of the HDL-associated antioxidant enzyme paraoxonase 1 (PON1) significantly increased (by 8%) after Hallawi date consumption.

17.3.5 PERSIMMONS

Persimmons (*Diospyros kaki* L.) originated in Japan. They are processed for use as a sweetening ingredient for baked products and fruit ice creams, jellies, and nectars in dry form. The crude plant extract is a complex mixture containing vitamins, *p*-coumaric acid, gallic acid, catechin, flavonoids, carotenoids, and condensed tannins, and it is used in its fresh form as a source of natural antioxidants (Dembitsky et al. 2011). Thus, Gorinstein et al. (2000) compared the hypolipidemic and antioxidant effects of two diets fortified with 7% whole dry persimmon and 7% phenol-free dry persimmon, respectively. The results of this experiment showed that both diets improved lipid levels, but only the diet supplemented with whole persimmon exerted an antioxidant effect. Therefore, the antioxidant effect of this fruit is associated mainly with the phenols it contains and not with the fiber. Katsube et al. (2004) studied the antioxidant activity of one astringent and one non-astringent persimmon by means of LDL oxidation and DPPH assays. In both methods, the astringent persimmon showed values (111 ± 1 and 88 ± 4 µmol of epigallocatechin gallate equivalent per gram of fresh weight, respectively) approximately two orders of magnitude higher than those of the non-astringent persimmon and approximately five or six times higher than the values observed in mulberries and blueberries. Persimmon peel was reported to act as a valuable source of antioxidants in the diabetic condition because it reduced oxidative stress induced by hyperglycemia (Yokozawa et al. 2007). Tian et al. (2012) evaluated the antioxidant activities of high molecular weight persimmon condensed tannin in an *ex vivo* tissue system and *in vivo*. An oral dose of high molecular weight condensed persimmon tannin at 200 or 400 mg/kg significantly prevented the bromobenzene-induced decrease in serum and liver SOD and GPx activities and decreased liver malondialdehyde levels in bromobenzene-treated mice. The results suggest that dietary high molecular weight condensed tannin from persimmon may provide protection from oxidative damage both *ex vivo* and *in vivo*.

17.3.6 CITRUS FRUITS

Citrus fruits are rich sources of vitamin C (ascorbic acid), an essential nutrient with well-described antioxidant properties. However, recent studies have demonstrated that citrus also contains other bioactive compounds, including flavonoids, coumarins, carotenoids, and limonoids, with potential health-promoting properties (Wilmsen, Spada, and Salvador 2005). Moreover, the main phytochemical compounds in citrus fruits are terpenes present in the essential oil, phenolic acids, and flavonoid compounds (Fernández-López et al. 2009). Within the flavonoids, hesperidin is the most abundant flavanone glycoside found in citrus. Citrus peels also contain other important flavonoids, such as narigin, narirutin, diosmin, and eriocitrin (Schieber, Stintzing, and Carle 2001; Fernández-López et al. 2007).

Recent studies have pointed to an interaction between the bioactive compounds present in citrus fruits and antioxidant activity. Using the thiobarbituric acid reactive substances (TBARS) assay, Londoño-Londoño et al. (2010) demonstrated that all flavonoid fractions (hesperidin, neohesperidin, diosmin, nobiletin, and tangeritin) present in orange peel were able to inhibit copper (Cu^{2+}) or peroxynitrite (ONOO$^-$) induced human LDL oxidation. Differences in the antioxidant activity of individual components from flavonoid fractions were also observed. Lo et al. (2010) reported that 3',4'-dihydroxy-5,6,7,8-tetramethoxyflavone (DTF), a major metabolite of nobiletin (a citrus polymethoxylated flavone), reduces LDL oxidation, attenuates monocyte differentiation into macrophage, and blunts the uptake of modified LDL by macrophage. The effect is different from that of nobiletin, from which DTF is derived. As mentioned above, hesperidin is the most abundant flavanone glycoside found in citrus peel. Hesperidin is reported to have the ability to inhibit copper-induced LDL oxidation (Cirico and Omaye 2006). Essential oils from lemon prevent LDL oxidation and are able to reduce plasmatic levels of cholesterol and triglycerides. The mechanism by which essential oils reduce LDL oxidation involves preventing the oxidation of intrinsic carotenoids of LDL (Milde, Elstner, and Graßmann 2007). Compounds present in lemon peel have been described as preventing LDL oxidation and reducing plaque formation, thus decreasing the risk of CVD (Takahashi et al. 2003).

17.3.7 Exotic Fruits

Besides their delicious taste and flavor, exotic fruits are an important source of bioactive compounds in the human diet; moreover, the consumption of exotic fruits is increasing in the domestic and international markets because of the growing recognition of their nutritional value (Loizzo et al. 2012).

Mango (*Mangifera indica* L.) is one of the most important tropical fruits. The consumption of mango could provide significant amounts of bioactive compounds to the human diet. The major polyphenols in mango in terms of antioxidative capacity and/or quantity are mangiferin, catechins, quercetin, kaempferol, rhamnetin, anthocyanins, gallic and ellagic acids, propyl and methyl gallate, benzoic acid and protocatechuic acid carotenoids, and vitamin C (González-Aguilar et al. 2008; Vijaya Kumar Reddy, Sreeramulu, and Raghunath 2010; Dembitsky et al. 2011). In a recent study, Robles-Sánchez et al. (2011) analyzed the antioxidant capacity of whole and fresh-cut mango and their influence on the serum antioxidant capacity and lipid profile of normolipidemic humans. These authors reported a significant effect on fasting plasma antioxidant capacity levels, measured as TEAC and ORAC, and concluded that the daily consumption of mango for 30 days induced significant effects on plasma antioxidant capacity. In another study, an increase in the antioxidant capacity of plasma was also found in rat diets supplemented with mango juice for 4 months (García-Solís, Yahia, and Aceves 2008).

Cherimoya (*Annona cherimola*) is a subtropical fruit tree indigenous to Ecuador and Peru, which is cultivated in Taiwan, Spain, and the south of Italy, too. This fruit is rich in health-promoting compounds, such as cherimoline, cherinonaine, kauranes, lignans, amides, acetogenins, lactam amide, purines, steroids, alkaloids, *p*-quinone, benzenoids, and polyamine (Chen et al. 1998, 1999). Little has been published concerning the antioxidant activity of cherimoya, although the antioxidant and cytoprotective properties of cherimoya pulp organic extracts were analyzed by Barreca et al. (2011). Their results clearly show that cherimoya has a high total phenol content, in particular, flavanols and procyanidins (dimers and trimers), and a high antioxidant potential against a great variety of radical reactive species. Gupta-Elera et al. (2011) analyzed the potential health benefits of cherimoya consumption by examining the antioxidant activity of its individual components, including skin, flesh, and juice. Initial analyses suggested that *A. cherimola* has strongly antioxidative properties and that the highest antioxidative potential is found in the juice followed by the skin. For these authors, the regular consumption of cherimoya may contribute to increasing the antioxidant capacity of human serum and may thereby help to prevent the development and progression of CVD, neurodegenerative diseases, cancer, and other diseases thought to be linked to oxidative stress.

Lychee (*Litchi chinensis*) polysaccharides from pulp tissue show potential antioxidant capacities. Thus, Kong et al. (2010) demonstrated that four polysaccharide-enriched fractions extracted from lychee pulp tissue exhibit dose-dependent free radical-scavenging activity. Guava (*Psidium guajava* L.) is an important fruit, and it is available all year round fresh and processed as juice. Guava fruit contains several phytochemicals with antioxidant activity. Jimenez-Escrig et al. (2001) evaluated the antioxidant activity of guava pulp and peel fractions, finding that all the fractions tested showed a remarkable antioxidant capacity, which was correlated with the corresponding TPC. A 1 g (dry matter) portion of peel contained DPPH and ferric reducing antioxidant power (FRAP) activities and the ability to inhibit copper-induced *in vitro* LDL oxidation, equivalent to 43, 116, and 176 mg of Trolox, respectively.

Longan (*Dimocarpus longan* Lour.) belongs to the *Sapindaceae* family and is a highly attractive fruit that is extensively distributed in the Southern part of China. Longan fruit pericarp contains high amounts of bioactive compounds, such as phenolic acids, flavonoids, hydrolysable tannins, and polysaccharides (Rangkadilok et al. 2007; Yang et al. 2008). When Prasad et al. (2009) determined the antioxidant activity of two extracts of longan fruit, the lipid peroxidation inhibitory activity of a high-pressure-assisted extract was higher at every concentration tested than the activity of a conventional extract, and its inhibitory activity was dose-dependent. The EC_{50} values for high-pressure-assisted and conventional extracts and butylated hydroxytoluene were 40.23, 58.03, and 17.45 µg/mL, respectively.

17.4   VEGETABLES

There is consensus among nutrition scientists that a high consumption of vegetables is associated with reduced risks of developing numerous diseases. Efforts to encourage higher vegetable consumption may be more successful if they mention the benefits associated with healthy vegetable-eating habits. Garlic, broccoli, tomatoes, carrots, Brussels sprouts, kale, cabbage, onions, cauliflower, and red beets are mentioned as being among the richest sources of antioxidants.

17.4.1 TOMATOES

Of all vegetables, the tomato (*Lycopersicon esculentum*) is both qualitatively and quantitatively one of the most important components of the Mediterranean diet. Tomatoes are mainly consumed as a raw staple food because of their desirable nutritional properties, but they are also increasingly used in many popular tomato products (Pérez-Conesa et al. 2009). More than 80% of tomatoes grown are consumed in the form of processed products, such as juice, soup, concentrate, dry-concentrate, sauce, puree, dry-tomato, ketchup, or paste (Kaur et al. 2008). Tomato foods contain bioactive compounds that have a protective effect against some diseases (Markovits, Ben Amotz, and Levy 2009). The most abundant bioactive compounds in tomatoes are lycopene, ascorbic acid, and α-tocopherol (Frusciante et al. 2007). A variety of epidemiological studies have suggested that the intake of lycopene-containing foods is inversely related to the incidence of LDL oxidation. Thus, several clinical trials have provided evidence that lycopene plays a pivotal role in lowering oxidative stress, in particular, in preventing the oxidation of LDL (Basu and Imrhan 2007). Ghaffari and Ghiasvand (2006) reported that lycopene suppressed the formation of TBARS and LDL–copper complex in a dose-dependent manner. Lycopene, at concentrations of 10, 50, and 100 µM, reduced the susceptibility of LDL to oxidative modification by approximately 31%, 67%, and 71%, respectively. Alshatwi et al. (2010) reported that tomato powder is more effective than lycopene-beadlet against lipid peroxidation in the liver as well as in preventing the rise in serum malondialdehyde when challenged with H_2O_2 feeding. Bose and Agrawal (2007) indicated that lycopene raised the concentration of glutathione, the most important antioxidant metabolite, which plays a major role in maintaining high concentrations of glutathione peroxidase activity. Glutathione peroxidase is the main enzyme involved in removing H_2O_2 generated from superoxide anions by superoxide dismutase.

17.4.2 GARLIC

Garlic (*Allium sativum*) has been cultivated since ancient times and has been used as a spice and condiment for many centuries. Garlic contains biologically active compounds that exert multiple beneficial effects on the human organism (Banerjee, Mukherjee, and Maulik 2003). Ninety-five percent of the sulfur in intact garlic cloves is found in two classes of compound in similar abundance: the *S*-alkylcysteine sulfoxides and the γ-glutamyl-*S*-alkylcysteines (Christian, Yvan, and Myriam 2011).

The antioxidant properties of garlic are well documented (Durak et al. 2004a,b; Gedik et al. 2005). Thus, Benjamin and Lau (2001) reported that several garlic compounds can effectively suppress LDL oxidation *in vitro*. Short-term supplementation of garlic in human subjects has demonstrated an increased resistance of LDL to oxidation. These data suggest that suppressing LDL oxidation may be one of the most powerful mechanisms that account for the anti-atherosclerotic properties of garlic. Durak et al. (2004a) reported that the ingestion of garlic extract leads to significantly lower plasma and erythrocyte malondialdehyde levels in patients even in the absence of any change in antioxidant enzyme activities. Their results also demonstrated that ingesting garlic extract prevented oxidation reactions by eliminating oxidant stress in blood samples from patients with atherosclerosis. Avci et al. (2008) reported that garlic significantly lowers plasma and erythrocyte malondialdehyde levels while increasing antioxidant enzyme activity in elderly subjects. The beneficial effects of aqueous garlic extract in the prevention of oxidative stress were associated with organosulfur compounds through reduced aortic NAD(P)H-oxidase activity and lipid peroxidation as recently demonstrated in an experimental model of metabolic syndrome induced by fructose administration (Vazquez-Prieto et al. 2010). Heidarian, Jafari-Dehkordi, and Seidkhani-Nahal (2011) reported that garlic supplementation potentially resulted in a significant increase in plasma antioxidant power and a decrease in plasma malondialdehyde levels in treated rats, suggesting that garlic might have antioxidant activities to produce such responses.

17.4.3 ONION

The onion (*Allium cepa* L.), a family of *Allium* plants, has been used in spice blends and foods, as flavoring, and as medicinal remedies. It is a versatile vegetable that is consumed fresh and as a processed product, in powdered form as a flavor enhancer and a dried form as a seasoning (Takahashi and Shibamoto 2008). The nutritional composition of onion is very complex. It has been shown to be one of the major sources of dietary flavonoids in many countries. More specifically, onion has been characterized for its flavonol quercetin and quercetin derivates (Roldán et al. 2008). Moreover, it is rich in other bioactive compounds, such as fructooligosaccharides and sulfur compounds. Sulfur-containing components in *Allium* species consist of volatiles (disulfides, trisulfides, etc.) and nonvolatiles (sulfur-containing amino acids). The volatile sulfur compounds, such as dialk(en)yl disulfides and dialk(en)yl trisulfides, are produced by the enzymatic reaction of alk(en)yl-L-cysteine sulfoxides with C-S lyase, followed by thermochemical reactions when *Allium* vegetables are cut or ruptured (Block et al. 1996). More recently, renewed attention has been paid to the antioxidant content of onions because many epidemiological studies have suggested that the regular consumption of onions in food is associated with the prevention of vascular and heart diseases through the inhibition of lipid peroxidation. For example, Nuutila et al. (2003) found an observable correlation between high radical-scavenging or antioxidant activity and high amounts of total phenolics and flavonoids in onion extracts, suggesting that the phenolic compounds of onion contribute to their antioxidative properties. Moreover, these authors showed that skin extracts of onion possessed the highest activities. Wang et al. (2005a) investigated the effects of aqueous extracts of Welsh onion green leaves on the oxidation of LDLs and the production of nitric oxide in macrophages. The results showed that aqueous extracts of Welsh onion green leaves in the range of 0.1–1.0 mg/mL inhibited LDL oxidation and scavenged ABTS$^{\bullet+}$ radicals in a cellular system. Gülsen, Makris, and Kefalas (2007) indicated that the dry outer layers of onion, which are wasted before food processing or cooking, contain large amounts of quercetin, quercetin glycoside, and their oxidative products, which are effective antioxidants against nonenzymatic lipid peroxidation and the oxidation of LDLs. Park et al. (2009) investigated the effects of onion, red onion, or quercetin oil plasma antioxidant vitamin on lipid peroxidation and leukocyte DNA damage in rats. The high fat-cholesterol diet resulted in significantly higher plasma lipid peroxidation, which decreased with onion, red onion, or quercetin supplementation.

17.5 OILS

The dietary sources of monounsaturated fatty acids, polyunsaturated fatty acids, and antioxidant compounds are numerous and mainly represented by different plant oils, such as sunflower, maize, argan, soya, olive, and others.

17.5.1 OLIVE OIL

Virgin olive oil is the most commonly used cooking fat in Mediterranean countries; it is produced in large quantities from the fruit *Olea europea* L. Virgin olive oil is produced from the first and second pressings of the olive fruit by the cold pressing method (where no chemicals and only a small amount of heat are applied) and is composed of a glycerol fraction (90%–99% of the olive fruit) and a nonglycerol or unsaponifiable fraction (0.4%–5.0% of the olive fruit) (Tripoli et al. 2005; Sánchez-Zapata and Pérez-Álvarez 2008). The biological benefits of olive oil consumption in preventing LDLs from oxidation could be linked both to its antioxidant content, mainly phenolic compounds and vitamin E, and to its high monounsaturated fatty acid content (Marrugat et al. 2004). The principal phenolic compounds present in olive oil are tyrosol, hydroxytyrosol, oleuropein glycoside, ferrulic acid, *p*-coumaric acid, cinnamic acid, *p*-hydroxybenzoic acid, gallic acid, caffeic acid, luteolin, apigenin, vanillic acid, and 3,4-dihydroxybenzoic acid (Ballus et al. 2011). A review of human intervention studies shows that olive polyphenols decrease the levels of oxidized-LDL in plasma and positively affect several biomarkers of oxidative damage.

Some studies have reported a good correlation between the lag time for LDL oxidation and the phenolic content of olive oil—a high level of association being observed with the α-tocopherol content and a lower level with the β-carotene content (Fito et al. 2000). Marrugat et al. (2004) suggested that the sustained consumption of phenol-rich olive oil was more effective in protecting LDL from oxidation and in raising HDL-C than olive oils with lower quantities of phenolics. Thus, urinary tyrosol and hydroxytyrosol increased, *in vivo* plasma oxidized LDL decreased, and the *ex vivo* resistance of LDL to oxidation increased with the phenolic content of the olive oil administered. Weinbrenner et al. (2004) reported a greater decrease in LDL oxidation concentrations following the consumption of olive oil with a high phenolic content compared to than obtained after consuming oil with a low phenolic content. Examining the role of the phenolic compounds from olive oil on postprandial oxidative stress and LDL antioxidant content, Covas et al. (2006) reported that all olive oils promoted postprandial oxidative stress indicated by increased levels of F2-isoprostanes; however, the degree of LDL oxidation decreased as the phenolic content of the administered oil increased. Dietary virgin olive oil phenols have also been shown to increase the resistance to LDL lipoprotein oxidation and oxidative DNA damage in humans (Salvini et al. 2006).

Nakbi et al. (2010) investigated the antioxidant properties of two varieties of olive oil (Chetoui and Chemlali) and the protective effect of phenolic extracts from these varieties against LDL oxidation *in vitro*. These authors reported that the highest antioxidant activity was that of Chetoui oil (78.56% vs. 37.23% of DPPH and 2.42 vs. 0.61 mmol Trolox/kg). Chetoui phenolic extract also had a significantly greater inhibitory effect on LDL oxidation than Chemlali phenolic extract. de la Torre-Carbot et al. (2010) found that the phenol concentration of olive oil modulates the phenolic metabolite content in LDL after sustained daily consumption. The inverse relationship of these metabolites with the degree of LDL oxidation supports the *in vivo* antioxidant role of olive oil phenolic compounds.

17.5.2 ARGAN OIL

The argan fruit (*Argania spinosa*) is rich in fat. Argan oil is very interesting because of its particular chemical properties. It is composed of 45% of monounsaturated fatty acids, 35% of polyunsaturated fatty acids, and 20% of saturated fatty acids. Moreover, this oil is rich in minor components, such as phytosterols, tocopherols, and phenolic compounds (Khallouki et al. 2003). Polyunsaturated fatty acids have a protective effect against oxidation as explained by the presence of the double bonds. Argan oil is rich in oleic and linoleic acids, which show low susceptibility to peroxidation (Berrougui et al. 2003). Also, argan oil is rich in phytosterols, which are known for their beneficial effects on lipid markers (Marangoni and Poli 2010). The hypocholesterolemic effect of argan oil may be a result of its high content of sterols in the minor compound fraction. Numerous studies have been conducted to evaluate the beneficial properties of virgin argan oil phenolic extracts in protecting human LDL against lipid peroxidation. Thus, Drissi et al. (2004) investigated the effect of regular virgin argan oil consumption on the lipid profile and antioxidant status in Moroccan subjects and the *in vitro* effect of argan oil on LDL peroxidation. These authors reported that plasma lipid peroxides were lower (58.3%) while the α-tocopherol concentration (13.4%) was higher in argan oil consumers than in nonconsumers. However, despite the levels of plasma antioxidants and lower levels of lipid peroxides in argan oil consumers, LDL oxidation susceptibility remained similar. A prospective Cherki et al. (2005) study showed that the everyday consumption of virgin argan oil has an LDL-cholesterol lowering and an antioxidant effect because the susceptibility of LDL to lipid peroxidation showed a significant increase in the lag phase, accompanied by a significant decrease in maximum diene production. These facts suggest that argan oil could play a role in CVD prevention by reducing the susceptibility of LDL to oxidation. Berrougui et al. (2006) evaluated LDL lipid peroxidation in the presence of argan oil by conjugated diene and malondialdehyde formation and vitamin E disappearance. These authors suggested that virgin argan oil provides a source of dietary phenolic antioxidants, which prevent CVDs by inhibiting LDL oxidation and enhancing reverse cholesterol transport. Ould Mohamedou et al. (2011) investigated the effect of argan oil consumption on serum lipids, apolipoproteins (AI and B), and LDL susceptibility to oxidation in type

2 diabetic patients. The susceptibility of LDL to lipid peroxidation was significantly reduced as seen from the 20.95% increase in the lag phase after argan oil consumption. This could be a result of the fact that isolated LDL particles from patients may be enriched with different antioxidants from argan oil, reducing their susceptibility to lipid peroxidation.

17.5.3　Coconut Oil

Coconut oil is believed to increase blood cholesterol because it mostly contains saturated fatty acids. Usually coconut oil is obtained by a drying process in which copra is exposed to very high temperatures or sunlight for several days until most of the moisture is removed. Such exposure to sunlight or high temperatures may inactivate the minor components, such as tocopherols, tocotrienols, and polyphenols (Wyatt, Carballido, and Mendez 1998). On the other hand, virgin coconut oil (VCO) extracted directly from coconut milk by a wet process at a controlled temperature may have more beneficial effects than copra oil (CO) because it retains most of the unsaponifiable components. Nevin and Rajmohan (2004) investigated the effect of the consumption of VCO by analyzing the preventive effect of the polyphenol fraction from test oils on the copper-induced oxidation of LDL and carbonyl formation. The results demonstrated the potential beneficial effect of VCO in lowering lipid levels in serum and tissues and in decreasing LDL oxidation by physiological oxidants as a result of reduced carbonyl formation. In a similar study, Nevin and Rajmohan (2006) analyzed the effect of VCO on the antioxidant enzyme activities and lipid peroxidation level in rats. VCO had higher levels of unsaponifiable components, which contained vitamin E and polyphenols, than refined CO. The lipoprotein levels and the conjugated dienes were significantly lower in the heart, liver, and kidneys of rats fed with VCO than in those fed with refined CO. Refined CO had a similar fatty acid composition to VCO. VCO also significantly increased the antioxidant enzyme activities and reduced the lipid peroxide content. Nagaraju and Belur (2008) studied the effects of feeding Wistar rats with blended and interesterified oils of coconut groundnut (GNO) or CO olive (OLO) oils on liver antioxidant enzyme activities and the susceptibility of LDL to oxidation. The results demonstrated that CO blended and interesterified with GNO or OLO enhanced hepatic antioxidant enzymes, decreased lipid peroxidation in liver, and reduced the susceptibility of LDL to oxidation.

17.6　CEREALS

Cereals, mainly barley, maize, rice, wheat, sorghum, millet, oat, rye, or triticale, play an important role in human nutrition. Whole-grain cereals contain a much wider range of compounds with potential antioxidant effects than refined cereals. These include polyphenols, especially phenolic acids, such as ferulic, vanillic, caffeic, syringic, sinapic, and p-coumaric acids; vitamin E (mainly in the germ); folates; minerals (iron, zinc) and trace elements (selenium, copper, and manganese); carotenoids; phytic acid; lignin; and other compounds, such as betaine, choline, sulfur amino acids, alkylresorcinols, and lignans found mainly in the bran fraction (Fardet, Rock, and Rémésy 2008). Epidemiological studies have clearly demonstrated that a diet containing whole-grain cereals can protect against metabolic disorders, such as CVDs (Anderson 2003). For example, Gray et al. (2002) reported that oats contain antioxidants, recoverable by 50% ethanol or isopropanol, which can protect LDL from oxidation *in vitro*. In terms of stabilizing LDL particles, this may be related to the tocol and/or phenolic alkyl conjugate content of the isopropanol polar extract. Chen et al. (2004) reported that no effect was observed on *ex vivo* resistance of LDL to Cu^{2+}-induced oxidation following oat bran consumption by hamsters but that the direct addition of oat phenolics inhibited *in vitro* Cu^{2+}-induced human plasma LDL oxidation and that this inhibition was dose-dependent. The protection against oxidation provided to LDL by cereal extracts can be extended to the lipids present in tissues. For Liu et al. (2011), the antioxidant ability of oats may stimulate the expression of antioxidant enzyme mRNA in a molecular mechanism. Wheat is a staple food for the majority of the world's population and serves as a source of potentially health-enhancing components. Yu, Zhou, and Parry (2005) examined bran extracts of Akron and Trego wheat for their inhibitory activities against lipid peroxidation in human LDL. These authors reported that all bran extracts significantly reduced lipid peroxidation in LDL. The greatest activity in suppressing LDL oxidation was detected in Akron bran (1.56 mg TBARS reduction/g bran), and the Trego bran showed the lowest activity (1.03 mg TBARS reduction/g bran). Liyana-Pathirana and Shahidi (2005) indicated that samples of wheat germ and bran possessed a higher total phenol content than whole grain and flour and demonstrated the greatest inhibition against LDL oxidation. These authors concluded that aqueous extracts of wheat contained phenolic compounds that contributed to total antioxidant activity, which was significantly enhanced when wheat samples were subjected to simulated gastrointestinal pH treatment prior to extraction. The low pH could have improved the extractability of the phenolic compounds from wheat. Aqueous methanolic extracts of whole kernels from six different barley cultivars were examined by Madhujith and Shahidi (2007) for their efficacy in the inhibition of Cu^{2+}-induced human LDL cholesterol oxidation. They found that barley extracts provided 19.64–33.93% inhibition against Cu^{2+}-induced human LDL cholesterol oxidation at a final concentration of 0.02 mg/mL. Parrado et al. (2003) showed that an extract of a rice bran fraction (a water-soluble oryzanol enzymatic extract) protected the proteins and lipids in rat brain homogenates from oxidation. Andreasen et al. (2001) determined the total phenol contents of the flour, whole grain, and bran of rye. The total phenol contents in whole grain and bran of rye were 5.6- and 14.8-fold, respectively, higher than that of rye flour. Moreover, the antioxidant activity of bran extracts against copper-induced oxidation of LDL was significantly higher than that of whole grain and flour.

17.7 LEGUMES

Legumes are rich source of proteins, dietary fiber, micronutrients, and bioactive phytochemicals. The nutritional value of legumes as a source of good-quality proteins and micronutrients in the daily diet is very significant, having the added advantage of being significantly cheaper than animal proteins. Supplementing cereal-based diets with legumes improves overall nutritional status and could be one of the best solutions for preventing the protein-calorie malnutrition observed in developing countries (Marathe et al. 2011). A variety of studies have observed the antioxidant activities of many legumes, such as yellow and green peas, chickpeas, lentils, common beans, fava beans, beach beans, and yellow and black soybeans (Luthria and Pastor-Corrales 2006; Xu and Chang 2007, 2008). The biologically active compounds of interest found in leguminous seeds come from many chemical classes and include phenolic acids and flavonoids as well as their derivatives, flavanols, flavan-3-ols, anthocyanins/anthocyanidins, condensed tannins, proanthocyanidins, tocopherols, and vitamin C (Amarowicz and Pegg 2008). Among flavonoids, isoflavones are the most abundant subclass in legumes (Rossi and Kasum 2002). Two extensively reported isoflavones are genistein and daidzein, which are found in legumes, such as soybeans and chickpeas (Marathe et al. 2011). Several studies have shown that soy protein containing isoflavones reduces the susceptibility of LDL cholesterol to oxidation. Anderson et al. (2000) determined that the amount of soy isoflavones needed to achieve all their potential benefits, including the reduced risk of certain cancers, was an average of 100–160 mg of isoflavones per day. Also, Jenkins et al. (2002) reported that high isoflavone intakes (168 mg/day isoflavones) may decrease the risk of CVD by reducing oxidized LDL in men and women. Yousef et al. (2004) showed that the formation of TBARS in the plasma and tissue of rabbits was significantly decreased by isoflavones. Soy protein, the soy-derived isoflavones genistein and daidzein, and the metabolite equol are hypothesized to impart antioxidants against oxidative stress (Heneman, Chang, and Prior 2007). Cell culture studies suggest that they may act by enhancing the cellular antioxidant network, inhibiting peroxynitrite-mediated LDL oxidation by delaying tyrosine nitration, and activating glutathione peroxidase (thereby increasing cellular levels of reduced glutathione) or inhibiting superoxide production and, thus, cell-mediated LDL modification (Lai and Yen 2002; Suzuki et al. 2002; Guo et al. 2002; Hwang et al. 2003). Interestingly, dark (red, bronze, and black) legumes, such as lentils, colored beans, and black soybeans, were seen to have a significantly higher phenolic content and antioxidant capacity than pale-colored (green, yellow, and white) legumes, such as yellow peas, green peas, and yellow soybeans (Xu, Yuan, and Chang 2007). *In vitro* extracts of black beans, black soybeans, lentils, and red kidney beans are more effective in inhibiting LDL oxidation than yellow soybeans (Takahashi et al. 2005).

17.8 NUTS AND SEEDS

Nuts are traditionally associated with the Mediterranean diet. Regular nut consumption, in moderate doses, has been proven to reduce the blood levels of total and LDL cholesterol, parameters that are associated with a lower incidence of cardiovascular and obesity-related diseases (Chen, Lapsley, and Blumberg 2006). These healthy effects are attributed, in addition to their lipid profile and other components, to the presence of antioxidant compounds (Wijeratne, Abou-Zaid, and Shahidi 2006). Nuts have different types of antioxidants. For instance, almonds contain phenolic acids and flavonoids, such as catechins, flavonols, and flavonones, in their aglycone and glycoside form (Bartolomé et al. 2010), and peanuts and pistachios contain flavonoids and have higher concentrations of resveratrol than other nuts (Chukwumah et al. 2012). Pistachios (seeds and skin) are a rich source of phenolic acids and flavonoid compounds (Tomaino et al. 2010). Walnuts contain a wide range of polyphenols and tocopherols, and cashews have alkyl phenols and tannins as their principal antioxidant compounds (Solar et al. 2006; Michodjehoun-Mestres et al. 2009). The phytochemicals contained in nuts could work in synergy with other important nut constituents to promote antioxidant activities. Thus, the beneficial effects of phenolics from nut products for the protection of DNA and the inhibition of human LDL oxidation have been reported. Kay et al. (2010) conducted a randomized, crossover controlled-feeding study to evaluate two doses of pistachios on serum antioxidants and biomarkers of oxidative status in 28 hypercholesterolemic adults. The authors demonstrated the beneficial effects of pistachios on multiple biomarkers of the oxidative state with significant decreases in serum oxidized-LDL in participants following the pistachio-enriched treatment diets relative to the control diet. Sari et al. (2010) investigated 32 healthy young men fed with a Mediterranean diet with pistachio replacing the monounsaturated fat content. These authors reported that the pistachio diet significantly decreased serum interleukin-6, the total oxidant status, lipid hydroperoxide, and malondialdehyde and increased superoxide dismutase.

Anderson et al. (2001) studied extracts from walnuts for their ability to inhibit *in vitro* plasma and LDL oxidation. These authors reported that 2,2'-azobis'(2-amidino propane) hydrochloride (AAPH)-induced LDL oxidation was significantly (38%) inhibited by the highest concentration (1.0 mmol/L) of walnut extract. In addition, copper-mediated LDL oxidation was inhibited by 84% in the presence of walnut extract with a modest but significant LDL α-tocopherol sparing effect observed. Plasma TBARS formation was significantly inhibited by walnut extracts. Wijeratne, Abou-Zaid, and Shahidi (2006) evaluated the antioxidant efficacy of defatted almond whole seed, brown skin, and green shell cover extracts in the inhibition of human LDL oxidation. These authors reported that brown skin extract at 50 mg/kg effectively inhibited copper-induced oxidation of human LDL cholesterol compared to whole seed and green shell cover extracts, which reached the same level of efficacy at 200 mg/kg. Chen et al. (2007) reported that almond-skin polyphenolics and quercetin reduce the oxidative modification of apo B-100 and stabilize LDL conformation in a dose-dependent manner, acting in an additive or synergistic fashion with vitamins C and E. As regards hazelnuts, Shahidi, Alasalvar, and Liyana-Pathirana (2007) reported that hazelnut skin at 50 mg/kg concentration effectively inhibited copper-induced oxidation of human LDL cholesterol (99%) compared to hazelnut kernel (42%) extracts, which reached the same level of efficacy (99%) at 100 mg/kg.

17.9 SPICES AND HERBS

Spices and aromatic herbs are an important part of human nutrition and have found a place in all cultures of the world. The literature describes how they impart flavor and reduce the need for salt and fatty condiments, improve digestion, and provide the organism with extra antioxidants that prevent the appearance of physiological and metabolic alterations (Perez-Alvarez, Fernández-López, and Sayas-Barberá 2002). In their composition, proteins, fiber, sugars, essential oils, minerals, and pigments besides bioactive compounds, such as phenolic acids, flavonoids, sterols, and coumarins, can be found (Viuda-Martos et al. 2007). The antioxidant activity of aromatic herbs, spices, essential oils, and their components has been the subject of many studies. For example, the antioxidant activities of 23 essential oils isolated from various spices and herbs were seen to inhibit the copper-catalyzed oxidation of human LDLs and were determined *in vitro* (Teissedre and Waterhouse 2000). The essential oil of thyme (which is rich in thymol, carvacrol, cuminol, or eugenol) showed a moderate inhibition of LDL oxidation (20%–27%) (Teissedre and Waterhouse 2000). Naderi et al. (2005) investigated the antioxidant effects of two spices, *Curcuma longa* and *Crocus sativus*, on LDL oxidation and the oxidation of cell membranes of liver hepatocytes. These authors reported that curcuma at a concentration of 10 µg/mL inhibited malondialdehyde formation by 28.8%, while the plant showed the greatest antioxidant effect on LDL oxidation at 1 µg/mL. Crocus has no clear inhibitory effect on malondialdehyde formation but has a minimal inhibitory effect on LDL oxidation. Hashim et al. (2005) evaluated the antioxidant potencies of polyphenolic compounds from *Coriandrum sativum* against hydrogen peroxide-induced oxidative damage in human lymphocytes. Treatment with polyphenolic fractions (50 µg/mL) increased the activities of antioxidant enzymes and glutathione content and reduced the levels of TBARS significantly. The observed reduction in lipid peroxides reflected lower peroxidative damage. Manjunatha and Srinivasan (2006) analyzed curcumin and capsaicin separately and together in rats, finding that, in both cases, LDL oxidation was inhibited and that the species acted synergically. Ahuja et al. (2006) reported that the active ingredients of spices, such as chile and turmeric (capsaicin and curcumin, respectively), have been seen to reduce the susceptibility of LDL to oxidation. They investigated the effects of different concentrations (0.1–3.0 µM) of capsaicin and curcumin on the copper-induced oxidation of serum lipoproteins and found that the oxidation of serum lipids was reduced by these compounds in a concentration-dependent manner. Kulišić, Kriško, and Dragović-Uzelac (2007) studied the antioxidative capacity of essential oils and aqueous infusions obtained from oregano, thyme, and wild thyme on the oxidation susceptibility of LDLs. The results indicate a dose-dependent protective effect of the tested essential oils and aqueous tea infusions on the copper-induced LDL oxidation. This protective effect of essential oils was attributed to the presence of phenolic monoterpenes, thymol, and carvacrol. The compounds present in myrtle (*Myrtus communis* L.) have been shown to significantly protect LDL from oxidative damage and to have a remarkable protective effect on the reduction of polyunsaturated fatty acids and cholesterol, inhibiting the increase of their oxidative products (Rosa et al. 2008).

17.10   BEVERAGES

Beverages are frequently used to deliver high concentrations of functional ingredients (e.g., sports and performance beverages, ready-to-drink teas, coffees, vitamin-enhanced water, soy beverages, and energy beverages). This is a result, in part, of their ease of delivery but also of the innate human requirement for fluid. Beverages represent an appropriate medium for the dissolution of functional components but also a convenient and widely accepted method of consumption (Wootton-Beard and Ryan 2011).

17.10.1 Tea

Approximately 3000 million kg of tea (*Camellia sinensis* L.) are produced and consumed each year, making it the second most popular beverage in the world (Khan and Mukhtar 2007), and as the popularity of tea has increased in unfermented (green tea), semi-fermented (oolong), and fermented (black tea) forms, the amount of another product of the tea plant, tea fruit, has greatly increased as well. Green tea polyphenols are composed of numerous types of catechins. The major catechins present in green tea are (–)-epigallocatechin 3-*O*-gallate (EGCG), (–)-gallocatechin 3-*O*-gallate (GCG), (–)-epicatechin 3-*O*-gallate (ECG), (–)-epigallocatechin (EGC), (+)-gallocatechin (GC), and (–)-epicatechin (EC) (Bajerska et al. 2011). Several interventional studies have demonstrated that habitual green tea consumption causes an increase in plasma antioxidant status and a quantitative reduction of free radical-induced markers of lipid peroxidation (Rietveld and Wiseman 2003; Sung et al. 2005; Ellinger et al. 2011). Thus, Yang and Koo (2000) demonstrated that tea and its catechin-rich fractions significantly prevented endothelial cell-induced LDL oxidation, because tea and its catechin-rich fraction reduced LDL oxidation and decreased its relative electrophoretic mobility in a dose-dependent way when compared to the oxidized LDL. In addition, lipid peroxidation products, TBARS, and cellular cholesterol were also significantly lowered in a dose-dependent manner. Nakagawa and Yokozawa (2002) reported that the regular consumption of green tea has an antioxidant effect because the tea can directly scavenge nitric oxide and superoxide anions, an action attributable to its tannin components, such as EGCG, GCG, ECG, EGC, GC, and EC. Sung et al. (2005) reported that the levels of oxidized LDL and soluble vascular cell adhesion molecule-1 (atherosclerotic biological markers) were significantly decreased after 4 weeks of green tea ingestion. Ostrowska and Skrzydlewska (2006) showed the ability of catechins and green tea to protect lipophilic antioxidants. The peroxidation of LDL is markedly inhibited by green tea extract and to a slightly weaker extent by catechins (EGCG in particular), as manifested by a decrease in the concentration of conjugated dienes, lipid hydroperoxides, malondialdehyde, and dityrosine and by an increase in the tryptophan content. Ellinger et al. (2011) reported that the regular consumption of green tea in amounts of at least 0.6–1.5 L/day may increase plasma antioxidant activity, reduce lipid (protein) peroxidation (especially the oxidation of LDL), and improve protection against DNA damage in healthy subjects.

17.10.2 Coffee

Coffee is a widely consumed beverage throughout the world. There are two species of coffee tree of commercial importance, *Coffea arabica* and *Coffea robusta*. The two species differ in the chemical composition of the green coffee bean. *Arabica* contains more lipids, and *robusta* contains more caffeine and sucrose as well as the antioxidant polyphenols chlorogenic acid and its derivatives (Parliament and Stahl 2005). The antioxidant capacity of brewed coffee is attributed both to its natural antioxidants (phenolic compounds, mainly chlorogenic acid and diterpenes, such as cafestol and kahweol) and roasting-induced antioxidants, such as melanoidins and other Maillard reaction products (Moreira et al. 2005; Crozier, Jaganath, and Clifford

2009). In recent years, there has been an increasing interest in the possible positive implications of coffee consumption for human health. It is well known that brewed coffee has very strong antioxidant activity. Thus, in a short-term study with 22 subjects and a control group, Esposito et al. (2003) found that 5 cups/day of unfiltered Italian-style coffee produced a significant 16% increase in plasma glutathione, a major *in vivo* antioxidant. No difference in plasma hydroperoxides or homocysteine (both prooxidants) was noted in this intervention study with a coffee intake that is considered average for the Italian population. Yukawa, Mune, and Otani (2004) investigated coffee consumption (24 g total per day) for 1 week. Fasting peripheral venous blood samples were taken at the end of each 1-week period. The LDL oxidation lag time was approximately 8% greater after the coffee-drinking period. Serum levels of total cholesterol and LDL-cholesterol and malondialdehyde as TBARS were significantly decreased after the coffee-drinking period. Finally, regular coffee ingestion may favorably affect cardiovascular risk status by modestly reducing LDL oxidation susceptibility and decreasing LDL-cholesterol and malondialdehyde. Natella et al. (2007) evaluated the effect of coffee consumption on the redox status of LDL as modulated by the possible incorporation of phenolic acids into the LDL. These authors reported that the resistance of LDL to oxidative modification increased significantly after coffee drinking (200 mL). The concentration in LDL of conjugated forms of caffeic, *p*-coumaric, and ferulic acids increased significantly after coffee drinking. The resistance of LDL to oxidative modification increased, probably as a result of the incorporation of coffee's phenolic acids into LDL.

17.10.3 MATE

Yerba mate (*Ilex paraguariensis*) is one of the most commercialized and widely consumed plants in South America, growing naturally or as a cultivated crop in Argentina, Brazil, Uruguay, and Paraguay. Mate beverages have been widely consumed for hundreds of years as infusions popularly known as chimarrão or tereré (both from dried green mate leaves) and mate tea (roasted mate leaves) (Gorzalczany, Filip, and Alonso 2001). Leaves from yerba mate are a potential source of polyphenols, such as phenolic acids, mainly chlorogenic and caffeic acids, which are also present in hot infusions made from either the dried green leaves or the roasted leaves (Bastos et al. 2007). In addition to polyphenols, yerba mate contains caffeine and saponins (Heck and Mejia 2007). The most notable of mate's biological activities is its high antioxidant capacity. Matsumoto et al. (2009) evaluated the antioxidant activity of mate tea on LDL from young female volunteers after acute and prolonged mate tea intake (1 week). They observed that prolonged mate tea consumption prevented LDL oxidation, expressed as diene conjugate formation, and prevented structural LDL Apo B changes when copper is the oxidative agent but not in the presence of other prooxidants, such as peroxynitrite and lipoxygenase. Arçaria et al. (2011) showed that chronic treatment with yerba mate for 60 days may improve the antioxidant capacity of the body and the resistance of LDL particles to oxidation. They indicated that (i) serum total antioxidant status, the enzymatic activity of erythrocytes, and Cu–Zn superoxide dismutase were increased; (ii) the oxidative susceptibility of LDL decreased; (iii) levels of TBARS, the products from lipid oxidation, were significantly reduced; and (iv) DNA resistance against H_2O_2-induced DNA strand breaks in lymphocyte human cells was increased. Additionally, the remarkable ability of yerba mate to inhibit *in vitro* lipid peroxidation of plasma and isolated LDL has been shown in several different oxidative systems, including transition metal ions, free radical generation, and the lipoxygenase enzyme (Filip, Sebastian, and Ferraro 2007). When da Silva et al. (2008) examined the acute effects of the consumption of mate infusion on *ex vivo* plasma, LDL oxidation, and plasma antioxidant capacity, they found that an intake of 500 mL of yerba mate infusion improved the antioxidant capacity and the resistance of plasma and LDL particles to *ex vivo* lipid peroxidation.

17.10.4 COCOA

Cocoa-derived foods, such as cocoa powders, chocolate, and other cocoa-related products, are polyphenol-rich foods derived from the fermented, roasted, and industrially processed seeds of *Theobroma cacao* L. (*Sterculiaceae*). The polyphenol content in cocoa-derived products is lower than that found in the raw material used in their production. The major flavan-3-ol enantiomer identified in unfermented, dried, unroasted cocoa beans is the (–)-epicatechin compound. However, during the processing of cocoa, a significant degradation of (–)-epicatechin and (+)-catechin compounds takes place (Schinella et al. 2010). Evidence based on epidemiological studies suggests that the consumption of cocoa-containing products increases plasma antioxidant capacity (Wan et al. 2001); inhibits oxidation of LDL particles in humans *ex vivo* (Osakabe et al. 2001); and reduces biomarkers of oxidation, such as F2-isoprostanes and malondialdehyde (Wiswedel et al. 2004). Some studies have shown that the consumption of cocoa powder significantly inhibits susceptibility of LDL to oxidation in healthy humans (Osakabe et al. 2001), and others show that cocoa products increase serum total antioxidant capacity and HDL-associated cholesterol (HDLc) concentrations but only modestly reduces LDL oxidation susceptibility (Mursu et al. 2004). Wan et al. (2001) reported that after cocoa supplementation for 4 weeks (22 g cocoa powder and 16 g dark chocolate), serum total antioxidant capacity increased and LDL oxidation susceptibility fell in 23 healthy subjects. Steinberg et al. (2002) demonstrated the ability of purified monomeric flavanols and oligomeric cocoa procyanidin fractions to delay the utilization of endogenous LDL α-tocopherol and to decrease the susceptibility of LDL to metal ion-dependent and metal ion-independent oxidation *in vitro*. Khan et al. (2012) showed that consumption of soluble cocoa powder over 4 weeks significantly increased plasma (HDLc) levels and decreased concentrations of oxidized LDL. In addition, these changes appeared to be associated with the increases in the urinary levels of phase II and microbial-derived metabolites of cocoa flavonoids, suggesting a relationship between the cocoa intake, changes in the lipid profile, and serum LDL-oxidized measurements.

17.11 ALCOHOLIC DRINKS

17.11.1 BEER

Beer is a traditional alcoholic beverage with few calories and no fat consumed in large amounts in almost all countries of the world. It contains organic acids and vitamins (from the malt), proteins, hops (a mild sedative and an appetite stimulant), and water. Beer has a higher nutritional value than other alcoholic beverages because of its minerals and essential nutrients, such as potassium, magnesium, calcium, and sodium. The use of cereals and malt to produce beer may also contribute to the ingestion of naturally occurring antioxidant compounds (Wei, Mura, and Shibamoto 2001; Girotti et al. 2002). There are many endogenous antioxidants including phenolic compounds and Maillard reaction products (Vanderhaegen et al. 2006). Approximately 80% of beer phenols are derived from malt and about 20% from hops. The most important phenolic compounds present in beer are phenolic acids (ferulic, cinnamic, chlorogenic, vanillic, gallic, caffeic, o-coumaric and p-coumaric, syringic), derivatives of flavan-3-ol (catechin, epicatechin, procyanidin, prodelphinidin), and flavonoglycosides (Gorjanovic et al. 2010). A variety of studies have pointed to the antioxidant activities of beers and their components. Thus, Ghiselli et al. (2000) reported that beer, which has a moderate antioxidant capacity coupled with a low ethanol content, is able to improve plasma antioxidant capacity without the negative effects produced by high doses of ethanol. In fact, although the amount of ethanol present in 500 mL of beer (approximately 18 g) did not induce any appreciable change in the markers of metabolic control, it facilitated the transfer of the antioxidant capacity from beer to body fluids, probably through the increased absorption of phenolic compounds. Miranda et al. (2000) reported that xanthohumol, the major prenylchalcone in hops and beer, was a much better antioxidant than vitamin E in cupric ion-catalyzed LDL oxidation. Vinson et al. (2003) carried out a study to analyze the antioxidant effect of two types of beer on animal models. Dark beer and a lager beer were given at two concentrations to cholesterol-fed hamsters, an animal model of atherosclerosis. At the high dose (1/2-diluted beer), lager significantly decreased cholesterol and triglycerides, and both beers acted as *in vivo* antioxidants by decreasing the oxidizability of lower-density lipoproteins. Gasowski et al. (2004) found that beer has a positive effect on the plasma lipid profile and the plasma antioxidant capacity. The degree of this positive influence of beer is directly related to the bioactive compounds in beer.

17.11.2 Wine

Wine is a complex matrix and may be considered as a phyto-complex to which ethanol has been added following natural fermentation. The last two decades have seen renewed interest in the health benefits of wine as documented by increasing research and several epidemiologic observations showing that moderate wine drinkers have lower mortality rates than heavy drinkers or teetotalers (Di Castelnuovo et al. 2002). Red wine contains a variety of polyphenols derived from the skin of the grapes, mainly flavonoids (such as quercetin, myricetin, catechin, and epicathechin), phenolic acids (mainly gallic, caffeic, and ferulic acid), stilbenes (as resveratrol), condensed tannins (mainly catechin and epicatechin polymers), and anthocyanins (such as cyanidin, malvidin, petunidin, delphinidin, peonidin, and pelargonidin) (Howard et al. 2002; Dudley et al. 2008; Rodrigo, Miranda, and Vergara 2011). Resveratrol is the most well-known polyphenolic compound occurring in grapes and wine. The level of resveratrol found in wine varies greatly but is generally more abundant in red grapes and red wine (Vingtdeux et al. 2008).

A large number of studies, both in experimental models and in humans, have been performed to ascertain the antioxidant properties of wine. Thus, red wine flavonoids have been found to increase the concentration of serum paraoxonase, which hydrolyzes LDL-associated lipid peroxides, therefore leading to a reduction of LDL oxidation (Aviram and Fuhrman 2002). Deckert et al. (2002) demonstrated that red wine polyphenolic compounds (RWPCs) can preserve normal vascular reactivity by acting at different stages of the cascade that leads to lipoprotein oxidation, endothelium dysfunction, and vasospasm. RWPCs can delay the utilization of α-tocopherol during the oxidation of LDL, reducing the concomitant formation of oxidation-derived lipid species, including 7-β-hydroxycholesterol and 7-ketocholesterol. Reduced *ex vivo* LDL oxidation after the consumption of red wine taken without meals was found by Covas et al. (2003). A decrease in the susceptibility of LDL to lipid peroxidation has been proposed as a reason for the lower incidence of atherosclerosis among red wine drinkers. Guarda et al. (2005) reported that the sustained consumption of red wine (250 mL/day) over 2 months—but not of water—decreased the DNA oxidative damage and increased plasma total antioxidant capacity. Tsang et al. (2005) observed that conjugated dienes and TBARS in copper-oxidized LDL were decreased after the daily consumption of 375 mL red wine for 2 weeks, while no effects where observed on LDL-TBARS.

17.12   CONCLUSIONS

An extensive body of scientific evidence indicates that diets rich in fruit, vegetables, legumes, whole grains, fish, low-fat dairy products, and monounsaturated fats are associated with a lower incidence of CVD, mainly through their influence on blood pressure, lipids, and lipoproteins levels as well as LDL oxidation. It is generally assumed that the main dietary constituents contribute to these protective effects. These constituents with functional properties are mainly composed of polyphenolic compounds in all forms (phenolic acids, flavonoids, anthocyanins, tannins, and so on). The protective effects could be a result of their properties as free radical scavengers, hydrogen-donating compounds, singlet oxygen quenchers, and/or metal ion chelators. It should be borne in mind that human diets are a complex mixture, which may contain a combination of stimulatory and inhibitory bioactive components. These may not only result in positive (synergistic) effects but also have negative (antagonistic) effects on the physiological effect of foods or diet. Unfortunately, there is little information to guide the public in selecting appropriate foods or diets and to avoid possible antagonisms.

REFERENCES

Ahuja, K. D. K., Kunde, D. A., Ball, M. J. et al. 2006. Effects of capsaicin, dihydrocapsaicin and curcumin on copper-induced oxidation of human serum lipids. *J Agric Food Chem* 54: 6436–6439.

Ali, S. S., Kasoju, N., Luthra, A. et al. 2008. Indian medicinal herbs as sources of antioxidants. *Food Res Int* 41: 1–15.

Allaith, A. A. 2005. *In vitro* evaluation of antioxidant activity of different extracts of *Phoenix dactylifera* L. fruits as functional foods. *Deutsch Lebensmitt Rundsch* 101: 305–308.

Alshatwi, A. A., Al Obaaid, M. A., Al Sedairy, S. A. et al. 2010. Tomato powder is more protective than lycopene supplement against lipid peroxidation in rats. *Nutr Res* 30: 66–73.

Amarowicz, R., Pegg, R. B. 2008. Legumes as a source of natural antioxidants. *Eur J Lipid Sci Technol* 110: 865–878.

Anderson, J. J. B., Adlercreutz, H., Barnes, S. et al. 2000. Appropriate isoflavone food fortification levels: Results of a consensus conference. Experimental Biology 2000, San Diego, CA, April 15–18.

Anderson, J. W. 2003. Whole grains protect against atherosclerotic cardiovascular disease. *Proceed Nutr Soc* 62: 135–142.

Anderson, K. J., Teuber, S. S., Gobeille, A. et al. 2001. Walnut polyphenolics inhibit *in vitro* human plasma and LDL oxidation. *J Nutr* 131: 2837–2842.

Andreasen, M. F., Landbo, A. K., Christensen, L. P. et al. 2001. Effects of phenolic rye (*Secale cereale* L.) extracts, monomeric hydroxycinnamates, and ferulic acid dehydrodimers on human low-density lipoprotein. *J Agr Food Chem* 49: 4090–4096.

Anoosh, E., Mojtab, E., Fatemeh, S. 2010. Study the effect of juice of two variety of pomegranate on decreasing plasma LDL cholesterol. *Proc Soc Behav Sci* 2: 620–623.

Arçaria, D. P., Porto, V. B., Varalda Rodrigues, E. R. et al. 2011. Effect of mate tea (*Ilex paraguariensis*) supplementation on oxidative stress biomarkers and LDL oxidisability in normo- and hyperlipidaemic humans. *J Function Foods* 3: 190–197.

Aruoma, O. I. 1998. Free radicals, oxidative stress, and antioxidants in human health and disease. *J Am Oil Chem Soc* 75: 199–212.

Avci, A., Atli, T., Erguder, I. B. et al. 2008. Effects of garlic consumption on plasma and erythrocyte antioxidant parameters in elderly subjects. *Gerontology* 54: 173–176.

Aviram, M., Fuhrman, B. 2002. Wine flavonoids protect against LDL oxidation and atherosclerosis. *Ann New York Acad Sci* 957: 146–161.

Aviram, M., Rosenblat, M., Gaitini, D. 2004. Pomegranate juice consumption for 3 years by patients with carotid artery stenosis reduces common carotid intima-media thickness, blood pressure and LDL oxidation. *Clin Nutr* 23: 423–433.

Bajerska, J., Wozniewicz, M., Jeszka, J. et al. 2011. Green tea aqueous extract reduces visceral fat and decreases protein availability in rats fed with a high-fat diet. *Nutr Res* 31: 157–164.

Balasundram, N., Sundram, K., Samman, S. 2006. Phenolic compounds in plants and agro-industrial byproducts: Antioxidant activity, occurrence, and potential uses. *Food Chem* 99: 191–203.

Baliga, M. S., Baliga, B. R. V., Kandathil, S. M. et al. 2011. A review of the chemistry and pharmacology of the date fruits (*Phoenix dactylifera* L.). *Food Res Int* 44: 1812–1822.

Ballus, C. A., Meinhart, A. D., Bruns, R. E. et al. 2011. Use of multivariate statistical techniques to optimize the simultaneous separation of 13 phenolic compounds from extra-virgin olive oil by capillary electrophoresis. *Talanta* 83: 1181–1187.

Bandyopadhyay, D., Chattopadhyay, A., Ghosh, G. et al. 2004. Oxidative stress-induced ischemic heart disease: Protection by antioxidants. *Curr Med Chem* 11: 369–387.

Banerjee, S. K., Mukherjee, P. K., Maulik, S. K. 2003. Garlic as an antioxidant: The good, the bad and the ugly. *Phytother Res* 17: 97–106.

Barreca, D., Laganà, G., Ficarra, S. et al. 2011. Evaluation of the antioxidant and cytoprotective properties of the exotic fruit *Annona cherimola* Mill. (*Annonaceae*). *Food Res Int* 44: 2302–2310.

Bartolomé, B., Monagas, M., Garrido, I. et al. 2010. Almond (*Prunus dulcis* (Mill.) D.A. Webb) polyphenols: From chemical characterization to targeted analysis of phenolic metabolites in humans. *Arch Biochem Biophys* 501: 124–133.

Bastos, D. H. M., Saldanha, L. A., Catharino, R. R. et al. 2007. Phenolic antioxidants identified by ESI-MS from yerba maté (*Ilex paraguariensis*) and green tea (*Camelia sinensis*) extracts. *Molecules* 12: 423–432.

Basu, A., Du, M., Leyva, M. et al. 2010. Blueberries decrease cardiovascular risk factors in obese men and women with metabolic syndrome. *J Nutr* 140: 1582–1587.

Basu, A., Imrhan, V. 2007. Tomatoes versus lycopene in oxidative stress and carcinogenesis: Conclusions from clinical trials. *Eur J Clin Nutr* 61: 295–303.

Ben Ammar, R., Bhouri, W., Ben Sghaier, M. et al. 2009. Antioxidant and free radical-scavenging properties of three flavonoids isolated from the leaves of *Rhamnus alaternus* L. (Rhamnaceae): A structure-activity relationship study. *Food Chem* 116: 258–264.

Benjamin, H., Lau, S. 2001. Suppression of LDL oxidation by garlic. *J Nutr* 131: 985–988.

Berrougui, H., Cloutier, M., Isabelle, M. et al. 2006. Phenolic-extract from argan oil (*Argania spinosa* L.) inhibits human low-density lipoprotein (LDL) oxidation and enhances cholesterol efflux from human THP-1 macrophages. *Atherosclerosis* 184: 389–396.

Berrougui, H., Ettaib, A., Herrera González, A. D. et al. 2003. Hypolipidemic and hypocholesterolemic effect of argan oil in Merioneshawi rats. *J Ethnopharmacol* 89: 15–18.

Block, E., Thiruvazhi, M., Toscano, J. P. et al. 1996. *Allium* chemistry: Structure, synthesis, natural occurrence in onion (*Allium cepa*), and reaction of 2,3-dimethyl-5,6-dithiabicyclo[2.1.1]hexane *S*-oxides. *J Am Chem Soc* 118: 2790–2798.

Borchani, C., Besbes, S., Masmoudi, M. et al. 2011. Effect of drying methods on physicochemical and antioxidant properties of date fibre concentrates. *Food Chem* 125: 1194–1201.

Bose, K. S., Agrawal, B. K. 2007. Effect of lycopene from cooked tomatoes on serum antioxidant enzymes, lipid peroxidation rate and lipid profile in coronary heart disease. *Singapore Med J* 48: 415–420.

Caillet, S., Côté, J., Doyon, G. et al. 2011. Antioxidant and antiradical properties of cranberry juice and extracts. *Food Res Int* 44: 1408–1413.

Carr, T. P., Jesch, E. D. 2006. Food components that reduce cholesterol absorption. *Adv Food Nutr Res* 51: 165–204.

Cerdá, B., Ceron, J. J., Tomas-Barberan, F. A. 2003. Repeated oral administration of high doses of pomegranate ellagitannin punicalagin to rats for 37 days is not toxic. *J Agr Food Chem* 51: 3493–3501.

Chau, C. F., Huang, Y. L., Lin, C. Y. 2004. Investigation of the cholesterol-lowering action of insoluble fibre derived from the peel of *Citrus sinensis* L. cv. Liucheng. *Food Chem* 87: 361–366.

Chen, C. Y., Chang, F. R., Chiu, H. F. et al. 1999. Aromin-A, an annonaceous acetogenins from *Annona cherimola*. *Phytochem* 51: 29–33.

Chen, C. Y., Chang, F. R., Yen, H. F. et al. 1998. Amides from stems of *Annona cherimola*. *Phytochem* 49: 1443–1447.

Chen, C. Y., Lapsley, K., Blumberg, J. 2006. A nutrition and health perspective on almonds. *J Sci Food Agr* 86: 2245–2250.

Chen, C. Y., Milbury, P. E., Chung, S. K. et al. 2007. Effect of almond skin polyphenolics and quercetin on human LDL and apolipoprotein B-100 oxidation and conformation. *J Nutr Biochem* 18: 785–794.

Chen, C. Y., Milbury, P. E., Kwak, H. K. et al. 2004. Avenanthramides and phenolic acids from oats are bioavailable and act synergistically with vitamin C to enhance hamster and human LDL resistance to oxidation. *J Nutr* 134: 1459–1466.

Cherki, M., Derouiche, A., Drissi, A. et al. 2005. Consumption of argan oil may have an antiatherogenic effect by improving paraoxonase activities and antioxidant status: Intervention study in healthy men. *Nutr Metab Cardiovasc Dis* 15: 352–360.

Christian, S., Yvan, N., Myriam, T. 2011. Nonvolatile *S*-Alk(en)ylthio-L-cysteine derivatives in fresh onion (*Allium cepa* L. cultivar). *J Agr Food Chem* 59: 9457–9465.

Chukwumah, Y., Walker, L., Vogler, B. et al. 2012. Profiling of bioactive compounds in cultivars of Runner and Valencia peanut market-types using liquid chromatography/APCI mass spectrometry. *Food Chem* 132: 525–531.

Cirico, T. L., Omaye, S. T. 2006. Additive or synergetic effects of phenolic compounds on human low density lipoprotein oxidation. *Food Chem Toxicol* 44: 510–516.

Clifford, M. N., Scalbert, A. 2000. Review: Ellagitannins—Nature, occurrence and dietary burden. *J Sci Food Agr* 80: 1118–1125.

Conforti, F., Sosa, S., Marrelli, M. et al. 2009. The protective ability of Mediterranean dietary plants against the oxidative damage: The role of radical oxygen species in inflammation and the polyphenol, flavonoid and sterol contents. *Food Chem* 112: 587–594.

Covas, M. I., de la Torre, K., Farre-Albaladejo, M. et al. 2006. Postprandial LDL phenolic content and LDL oxidation are modulated by olive oil phenolic compounds in humans. *Free Radic Biol Med* 40: 608–616.

Covas, M. I., Konstantinidou, V., Mysytaki, E. et al. 2003. Postprandial effects of wine consumption on lipids and oxidative stress biomarkers. *Drugs Exp Clin Res* 29: 217–223.

Crespo, I., García-Mediavilla, M. V., Almar, M. et al. 2008. Differential effects of dietary flavonoids on reactive oxygen and nitrogen species generation and changes in antioxidant enzyme expression induced by pro-inflammatory cytokines in Chang liver cells. *Food Chem Toxicol* 46: 1555–1569.

Crozier, A., Jaganath, I., Clifford, M. 2009. Dietary phenolics: Chemistry, bioavailability and effects on health. *Nat Prod Rep* 26: 1001–1043.

da Silva, E. L., Neiva, T. J. C., Shirai, M. et al. 2008. Acute ingestion of yerba mate infusion (*Ilex paraguariensis*) inhibits plasma and lipoprotein oxidation. *Food Res Int* 41: 973–979.

Dammak, I., Abdallah, F. B., Boudaya, S. et al. 2007. Date seed oil limit oxidative injuries induced by hydrogen peroxide in human skin organ culture. *Biofactors* 29: 137–145.

de la Torre-Carbot, K., Chavez-Servin, J. L., Jauregui, O. et al. 2010. Elevated circulating LDL phenol levels in men who consumed virgin rather that refined olive oil are associated with less oxidation of plasma LDL. *J Nutr* 140: 501–508.

de Nigris, F., Williams-Ignarro, S., Botti, C. et al. 2006. Pomegranate juice reduces oxidized low-density lipoprotein down regulation of endothelial nitric oxide synthase in human coronary endothelial cells. *Nitric Oxide* 15: 259–263.

de Souza, M. O., Silva, M., Silva, E. et al. 2010. Diet supplementation with açai (*Euterpe oleracea* Mart) pulp improves biomarkers of oxidative stress and serum lipid profiles in rats. *Nutrition* 26: 804–810.

Deckert, V., Desrumaux, C., Athias, A. et al. 2002. Prevention of LDL α-tocopherol consumption, cholesterol oxidation, and vascular endothelium dysfunction by polyphenolic compounds from red wine. *Atherosclerosis* 165: 41–50.

Dembitsky, V. M., Poovarodom, S., Leontowicz, H. et al. 2011. The multiple nutrition properties of some exotic fruits: Biological activity and active metabolites. *Food Res Int* 44: 1671–1701.

Di Castelnuovo, A., Rotondo, S., Iacoviello, L. et al. 2002. Meta-analysis of wine and beer consumption in relation to vascular risk. *Circulation* 105: 2836–2844.

Dongowski, G. 2007. Interactions between dietary fibre-rich preparations and glycoconjugated bile acids *in vitro*. *Food Chem* 104: 390–397.

Drissi, A., Girona, J., Cherki, M. et al. 2004. Evidence of hypolipemiant and antioxidant properties of argan oil derived from the argan tree (*Argania spinosa*). *Clin Nutr* 23: 1159–1166.

Dudley, J. I., Lekli, I., Mukherjee, S. et al. 2008. Does white wine qualify for French paradox? Comparison of the cardioprotective effects of red and white wines and their constituents: Resveratrol, tyrosol, and hydroxytyrosol. *J Agr Food Chem* 56: 9362–9373.

Durak, I., Aytaç, B., Atmaca, Y. et al. 2004a. Effects of garlic extract consumption on plasma and erythrocyte antioxidant parameters in atherosclerotic patients. *Life Sci* 75: 1959–1966.

Durak, I., Kavutcu, M., Aytaç, B. et al. 2004b. Effects of garlic extract consumption on blood lipid and oxidant/antioxidant parameters in humans with high blood cholesterol. *J Nutr Biochem* 15: 373–377.

Egües, I., Sanchez, C., Mondragon, I. 2012. Antioxidant activity of phenolic compounds obtained by autohydrolysis of corn residues. *Indust Crops Prod* 36: 164–171.

El Gharras, H. 2009. Polyphenols: Food sources, properties and applications—A review. *Int J Food Sci Technol* 44: 2512–2518.

Ellinger, S., Müller, N., Stehle, P. et al. 2011. Consumption of green tea or green tea products: Is there an evidence for antioxidant effects from controlled interventional studies? *Phytomedicine* 18: 903–915.

Esposito, F., Morisco, F., Verde, V. et al. 2003. Moderate coffee consumption increases plasma glutathione but not homocysteine in healthy subjects. *Aliment Pharmacol Ther* 17: 595–601.

Fardet, A., Rock, E., Rémésy, C. 2008. Is the *in vitro* antioxidant potential of whole-grain cereals and cereal products well reflected *in vivo*? *J Cereal Sci* 48: 258–276.

Fernández-López, J., Sendra-Nadal, E., Navarro, C. et al. 2009. Storage stability of a high dietary fibre powder from orange by-products. *Int J Food Sci Technol* 44: 748–756.

Fernández-López, J., Viuda-Martos, M., Sendra, E. et al. 2007. Orange fibre as potential functional ingredient for dry-cured sausages. *Eur Food Res Technol* 226: 1–6.

Filip, R., Sebastian, T., Ferraro, G. 2007. Effect of Ilex extracts and isolated compounds on peroxidase secretion of rat submandibulary glands. *Food Chem Toxicol* 45: 649–655.

Fito, M., Covas, M. I., Lamuela Raventos, R. M. et al. 2000. Protective effect of olive oil and its phenolic compounds against low-density lipoprotein oxidation. *Lipids* 35: 633–638.

Frusciante, L., Carli, P., Ercolano, M. R. et al. 2007. Antioxidant nutritional quality of tomato. *Mol Nutr Food Res* 51: 609–617.

García-Solís, P., Yahia, E. M., Aceves, C. 2008. Study of the effect of 'Ataulfo' mango (*Mangifera indica* L.) intake on mammary carcinogenesis and antioxidant capacity in plasma of N-methyl-N-nitrosourea (MNU)-treated rats. *Food Chem* 111: 309–315.

Gasowski, B., Leontowicz, M., Leontowicz, H. et al. 2004. The influence of beer with different antioxidant potential on plasma lipids, plasma antioxidant capacity, and bile excretion of rats fed cholesterol-containing and cholesterol-free diets. *J Nutr Biochem* 15: 527–533.

Gedik, N., Kabasakal, L., Sehirli, O. et al. 2005. Long-term administration of aqueous garlic extract (AGE) alleviates liver fibrosis and oxidative damage induced by biliary obstruction in rats. *Life Sci* 76: 2593–2606.

Ghaffari, M. A., Ghiasvand, T. 2006. Effect of lycopene on formation of low density lipoprotein-copper complex in copper peroxidation of low-density lipoprotein, as *in vitro* experiment. *Iran Biomed J* 10: 191–196.

Ghiselli, A., Natella, F., Guidi, A. et al. 2000. Beer increases plasma antioxidant capacity in humans. *J Nutr Biochem* 11: 76–80.

Gil, M. I., Tomas-Barberan, F. A., Hess-Pierce, B. et al. 2000. Antioxidant activity of pomegranate juice and its relationship with phenolic composition and processing. *J Agr Food Chem* 48: 4581–4589.

Girotti, S., Bolelli, L., Fini, F. et al. 2002. Chemiluminescent determination of antioxidant capacity of beverages. *Italian J Food Sci* 14: 113–122.

González-Aguilar, G. A., Celis, J., Sotelo-Mundo, R. R. et al. 2008. Physiological and biochemical changes of different fresh-cut mango cultivars stored at 5°C. *Int J Food Sci Techno* 43: 91–101.

Gorinstein, S., Kulasek, G. W., Bartnikowska, E. et al. 2000. The effects of diets, supplemented with either whole persimmon or phenol-free persimmon, on rats fed cholesterol. *Food Chem* 70: 303–308.

Gorjanovic, S. Z., Novakovic, M. M., Potkonjak, N. I. et al. 2010. Application of a novel antioxidative assay in beer analysis and brewing process monitoring. *J Agr Food Chem* 58: 744–751.

Gorzalczany, S., Filip, R., Alonso, M. 2001. Choleretic effect and intestinal propulsion of mate (*Ilex paraguariensis*) and its substitutes or adulterants. *J Ethnopharmacol* 75: 291–294.

Gray, D. A., Clarke, M. J., Baux, C. et al. 2002. Antioxidant activity of oat extracts added to human LDL particles and in free radical trapping assays. *J Cereal Sci* 36: 209–218.

Griendling, K. K., FitzGerald, G. A. 2003. Oxidative stress and cardiovascular injury: Part II: Animal and human studies. *Circulation* 108: 2034–2040.

Guarda, E., Godoy, I., Foncea, R. et al. 2005. Red wine reduces oxidative stress in patients with acute coronary syndrome. *Int J Cardiol* 104: 35–38.

Gülsen, A., Makris, D. P., Kefalas, P. 2007. Biomimetic oxidation of quercetin: Isolation of a naturally occurring quercetin heterodimer and evaluation of its *in vitro* antioxidant properties. *Food Res Int* 40: 7–14.

Guo, Q., Rimbach, G., Moini, H. et al. 2002. ESR and cell culture studies on free radical-scavenging and antioxidant activities of isoflavonoids. *Toxicology* 79: 171–180.

Gupta-Elera, G., Garrett, A. R., Martínez, A. et al. 2011. Antioxidant properties of the cherimoya (*Annona cherimola*) fruit. *Food Res Int* 44: 2205–2209.

Hasan, N. S., Amom, Z. H., Nor, A. I. et al. 2010. Nutritional composition and *in vitro* evaluation of the antioxidant properties of various dates extracts (*Phoenix dactylifera* L.) from Libya. *Asian J Clin Nutr* 2: 208–214.

Hashim, M. S., Lincy, S., Remya, V. et al. 2005. Effect of polyphenolic compounds from *Coriandrum sativum* on H_2O_2-induced oxidative stress in human lymphocytes. *Food Chem* 92: 653–660.

Hassan, F. A., Ismail, A., Azizah Hamid, A. A. et al. 2011. Characterization of fibre-rich powder and antioxidant capacity of *Mangifera pajang* K. fruit peels. *Food Chem* 126: 283–288.

Hassan, H. A., Abdel-Aziz, A. F. 2010. Evaluation of free radical-scavenging and antioxidant properties of blackberry against fluoride toxicity in rats. *Food Chem Toxicol* 48: 1999–2004.

Hassan, H. A., Yousef, M. I. 2009. Mitigating effects of antioxidant properties of blackberry juice on sodium fluoride induced hepatotoxicity and oxidative stress in rats. *Food Chem Toxicol* 47: 2332–2337.

Heck, C. I., Mejia, E. G. 2007. Yerba mate tea (*Ilex paraguariensis*): A comprehensive review on chemistry, health implications, and technological considerations. *J Food Sci* 12: 138–151.

Heggen, E., Granlund, L., Pedersen, J. I. et al. 2010. Plant sterols from rapeseed and tall oils: Effects on lipids, fat-soluble vitamins and plant sterol concentrations. *Nutr Metabol Cardiovasc Dis* 20: 258–265.

Heidarian, E., Jafari-Dehkordi, E., Seidkhani-Nahal, A. 2011. Effect of garlic on liver phosphatidate phosphohydrolase and plasma lipid levels in hyperlipidemic rats. *Food Chem Toxicol* 49: 1110–1114.

Heneman, K. M., Chang, H. C., Prior, R. L. 2007. Soy protein with and without isoflavones fails to substantially increase postprandial antioxidant capacity. *J Nutr Biochem* 18: 46–53.

Howard, A., Chopra, M., Thurnham, D. et al. 2002. Red wine consumption and inhibition of LDL oxidation: What are the important components? *Med Hypoth* 59: 101–104.

Hu, F. B. 2003. Plant-based foods and prevention of cardiovascular disease: An overview. *Am J Clin Nutr* 7: 544–551.

Hwang, J., Wang, J., Morazzoni, P. et al. 2003. The phytoestrogen equol increases nitric oxide availability by inhibiting superoxide production: An antioxidant mechanism for cell-mediated LDL modification. *Free Radic Biol Med* 4: 1271–1282.

Ignarro, L. J., Byrns, R. E., Sumi, D. et al. 2006. Pomegranate juice protects nitric oxide against oxidative destruction and enhances the biological actions of nitric oxide. *Nitric Oxide* 15: 93–102.

Jenkins, D. J., Kendall, C. W., Jackson, C. J. et al. 2002. Effects of high-and low-isoflavone soyfoods on blood lipids, oxidized LDL, homocysteine, and blood pressure in hyperlipidemic men and women. *Am J Clin Nutr* 76: 365–372.

Jiao, H. J., Wang, S. Y. 2000. Correlation of antioxidant capacities to oxygen radical scavenging enzyme activities in blackberry. *J Agr Food Chem* 48: 5672–5676.

Jiao, Z., Liu, J., Wang, S. 2005. Antioxidant activities of total pigment extract from blackberries. *Food Technol Biotechnol* 43: 97–102.

Jiménez-Escrig, A., Rincón, M., Pulido, R. et al. 2001. Guava fruit (*Psidium guajava* L.) as a new source of antioxidant dietary fiber. *J Agr Food Chem* 49: 5489–5493.

Kartal, N., Sokmen, M., Tepe, B. et al. 2007. Investigation of the antioxidant properties of *Ferula orientalis* L. using a suitable extraction procedure. *Food Chem* 100: 584–589.

Katsube, T., Tabata, H., Ohta, Y. et al. (2004). Screening of antioxidant activity in edible plant products: Comparison of low-density lipoprotein oxidation assay, DPPH radical scavenging assay, and Folin-Ciocalteu assay. *J Agr Food Chem* 52: 2391–2396.

Kaur, D., Wani, A. A., Oberoi, D. P. S. et al. 2008. Effect of extraction conditions on lycopene extractions from tomato processing waste skin using response surface methodology. *Food Chem* 108: 711–718.

Kay, C. D., Gebauer, S. K., West, S. G. et al. 2010. Pistachios increase serum antioxidants and lower serum oxidized-LDL in hypercholesterolemic adults. *J Nutr* 140: 1093–1098.

Khallouki, F., Younos, C., Soulimani, R. et al. 2003. Consumption of argan oil (Morocco) with its unique profile of fatty acids, tocopherols, squalene, sterols and phenolic compounds should confer valuable cancer chemopreventive effects. *Eur J Cancer Prevent* 12: 67–75.

Khan, N., Monagas, M., Andres-Lacueva, C. et al. 2012. Regular consumption of cocoa powder with milk increases HDL cholesterol and reduces oxidized LDL levels in subjects at high-risk of cardiovascular disease. *Nutr Metabol Cardiovasc Dis* 22: 1046–1053.

Khan, N., Mukhtar, H. 2007. Tea polyphenols for health promotion. *Life Sci* 81: 519–533.

Kilani-Jaziri, S., Neffati, A., Limem, I. et al. 2009. Relationship correlation of antioxidant and antiproliferative capacity of *Cyperus rotundus* products towards K562 erythroleukemia cells. *Chem Biol Int* 181: 85–94.

Kim, N. D., Mehta, R., Yu, W. et al. 2002. Chemopreventive and adjuvant therapeutic potential of pomegranate (*Punica granatum*) for human breast cancer. *Breast Cancer Res Treatment* 71: 203–217.

Kim, S. S., Oh, O. J., Min, H. Y. et al. 2003. Eugenol suppresses cyclooxygenase-2 expression in lipopolysaccharide-stimulated mouse macrophage RAW264.7 cells. *Life Sci* 73: 337–348.

Kong, F., Zhang, M., Liao, S. et al. 2010. Antioxidant activity of polysaccharide-enriched fractions extracted from pulp tissue of *Litchi chinensis* Sonn. *Molecules* 15: 2152–2165.

Kritchevsky, D., Chen, S. C. 2005. Phytosterol health benefits and potential concerns: A review. *Nutr Res* 25: 413–428.

Kulišić, T., Kriško, A., Dragović-Uzelac, V. 2007. The effects of essential oils and aqueous tea infusions of oregano (*Origanum vulgare* L. spp. *hirtum*), thyme (*Thymus vulgaris* L.) and wild thyme (*Thymus serpyllum* L.) on the copper-induced oxidation of human low-density lipoproteins. *Int J Food Sci Nutr* 58: 87–93.

Lai, H. H., Yen, G. C. 2002. Inhibitory effect of isoflavones on peroxynitrite mediated low-density lipoprotein oxidation. *Biosci Biotechnol Biochem* 66: 22–28.

Lau, F. C., Joseph, J. A., McDonald, J. E. 2009. Attenuation of iNOS and COX_2 by blueberry polyphenols is mediated through the suppression of NF-κB activation. *J Funct Foods* 1: 274–283.

Lim, Y. Y., Lim, T. T., Tee, J. J. 2007. Antioxidant properties of several tropical fruits: A comparative study. *Food Chem* 103: 1003–1008.

Liu, S., Yang, N., Hou, Z. H. et al. 2011. Antioxidant effects of oats avenanthramides on human serum. *Agr Sci China* 10: 1301–1305.

Liyana-Pathirana, C. M., Shahidi, F. 2005. Antioxidant activity of commercial soft and hard wheat (*Triticum aestivum* l.) as affected by gastric pH conditions. *J Agr Food Chem* 53: 2433–2440.

Lo, Y. H., Pan, M. H., Li, S. et al. 2010. Nobiletin metabolite, 3′,4′-dihydroxy-5,6,7,8-tetramethoxyflavone, inhibits LDL oxidation and down-regulates scavenger receptor expression and activity in THP-1 cells. *Biochim Biophys Acta* 1801: 114–126.

Loizzo, M. R., Tundis, R., Bonesi, M. et al. 2012. Radical scavenging, antioxidant and metal chelating activities of *Annona cherimola* Mill. (Cherimoya) peel and pulp in relation to their total phenolic and total flavonoid contents. *J Food Compos Anal* 25: 179–184.

Londoño-Londoño, J., Rodrigues de Lima, V., Lara, O. et al. 2010. Clean recovery of antioxidant flavonoids from citrus peel: Optimizing an aqueous ultrasound-assisted extraction method. *Food Chem* 119: 81–87.

Luthria, D. L., Pastor-Corrales, M. A. 2006. Phenolic acids content of fifteen dry edible bean (*Phaseolus vulgaris* L.) varieties. *J Food Comp Anal* 19: 205–211.

Madhujith, T., Shahidi, F. 2007. Antioxidative and antiproliferative properties of selected barley (*hordeum vulgarae* l.) cultivars and their potential for inhibition of low-density lipoprotein (LDL) cholesterol oxidation. *J Agr Food Chem* 55: 5018–5024.

Maiani, G., Caston, M. J., Catasta, G. et al. 2009. Carotenoids: Actual knowledge on food sources, intakes, stability and bioavailability and their protective role in humans. *Mol Nutr Food Res* 53: 194–218.

Manach, C., Scalbert, A., Morand, C. et al. 2004. Polyphenols: Food sources and bioavailability. *Am J Clin Nutr* 79: 727–747.

Manjunatha, H., Srinivasan, K. 2006. Protective effect of dietary curcumin and capsaicin on induced oxidation of low-density lipoprotein, iron-induced hepatotoxicity and carrageenan-induced inflammation in experimental rats. *FEBS J* 273: 4528–4537.

Marangoni, F., Poli, A. 2010. Phytosterols and cardiovascular health. *Pharmacol Res* 61: 193–199.

Marathe, S. A., Rajalakshmi, V., Jamdar, S. N. et al. 2011. Comparative study on antioxidant activity of different varieties of commonly consumed legumes in India. *Food Chem Toxicol* 49: 2005–2012.

Marín, F. R., Martínez, M., Uribesalgo, T. et al. 2001. Changes in nutraceutical composition of lemon juices according to different industrial extraction systems. *Food Chem* 78: 319–324.

Markovits, N., Ben Amotz, A., Levy, Y. 2009. The effect of tomato-derived lycopene on low carotenoids and enhanced systemic inflammation and oxidation in severe obesity. *Israel Med Ass J* 11: 598–601.

Marrugat, J., Covas, M. I., Fito, M. et al. 2004. Effects of differing phenolic content in dietary olive oils on lipids and LDL oxidation—a randomized controlled trial. *Eur J Nutr* 43: 140–147.

Matsumoto, R. L. T., Mendonça, S., de Oliveira, D. M. et al. 2009. Effects of maté tea intake on *ex vivo* LDL peroxidation induced by three different pathways. *Nutrients* 1: 18–29.

Mello, L. D., Kubota, L. T. 2007. Biosensors as a tool for the antioxidant status evaluation. *Talanta* 72: 335–348.

Mertens-Talcott, S. U., Rios, J., Jilma-Stohlawetz, P. et al. 2008. Pharmacokinetics of anthocyanins and antioxidant effects after the consumption of anthocyanin-rich açai juice and pulp (*Euterpe oleracea* Mart.) in human healthy volunteers. *J Agr Food Chem* 56: 7796–7802.

Michodjehoun-Mestres, L., Souquet, J. M., Fulcrand, H. et al. 2009. Characterisation of highly polymerised prodelphinidins from skin and flesh of four cashew apple (*Anacardium occidentale* L.) genotypes. *Food Chem* 114: 989–995.

Milan, K. S. M., Dholakia, H., Tiku, P. K. et al. 2008. Enhancement of digestive enzymatic activity by cumin (*Cuminum cyminum* L.) and role of spent cumin as a bionutrient. *Food Chem* 110: 678–683.

Milde, J., Elstner, E. F., Graßmann, J. 2007. Synergistic effects of phenolics and carotenoids on human low-density lipoprotein oxidation. *Mol Nutr Food Res* 51: 956–961.

Miranda, C. L., Stevens, J. F., Ivanov, V. et al. 2000. Antioxidant and prooxidant actions of prenylated and nonprenylated chalcones and flavanones *in vitro*. *J Agr Food Chem* 48: 3876–3884.

Moreira, D. P., Monteiro, M. C., Ribeiro-Alves, M. et al. 2005. Contribution of chlorogenic acids to the iron-reducing activity of coffee beverages. *J Agr Food Chem* 53: 1399–1402.

Mursu, J., Voutilainen, S., Nurmi, T. et al. 2004. Dark chocolate consumption increases HDL cholesterol concentration and chocolate fatty acids may inhibit lipid peroxidation in healthy humans. *Free Radic Biol Med* 37: 1351–1359.

Naderi, G. A., Sedigheh, A., Taher, M. A. et al. 2005. Antioxidant effect of turmeric and saffron on the oxidation of hepatocytes, LDL and non-enzymatic glycation of hemoglobin. *J Med Plants* 4: 29–35.

Nagaraju, A., Belur, L. R. 2008. Rats fed blended oils containing coconut oil with groundnut oil or olive oil showed an enhanced activity of hepatic antioxidant enzymes and a reduction in LDL oxidation. *Food Chem* 108: 950–957.

Nakagawa, T., Yokozawa, T. 2002. Direct scavenging of nitric oxide and superoxide by green tea. *Food Chem Toxicol* 40: 1745–1750.

Nakbi, A., Issaoui, M., Dabbou, S. et al. 2010. Evaluation of antioxidant activities of phenolic compounds from two extra virgin olive oils. *J Food Compos Anal* 23: 711–715.

Natella, F., Nardini, M., Belelli, F. et al. 2007. Coffee drinking induces incorporation of phenolic acids into LDL and increases the resistance of LDL to *ex vivo* oxidation in humans. *Am J Clin Nutr* 86: 604–609.

Navarro-González, I., García-Valverde, V., García-Alonso, J. et al. 2011. Chemical profile, functional and antioxidant properties of tomato peel fiber. *Food Res Int* 144: 1528–1535.

Nevin, K. G., Rajmohan, T. 2004. Beneficial effects of virgin coconut oil on lipid parameters and *in vitro* LDL oxidation. *Clin Biochem* 37: 830–835.

Nevin, K. G., Rajmohan, T. 2006. Virgin coconut oil supplemented diet increases antioxidant status in rats. *Food Chem* 99: 260–266.

Noziere, P., Graulet, B., Lucas, A. 2006. Carotenoids for ruminants: From forages to dairy products. *Animal Feed Sci Technol* 131: 418–450.

Nuutila, A. M., Puupponen-Pimiä, R., Aarni, M. et al. 2003. Comparison of antioxidant activities of onion and garlic extracts by inhibition of lipid peroxidation and radical scavenging activity. *Food Chem* 81: 485–493.

Osadee Wijekoon, M. M. J., Bhat, R. A., Karim, A. A. 2011. Effect of extraction solvents on the phenolic compounds and antioxidant activities of bunga kantan (*Etlingera elatior* Jack.) inflorescence. *J Food Compos Anal* 24: 615–619.

Osakabe, N., Baba, S., Yasuda, A. et al. 2001. Daily cocoa intake reduces the susceptibility of low-density lipoprotein to oxidation as demonstrated in healthy human volunteers. *Free Radic Res* 34: 93–99.

Ostrowska, J., Skrzydlewska, E. 2006. The comparison of effect of catechins and green tea extract on oxidative modification of LDL *in vitro*. *Adv Med Sci* 51: 298–303.

Ould Mohamedou, M. M., Zouirech, K., El Messal, M. et al. 2011. Argan oil exerts an anti-atherogenic effect by improving lipids and susceptibility of LDL to oxidation in type 2 diabetes patients. *Int J Endocrinol* 2011: 1–8.

Pacheco-Palencia, L., Duncan, C. E., Talcott, S. T. 2009. Phytochemical composition and thermal stability of two commercial açai species, *Euterpe oleracea* and *Euterpe precatoria*. *Food Chem* 115: 1199–1205.

Park, J. H., Seo, B. Y., Lee, K. H. et al. 2009. Onion supplementation inhibits lipid peroxidation and leukocyte DNA damage due to oxidative stress in high fat-cholesterol fed male rats. *Food Sci Biotechnol* 18: 179–184.

Parliament, T. H., Stahl, H. B. 2005. What makes the coffee smell so good? *Chem Technol* 25: 38–47.

Parrado, J., Miramontes, E., Jover, M. et al. 2003. Prevention of brain protein and lipid oxidation elicited by a water-soluble oryzanol enzymatic extract derived from rice bran. *Eur J Nutr* 42: 307–314.

Perez-Alvarez, J. A., Aleson-Carbonell, L. 2003. Origen y aspectos genéricos de la dieta Mediterránea. In *Alimentos funcionales y dieta Mediterranea*. Ed. J. A. Perez-Alvarez, J. Fernández-López, and E. Sayas-Barberá, 1–25. Orihuela: Universidad Miguel Hernández.

Pérez-Álvarez, J. A., Fernández-López, J., Sayas-Barberá, E. 2002. Especias. In *Fundamentos tecnológicos y nutritivos de la dieta Mediterranea*, Ed. J. A. Pérez-Alvarez, E. Sayas-Barberá, and J. Fernández-López, 103–119. Elche: Universidad Miguel Hernández.

Pérez-Conesa, D., García-Alonso, J., García-Valverde, V. et al. 2009. Changes in bioactive compounds and antioxidant activity during homogenization and thermal processing of tomato puree. *Innov Food Sci Emerg Technol* 10: 179–188.

Poiroux-Gonord, F., Bidel, L. P. R., Fanciullino, A. L. et al. 2010. Health benefits of vitamins and secondary metabolites of fruits and vegetables and prospects to increase their concentrations by agronomic approaches. *J Agr Food Chem* 58: 12065–12082.

Porgali, E., Büyüktuncel, E. 2012. Determination of phenolic composition and antioxidant capacity of native red wines by high performance liquid chromatography and spectrophotometric methods. *Food Res Int* 45: 145–154.

Pozo-Insfran, D. D., Brenes, C. H., Talcoot, S. T. 2004. Phytochemical composition and pigment stability of açai (*Euterpe oleracea* Mart.). *J Agr Food Chem* 52: 1539–1545.

Prasad, K. N., Hao, J., Shi, J. et al. 2009. Antioxidant and anticancer activities of high pressure-assisted extract of longan (*Dimocarpus longan* Lour.) fruit pericarp. *Innov Food Sci Emerg Technol* 10: 413–419.

Rangkadilok, N., Sitthimonchai, S., Worasuttayangkurn, L. et al. 2007. Evaluation of free radical scavenging and antityrosinase activities of standardized longan fruit extract. *Food Chem Toxicol* 45: 328–336.

Razali, N., Mat-Junit, S., Abdul-Muthalib, A. F. 2012. Effects of various solvents on the extraction of antioxidant phenolics from the leaves, seeds, veins and skins of *Tamarindus indica* L. *Food Chem* 131: 441–448.

Ribayo-Mercado, J. D., Solon, S. F., Tang, G. et al. 2000. Bioconversion of plant carotenoids to vit-A in Filipino school-aged children varies inversely with vit-A status. *Am J Clin Nutr* 72: 455–465.

Riboli, E., Norat, T. 2003. Epidemiologic evidence of the protective effect of fruit and vegetables on cancer risk. *Am J Clin Nutr* 78: 559–569.

Riccioni, G. 2009. Carotenoids and cardiovascular disease. *Curr Atherosclerosis Rep* 11: 434–439.

Rietveld, A., Wiseman, S. 2003. Antioxidant effects of tea: Evidence from human clinical trials. *J Nutr* 133: 3285–3292.

Robles-Sánchez, M., Astiazarán-García, H., Martín-Belloso, O. et al. 2011. Influence of whole and fresh-cut mango intake on plasma lipids and antioxidant capacity of healthy adults. *Food Res Int* 44: 1386–1391.

Rodrigo, R., Miranda, A., Vergara, L. 2011. Modulation of endogenous antioxidant system by wine polyphenols in human disease. *Clin Chim Acta* 412: 410–424.

Roldán, E., Sánchez-Moreno, C., de Ancos, B. et al. 2008. Characterisation of onion (*Allium cepa* L.) byproducts as food ingredients with antioxidant and anti-browning properties. *Food Chem* 108: 907–916.

Rosa, A., Melis, M. P., Deiana, M. et al. 2008. Protective effect of the oligomeric acylphloroglucinols from *Myrtus communis* on cholesterol and human low-density lipoprotein oxidation. *Chem Phys Lipids* 155: 16–23.

Rossi, J. A., Kasum, C. M. 2002. Dietary flavonoids: Bioavailability, metabolic effects and safety. *Ann Rev Nutr* 22: 19–34.

Salvini, S., Sera, F., Caruso, D. et al. 2006. Daily consumption of a high-phenol extra-virgin olive oil reduces oxidative DNA damage in postmenopausal women. *Br J Nutr* 95: 742–751.

Sánchez-Quesada, J. L., Benitez, S., Ordoñez-Llanos, J. 2004. Electronegative low-density lipoprotein. *Curr Opin Lipidol* 15: 29–35.

Sánchez-Zapata, E., Pérez-Álvarez, J. A. 2008. El aceite de oliva un alimento funcional. *Alimentac Equip Tecnol* 233: 33–35.

Sari, I., Baltaci, Y., Bagci, C. et al. 2010. Effect of pistachio diet on lipid parameters, endothelial function, inflammation, and oxidative status: A prospective study. *Nutrition* 26: 399–404.

Saura-Calixto, F., Goñi, I. 2009. Definition of the Mediterranean diet base on bioactive compounds. *Crit Rev in Food Sci Nutr* 49: 145–152.

Schauss, A. G., Wu, X., Prior, R. L. et al. 2006a. Antioxidant capacity and other bioactivities of the freeze-dried Amazonian palm berry, *Euterpe oleraceae* mart (açai). *J Agr Food Chem* 54: 8604–8610.

Schauss, A. G., Wu, X., Prior, R. L. et al. 2006b. Phytochemical and nutrient composition of the freeze-dried Amazonian palm berry, *Euterpe oleraceae* Mart. (Açai). *J Agr Food Chem* 54: 8598–8603.

Schieber, A., Stintzing, F. C., Carle, R. 2001. Byproducts of plant food processing as a source of functional compounds: Recent developments. *Trends Food Sci Technol* 12: 401–413.

Schinella, G., Mosca, S., Cienfuegos-Jovellanos, E. et al. 2010. Antioxidant properties of polyphenol-rich cocoa products industrially processed. *Food Res Int* 43: 1614–1623.

Seeram, N. P. 2006. Berries. In *Nutritional Oncology*, Ed. D. Heber, G. Blackburn, V. L. W. Go, and J. Milner, 615–625. 2nd ed. London: Academic Press.

Seeram, N. P. 2008. Berry fruits for cancer prevention: Current status and future prospects. *J Agr Food Chem* 56: 630–663.

Seeram, N., Lee, R., Hardy, M. et al. 2005. Rapid large-scale purification of ellagitannins from pomegranate husk, a byproduct of the commercial juice industry. *Separat Purificat Technol* 41: 49–55.

Sezer, E. D., Akçay, Y. D., İlanbey, B. et al. 2007. Pomegranate wine has greater protection capacity than red wine on low-density lipoprotein oxidation. *J Med Food* 10: 371–374.

Shahidi, F., Alasalvar, C., Liyana-Pathirana, C. M. 2007. Antioxidant phytochemicals in hazelnut kernel (*Corylus avellana* L.) and hazelnut byproducts. *J Agr Food Chem* 55: 1212–1220.

Shi, H. L., Noguchi, N., Niki, E. 2001. Introducing natural antioxidants. In *Antioxidants in food: practical applications*, Ed. J. Pokorny, N. Yanishlieva, and M. Gordon, 147–158. Cambridge: Woodhead Publishing.

Solar, A., Colarič, M., Usenik, V. et al. 2006. Seasonal variations of selected flavonoids, phenolic acids and quinones in annual shoots of common walnut (*Juglans regia* L.). *Plant Sci* 170: 453–461.

Sreeramulu, D., Raghunath, M. 2010. Antioxidant activity and phenolic content of roots, tubers and vegetables commonly consumed in India. *Food Res Int* 43: 1017–1020.

Stanner, S. A., Hughes, J., Kelly, C. N. et al. 2004. A review of the epidemiological evidence for the "antioxidant hypothesis". *Publ Health Nutr* 7: 407–422.

Steinberg, F. M., Holt, R. R., Schmitz, H. H. et al. 2002. Cocoa procyanidin chain length does not determine ability to protect LDL from oxidation when monomer units are controlled. *J Nutr Biochem* 13: 645–652.

Steinbrenner, H., Sies, H. 2009. Protection against reactive oxygen species by selenoproteins. *Biochim Biophys Acta* 1790: 1478–1485.

Stowe, C. B. 2011. The effects of pomegranate juice consumption on blood pressure and cardiovascular health. *Complement Ther Clin Pract* 17: 113–115.

Sung, H., Min, W. K., Lee, W. et al. 2005. The effects of green tea ingestion over four weeks on atherosclerotic markers. *Ann Clin Biochem* 42: 292–297.

Suzuki, K., Koike, H., Matsui, H. et al. 2002. Genistein, a soy isoflavone, induces glutathione peroxidase in the human prostate cancer cell lines LNCaP and PC-3. *J Cancer* 99: 846–852.

Szajdek, A., Borowska, E. 2008. Bioactive compounds and health-promoting properties of berry fruits: A review. *Plant Foods Hum Nutr* 63: 147–156.

Takahashi, M., Shibamoto, T. 2008. Chemical compositions and antioxidant/anti-inflammatory activities of steam distillate from freeze-dried onion (*Allium cepa* L.) sprout. *J Agr Food Chem* 56: 10462–10467.

Takahashi, R., Ohmori, R., Kiyose, C. et al. 2005. Antioxidant activities of black and yellow soybeans against low-density lipoprotein oxidation. *J Agr Food Chem* 53: 4578–4582.

Takahashi, Y., Inaba, N., Kuwahara, S. et al. 2003. Antioxidative effect of citrus essential oil components on human low-density lipoprotein *in vitro*. *Biosci Biotechnol Biochem* 67: 195–197.

Teissedre, P. L., Waterhouse, A. L. 2000. Inhibition of oxidation of human low-density lipoproteins by phenolic substances in different essential oils varieties. *J Agr Food Chem* 48: 3801–3805.

Thomas, S. R., Davies, M. J., Stocker, R. 1998. Oxidation and antioxidation of human low-density lipoprotein and plasma exposed to 3-morpholinosydnonimine and reagent peroxynitrite. *Chem Res Toxicol* 11: 484–494.

Tian, Y., Zou, B., Li, C. M. et al. 2012. High molecular weight persimmon tannin is a potent antioxidant both ex vivo and *in vivo*. *Food Res Int* 45: 26–30.

Tomaino, A., Martorana, M., Arcoraci, T. et al. 2010. Antioxidant activity and phenolic profile of pistachio (*Pistacia vera* L., variety Bronte) seeds and skins. *Biochimie* 92: 1115–1122.

Trinidad, T. P., Mallillin, A. C., Valdez, D. H. et al. 2006. Dietary fiber from coconut flour: A functional food. *Innovat Food Sci Emerg Technol* 7: 302–317.

Tripoli, E., Giammanco, M., Tabacchi, G. et al. 2005. The phenolic compounds of olive oil: Structure, biological activity and beneficial effects on human health. *Nutr Res Rev* 18: 98–112.

Tsang, C., Higgins, S., Duthie, G. G. et al. 2005. The influence of moderate red wine consumption on antioxidant status and indices of oxidative stress associated with CHD in healthy volunteers. *Br J Nutr* 93: 233–240.

Valsta, L. M., Lemström, A., Ovaskainen, M. L. et al. 2004. Estimation of plant sterol and cholesterol intake in Finland: Quality of new values and their effect on intake. *Br J Nutr* 92: 671–678.

Vanderhaegen, B., Neven, H., Verachtert, H. et al. 2006. The chemistry of beer aging: A critical review. *Food Chem* 95: 357–381.

Vayalil, P. K. 2002. Antioxidant and antimutagenic properties of aqueous extract of date fruit (*Phoenix dactylifera* L. Arecaceae). *J Agr Food Chem* 50: 610–617.

Vazquez-Prieto, M. A., González, R. E., Renna, N. F. et al. 2010. Aqueous garlic extracts prevent oxidative stress and vascular remodeling in an experimental model of metabolic syndrome. *J Agr Food Chem* 58: 6630–6635.

Vijaya Kumar Reddy, C., Sreeramulu, D., Raghunath, M. 2010. Antioxidant activity of fresh and dry fruits commonly consumed in India. *Food Res Int* 43: 285–288.

Vingtdeux, V., Dreses-Werringloer, U., Zhao, H. et al. 2008. Therapeutic potential of resveratrol in Alzheimer's disease. *BMC Neurosci* 9: 1–6.

Vinson, J. A., Mandarano, M., Hirst, M. et al. 2003. Phenol antioxidant quantity and quality in foods: Beers and the effect of two types of beer on an animal model of atherosclerosis. *J Agr Food Chem* 51: 5528–5533.

Viuda-Martos, M., Ruiz-Navajas, Y., Fernández-López, J. et al. 2007. Chemical composition of the essential oils obtained from some spices widely used in Mediterranean region. *Acta Chim Slov* 54: 921–926.

Viuda-Martos, M., Ruiz-Navajas, Y., Fernández-López, J. et al. 2011. Spices as functional food. *Crit Rev Food Sci Nutr* 51: 13–28.

Wan, Y., Vinson, J. A., Etherton, T. D. et al. 2011. Effects of cocoa powder and dark chocolate on LDL oxidative susceptibility and prostaglandin concentrations in humans. *Am Clin Nutr* 74: 596–602.

Wang, B. S., Chen, J. H., Liang, Y. C. et al. 2005a. Effects of Welsh onion on oxidation of low-density lipoprotein and nitric oxide production in macrophage cell line RAW 264.7. *Food Chem* 91: 147–155.

Wang, S. Y., Ballington, J. R. 2007. Free radical scavenging capacity and antioxidant enzyme activity in deerberry (*Vaccinium stamineum* L.). *LWT-Food Sci Technol* 40: 1352–1361.

Wang, S. Y., Feng, R., Lu, Y. et al. 2005b. Inhibitory effect on activator protein-1, nuclear factor-kappaB and cell transformation by extracts of strawberries (*Fragaria* x *ananassa* Duch.). *J Agr Food Chem* 53: 4187–4193.

Wasseem, R., Mira, M., Hamutal, B. N. et al. 2009. Effects of date (*Phoenix dactylifera* L., Medjool or Hallawi variety) consumption by healthy subjects on serum glucose and lipid levels and on serum oxidative status: A pilot study. *J Agr Food Chem* 57: 8010–8017.

Wei, A., Mura, K., Shibamoto, T. 2001. Antioxidative activity of volatile chemicals extracted from beer. *J Agr Food Chem* 49: 4097–4101.

Weinbrenner, T., Fito, M., de la Torre, R. et al. 2004. Olive oils high in phenolic compounds modulate oxidative/antioxidative status in men. *J Nutr* 134: 2314–2321.

Wijeratne, S. S. K., Abou-Zaid, M. M., Shahidi, F. 2006. Antioxidants polyphenols in almond and its coproducts. *J Agr Food Chem* 54: 312–318.

Wilmsen, P. K., Spada, D. S., Salvador, M. 2005. Antioxidant activity of the flavonoid hesperidin in chemical and biological systems. *J Agr Food Chem* 53: 4757–4761.

Wiswedel, I., Hirsch, D., Kropf, S. et al. 2004. Flavanol-rich cocoa drink lowers plasma F(2)-isoprostane concentrations in humans. *Free Radic Biol Med* 37: 411–421.

Wootton-Beard, P. C., Ryan, L. 2011. Improving public health? The role of antioxidant-rich fruit and vegetable beverages. *Food Res Int* 44: 3135–3148.

Wyatt, C. J., Carballido, S. P., Mendez, R. O. 1998. α-Tocopherol content of selected foods in Mexican diet. *J Agr Food Chem* 46: 4657–4661.

Xie, C., Kang, J., Burris, R. et al. 2011. Açaí juice attenuates atherosclerosis in ApoE deficient mice through antioxidant and anti-inflammatory activities. *Atherosclerosis* 216: 327–333.

Xu, B. J., Chang, S. K. C. 2007. A comparative study on phenolic profiles and antioxidant activities of legumes as affected by extraction solvents. *J Food Sci* 72: 159–166.

Xu, B. J., Chang, S. K. C. 2008. Total phenolics, phenolic acids, isoflavones and anthocyanins and antioxidant properties of yellow and black soybeans as affected by thermal processing. *J Agr Food Chem* 56: 7165–7175.

Xu, B. J., Yuan, S. H., Chang, S. K. C. 2007. Comparative analyses of phenolic composition, antioxidant capacity, and color of cool season legumes and other selected food legumes. *J Food Sci* 72: 167–177.

Yang, B., Zhao, M., Shi, J. et al. 2008. Effect of ultrasonic treatment on the recovery and DPPH radical scavenging activity of polysaccharides from longan fruit pericarp. *Food Chem* 106: 685–690.

Yang, T. T. C., Koo, M. W. L. 2000. Inhibitory effect of Chinese green tea on endothelial cell-induced LDL oxidation. *Atherosclerosis* 148: 67–73.

Yokozawa, T., Kim, Y. A., Lee, Y. A. et al. 2007. Protective effects of persimmon peel polyphenol against high glucose-induced oxidative stress in LLC-PK1 cells. *Food Chem Toxicol* 45: 1979–1987.

Yousef, M. I., Kamel, K. I., Esmail, A. M. et al. 2004. Antioxidant activities and lipid lowering effects of isoflavone in male rabbits. *Food Chem Toxicol* 42: 1497–1503.

Yu, L., Zhou, K., Parry, J. W. 2005. Inhibitory effects of wheat bran extracts on human LDL oxidation and free radicals. *LWT-Food Sci Technol* 38: 463–470.

Yukawa, G. S., Mune, M., Otani, H. 2004. Effects of coffee consumption on oxidative susceptibility of low-density lipoproteins and serum lipid levels in humans. *Biochemistry* 69: 70–74.

Zhou, H. C., Lin, Y. M., Wei, S. D. et al. 2011. Structural diversity and antioxidant activity of condensed tannins fractionated from mangosteen pericarp. *Food Chem* 129: 1710–1720.

18 Concluding Remarks

Grzegorz Bartosz and Izabela Sadowska-Bartosz

One of the main processes occurring in food is its oxidation, which, in a vast majority of cases, leads to the deterioration of its quality (some interesting exceptions to this rule have been discussed in this book). The content of antioxidants is thus of primary concern for food preparation and storage, and in cases when endogenous antioxidants may be insufficient, the addition of exogenous compounds or antioxidant supplementation in animals, which will be the source of food products, is often implemented.

Estimation of the antioxidant content of food is a nontrivial problem. The idea of measurement of the resultant activity of all antioxidants present in the sample studied was put forward long ago (Burlakova et al. 1965; Wayner et al. 1985) based on the chemical definition of antioxidants as substances that "when present at low concentrations compared to those of an oxidizable substrate, significantly delay or prevent oxidation of that substrate" (Halliwell 1995). The common principle gave rise to a variety of methods of estimation of total antioxidant capacity (TAC), which, based on different principles, are not easily comparable (Bartosz 2003, 2010). The challenging idea of building a database of TAC of foods (Wu et al. 2004) is also not free from difficulties as the TAC of plant materials strongly depends on the conditions of growth, ripening, and storage. For example, extracts from oregano plants harvested at the end of the flowering stage in July show the highest antioxidant capacity compared to herbs harvested at other stages (Ozkan, Baydar, and Erbas 2010). Moreover, the commonly used TAC assays are suited to the determination of activities of water-soluble antioxidants and may not be completely relevant to a complex multiphase material, such as food. In many cases, the nature of the antioxidants is of essential importance. This is important especially with respect to food, because antioxidants may differ considerably in bioavailability; the mere value of TAC does not provide such information.

Antioxidants are only the passive side of the oxidation problem in food; the active side includes prooxidants, both endogenous and external. The control of the content, state, and reactivity of prooxidants present in food and of external factors, such as light, salt, heat, radiation, and chemical additives, is of equal importance for the preservation of desired food quality. It should be considered that there is no clear-cut borderline between prooxidants and antioxidants. Virtually all antioxidants can have prooxidant activity under certain conditions; in particular, they may reduce transition metal ions, especially iron, to the forms able to enter the Fenton reaction:

$$\text{Antioxidant} - \text{H} + \text{Metal}^{n+1} \rightarrow \text{Antioxidant}^{\bullet} + \text{Metal}^{n+} + \text{H}^+$$

$$\text{Metal}^{n+} + \text{H}_2\text{O}_2 \rightarrow \text{Metal}^{n+1} + \text{HO}^{\bullet} + \text{HO}^-$$

Such behavior has been demonstrated by many authors for ascorbic acid (Stadtman 1991; Du, Cullen, and Buettner 2012) but is equally true for other antioxidants (Novellino, Napolitano, and Prota 1999; Perron and Brumaghim 2009; Maurya and Devasagayam 2010). A list of 14 phenolic acids that are considered to be antioxidants but under certain conditions behave as prooxidants has recently been published (Yordi et al. 2012). It should taken into account, however, that prooxidant effects can be beneficial because the imposition of a mild degree of oxidative stress might raise the levels of antioxidant defense and xenobiotic-metabolizing enzymes, leading to overall cytoprotection (Halliwell 2008).

Moreover, it should be kept in mind that compounds considered to be antioxidants (especially flavonoids) have many other biological activities apart from a direct antioxidant action, and their beneficial effects cannot always be ascribed to the latter (Fraga et al. 2010; Mandel et al. 2011; Węgrzyn 2012). For example, polyphenols activate and enhance endothelial nitric oxide synthase (eNOS) expression by several signaling pathways, increase glutathione (GSH), and inhibit ROS-producing enzymes, such as NADPH and xanthine oxidases. These pathways lead to improved endothelial function, subsequent normalization of vascular tone, and an overall antihypertensive effect. In practice, diets, such as the Mediterranean responsible for French paradox phenomenon; light or moderate red wine consumption; supplementation with polyphenols such as resveratrol or quercetin; and also experimental and clinical trials applying the above-mentioned have coincided in the antihypertensive effect of polyphenols, either in prevention or in therapy. However, further trials are yet needed to fully assess the molecular mechanisms of action and the appearance of adverse reactions (Rodrigo et al. 2012).

In recent years, it has become increasingly obvious that an important facet of the homeostasis is redox homeostasis of the body. The redox status of cells and extracellular compartments can be precisely defined by the values of redox potentials of appropriate redox systems, mainly the glutathione redox couple (Jones et al. 2000; Schafer and Buettner 2001; Buettner, Wagner, and Rodgers 2011). These redox potentials are kept within surprisingly narrow limits and shift toward higher values in the course of aging (Sohal and Orr 2012). More generally, the redox status is characterized by levels of antioxidants; activities of antioxidant enzymes; the rate of production of ROS or RNS; or, indirectly, by the level of markers of oxidative damage to macromolecules and consumption of antioxidants.

One of the main factors that may influence redox homeostasis is food. Postprandial changes in the TAC of blood plasma after food ingestion have been reported, and it was demonstrated that food rich in antioxidants can prevent a postprandial decrease in TAC induced especially by fat-rich meals (Natella et al. 2002; Burton-Freeman 2010; Blacker et al. 2012). As blood plasma TAC, contributed mainly by uric acid and protein plasma thiols, is a parameter that is rather insensitive to ingestion of individual antioxidants, its changes suggest that other parameters may be subject to much more significant alterations.

The problem with many antioxidants, especially flavonoids, is their limited bioavailability. However, even micromolar concentrations of food components, although not influencing TAC significantly, may have significant biological (including antioxidant) effects, related, for example, to effects on gene expression, specific receptors, and modifications of the cellular epigenome (Rodrigo, Miranda, and Vergara 2011; Malireddy et al. 2012; Murakami and Ohnishi 2012). Moreover, even if not ingested, antioxidants can affect the redox environment of the intestine preventing oxidative damage to enterocytes and modulating or preventing intestinal inflammation (Halliwell 2007; Biasi et al. 2011). Active compounds contained in garlic, mainly *S*-allylcysteine, were reported to increase glutathione levels and augment the activities of catalase and glutathione peroxidase in the liver and kidneys; activate the Nrf2 transcription factor and decrease NF-κB activation; and inhibit NADPH oxidase, inducible nitric oxide synthase, and cyclooxygenase (Colín-González et al. 2012). These effects seem to be more important than the direct antioxidant activity of these compounds. Flavonoids, as well, can have multiple biological functions besides antioxidant activity, such as affecting the enzyme activity of cyclooxygenases and lipoxygenases (Virgili and Marino 2008).

Polyphenols can also activate the SIRT1 protein, resulting in cell proliferation and cell survival. Cellular substrates of SIRT1 include the tumor suppressor p53, the transcription factor NF-κB, the forkhead box class O (FoxO) family of transcription factors, the peroxisome proliferator activated receptor (PPAR)-γ, the PPAR-γ coactivator 1α (PGC-1α), and the endothelial nitric oxide synthase (eNOS) (Vauzour 2012).

Numerous studies have demonstrated the occurrence of oxidative stress in a variety of diseases. Reactive oxygen species have been linked to many severe diseases, such as cancer; cardiovascular diseases, including atherosclerosis and stroke; neurological disorders; renal disorders; liver disorders; hypertension; rheumatoid arthritis; adult respiratory distress syndrome; autoimmune deficiency diseases; inflammation; degenerative disorders associated with aging; diabetes mellitus; diabetic complications; cataracts; obesity; autism; Alzheimer's, Parkinson's, and Huntington's diseases; vasculitis; glomerulonephritis; lupus erythematous; gastric ulcers; hemochromatosis; and preeclampsia, among others (Carocho and Ferreira 2012). It is not obvious whether this oxidative stress is a consequence or a cause of these diseases, although, in many cases, convincing evidence has been accumulated for the role of reactive oxygen species in the pathogenesis of diseases. These data strongly contributed to the broad interest in antioxidants, antioxidant-rich foods, and functional foods enriched with antioxidants. However, results of epidemiological studies and antioxidant supplementation studies have brought disappointing results in a considerable fraction of cases, pointing to the considerable differences between the unequivocal effects of *in vitro* studies of antioxidants and their *in vivo* effects. For instance, β-carotene has shown no effect in preventing lung cancer when applied in population-based trials but provoked a significant increase in cancer in heavy smokers (Omenn 2007; Goodman et al. 2004).

One of the main reasons for antioxidant supplementation has been the belief that antioxidants retard aging. This belief stemmed from the free radical theory of aging, proposed originally by Harman (1956) and subject to later modifications. If damage to macromolecules inflicted by free radicals and other ROS is the cause of aging, enhancement of antioxidant defense should be a simple means of lifespan prolongation. This prediction has been tested by many researchers, and the results did not meet expectations, showing generally no effect or moderate effects of supplementation of experimental animals with antioxidants or genetic manipulations (overexpression of main antioxidant enzymes). These findings prompted various researchers to put in doubt the validity of the free-radical hypothesis of aging (Gems and Doonan 2009; Pérez et al. 2009). However, many findings are in agreement with the free radical theory of aging, especially when the complex role of ROS in the organism and the phenomenon of redox homeostasis are taken into account. ROS, apart from being damaging agents, also play a role in intracellular and intercellular signaling, especially mediating the action of some cytokines and growth factors (Bartosz 2009). Therefore, their total elimination is neither desirable nor possible. Instead, the beneficial action of food components is nowadays expected to directly target and enhance intrinsic cytoprotective mechanisms, including modulation of the expression of genes involved in the detoxification of xenobiotics and their metabolites, genes involved in the synthesis and regulation of intrinsic antioxidants and antioxidant enzymes, genes involved in the regulation of inflammation, and vitagenes (Mastaloudis and Wood 2012).

Taking into account the profound physiological relevance of antioxidants, it seems obvious that more detailed studies on absorption, nutrikinetics, clinical effects, and toxicity of continuous ingestion seem necessary (Davies, Greenacre, and Lockwood 2005; Berger et al. 2012). Seemingly, there is still a long road to travel before the action of antioxidants is fully understood. It should be kept in mind that laboratory mice are more sensitive to dietary antioxidants than humans, so the results of animal experiments cannot be easily extrapolated onto humans. Another limitation regarding antioxidant research is cell cultures because, in many cases, the antioxidants tested *in vitro* react with the medium or are neutralized very quickly, thus leading to erroneous results that are usually overlooked by peer review (Halliwell 2006; Gutteridge and Halliwell 2010).

Antioxidants do have an impact on our health, but the big question is the method of administration (food vs. supplements) and quantity, which might be debatable. The fact that potent antioxidants *in vitro* may not have any effect *in vivo* should not discourage further research but rather stimulate it (Devasagayam et al. 2004). In view of the conflicting evidence concerning the potential benefit of higher intake of, especially, single antioxidants, some authors suggest that a permanent intake of nonphysiological dosages of isolated antioxidants should not be recommended to healthy consumers. This must not be confused with a high intake of fruits and vegetables, which is considered safe and beneficial (Berger et al. 2012).

It should be considered that some fruits and vegetables are better than others in this respect, taking into account the content of biologically active phytonutrients. Therefore, detailed studies of the composition and effects of the consumption of various fruits and vegetables, including those that are not commonly consumed, may provide important indications for the healthy foods and diet that may alleviate pathologies.

The analysis of the physiological effects of food sometimes brings unexpected findings. Epidemiological evidence demonstrates that higher consumption of vegetables confers a protective effect against the risk of cardiovascular disease, mainly by augmenting the bioavailability of the vasodilatory nitric oxide and preventing hypertension. Classically, vascular endothelium has been believed to be the sole source of bioactive NO in the vasculature. Emerging data, however, underscores the significance of the nitrate–nitrite pathway in which endogenous nitrate undergoes a reduction to nitrite and then to NO in various tissues, including blood, resulting in the production of bioactive NO. Consumption of vegetables is the source of approximately 80%–85% of daily nitrate in humans, thereby establishing inorganic nitrate as a promising factor in the cardiovascular health benefits of vegetables (Machha and Schechter 2012).

All these examples posed to the value of food science the necessity of detailed analysis of food components, including food prooxidants and antioxidants and their physiological effects. Such studies can bring completely new information, rationalizing food consumption for the sake of maintenance and improvement of the redox homeostasis of the body, contributing to the beneficial health effects of the proper diet.

REFERENCES

Bartosz, G. 2003. Total antioxidant capacity. *Adv Clin Chem* 37: 219–292.

Bartosz, G. 2009. Reactive oxygen species: Destroyers or messengers? *Biochem Pharmacol* 77: 1303–1315.

Bartosz, G. 2010. Non-enzymatic antioxidant capacity assays: Limitations of use in biomedicine. *Free Radic Res* 44: 711–720.

Berger, R. G., S. Lunkenbein, A. Ströhle, and A. Hahn. 2012. Antioxidants in food: Mere myth or magic medicine? *Crit Rev Food Sci Nutr* 52: 162–171.

Biasi, F., M. Astegiano, M. Maina, G. Leonarduzzi, and G. Poli. 2011. Polyphenol supplementation as a complementary medicinal approach to treating inflammatory bowel disease. *Curr Med Chem* 18: 4851–4865.

Blacker, B. C., S. M. Snyder, D. L. Eggett, and T. L. Parker. 2012. Consumption of blueberries with a high-carbohydrate, low-fat breakfast decreases postprandial serum markers of oxidation. *Br J Nutr* 31: 1–8.

Buettner, G. R., B. A. Wagner, and V. G. Rodgers. 2011. Quantitative redox biology: An approach to understand the role of reactive species in defining the cellular redox environment. *Cell Biochem Biophys* Dec 9. [Epub ahead of print].

Burlakova, E. B., N. M. Dziuba, N. P. Palmina, and N. M. Emanuél. 1965. Antioxidative activity of lipids of mouse liver in radiation disease and reinoculation leucosis, and the effect of inhibitors of free-radical reactions. *Dokl Akad Nauk SSSR* 163: 1278–1281.

Burton-Freeman, B. 2010. Postprandial metabolic events and fruit-derived phenolics: A review of the science. *Br J Nutr* 104: Suppl 3: S1–S14.

Carocho, M., and I. C. Ferreira. 2012. A review on antioxidants, prooxidants and related controversy: Natural and synthetic compounds, screening and analysis methodologies and future perspectives. *Food Chem Toxicol* 51C: 15–25.

Colín-González, A. L., R. A. Santana, C. A. Silva-Islas, M. E. Chánez-Cárdenas, A. Santamaría, and P. D. Maldonado. 2012. The antioxidant mechanisms underlying the aged garlic extract- and S-allylcysteine-induced protection. *Oxid Med Cell Longev* 2012: 907162.

Davies, E., D. Greenacre, and G. B. Lockwood. 2005. Adverse effects and toxicity of nutraceuticals. *Rev Food Nutr Toxicol* 3: 165–195.

Devasagayam, T. P., J. C. Tilak, K. K. Boloor, K. S. Sane, S. S. Ghaskadbi, and R. D. Lele. 2004. Free radicals and antioxidants in human health: Current status and future prospects. *J Assoc Phys India* 52: 794–804.

Du, J., J. J. Cullen, and G. R. Buettner. 2012. Ascorbic acid: Chemistry, biology and the treatment of cancer. *Biochim Biophys Acta* 1826: 443–457.

Fraga, C. G., M. Galleano, S. V. Verstraeten, and P. I. Oteiza. 2010. Basic biochemical mechanisms behind the health benefits of polyphenols. *Mol Aspects Med* 31: 435–445.

Gems, D., and R. Doonan. 2009. Antioxidant defense and aging in C. elegans: Is the oxidative damage theory of aging wrong? *Cell Cycle* 8: 1681–1687.

Goodman, G. E., M. D. Thornquist, J. Balmes, M. R. Cullen, F. L. Meyskens Jr., G. S. Omenn, B. Valanis, and J. H. Williams Jr. 2004. The Beta-Carotene and Retinol Efficacy Trial: Incidence of lung cancer and cardiovascular disease mortality during 6-year follow-up after stopping beta-carotene and retinol supplements. *J Natl Cancer Inst* 96: 1743–1750.

Gutteridge, J. M., and B. Halliwell. 2010. Antioxidants: Molecules, medicines, and myths. *Biochem Biophys Res Commun* 393: 561–564.

Halliwell, B. 1995. Antioxidant characterization: Methodology and mechanism. *Biochem Pharmacol* 49: 1341–1348.

Halliwell, B. 2006. Reactive species and antioxidants: Redox biology is a fundamental theme of aerobic life. *Plant Physiol* 141: 312–322.

Halliwell, B. 2007. Dietary polyphenols: Good, bad, or indifferent for your health? *Cardiovasc Res* 73: 341–347.

Halliwell, B. 2008. Are polyphenols antioxidants or pro-oxidants? What do we learn from cell culture and in vivo studies? *Arch Biochem Biophys* 476: 107–112.

Harman, D. 1956. Aging: A theory based on free radical and radiation chemistry. *J Gerontol* 11: 298–300.

Jones, D. P., J. L. Carlson, V. C. Mody, J. Cai, M. J. Lynn, and P. Sternberg. 2000. Redox state of glutathione in human plasma. *Free Radic Biol Med* 28: 625–635.

Machha, A., and A. N. Schechter. 2012. Inorganic nitrate: A major player in the cardiovascular health benefits of vegetables? *Nutr Rev* 70: 367–372.

Malireddy, S., S. R. Kotha, J. D. Secor, T. O. Gurney, J. L. Abbott, G. Maulik, K. R. Maddipati, and N. L. Parinandi. 2012. Phytochemical antioxidants modulate mammalian cellular epigenome: Implications in health and disease. *Antioxid Redox Signal* 17: 327–339.

Mandel, S. A., T. Amit, O. Weinreb, and M. B. Youdim. 2011. Understanding the broad-spectrum neuroprotective action profile of green tea polyphenols in aging and neuro-degenerative diseases. *J Alzheimers Dis* 25: 187–208.

Mastaloudis, A., and S. M. Wood. 2012. Age-related changes in cellular protection, purification, and inflammation-related gene expression: Role of dietary phytonutrients. *Ann N Y Acad Sci* 1259: 112–120.

Maurya, D. K., and T. P. Devasagayam. 2010. Antioxidant and prooxidant nature of hydroxy-cinnamic acid derivatives ferulic and caffeic acids. *Food Chem Toxicol* 48: 3369–3373.

Murakami, A., and K. Ohnishi. 2012. Target molecules of food phytochemicals: Food science bound for the next dimension. *Food Funct* 3: 462–476.

Natella, F., F. Belelli, V. Gentili, F. Ursini, and C. Scaccini. 2002. Grape seed proanthocyanidins prevent plasma postprandial oxidative stress in humans. *J Agric Food Chem* 50: 7720–7725.

Novellino, L., A. Napolitano, and G. Prota. 1999. 5,6-Dihydroxyindoles in the fenton reaction: A model study of the role of melanin precursors in oxidative stress and hyperpigmentary processes. *Chem Res Toxicol* 12: 985–992.

Omenn, G. S. 2007. Chemoprevention of lung cancers: Lessons from CARET, the beta-carotene and retinol efficacy trial, and prospects for the future. *Eur J Cancer Prev* 16: 184–191.

Ozkan, G., H. Baydar, and S. Erbas. 2010. The influence of harvest time on essential oil composition, phenolic constituents and antioxidant properties of Turkish oregano (*Origanum onites* L.). *J Sci Food Agric* 90: 205–209.

Pérez, V. I., A. Bokov, H. Van Remmen, J. Mele, Q. Ran, Y. Ikeno, and A. Richardson. 2009. Is the oxidative stress theory of aging dead? *Biochim Biophys Acta* 1790: 1005–1014.

Perron, N. R., and J. L. Brumaghim. 2009. A review of the antioxidant mechanisms of polyphenol compounds related to iron binding. *Cell Biochem Biophys* 53: 75–100.

Rodrigo, R., D. Gil, A. Miranda-Merchak, and G. Kalantzidis. 2012. Antihypertensive role of polyphenols. *Adv Clin Chem* 58: 225–254.

Rodrigo, R., A. Miranda, and L. Vergara. 2011. Modulation of endogenous antioxidant system by wine polyphenols in human disease. *Clin Chim Acta* 412: 410–424.

Schafer, F. Q., and G. R. Buettner. 2001. Redox environment of the cell as viewed through the redox state of the glutathione disulfide/glutathione couple. *Free Radic Biol Med* 30: 1191–1212.

Sohal, R. S., and W. C. Orr. 2012. The redox stress hypothesis of aging. *Free Radic Biol Med* 52: 539–555.

Stadtman, E. R. 1991. Ascorbic acid and oxidative inactivation of proteins. *Am J Clin Nutr* 54: 1125S–1128S.

Vauzour, D. 2012. Dietary polyphenols as modulators of brain functions: Biological actions and molecular mechanisms underpinning their beneficial effects. *Oxid Med Cell Longev* 2012: 914273.

Virgili, F., and M. Marino. 2008. Regulation of cellular signals from nutritional molecules: A specific role for phytochemicals, beyond antioxidant activity. *Free Radic Biol Med* 45: 1205–1216.

Wayner, D. D., G. W. Burton, K. U. Ingold, and S. Locke. 1985. Quantitative measurement of the total, peroxyl radical-trapping antioxidant capability of human blood plasma by controlled peroxidation: The important contribution made by plasma proteins. *FEBS Lett* 187: 33–37.

Węgrzyn, A. 2012. Gene expression-targeted isoflavone therapy. *IUBMB Life* 64: 307–315.

Wu, X., L. Gu, J. Holden, D. B. Haytowitz, S. E. G. Gebhardt, G. Beecher, and R. L. Prior. 2004. Development of a database for total antioxidant capacity in foods: A preliminary study. *J Food Comp Anal* 17: 407–422.

Yordi, E. G., E. M. Pérez, M. J. Matos, and E. U. Villares. 2012. Structural alerts for predicting clastogenic activity of pro-oxidant flavonoid compounds: Quantitative structure–activity relationship study. *J Biomol Screen* 17: 216–224.

Index

Page numbers followed by f and t indicate figures and tables, respectively.

Printed and bound by CPI Group (UK) Ltd, Croydon, CR0 4YY

21/10/2024

01777083-0020